MEDICAL HISTORY OF CONTRACEPTION

TO

SORANOS
(98–138)

most brilliant gynecologist of antiquity, whose originality and distinguished career illumined a future
path of medicine for nearly two thousand years.

"The farther a notion reaches back into primitive times for its origin, the more universal must be its extent, and its power in history is rooted in this universality."

(Lippert, *Kulturgeschichte*. Quoted by Sumner and Keller, *The Science of Society*, ii, 1465–6.)

PREFACE TO THE PAPERBACK EDITION

NORMAN HIMES's *Medical History of Contraception* represents the only large-scale effort in the English language, and indeed in any language, to fully document man's attempts to control his fertility from prehistoric to modern times. This lively and comprehensive account of man's ambivalent relationship to his own reproductive capacity is as important and readable today as it was thirty years ago, when it was first published. It is a well-deserved tribute to its author that it is now being republished in its entirety in a paperback edition.

Every field of endeavor has its own history. Fortunately for us, Norman Himes's thorough study of the history of contraception has resulted in a document which is both scholarly and literary. Although the title states that it is a medical history, the book itself covers the anthropologic, economic, and sociologic aspects as well. As a reference work, it has saved busy scholars countless hours of digging for obscure sources. As a work of history, it has made the experience of workers in the field of birth control so much more vivid and meaningful.

The central theme of the book is the concept that birth control represents the ageless struggle of mankind to achieve "adequate parenthood." It is Mr. Himes's contention that the birth-control propagandists of the nineteenth century served merely to crystallize the public demand associated with such factors as industrialization, urbanization, lessened ecclesiastical authority, and greater freedom for women. He rightly predicted that the democratization of contraceptive practice, which was in his day limited even within the Western world, would, in the twentieth century, be diffused throughout the Orient. And, in fact, the first major national family-planning programs in the world were those of India, Pakistan, Korea, and Taiwan. The roster of other developing countries undertaking, during the 1960's, either an official family-planning program or a major governmental involvement in family planning includes: Ceylon, Iran, Malaysia, Hong Kong, Singapore, and Turkey in Asia; Mauritius, Morocco, Tunisia, and the United Arab Republic in Africa; Chile, Colombia, the Dominican Republic, Honduras, Jamaica, and Trinidad and Tobago in the Western Hemisphere. The list can be considerably expanded if it were to include countries with some governmental activity in family planning, although on a limited scale.

The bibliography of some 1,500 items at the end of this volume is unique for the period covered. The listing is both comprehensive and selective in the best sense, and a code is provided for the location of rare items.

This volume brings the history of birth-control endeavor up to the 1930's. Such dramatic changes in contraceptive techniques and practices as the development and widespread use of the rhythm method, oral contraceptives, and intrauterine devices, were still beyond the horizon. A new Norman Himes is urgently needed today to record as vividly and in as scholarly a manner as he did the development of new contraceptive techniques; the emphasis on statistical evaluation of the safety, effectiveness, and acceptability of contraceptive methods; and the growing public awareness that a balance will have to be achieved between population growth and social and economic development.

CHRISTOPHER TIETZE, M.D.
The Population Council

FOREWORD

TIMELY and welcome is this first thorough study of the history of control of conception. Its broad range is in no wise restricted by the word "medical" in the title, because social and economic implications can no more be disregarded within this area than they can be in the diagnosis and treatment of disease or in any other section of preventive medicine.

Perhaps the most striking feature of this assembly of activities and of attitudes, ancient and modern, is the evidence of the universality of the striving toward a given end. In virtually every culture which is of historic importance the author discovers the presence of a *desire* to control fertility by artificial means. It has been common knowledge that early peoples scorned sterility. It has not been generally recognized that they sought at the same time to avoid excessive production of progeny. Among other means toward limiting undue numbers, it is shown that disproportionate attention has been focussed on abortion and infanticide, and relatively little heed has been given to the more elusive evidence bearing on widespread and consistent *groping* toward artificial control of conception. Whereas advances made in the process of civilization are forever characterized by economy of effort, abortion and infanticide are conspicuous examples of extravagant waste. If progress means anything, it means prevention curtailing destruction.

It is noteworthy that this volume represents one of the first attempts to apply to the history of medicine the sociological methodology of Pareto. In his *Trattato di Sociologia Generale*, which is in these days under constant discussion, the famous Italian has shown quite conclusively that if we are to build up social generalizations and arrive at concepts of uniform general principles in human conduct, it is important to study, not alone our own brief culture, but the facts of all cultures throughout the entire range of social evolution.

Dr. Himes sees sociology as a science whose business it is to construct generalizations built on the broadest foundations, and he is of the opinion that not a few of his colleagues err in method when they attempt to generalize on a basis of studies of conduct as seen in contemporary urban society, and on this basis almost alone; whereas such a society is a mere end product of human evolution.

If we apply this point of view to the physician's section of service to the community, it is evident that for contemporary medicine the need of the wide perspective involved in historical review is as great as for the student of the whole field of human conduct. Moreover, perspectives of research on control of conception show reason for hope of fresh discovery.

Fearless investigation is in line with the best traditions of medicine; that is, with its traditions since it emerged from magic, and, in most of its departments, from the domination of dogma, and before it acquired, in places, the infusion of commercialism. By assuming its share of the responsibility for discoveries in control of conception and for instruction wherever instruction is needed, medicine might give pause to the accusation that in some matters social and crucial its official organized societies are not leaders but laggards, nearly as timid as organized legal bodies. With their charters as agencies created for service to humanity in trouble, we have a right to look to them for active participation in study and in counsel.

Toward any inquiry bearing on these importunate problems the author tenders material of high present and potential value, reaching back as it does to the uttermost edge of social origins, so little known, and forward to the very brink of the future, even less knowable. For the collection of the mass of data—and speculation—embodied in this book, and particularly for the stimulus to thought which it provokes on many lines, the science and art of medicine should express its obligation. This gratitude may well be shared by students of population and workers on very many of the social problems in which control of the number and the quality of progeny play a part.

ROBERT L. DICKINSON, M.D., F.A.C.S.

INTRODUCTION

A PRESENTATION addressed to physicians by a non-medical writer calls for a word of explanation. I was asked by the National Committee on Maternal Health, Inc. to prepare a few chapters on the history of conception control for a medical source book which would deal exhaustively with the control of human fertility, sterility, abortion, sterilization, etc.; and a grant-in-aid of research to the amount of one thousand dollars was made to me for that purpose. Presumably the committee honored me with the request because it knew that I had, as an economist and sociologist, devoted the preceding five or six years to a study of the economic and social history of birth control. Though, as a fellow of the Social Science Research Council, I had made in 1926–27 a study of the work of the English birth-control clinics, I had steadfastly up to this time refrained from discussing in my published papers the medical aspects of the subject, realizing that my province lay elsewhere. When the Committee made its request, however, I accepted gladly for several reasons: (1) It was clear that here was a significant hiatus in knowledge that needed filling. (2) No physician or medical historian appeared on the scene willing to expend the required effort. (3) There was the realization that, while I had no medical training, the final report would be scanned by a highly competent medical editorial board. Had not Hippocrates declared that the good physician will not hesitate to learn from the layman in those instances in which, through peculiar circumstances, he happens to have specialized information? The publication of a medical history by a sociologist proceeds from no desire to usurp a medical function but rather from a sincere effort to contribute some measure of perspective toward the understanding of a human problem which, after all, has implications not alone for medicine but for human biology, for economics, sociology, jurisprudence, and many other fields of human knowledge and endeavor.

It is commonly supposed, even in well-informed circles, that birth control is very recent, ultra-modern. This is an error—as this book aims to show. Just how old is it? The man or woman on the street usually thinks of it as having its origin in a public agitation led by Margaret Sanger or Marie Stopes. The better informed have recalled perhaps the notoriety achieved by the so-called Knowlton trial in England in 1877–78. Then Professor James A. Field pushed back the boundaries of our knowledge by tracing the public educational work of Francis Place in England in 1822 and the years immediately following. A few Continental writers have made passing reference to older authors who treated the subject; but, in general, published works, including histories of medicine, have been conspicuously silent on the early history.

Hence this book. To be sure, there have occasionally appeared would-be wiseacres who, with a wave of the hand, asserted the antiquity of birth-control practices; but when pressed for evidence, it proved lacking. In this book I have tried to make a beginning in collecting the evidence. Though science consists, in part, of a body of well-founded generalizations about given phenomena, I have tried to refrain from premature generalizations. Doubtless I have not altogether succeeded in doing so. If, on the other hand, the few conclusions I have drawn stimulate others to amend them; if they are used eventually to throw light on significant theoretical questions, I shall be amply repaid.

For reasons which appear in due course, it is important to know in what respects conception control—or the use of given anti-conceptional measures —is old or new. This book ventures an answer.

An essential purpose is, further, to demonstrate that contraception, as only one form of population control, is a social practice of much greater historical antiquity, greater cultural and geographical universality than commonly supposed even by medical and social historians. Contraception has existed in some form throughout the entire range of social evolution, that is, for at least several thousand years. The *desire for*, as distinct from the *achievement of*, reliable contraception has been characteristic of many societies widely removed in time and place. Moreover, this desire for controlled reproduction characterizes even those societies dominated by mores and religious codes demanding that people "increase and multiply."

To state this sociological and theoretical purpose another way, in the terminology of Vilfredo Pareto, the great Italian sociologist, one of my objects has been to show that contraception is a social practice repeated in space (i.e., in various cultures) and time (i.e., not an ephemeral phenomenon) and, as such, one of several social phenomena peculiarly worthy of scientific sociological inquiry. Ephemeral, non-repeated phenomena are much less worthy of scientific inquiry.

That the members of cultures disdaining sterility, for example, most primitive peoples, the ancient Hebrews, and modern Orientals, have longed for controlled reproduction is a cultural fact which has not heretofore been realized sufficiently. This survey seems to show that men and women have always longed for both fertility and sterility, each at its appointed time and in its chosen circumstances. *This has been a universal aim, whether people have always been conscious of it or not.* Despite the antiquity of some anti-conceptional techniques, it seems abundantly clear from what follows that *only within the last century do we find any organized, planned effort to help the masses to acquire a knowledge of contraception.* It would seem as if the striving were toward adequate parenthood together with control of conception; toward fertility or sterility, each in its appointed time or place, according to the circumstances of each case.

This universal aim is not only old, but in the early period the adjustments which population control effected were much more spontaneous, unconscious and automatic than in Western societies since 1800. We need to recognize that population adjustments, like all social institutional adjustments, are in the main automatic. They operate, whatever direction they take, because various pressures, economic, psychic, social are set up when some change causes a maladjustment. They are a consequence of needs. Since needs vary from time to time, so likewise do population adjustments. This is true now as indeed it has always been true; but with this qualification: since knowledge is ordinarily cumulative we ought to be able to make some adaptations a little more intelligently than our predecessors. Within recent centuries there seems to have been an increase of what Ross has aptly called "adaptive fertility."

It would be incorrect to conclude, as at least one prominent American demographer has done, that the modern birth-control movement, as a social demand or a social movement, is chiefly a response of the populace to the teachings of birth-control propagandists. It ante-dates the alleged cause, as this book well demonstrates. Conception control is older than propaganda movements. No one has ever found evidence of an organized birth-control propaganda prior to that conducted by Francis Place in 1822. The birth strikes of antiquity, suggested by the lamentations of such writers as Polybius, cannot logically be introduced as evidence to the contrary. The fact is that people adjust to most pressures unconsciously, by trial and failure, trial and success.

I conceive of population movements as adaptations—or, in the jargon of the sociologists—as accommodations. They are equilibria and disequilibria phenomena much as most economic phenomena, properly interpreted, are. Usually they are moving equilibria. The value of this way of looking at the facts will be considered in a subsequent volume. Here I simply call attention to the fact in order that the reader may ascertain my point of view. More immediately relevant is the consideration that, if my contentions are sound, the present birth-control "plague" is not caused by the propagandists, but is rather a response to a universal desire, a way out of certain maladjustments. Let us "blame" the people, if anyone is to be "blamed," but not the "propagandists." *They have merely crystallized a discontent—or, if you will, a constructive desire—which dates from pre-history*. To accept a contrary view is to flout the facts of history.

My thesis that birth control is an automatic adjustment does not deny that particular individuals may have been influential, especially since 1800, in arousing the interest of the populace in this question. Such, indeed, is the fact. But this is quite different from alleging that birth control has become popular because of the "propagandists."

My study does not support the thesis that those cultures which employed anti-conceptional practices died out because of it.

From the universality and antiquity of anti-conception I infer that it fulfills some fundamental human need. It has shown great sticking power. It has not only survived; it has grown increasingly strong.

It is worth while to study quite for their own sake, as an effort in pure science, the contraceptive techniques, now bizarre and pathetically ineffective or injurious, now strangely ingenious, original and workable, that man has gropingly hit upon to realize the universal aim of controlled paternity. Even if no generalizations emerged, such fact gathering is important in itself; for one will search histories of medicine in vain for any account of this neglected subject. The few accounts that have appeared are, at best, sketchy.

The present volume stresses the medical aspects of the history of contraception. A succeeding volume will trace the social and economic development of birth control, while another will be devoted to the relation of birth control to certain fundamental aspects of modern population theory.

It is imperative for several reasons that detailed consideration be given to the exact methods of prevention. There is only one way to do this—to dig the facts from the original sources; and to see, in so far as it may be possible, our problem whole, that is, through the entire range of social evolution from primitive societies to our day. Only by ascertaining the exact nature of the techniques used can we hope to essay even a tentative judgment of the effectiveness of anti-conceptional methods. Bowdlerized, euphemistic statements to the effect that this or that social group knew and practised contraception are virtually useless. We want to know the techniques in order to compare and trace them historically, in order to study their effectiveness; for their clues to the biochemist searching for new methods to prevent disease. Readers unaccustomed to the perusal of medical literature, must, therefore, be prepared to meet with evidence shocking to their aesthetic senses, techniques in some instances revolting. But the path of science is sometimes a narrow and unpleasant one. Moreover, approval or disapproval of such practices is not in question.

Certain special difficulties encountered in the study may interest the reader. All of the chief American libraries, whether the Library of Congress, the New York Public Library, or the Harvard and Yale libraries, or such medical libraries as that of the New York Academy of Medicine, the Boston Medical Library, the Surgeon General's Library, etc., are definitely limited in source material. Speaking generally, American libraries possess few works on the sexual life of peoples in various cultures at different times. My personal private collection at considerable expense has helped. Source material, even when possessed by American libraries, is sometimes intentionally left uncatalogued. This is true more especially of the public libraries. Librarians of such institutions not infrequently find that they must, in deference to public opinion, restrict the circulation of even the most innocuous books. In the instance of books of genuine scientific value, failure to catalogue them in the index generally available to the public sometimes seriously interferes with scientific work. Yet responsibility lies more perhaps with the community than with the librarian. Few have had direct access to the files in the Director's Office at the Boston Public Library, of "books not in the library." Even the British Museum has a special cabinet for certain books; and to secure access to these requires not only serious purpose but tact, patience, and persistence. Some amusing stories could be related of these experiences.

The second difficulty has been the almost total lack of reliable secondary sources where one could find leads to the original data. There are, of course, some exceptions to this, but in general, the few accounts at present existing are, almost without exception, not only inaccurate factually, but improperly documented.

This historical account is less complete than it ought to be; but the reader will realize that searching for evidence on early contraceptive mechanisms has proved a very time-consuming process. It is a search for needles in haystacks. Especially is this true of the literature published prior to 1800, which is rarely indexed. The few relevant lines are often lost in hundreds of pages. Anthropological sources are invariably badly indexed, save in the instance of a few recently published accounts. Small wonder, then, that this volume omits much when one contemplates what it should ideally contain. Had funds for research been available much more could have been done. But no foundation could be interested in the project.

It is no part of my present purpose to discuss the desirability or undesirability of conception control in our culture or any other culture. This is a report and an interpretation, not a case for contraception. Only rarely will one find evaluation, and that is confined mainly to the question of the effectiveness of the techniques reported. In the latter parts of this work, the task is a different one. There, critical evaluation is an essential part of my purpose.

It should be borne clearly in mind by reviewers as well as readers that while the present work touches on recent events of medical interest, it is a *history*, not a running commentary on *contemporary* affairs. Enough material on recent events has been inserted to bring certain lines of thought down to date. But many other interesting phases have had to be omitted for lack of space or because they could be considered more appropriately in another volume. Many questions in readers' minds will not, therefore, be answered in this book. This policy has been deliberately adopted. The present work does not pretend to be a general treatise on birth control. It should be judged accordingly, especially by reviewers. History is not a record of contemporary events. I have made an exception in the case of the clinics, and more briefly in a few other instances, because the development and spread of birth-control clinics are perhaps the chief product of a century of agitation to democratize contraceptive knowledge.

From the first I have operated on the principle that it is impossible to understand the modern social significance of a world force like birth control without a well-rounded conception of its historical development. In this, as in other instances, the longest way round is the surest, if not the shortest, way home. It is often so in science. It is axiomatic with me that the economics and sociology of this subject will never be properly understood until its history is fairly accurately and fully explored. Accordingly, I hope that this book will assist in laying the historical foundation for further theoretical work, some of which I plan to undertake myself in a later volume.

To some people this book will lack proper perspective because some sub-topics they think important are touched upon lightly or hardly at all. They will look up "Holland" or "Soviet Russia" or popularly-known surnames in the index, and, finding nothing or few references, will conclude that there are important omissions. So there are, as I have already admitted. Yet the above remarks are pertinent in this connection. Again I must say, this is not a record of contemporary events. Nor is it a social and economic history of the subject except very incidentally. It is essentially a history of contraceptive technique.

In general the book is divided into six Parts. The first Part dealing with "Contraceptive Technique Before the Dawn of Written History" is essentially an analysis of contraceptive methods employed by various preliterate peoples in various parts of the world. Part Two on "Contraceptive Technique in Antiquity (Western World)" traces the techniques developed by the Egyptians (Chapter II), by Greek and Roman writers (Chapter IV), as well as those found in the Bible and Talmud (Chapter III). Part Three deals with Oriental Civilizations—India, China and Japan. ` Part Four, on "Technique in the West During the Middle Ages and Early Modern Times," consists of Chapters VI, VII, and VIII. The first is devoted to the rise, flowering and decline of Islamic contraceptive medicine, a civilization whose contribution to the development of medicine in general has been all too little studied. There would be a marked hiatus in this chronicle if some attention were not devoted to the development of folk medicine. This is rather a loose classification, and includes the observations of Casanova. Such European folk beliefs from 1400 on are studied in Chapter VII. It may seem odd that we have no thorough study of the history of the condom or sheath, which has done so much, especially in the last century, to revolutionize the sexual relations of Western civilization. This gap has seemed to me altogether amazing; hence an attempt to gather the evidence in Chapter VIII. No doubt lacunae still remain to be filled.

Part Five (Chapters IX–XII) is essentially a review of the contraceptive literature of the nineteenth century stressing the techniques recommended, and an attempt to evaluate the importance and influence of each writer. The account is chronological, begins with the early Neo-Malthusians, notably Place and Carlile, jumps to the U. S. A. to scan the early beginnings there in the work of Robert Dale Owen and Dr. Charles Knowlton, and oscillates between England and the United States in tracing the more important developments of medical interest. Though this Part contains the first thorough, systematic treatment of contraceptive development in the English speaking world during the nineteenth century, I am conscious of many gaps. Concerning developments in Germany it has been possible merely to call attention to a portion of the large literature in that language, though probably mention has been made either in the text or in the bibliography of nearly all the authors who have written special pamphlets, books or articles on technique. The reader should again recall that the literature on social theory will receive a place elsewhere.

In this Part much is made of two central theses: improvement in technique over preceding centuries; increasing diffusion, democratization or socialization of this knowledge. *Socialization of contraceptive knowledge is the central feature of contraceptive history during the nineteenth century.*

Chapter XIII reviews briefly the clinical and statistical evidence supporting further the thesis that the central trend of recent years has been the socialization of birth-control knowledge. Some theoretical consequences of this diffusion are then traced (Chapter XIV).

Following a "Conclusion" (Chapter XV), there is a Bibliography, concerning the scope of which the Note preceding it should be read.

The terms contraception, anti-conception, and birth control are used herein as synonymous with the prevention of conception, that is, preventing spermatozoa from reaching the ovum. This implies normal coitus and rules out such variant practices as anal and oral coitus which have been considered by some as birth-control practices.

I am under no illusions regarding the completeness of this account. I have more than a suspicion that it lacks a perspective which the history should, and doubtless will have when more is known about it. For instance, I have constantly had to check a tendency to pay little attention to the well-known figures, especially the recent ones and those still living, and to delve into the contributions and ideas of obscure figures whose names have not heretofore appeared in the literature. Hence I had found myself omitting Margaret Sanger in the U. S. A., Dr. Aletta Jacobs of Holland, and Professor Grotjahn of Germany, etc. This proceeded not from a failure to recognize their importance, but rather from these circumstances: Nearly everyone who pretends to any elementary knowledge of this subject knows of these individuals; secondly, they are too close to us for altogether objective treatment; thirdly, they are more accurately described as contemporaries than as historical figures; fourthly, the significance of some leaders not dealt with fully in the present volume attaches more closely to the social history of the movement. Grotjahn and Sanger have influenced social policies. Despite these circumstances the MS. has latterly been revised to include, at least in some measure, mention of these figures.

Readers who therefore turn to the *Index of Names* and fail to find mentioned some familiar friends should bear in mind the circumstances mentioned above; also the fact that a later volume will include many more names not included in this volume. Most scholars do not realize that investigation of this subject is as yet too young to enable us to see the broad outlines of development with such perfect perspective as to give each person his due share of credit—no more and no less. Doubtless too much space has been devoted to some figures, not enough to others. But space given is not to be considered a fit criterion of historical importance.

NORMAN E. HIMES.

Colgate University,
Hamilton, New York.

ACKNOWLEDGMENTS

THIS research had not proceeded far when it became clear that it led into such diverse areas of knowledge as to require the assistance of experts. This has seemed the only sound policy to pursue, for the inquiry takes the investigator not only into anthropology, economics, and sociology, but into Egyptology, and the Oriental languages, many untrodden bypaths of historical medicine, into philology, bacteriology, and biochemistry, into the history of the cultural life of various peoples in widely divergent epochs of time, into the most obscure areas of botany, materia medica, as well as into the chemical theory of contraception, etc. No single individual is an authority on the interpretation of Egyptian, Sanskrit, Persian, Arabic, Hebrew, and Chinese texts. Since such an inquiry is beyond the scope of any one scholar, I naturally owe much to others.

There has been aid from anthropologists, ethnographers, and medical historians of the highest competence from Bombay and Belgium to Boston. Their assistance is acknowledged below, as well as in appropriate parts of the text, and in footnotes attached to each chapter.

To Michael J. Hagerty of the University Library, University of California, who searched the original texts of certain ancient Chinese medical works, and to Dr. Solomon Gandz, Talmudic scholar, and until recently Librarian of the Rabbi Isaac Elchanan Theological Seminary and Yeshiva College, New York City, who prepared the draft of the greater part of the chapter on the ancient Hebrews, I owe much. I am also indebted to Mr. Arthur W. Hummel, Chief of the Division of Chinese Literature, Library of Congress, who enlisted the coöperation of Mr. Hagerty. Were it not for Dr. Max Meyerhof, M.D., of Cairo, the great Arabic scholar, my chapter on Islamic contraceptive medicine would have been very slender indeed. He has imparted unstintingly the fruits of his erudition. I am indebted to Dr. Cyril Elgood of Wareham, Dorset, England, for translating a portion of his Persian MS. copy of Ibn al-Jurjānī's *Dhakhīra*.

I owe a special debt to Professor J. P. Kleiweg de Zwaan, Director of the Colonial Institute, Amsterdam, Holland, for much material and for further leads on contraceptive practices employed by the natives of Sumatra, Java, and neighboring territory. My friend, Mr. M. van Stappen, a mechanical engineer of Worcester, Massachusetts, has been of indispensible assistance by translating and abstracting material in the Dutch language and in preparing four drawings.

Dr. M. Moïssidès of Athens, Greece, patiently copied for me the relevant passages in the French edition by Dr. Zervos of the French text of Aëtios; which I publish within in English, I believe for the first time. The Zervos edition of Aëtios' treatise on the diseases of women was not available in the United States. Hence, I am very grateful to Dr. Moïssidès. Mr. R. D. Karvé of Bombay, India, searched the Sanskrit text of the *Bridhadyôgatarangini*. In connection with Egyptian texts, thanks are also due to Dr. James H. Breasted, Director, and Dr. Robert J. Barr, Assistant to the Director, respectively, of the Oriental Institute, Chicago.

When, in the summer of 1930, work on the medical section of this work was begun, individual letters were sent to forty leading medical historians in various parts of the world requesting leads to works antedating 1800 that might throw light on the medical history of contraception. This list was secured by the National Committee on Maternal Health from the New York Academy of Medicine and other organizations. On it were placed only those medical historians who had achieved some eminence for their wide learning in their field. No helpful replies were received—impressive evidence of the present state of knowledge in this field—save from Dr. Isador Fischer of Vienna, Dr. R. de Waard of Groningen, Holland, and Dr. Paul Delaunay of Le Mans, Sarthe, France. These gentlemen I found informed and coöperative. It is safe to say that medical historians have given practically no attention to our subject. The histories of medicine almost without exception neglect it.

Certain anthropologists and ethnographers have been more informed and coöperative. Special thanks are due Dr. Frans M. Olbrechts of the Musées Royaux et d'Histoire in Brussels. Professor W. Lloyd Warner, formerly of Harvard and now at Chicago, secured for me by correspondence two or three statements from American anthropologists; while one of his students, Mr. Lloyd Cabot Briggs, culled certain references from Westermarck on African practices. A few leads were received by reading in manuscript Mr. Herbert Aptekar's *Anjea*. But as in the instance of other secondary sources (e.g., Ploss-Bartels, *Das Weib*), an effort has been made to trace all references to the original observer or recorder. However, I was not always successful for the library reasons mentioned on page xv.

I wish to acknowledge the value of criticisms of the chapter on preliterate society received from Dr. Ralph Linton of the Department of Anthropology, University of Wisconsin, and from Dr. A. R. Radcliffe-Brown of the Department of Anthropology, University of Chicago.

Professor Frank H. Hankins, Professor J. J. Spengler, Dr. Solomon Gandz, and Dr. Louise Stevens Bryant have kindly read the entire typescript at some stage, and offered thoughtful suggestions. Dr. Robert L. Dickinson,

Chairman of the Executive Committee of the National Committee on Maternal Health, has kindly and carefully read the medical portions.

Such generous coöperation is rather unusual even in a scientific project. Specialists of the highest standing have given unstintingly of their time. This help, full in measure and high in quality, it will be impossible to repay.

Numerous are the library workers to whom I owe thanks. Among them are the staffs at the British Museum and at Harvard University. The Misses Lotta M. McCrea, May Walker and Muriel A. Ballard at the Boston Medical Library were very patient in bringing me countless volumes of old medical periodicals and other tomes—this under conditions which were very trying (new stacks, but inadequate funds for storing, indexing, etc.). The librarians at Clark and Colgate Universities secured some otherwise inaccessible works through the inter-library loan service.

I wish to make special acknowledgment here of the brilliant work on the medical history of contraception given us in 1898 by the German worker, Dr. Felix Freiherr von Oefele, and translated into Dutch by Dr. Rutgers (see Bibliography). It seems desirable to mention von Oefele's name here not only because his articles furnished valuable leads to the present writer, but because, with the exception of one citation in the modern literature, his name has fallen completely into oblivion; and this obscurity is most unmerited.

Without the loyal and steadfast coöperation of my wife, the completion of the work would have been well-nigh impossible. She not only typed half a dozen drafts of the manuscript, but freely offered wise counsel on many difficult points.

I wish also to remember those friends and former teachers who, though they have given no direct assistance, have seemed, through their sympathy, to have lent encouragement to an inquiry hardly as yet established as altogether legitimate. Among these sympathetic on-lookers have been some of my former teachers at Harvard, Professors T. N. Carver, E. A. Hooton, A. P. Usher and F. W. Taussig. Mention should also be made of Dr. E. B. Wilson of the Harvard School of Public Health, and my friend, Dr. Carl Joslyn of the Department of Sociology. It was that erudite and broadminded teacher of the history of economic theory, the late Professor Allyn Young, who, by a casual remark in a lecture, called my attention to the pioneer inquiries of the late Professor James A. Field, and who, together with the stimulus received in Professor Carver's seminary on agricultural economics—which that year discussed the relation of population to food supply—started me on my way toward inquiring into the whole domain of population problems. My indebtedness to Carver, Young, and Field is considerable.

Among the other "silent assistants" I should mention the late Graham Wallas, fatherly tutor and guide to American students studying in England, Professor H. J. Laski, Dr. Geoffrey May, formerly of the Russell Sage Foundation, of the Institute of Law, The Johns Hopkins University, and now a social-work executive in Richmond, Virginia; Professors Earl J. Hamilton and William McDougall of Duke University, and even more particularly Professors A. B. Wolfe of Ohio State University and E. A. Ross of Wisconsin. These men, whether they were conscious of it or not, have helped me to push an inquiry which, as I have indicated before, is hardly yet established as respectable or legitimate. Needless to say, for the shortcomings of this book the responsibilities are mine alone.

The author index was made by two of my students, Mr. F. W. Haines and Mr. E. E. Evans.

Most important of all, this book might never have been published, at least not as soon as it has been, if the National Committee on Maternal Health had not secured a substantial grant in aid of publication.

NORMAN E. HIMES.

Colgate University,
Hamilton, New York.

CONTENTS

BIBLIOGRAPHY

LIST OF FIGURES

LIST OF TABLES

PART ONE

CONTRACEPTIVE TECHNIQUE BEFORE THE DAWN OF WRITTEN HISTORY

CHAPTER I

PRELITERATE SOCIETIES

§1 CONTRACEPTION NOT THE CHIEF POPULATION CONTROL IN PRELITERATE
SOCIETIES

MAN'S attempts to control the increase in his numbers reach so far back into the dim past that it is impossible to discern their real origin. Some forms of limitation on the rate of increase are undoubtedly as old as the life history of man.[1] The fact of widespread limitation of population by primitive peoples was an established fact of ethnography and anthropology long before Carr-Saunders published his well-known and excellent study. See, for example, the works of Nieboer,[2] Ploss,[3] Westermarck,[4] Lippert,[5] Gerland,[6] Sutherland,[7] Lasch,[8] and others.

Occupying a central place among the early checks were the "positive," or death-producing, checks—disease, especially epidemic diseases and those whose spread was promoted owing to an absence of modern sanitation and the control factors introduced later by the development of preventive medicine; famine and a host of factors limiting the food supply; war, child mortality, human sacrifice, feuds, the deliberate killing or desertion of the aged, and witchcraft. Infanticide was, of course, the rule among a large number of tribes. Catastrophes such as floods, earthquakes, cyclones, and tornadoes must have played a very small rôle, even as they do in our day.

[1] See the accounts in A. M. Carr-Saunders, *The Population Problem.* Oxford: Clarendon Press, 1922. William G. Sumner, A. G. Keller, Maurice Davie, *The Science of Society.* New Haven: Yale University Press, 1927. See especially vol. i, ch. ii. Hannibal G. Duncan, *Race and Population Problems.* New York: Longmans, 1929, chs. xvi, xvii. Edward B. Reuter, *Population Problems.* Philadelphia: Lippincott, 1923, ch. viii. Carr-Saunders and Sumner, Keller and Davie are strongest in the use of primary sources. Warren S. Thompson, *Population Problems.* New York: McGraw-Hill. New ed., 1935.

[2] H. J. Nieboer, "Die Bevölkerungsfrage bei den Naturvölkern," *Korrespondenz-Blatt der deutschen Gesellschaft für Anthropologie,* xxxiv (1903), 143–150.

[3] Heinrich Ploss, *Das Kind in Brauch und Sitte der Völker* (2 Aufl.), ii, 251–261. *Das Weib* (4 Aufl.), i, 646–651, 656–662. *Die Medizin der Naturvölker.*

[4] Edward Westermarck, *History of Human Marriage,* pp. 312–3.

[5] Julius Lippert, *Kulturgeschichte der Menschheit,* i, 207–216.

[6] G. Gerland, *Über das Aussterben der Naturvölker,* pp. 50–62.

[7] A. Sutherland, *The Origin and Growth of the Moral Instinct,* i, 114–130.

[8] Richard Lasch, "Über Vermehrungstendenz bei den Naturvölkern," *Ztschr. f. Sozialwissensch.,* v (1902), 81–95; 162–169.

The chief "preventive" or birth-limiting check in primitive society was abortion. Anthropological monographs make frequent references to the crude practices of various peoples scattered all over the globe; and the literature on the subject is enormous.[9] Other preventive measures were: delayed marriage and celibacy, both almost negligible among primitive peoples; sex tabus limiting the time and frequency of connection, pre-puberty coition, sex perversions (more or less neglected by most writers), prolonged lactation, and conception control, both magical and rational.[10]

It is with the last of these only, with contraception, that we are here concerned. A mere enumeration, as above, of the population checks operating among contemporary primitive tribes and, therefore, by inference, among our more distant ancestors, suggests, and correctly, that conception control played but a small part in limiting the growth of numbers.[11] It seems clearly established that infanticide and abortion were much more frequently practised than conception control. In surveying, therefore, in the account that follows, the magical and rational methods of conception control employed by preliterate peoples, the relative infrequency of such practices should be borne in mind. On the other hand, we should have a larger number of data on conception control among primitive peoples had the earlier reporters taken more pains to get at the facts of the sex life of the groups studied. More concerted efforts in this direction are now being made by some of the younger anthropologists, though even their results have not always been enlightening.

Let us now survey by continents the contraceptive practices of primitive

---

[9] See the art. on "Abortion" in *Encyclopedia of the Social Sciences*. Also Gustav J. A. Witkowski, *Histoire des Accouchements chez tous les Peuples*. Paris, no date. A good account of abortion among primitive peoples is to be found in the literature cited in the first note.

[10] A word of explanation is required regarding the use within of the terms "magical" and "rational." They stand in the author's mind as a contrast, though he realizes that primitive and folk magic are often based upon reasoned—incorrectly reasoned—inductions or deductions. To that extent they partake of the rational; but such inferences are usually non-logical. An act may be said to be non-logical if it is not capable of inducing the result intended by the act. When primitive women, therefore, drink a decoction, or subject themselves to rites by medicine men to prevent pregnancy, these are referred to as magical, i.e., non-logical. The term "ineffective" is sometimes used also, though in many instances this term is avoided, because it places upon the author the burden, onerous in some cases, of finally passing upon the effectiveness of given contraceptive practices.

[11] H. J. Nieboer, *op. cit.*, p. 147. Nieboer's account contains a good, though undocumented, summary of population checks among primitive peoples. *Cf.*, Carr-Saunders, *op. cit.* Bloch [i.e., Dühren] exaggerates when he says that, among primitive races, measures for the prevention of conception "are widely employed." Iwan Bloch (pseud. for Eugen Dühren), *The Sexual Life of our Times*. Trans. by Eden and Cedar Paul from 6th German ed., p. 696.

peoples in widely scattered portions of the globe in order to determine (a) the mechanisms by which conception control is accomplished, (b) the degree of geographical universality of such practices, and where possible, the frequency with which they are employed. There will be occasion to note that the practices differ considerably in effectiveness and in the degree of rationality upon which they are based. Attention will be directed first to the continent of Africa.

§2 AFRICA

(2a) South Africa

Reports are available of magical and rational means of controlling conception used by the members of African tribes. Junod,[12] for example, states that the Thonga prevent conception by what seems to be *coitus interruptus*.[13] Upon the birth of a child, abstention from intercourse is enjoined. On the day when the child begins to crawl, however, a ceremonial rite is performed; and the parents "must [on the same day] have sexual intercourse, but in such a way that the mother will not become pregnant."[14] After this rite has been performed the child is considered as a grown-up, full member of the family or tribe. The parents may once more have conjugal intercourse regularly, though they must again avoid conception until the child is weaned. The passage referred to, *semine non immisso*, may refer to *coitus reservatus*; but it would seem more likely that the practice is *coitus interruptus*. While the purpose is apparently religious rather than economic, one wonders whether this birth-limiting method is employed by the Thonga only upon such ceremonial occasions. Our informant does not suggest that the practice is general. It is also quite possible that the practice has fundamentally an economic basis, though to external appearances the motive may appear religious or ceremonial.

Knowledge of this method seems to extend throughout South Africa,[15] the Congo,[16] in what was formerly German East Africa[17], and elsewhere.

[12] Henri A. Junod, *Life of a South African Tribe*, i, 55.

[13] "Semine non immisso. Ad hoc, marito sperma foras spargendum est (a nga mu weleri): hic est coitus rite factus et quasi lustralis. Inde, uxor in manus utriusque sordes (thyaka ra bona) sumit, quibus umbilicum illinit." *Op. cit.*, i, 488. [Without letting the semen in—that is, the man should emit the spermatozoa outside. This is coitus ritualistically performed like a ceremony of purification. Subsequently the woman takes in both hands her garment with which she smears her navel.]

[14] *Op. cit.* p. 55.

[15] Junod, *op. cit.*

[16] Adolphe Louis Cureau, *Les Sociétés primitives de l'Afrique Équatoriale* (Paris: A. Colin, 1912), p. 189.

[17] Friedrich Fülleborn, "Das deutsche Nyassa und Rowuma- Gebiet," *Deutsch Ost-Afrika*, ix (1906), 552, note.

(2b) *East Africa*

Thompson reports that an East African tribe, the Masai, practice withdrawal, the apparent reason for the custom being a disapprobation of extramarital pregnancy.[18]

Among the Nandi[19] "Girls must be careful not to go to the warriors' huts for some days afterwards [i.e., after menstruation] for fear of becoming pregnant after intercourse with the men." Here reliance seems to be placed upon an infertile period rather well chosen. The reason for avoiding pregnancy in this case is that it is frowned upon in unmarried girls, although it does not seem to result in any very formidable degree of disgrace or punishment. In German East Africa, says Fülleborn, there are long sleeping houses where all young people of both sexes sleep. Intercourse is allowed, but conception must be avoided.[20] This is done by the boys emitting their semen not intravaginally but between the partner's legs.[21]

Probably less effective because more magical is the method used by Yao women to prevent conception. According to Weule,[22] women who wish to prevent impregnation get into touch with a person who knows something about knot-tying. The "fundi" goes into the woods, seeks out two kinds of bark, and twists them into a cord. Into the cord he rubs the yolk of an egg. In the cord he ties three knots, saying as he does so: "Tree you are called so and so; and you, so and so. Out of you (egg) arises life. But, from now on I want no more life." As he says this, he ties the last knots in the cord, which is then worn by the native woman. Thereafter the curse of sterility will remain constantly with the Yao woman until, when she desires to become pregnant again, she unties the knots in the cord, places it in water, and drinks it. The cord is then thrown away. Roots, laid

[18] Joseph Thompson, *Through Masai Land*. In the Appendix Thompson says: "Mulierem gravidam, neque alicujus viri matrimonium tenentem, interficiunt Masaei, quum prium patet eam concepisse. Quod ne occidat, dum bellatores juvenes innuptaeque puellae amori venerio inter se indulgent, viris hoc curae est in coitu, ut ante semen emissum penem extrahant." Translation: The Masai kill a pregnant woman who is unmarried, as soon as it is clear that she is pregnant. To prevent this, while young warriors and unmarried girls are indulging in love making, the men take care during coitus to withdraw the penis before the emission of the semen.

[19] A. C. Hollis, *The Nandi*, p. 82.

[20] Fülleborn, *Deutsch-Ost-Afrika*, ix, 552. "So lange die jungen Paare hier wohnen, ist Nachkommenschaft natürlich nicht erwünscht; stellt sich diese dennoch ein, so gilt es aber nicht als Schande."

[21] Fülleborn says: "Ne fiat conceptio, juvenes coitum non in vaginas virginum, sed solum inter crura facere dicuntur." P. 552, note.

[22] Karl Weule, "Wissenschaftliche Ergebnisse meiner ethnogr. Forschungsreise in den Südosten Deutsch-Ostafrikas," *Mitt. a. d. D. Schutzgeb. Erg.* Heft 1, Berlin, 1908. See p. 61. Cited by H. Fehlinger, *Geschlechtsleben*.

under the head at night, are also used by the same people for the prevention of conception. As in the instance of many other tribes of preliterate people, one may infer from the frequency of abortion among them, that the ultimate reliance of the tribe is not upon contraception as a population control. Besides the sap of plants, Yao women use mechanical methods of abortion. Such interference, as is generally the case among primitive women, is not considered reprehensible as it is in our own culture.

Among the Amhara, or Abyssinians, those women not living on friendly terms with their husbands, and who therefore wish to avoid children by them, as well as prostitutes, attempt prevention by means of a magical medicine called *tongai*, prepared by medicine men. Tampons are ostensibly not used, although in some instances *coitus interruptus* is resorted to.[23] Our informant, Bieber, had contended in a previous article on "Sex Life in Ethiopia," that the Ethiopians had no conception of the physical proceedings during coitus,[24] and that they believed that impregnation happened quite automatically, or as the natives said, "without one knowing how God brought it about;" and that the Abyssinian women, when they wished to prevent conception for any reason, were accustomed to apply to the medicine man or priest, who gave them a medicine prepared from an unknown plant kept secret by the medicine men.

The following report on Madagascar is of interest not so much for the negative evidence it contains, as for its vividness in portraying the methods of control adopted by primitives when contraception is absent:

I believe that no contraceptive measures were practiced in Madagascar [writes Dr. Ralph Linton], although my information is not complete for all tribes. Even at the present time, the semi-civilized Hova do not know any. I can speak with authority on this, for several native women asked my wife how she had limited her family to one child, and expressed a desire for small families. In pre-European times this tribe would have considered any contraceptives as useless, *a priori*, for they held that after the first intercourse a woman would continue to bear children, whether she had intercourse or not.

Population was limited somewhat by the universal rule that a husband must abstain from cohabiting with his wife during a period of three to six months after a birth. This is still rigidly observed even by those who are civilized and Christian. Abortion was practised by unmarried mothers, but was rare, and the methods

[23] Friedrich J. Bieber, "Neue Forschungen über das Geschlechtleben in Äthiopien," *Anthropophyteia*, viii, 188.

[24] Friedrich J. Bieber, "Geschlechtsleben in Äthiopien," *Anthropophyteia*, v, 45–99. See especially p. 63. The Ethiopian kingdom comprises at present the northeastern African highland. This plain of approximately two million square kilometers contains fifteen million inhabitants of twenty or more racial branches or stems. In number and significance the greatest of these are the Amhara, or Abyssinians, the Agau, the Galla, the Kiffitscho, and the Ameti.

apparently not very effective. I believe that they consisted of herb remedies, but obtained no exact information.

Infanticide was extremely common in Madagascar. All children born on certain unlucky days were put to death to prevent them from bringing bad luck to their families. I do not think that there was any idea of limiting population in it, but the losses were severe. In at least one tribe all children born on three days in each week were killed. The child was killed immediately after birth, being dropped into a jar of boiling water head down, or buried in an ant hill.[25]

(2c) North Africa

North African tribes also make efforts to avoid pregnancy. According to an unpublished report by Dr. Walter B. Cline, it is the custom among the natives of the Oasis of Sima in the Lybian Desert, to drink infusions of gunpowder. This may be employed, of course, as an evacuant. But the foam from a camel's mouth is also supposed to be efficacious in preventing pregnancy. Perhaps the most frequent practice is to wear around the waist a Koranic formula sewn up in a little leather bag. The reasons for prevention seem to be personal and economic. The Swahili of Morocco, on the occasion of the ceremonial defloration of a girl, practise what one guesses to be withdrawal.[26]

Coon tells us[27] that among the Riffian Hill Tribes there is a market, exclusively used by women, which takes place weekly. Men are excluded from it, and any caught there are severely punished. Here are freely sold "magico-medico materials which are supposed to act as contraceptives and to produce abortions." It has been impossible to identify these herbs, inasmuch as the sale and possession of them is kept secret. Use of them is considered ample reason for divorce. In fact, a husband, if he could catch his wife practising contraception, would probably kill her.

[25] Letter of Dr. Ralph Linton to W. Lloyd Warner. Used by permission.

[26] "I am told," says Westermarck, "that in Andjra there are bridegrooms who take care that no offspring can result from the defloration of the bride, since many people believe that the child would be diseased if the semen came into contact with the hymeneal blood; whilst others maintain that the child will be all right if only the bride and bridegroom avoid cleaning themselves with the same towel." Edward Westermarck, *Marriage Ceremonies in Morocco*, pp. 265–266. The same passage appears in Westermarck's paper on "Beliefs Relating to Sexual Matters in Morocco" in *Verhand. I. Internat. Cong. f. Sexualforschung*, v. 163–169. See p. 167.

Probably the withdrawal is unnecessary if the girl has just passed puberty. In the Talmud, we may add, the belief is commonly expressed that a girl *cannot* become pregnant after the first coitus, on the occasion of defloration. This fits in well with the modern scientific view that there is an important distinction between puberty and sexual maturity. Hartman argues that there is a gap of three years after puberty when the girl is sterile. See Carl G. Hartman, "On the Relative Sterility of the Adolescent Organism," *Science*, lxxiv (1931), 226–227. Compare discussion below in §6.

[27] Carleton S. Coon, *Tribes of the Rif*, p. 110.

A curious magical practice employed by the Aiṭ Sáddĕn of Morocco is reported by Westermarck as follows:

Among the Aiṭ Sáddĕn the sterilizing effect attributed to a corpse may induce some woman who is anxious to avoid pregnancy—as a girl who has had sexual intercourse—to remain behind after a burial when the other people have left the grave, in order to avert the event she fears by stepping three times over the grave; but all the steps must be made in the same direction, since otherwise the return step would counteract the effect of the earlier step.[28]

The same reporter informs us that a kind of preventive magic or witchcraft called $t^s q\bar{a}f$ is supposed to cause barrenness.

Among the Aiṭ Sáddĕn, for example, water which has been used for the washing of a dead person is secretly given to a woman to drink in order to make her infertile. In Andjra a woman is for the same purpose made to eat some bread into which has been put a piece of a honeycomb containing a few dead bees. In Agui, if a man desires to have sexual intercourse with a certain woman, but she objects, he takes revenge in the following manner: he chars the hoof-parings of a mule, grinds them together with barley or wheat, makes bread of the flour, and gives the bread to the woman to eat, with the result that she will become as sterile as is the mule. At Fez a man prevents intercourse with a woman from resulting in pregnancy by eating the oviduct ($w\mathring{a}lda$) of a hen which he has boiled after first making a knot in it; and it is said that the woman will remain sterile for ever.[29]

The tying of the knot is, of course, symbolic magic.[30] In the same town (Fez) a woman is supposed to be prevented from becoming pregnant by being made to eat castor beans ($\d{h}abb \; l\text{-}\d{h}\acute{a}rwa'$), one for each year that she desires to be free from pregnancy. The same procedure is followed by women of their own volition, when they desire to avoid pregnancy.[31] Another ritual practised in Morocco is of some interest: A stone called 'ain l-horr is worn in a ring of silver or gold. It is believed that "if a man wears such a ring round his finger when he has conjugal intercourse with his wife, and turns the stone towards the next finger, no offspring will result from the connection."[32]

(2d)   West Africa

At least one primitive group in West Africa, the Dahomey, resort to the prevention of conception by a method more rational than the above. The Dahomey use a tubercled root in crushed form applied as a plug intra-

---

[28] Westermarck, *Ritual and Belief in Morocco*, ii, 557.

[29] *Ibid.*, i, 575–576.

[30] For similar practices, *cf.*, ch. vii *infra*.

[31] Westermarck, i, 576. *Cf.*, chapters ii and iv.

[32] *Ibid.*, i, 459.

vaginally.   This would seem to be a logical inference from the statement of the observer.[33]

(2e) Central Africa

Perhaps the most interesting and complete single report on the prevention of conception among primitive people in Africa is that of Masters, who states that among the Bapindas and Bambundas and other tribes of the Kasai Basin in Central Africa, drastic measures are used to occlude the *os uteri*.[34] The desire is generally prevalent among the women not to have a child more frequently than once every three years.   "To prevent the possibility of this, native remedies are taken by the mouth, but more frequently the vagina is plugged with rags or finely chopped grass.   As can well be imagined, the results are often diastrous to the female in question: Constipation, or rather, physical retention of fæces, with tenesmus; retention of urine with incontinence and uræmia are common, not to mention the ascending of the local infection to the genital organs and kidneys."   Masters cites three cases; but inasmuch as the third deals only with abortion, it is not included here.

(2f) Case Histories of Contraception Among Natives

Case One

A native female, aged about 35, was admitted to the hospital moribund.   There was a history of constipation for eight days, and of urinary retention for several days with slight incontinence.   There was marked abdominal pain and increasing drowsiness for six days.   The bladder was distended nearly to the sternum and there was free fluid in the peritoneal cavity.   The "husband" emphatically refused permission to examine the patient *p.v.*, as did also a crowd of women who had accompanied her to the hospital.   They threatened to remove the patient by force if the attempt were made.   Purgatives were given and a large amount of faecal material was passed.   It was not possible to pass a catheter.   The patient died in twenty-four hours and a partial *post-mortem* examination was done.   The vagina was found to be very firmly plugged with a cloth which was about half the size of a man's closed hand.   This pressed upon the rectum behind, causing retention of faeces and occluded the urethra against the pubis in front.   Urine came away freely when the cloth was removed; there was no stricture.   The cloth was replaced and the abdomen opened.   The bladder, ureters and the pelves of the kidneys were distended with urine and the abdominal cavity contained about 1 litre of fluid of the same nature as the urine, but no rupture of the bladder could be found.

[33] Édouard Binet, "Observations sur les Dahoméens," in *Bulletins et Mémoires de la Société d'Anthropologie de Paris*.   5ᵉ Series, i (1900), 244–252.   He says (p. 251) "Le *Beybe* (nagos) est une racine tuberculeuse qui, écrasée, est employée sous forme du cataplasmes pour l'usage secret des femmes."

[34] Walter E. Masters, "The Prevention of Conception Amongst the Natives of the Kasai Basin, Central Africa," *Jour. Trop. Med. and Hyg.*, xix (1916), 90–91.   Masters was a medical officer in the Kwango District, Central Africa.

The withdrawal of the cloth would certainly have saved the woman's life. The "husband" and the other women denied any knowledge of the cloth plug.[35]

Case Two

A native female, aged about 30, was brought to the hospital by the "husband" and a crowd of women who desired to be present to the last. The "husband" stated that the woman had been ill for one month and had been dying for six hours. There was retention of faeces with tenesmus and retention of urine with incontinence. There was great abdominal pain and marked exhaustion. An examination was permitted. The bladder was distended to just above the umbilicus; the vagina was plugged hard with finely chopped grass and made into a pulp. The rectum was pressed backwards and the urethra forwards, as in the former case. The urethra was prolapsed and looked like a "red cherry" at the urinary orifice. The grass plug was removed and the urine flowed in a good current. The bowels acted regularly, there being no real need for purgatives.

Two days later, when visiting the wards, the patient, who had made remarkable progress, did not seem so well. Upon examination a cloth was found tightly wedged in the vagina "to prevent the urine from dribbling away." This cloth had been torn from her loin-cloth and put into position surreptitiously. An attendant was placed in charge of her and in ten days she was discharged well, the prolapse having much improved without an operation. She was two months pregnant.[36]

These seem to be the only known detailed case reports by a physician observing the operation of contraception among a primitive people. There are other reports by physicians (e.g., see M. C. Kahn's report on the Djukas below); but such reports almost never give actual observation of use, and rarely appraise either frequency of use or its general effectiveness. Probably these African cases would never have come to the attention of Masters had not congestion resulted from abuse of, or from defects in, the method. It may be observed here parenthetically that the wedging of grass into the vagina is reminiscent of the practice, still used in certain portions of Japan, of occluding the *os* by stuffing the vagina with wads of bamboo paper (see page 126).

Cureau reports that "onanism,"[37] by which I gather that he means *coitus interruptus*, "is well known to exist everywhere" in Central Africa.[38]

Slaves among the Baholoholo, who live in the Congo region of Africa, take herbs given them by the medicine man to prevent the conception of

---

[35] *Ibid*. p. 90.

[36] *Ibid*.

[37] This word will not be used by those who have respect for accurate terminology. It is ambiguous. Sometimes it is used to mean masturbation, at other times *coitus interruptus*.

[38] Adolphe L. Cureau, *Savage Man in Central Africa* (Eng. trans. by E. Andrews. London: Unwin, 1915), pp. 166–7. P. 189 in the French edition. Cureau reports that sexual perversions are also prevalent in Central Africa—which is probably true. But some of Cureau's statements need discounting.

children condemned to a life of slavery.[39]   In view of the fact that the secret seems to be in the hands of medicine men, and is probably of doubtful effectiveness, one might be safe in inferring that it is not a consequence of contact with white men.

We may conclude, therefore, regarding Africa, that although contraception was not the chief check (abstention from intercourse, for example, being much more frequent), it was not totally absent.   As we shall see later, Carr-Saunders is in error in stating that among the primitive races "there is no evidence of the existence of any practice that renders sexual intercourse fruitless"[40] except among African tribes who use *coitus interruptus*.   On the other hand, Masters is doubtless generalizing from his few cases, and certainly stating the case too strongly, when he says that "the prevention of conception is practised by civilized as well as uncivilized people perhaps the whole world over."[41]

§3   NORTH AMERICA

Judging by the paucity of reports,[42] the primitive tribes of North America seem to have practised contraception but little.   Dr. Clark Wissler ventures the opinion, however, that "thirty or forty years ago there was not an American Indian tribe among whom medicine men did not possess several kinds of magical formulae for preventing childbirth."[43]   If this position is well taken—and Dr. Wissler is usually considered an authority on American Indians—I am not aware what the *published* evidence is in support of the view.   Ashe states[44] that the girls of the Shawnee Indians "drink the juice of a certain herb which prevents conception, and often renders them barren through life."   Other Indian tribes believe that sterility can be artificially induced; but the few practices that exist seem to be magical rather than genuinely effective methods.

The following report by Hrdlička, on magical contraception among the Indians of Southwestern United States and Northern Mexico, is of interest not simply for its essentially magical nature, but for the reasoning of the Indian mother reported in this account.

There is a very general belief among the Indians visited that sterility may be artificially induced.   To produce this result the women desiring to have no more

[39] Schmidt in Cyrille Van Overbergh's *Collection de Monographies Ethnographiques*, vol. ix.   *Cf.*, Herbert Aptekar, *Birth Control Review*, July, 1930, p. 203.

[40] *Population Problems*, p. 177.

[41] *Op. cit.*, p. 90.

[42] This is not a reliable criterion since some instances of contraceptive practices were doubtless overlooked by observers; but there is no way of allowing for this factor.

[43] Herbert Aptekar, *Anjea*, p. 111.

[44] T. Ashe, *Travels in America* (London, 1808), p. 272.

children take internally certain harmless substances, . . . which to the Indians are representative of sterility. The San Carlos Apache believe that artificial sterility can be induced, but the means is not generally known. It is supposed to be some variety of root. One of the women applied to the writer for a "medicine to make her have no more children." When questioned as to the propriety of such a proceeding, the answer was that when one child after another is born and dies, or when a number of children, one after another, are born dead, something should be done to end this unfortunate state of affairs.

Among the White Mountain Apache a woman desiring to have no children, or to stop bearing, swallows now and then a little of the red burned earth from beneath the fire. This means, which is much believed in, is used mostly by the dissolute unmarried, but also by sickly or very poor married women. Some of the Huichol women drink a decoction of a certain plant to prevent childbearing. Cora women, for the same purpose, take internally the scrapings of the male deer horn.[45]

According to Olbrechts,[46] the Cherokee Indians of western North Carolina, are not ignorant of contraception, though abortion is unknown. These Indians who inhabit the Great Smoky Mountain region, are not completely isolated, since they have slight contact with some poor whites. But there is no reason to believe that they have received any contraceptive instruction from that source. Furthermore, Olbrechts avows that the Cherokee "still cling to their aboriginal beliefs and customs with a tenacity which is unequalled by any of the other Indians living on reservations East of the Mississippi."

Cherokee women desiring to remain sterile chew and swallow for four consecutive days the roots of spotted cowbane (*Cicuta maculata*; other common names are musquash root and beaver's poison. The Cherokee name is thiliyusti).[47] They believe that "if a woman uses this [recipe], she will become sterile forever."

Olbrechts' chief informant (a prominent medicine man, holding a leading position in the tribal organization, twice married, and a high school graduate) knew, however, of no case in which the recipe had been used. But he

---

[45] Aleš Hrdlička, *Physiological and Medical Observations among the Indians of Southwestern United States and Northern Mexico.* Smithsonian Institution, Bureau of American Ethnology, Bull. 34 (Washington: Gov. Prtg Off. 1908), p. 165. *Cf.*, *J. A. M. A.*, cxix, 1665.

[46] Frans M. Olbrechts, "Cherokee Belief and Practice with Regard to Childbirth," *Anthropos*, xxvi (1931), 17–34. *Cf.*, James Mooney and Frans M. Olbrechts, *The Swimmer Manuscript. Cherokee Sacred Formulas and Medicinal Prescriptions.* Smithsonian Institution. Bur. Amer. Ethnol. Bull. 99 (1932), p. 117.

[47] *Anthropos*, xxvi, 19. Olbrechts says that the plant used by the Cherokee as a contraceptive closely resembles, at an early period of its growth, parsley (*Petreselinum sativum*), and cites von Hovorka and Kronfeld [*op. cit.*, (1908), i, 170] for evidence that parsley is still popular in several European countries as an abortifacient. It is still used as an emmenagogue [U. S. Disp. 19th ed. (1907), p. 1393, cited by Olbrechts]. For the use of parsley in folk medicine, see p. 170.

imagined it might be used by women who could not keep their children alive, or when parturition would endanger the mother's life. But even in these instances, the medicine man alleged, the Cherokee woman would not use the contraceptive, inasmuch as women would as soon die in childbirth as live without children. "There is a vague hint by some of the informants at the possibility of promiscuous women using this drug, especially if they are married, so that there can be no material proof of their misbehavior. But substantial evidence to prove this impression could not be given."[48] Other informants concurred with the medicine man in declaring they knew of no case of actual use; and agreed that, from the standpoint of morals, the use of contraceptives was "nothing less than a crime."

It is possible that the medicine man was withholding complete information from the inquirer.[49] But whether this is so or not, it is interesting to observe the recognition by this medicine man of modern indications for contraception (sickly children, danger of mother's death in parturition). The rationality of the reasoning involved may be compared to that shown by the Southwest Indians as reported above by Hrdlička.

What of the effectiveness of the recipe? It is highly probable that it was useless; for no drug has yet been discovered which, when taken by the mouth, will induce temporary sterility.

Vague, and possibly a little exaggerated, is the report of Currier (1891) that

We find the same tricks and crimes accompanying conception and gestation among Indians that are common everywhere. Nor is it probable that their ideas upon these matters are borrowed from civilization. Everywhere, in all grades of society, there seems to be an inherent desire with a certain number of women to avoid the cares and responsibilities of maternity.

Among the Quapaws the child-bearing period ends at thirty-five to forty. They occasionally use means to prevent conception. . . .

The Neah Bay (Washington) women drink a decoction of an herb (the name of which my correspondent did not know) to prevent conception, but the very young women are eager to become impregnated, that they may not be compelled to go to the Government school.[50]

Writing of the Isleta Indians in New Mexico, Parsons observes that women not wanting a child, or not desiring additional children, especially if they have suffered during parturition, "will apply to a member of one of the medicine societies, to whom a buckskin, flax cloth, a belt, and cotton

---

[48] *Anthropos*, xxvi, 19. Bur. Amer. Ethnol., Bull. 99, p. 117.

[49] Concerning the secrecy of the Cherokee on this point, Olbrechts observes: "I am inclined to think that the Cherokee hold the only [contraceptive] means known to them from the white settlers."

[50] A. F. Currier, *Trans. Amer. Gyn. Soc.*, xvi (1891), 277–278.

will be given.   Two women were cited as having no children after three or
four years of marriage, thanks to their medicine man."[51]   Probably Parsons
is here reporting the views of the women themselves, rather than vouching
for the effectiveness of any magical or rational contraceptive method.   Parsons continues:

If a woman does not wish to conceive she will not have intercourse for nine days
after menstruation . . . nor during pregnancy, nor for six months after child birth.
At least in theory.   A case was cited of a man who sought intercourse 10 days
after his child's birth; his wife wept, thinking she would conceive, and her mother
scolded her husband.   At [the time of the] first menstruation a medicine may be
given a girl which will preclude child bearing. . . . Lucinda had ceased menstruating at the age of 35.   An "old man" said she was too young for that and offered to
bring the function on again, but she refused.   In speaking of her daughter's
family, Lucinda opined that two children were enough for her daughter to have.[52]

This report is of interest chiefly for the early reference to a sterile period.
Anthropologists often interpret such conduct as purely ceremonial.   It is
clear in this instance, however, as it is in many others, that the real motive
lying behind it is population regulation.   The fact that Lucinda did not
care to be relieved of the suppression of the menses is further evidence that
she found sterility rather agreeable.   In the last sentence of the quoted
passage the idea is also clear that Lucinda believed in birth regulation for
her daughter.   This is only one more illustration of many that might be
cited to demonstrate that the desire for controlled fertility is very prevalent
among primitive peoples.

Concerning the Pueblo Indians, Aberle reports[53] that "Twenty representative informants were unanimous in saying that no contraceptive measures
were used by the women of these pueblos."   The older women are eager
for the younger women to have as many children as possible.   As is usual
among primitive peoples, the young women want offspring, and take pride
in their fruitfulness.[54]   No instance of sterility was found by Aberle; and
induced abortion is reported as infrequent.

[51] Elsie Clews Parsons, "Isleta, New Mexico," 47th Ann. Rpt. Bur. Amer. Ethnol.,
p. 213.

[52] *Ibid.*

[53] S. B. D. Aberle, "Frequency of Pregnancies and Birth Interval Among Pueblo
Indians," *Amer. Jour. Phys. Anthrop.*, xvi (1931), 63–80.   See especially p. 68.

[54] There are few Pueblo Indian women who have reached the age of thirty who have
not had one or two pregnancies—a striking contrast to the situation among native-born
white women in the United States.   In this sample studied by Aberle, the average age at
which the Pueblo woman had her first child was 17.8 years.   The average age of the mother
at the birth of the last child was 35.8 years.   The reproductive span averaged eighteen
years.

For another interesting recent study of vital statistics among a primitive people see

Such a negative report, unlike most negative reports, has value because it shows that the investigator was looking for what she did not find. Most anthropological reports, especially the early ones, are valueless from our point of view because, though they rarely refer to contraceptive practices among the primitive peoples observed, one cannot deduce from this fact that no contraceptive knowledge exists. Only when there is an explicitly negative statement can we have confidence in the report; and not always then.

Other than the aborigines inhabiting what is now the Continental United States, the chief native groups of North America were perhaps the Esquimaux and the Mayas. A survey of the literature on the former reveals no report of genuinely contraceptive practices; this is confirmed by Dr. Franz Boas.[55] However, Ratzel avows that the Eskimo mothers[56] of Baffin Land and American Indian mothers[57] were accustomed to prolong the suckling of their children with the *intention* of keeping the family small. While there is probably no doubt about the fact, it is quite possible that investigators have read into this conduct a motive of which the women were not conscious. Dr. Ralph L. Roys, an authority on the ethno-botany of the Mayas, finds no evidence that the native Maya doctors (called *ah-men*, or yerbatero in Spanish) had any knowledge of contraception.[58]

We thus conclude that American tribes had no effective methods of preventing conception; that, like other preliterate groups, they relied for the regulation of family size more upon abortion, infanticide and periods of tabued intercourse than on methods preventing conception. But it should be noted that an absence of contraceptive knowledge among North American natives does not mean uncontrolled family size.

Hortense Powdermaker, "Vital Statistics of New Ireland (Bismarck Archipelago) as Revealed in Genealogies," *Human Biology*, iii (1931), 351–375. The people studied by Powdermaker have had practically a stable birth rate for three generations; an average of 2.6 children per woman, or 2.9 per fertile woman. The modal number was three, the next largest groups being four and two respectively. The fertility of these people is thus about equal to that of native-born whites in the United States. Powdermaker discusses the causes of population decline. These are probably associated with the fact that a larger proportion of the offspring in more recent generations is dying in infancy, and consequently do not have an opportunity to reproduce themselves.

An interesting older study of depopulation in the Marquesas is that of Tautain in *L'Anthropologie*, ix (1898), 298–318; 418–426.

[55] Letter to the author.

[56] Friedrich Ratzel. *Völkerkunde*, Leipzig, 1877–88. English translation by A. J. Butler as *History of Mankind* (London, 1896–1898, 3 Vols.), ii, 106.

[57] *Ibid.*, ii, 126.

[58] Letter to the author, dated Dec. 21, 1931.

§4 SOUTH AMERICA

References to contraceptive methods employed by native peoples in South America are few;[59] but they manifest ingenuity.

Karsten writes[60] as follows of the Canelos Indian women of Ecuador:

> In order to be able to cohabit with a man without getting pregnant the Canelos women are in the habit of taking a medicine prepared from the small *piripiri* plant.[61] The root knots of the plant are crushed and soaked in water, and the woman takes a quantity of this drink. Afterwards she has to eat only roasted plantain without salt and small birds of the forest. If she infringes these rules of diet, she is believed to be particularly exposed to the very danger against which the *piripiri* drink was to protect her.[62]

Presumably, if the woman gets pregnant, it can always be countered that she failed to respect the food tabus.

More effective is a douche solution containing lemon juice "mixed with a decoction of the husks of mahogany nut." This is reported[63] in use by the Negro women of Guiana or Martinique. One cannot be certain from the original account which place is referred to.

This ought to be reliable provided enough lemon juice is used. For one or two tablespoons in a quart of water is an effective spermicide.[64] Lemon juice is about five per cent citric acid, which immobilizes sperms immediately at 1 to 1,000. Mahogany husks may also have an astringent effect. One wonders whether the Negro women reported to use this have come in contact with whites. If not, this is probably the only case on record of a primitive group using this particular spermicidal agent. And it is the first known anticipation of a more elaborate, still more ingenious technique re-

---

[59] Even though its title would suggest otherwise, the following source contained nothing on the subject: J. I. Sacón ["Malthusianism as Practised by South American Indians"] *El Hôpital Argentino*, iii, 876–879 (March 15, 1933). Despite the rarity of reports on contraception among South American natives, we know that the ancient races of Peru practised oral and anal coitus, as shown by surviving pottery. We are not here concerned with perversions, but we may note that they had a birth-limiting effect even when the intent was only to secure pleasure. It is probable that anal and oral coitus are as old as man. The earliest literature mentions them. In the Quran and Talmud anal coitus with one's own wife, though morally objectionable, is not forbidden legally. *Cf.*, Lauterbach.

[60] Rafael Karsten, "Contributions to the Sociology of the Indian Tribes of Ecuador. Three Essays," *Acta Academiae Aboensis. Humaniora* Åbo: Åbo Akademi, 1920, No. 3.

[61] Karsten informs us in a note that "Of the plant *piripiri* there are four varieties, which are distinguished by their different sizes, and all of which are used by the Indians for different superstitious purposes."

[62] *Ibid.*, p. 71.

[63] French Army Surgeon [Dr. Jacobus X], *Untrodden Fields of Anthropology* (Paris, 1898), i, 257.

[64] Dickinson and Bryant, *Control of Conception*, p. 42.

ported by Casanova[65] in the eighteenth century. This consisted in cutting a lemon in half, extracting most of the juice, the disk being used as a cervical cap. This is a direct forerunner of the modern cap method (pessary, spermicidal paste or jelly).

Perhaps equally effective is the contraceptive means known to some Djukas. This interesting group has recently been studied objectively by Dr. Morton C. Kahn,[66] a bacteriologist connected with Cornell Medical College in New York. The Djuka, which consist of six tribes, are the Bush Negroes of Dutch Guiana, South America. They are descendants of slaves who escaped from African slave ships and who, finding conditions in Guiana similar to their African homeland, have successfully established their own communities, and have thrived. They now number about 20,000. The Dutch, unable to subjugate these vigorous people in a series of long, bloody wars, granted them their autonomy. Today the Djukas are one of the very few primitive groups bargaining and entreating politically with the white man on a more or less equal plane.

From the standpoint of numbers, these people are maintaining themselves. The number of offspring ranges from 0–12 per mother with the average two or three.[67] There is a low infant, but high child mortality. Abstention from intercourse, and nursing for two years after the birth of a child are common. Abortion is also practised. Kahn also states that impotence is common,[68] and that the natives have a knowledge of aphrodisiacs.[69]

More interesting are the unpublished details of the contraceptive discovered by Kahn.[70] Native women sometimes insert into the vagina an okra-like seed pod about five inches long from which one end is snipped off. The intact end probably lies against the cervix, or in the posterior fornix, the open end receiving the penis. This is, therefore, a kind of vegetable

[65] *Mémoires de Casenova de Seingalt* (Paris: Librairie Garnier Frères) v, 77.

[66] Morton C. Kahn, *Djuka. The Bush Negroes of Dutch Guiana.* New York: Viking, 1931.

[67] *Ibid.*, p. 127.

[68] *Ibid.*, p. 124.

[69] *Ibid.*, p. 125. Dr. Kahn writes me that the natives "drink an infusion of a bush vine known as 'Debbil Dour' which is supposed to give them erections of long duration. The males also insert fragments of a reed known as the mucca-mucca in the urethra. This acts as an irritant, and is also designed to bring about erections of long duration. There is probably some such property in the second named substance, and certain white physicians of the colonies tell me that a properly made infusion of Debbil Dour will accomplish the same thing. I have no first-hand information concerning either preparation, however. The Djukas are highly promiscuous sexually, intercourse before marriage and adultery being the general practice." The families are small, chiefly because of a high mortality.

[70] Letters to author dated October 14 and November 13, 1931.

condom held in place by the vagina. Dr. Kahn's informants were medicine men who furnished oral reports. On his next trip Dr. Kahn has promised to bring back specimens for botanical indentification, and to secure photographs. It is not known how widely this custom is practised. My informant "heard of it only two or three times." He observed no actual use. However, since the Djukas are highly promiscuous sexually, and since intercourse before marriage and adultery are the common practice, it would seem reasonable to infer that population is controlled not only through abortion and high mortality, but perhaps through contraception as well.

The paucity of reports concerning American natives would lead one to the tentative conclusion that contraception was much less frequently resorted to in North and South America than in Africa and Australasia. If this is so, it is an interesting and perhaps significant anthropological fact. Many of the American natives, who perhaps migrated from Eastern, Central and Northeastern Asia across the Behring Straits to our Continent, seem to have brought little or no contraceptive knowledge with them. At least the scanty evidence at present available seems to point to the tenability of such a principle.

§5 AUSTRALASIA (AUSTRALIA, NEW ZEALAND, POLYNESIA, MELANESIA, MALAY ARCHIPELAGO, ETC.)

Pitt-Rivers many years ago noted that "European observers, such as missionaries and government officials, have often supposed that some mysterious contraceptive drug was used by the unmarried girls [of Oceania]. Native herbs and roots, mixed together with all manner of magical substances, such as spider's eggs, skins of snakes, etc., are as a matter of fact made into concoctions and drunk by girls with this idea. I have myself [continues Pitt-Rivers] collected such recipes from Melanesian and Papuan sorcerers and old women, but there is no reason to suppose that they have any physical effect.... No medical analyst to whom I have submitted several of these prescriptions has, however, found any reason to credit these concoctions with any of their supposed physical properties."[71]

[71] G. H. L. Pitt-Rivers, *The Clash of Culture and the Contact of Races* (London: Routledge, 1927, pp. 312), p. 132 n. and p. 148 n. Pitt-Rivers' psychological theory of the decline in native numbers as being due to a decline in desire to live, seems questionable, if not unsound; likewise questionable is his theory that promiscuity sterilizes by immunizing the effect of the sperm of one male upon that of another. Dr. Robert L. Dickinson informs me that the view is commonly held that frequent coitus renders couples sterile through absorption of the semen. However, Dr. Katharine Bement Davis, whose study of the sexual life of 1000 married women of the higher class in America is well-known, made especially for Dr. Dickinson a study of those cases having intercourse daily or oftener. No relative infertility was found as characterizing these sexual athletes. Thus frequent

A form of magical contraception exists among the Sinaugolo in British New Guinea; for Seligmann writes that in that locality "There is generally a woman in the village or one of the surrounding villages who is supposed to be gifted with a power, inherited from her mother, of causing women to become *hageabani*, literally incapable of having more children. Suppose a woman considers [that] she has [had] enough children; she will by stealth seize an opportunity of consulting such a woman, and will pay her for her services. The woman gifted with the power sits down behind, and as close as possible to, her patient, over whose abdomen she makes passes while muttering incomprehensible charms. At the same time herbs or roots are burnt, the smoke of which the patient inhales."[72] The report is of interest chiefly as showing the desire in New Guinea for prevention. The method could scarcely have been effective.

Krieger reports that in what was known as German New Guinea means for preventing conception are known;[73] but he furnishes no details. He avows that though sterility is uncommon, and though the natives like children, they "raise not more than three, chiefly from fear of lack of sufficient nourishment, or because it is inconvenient or wearisome to raise them."[74] Abortion, as well as contraception is practised; and the fact that twins are scarce suggests resort to infanticide. It is abundantly clear that many primitive peoples thought in Malthusian terms long before Malthus. The women of preliterate society knew all about Malthus' main point: that too rapid increase endangered support. Malthus' *Essay* was essentially a learned inductive proof of an obvious thesis long understood and long acted upon.[75]

Kiwai Papuan women, natives also of New Guinea, "who do not want a child, wear a rope tied very tightly round the waist, particularly during the sexual act, after which they also wash carefully."[76] The use of the rope is clearly magical; washing the vulva, however, partakes of the effective. The procedure might include the vagina in which case it would probably be

---

coitus, as practised by many preliterate peoples cannot, it would seem, be held responsible for the relatively small rate of births sometimes found by ethnographers. This would seem to have a bearing on the discussion of points raised by Malinowski and others (see *infra* pp. 29–40).

[72] *Jour. Anthrop. Inst.*, xxxii (1902), 303. Punctuation altered.

[73] M. Krieger, *Neu-Guinea* (Berlin, 1899), p. 165.

[74] *Ibid.*, p. 165. Punctuation mine.

[75] This is not to suggest that all checks were *consciously* adopted to control population. Sometimes they were accidentally hit upon, proved worthwhile, were selected for survival and became traditional.

[76] Gunnar Landtmann, *The Kiwai Papuans of British New Guinea* (London: Macmillan, 1927), p. 229.

more effective. Older women, considered experts in conception control and in procuring abortion, warn the younger women not to dabble with these matters on their own account because of the risk to their lives.

The natives of Torres Straits, just south of New Guinea, have a magical rite for producing temporary sterility by burying an unknown object called *gab* in a termite's nest, where it is left to rot. Seligmann has made several unsuccessful attempts to ascertain the meaning of this word. Ordinarily it means womb, but in one instance it seems to refer to after-birth.

Concerning the natives of Torres Straits Bruce reports through Haddon that, while no operation is known designed to induce sterility, and while no diet is adopted as a check, the

old women may give to young women the young leaves of the *argerarger* (Callicarpa sp.), a large tree, of which the fruit is inedible; *sòbe* (Eugenia, near E. chisiacfolia), a large tree with edible fruit; and *bok*, a large shrub. The young leaves of these trees are well chewed and the juice swallowed, until they feel that their bodies are wholly saturated with the juice. The process takes some time, but when their system is thoroughly impregnated, they are supposed to be proof against fecundity and can go with men indefinitely. Both men and women strongly believe [sic] in the efficacy of these leaves.[77]

Haddon adds that sterile women tell their husbands they use these plants as a preventive; and they are believed.

Other tribes use this method. Brown reports[78] that the native women of New Britain (in the Territory of New Guinea just east of Papua) eat the leaves of an unknown plant to prevent conception.

One wonders how much to credit the report of Riedel[79] that when the native women of the Island of Buru in the Moluccas (Malay Archipelago) have coitus with strange men "they maintain a passive and indifferent state for the purpose of avoiding impregnation." It is certain that this practice dates back to antiquity in the West, and quite far back in Chinese history —the Chinese call the practice Kong-fou—but this is the only report of it among primitives that the literature reveals. If the report is to be credited, this technique takes rank for antiquity with *coitus interruptus*. Perhaps the anthropologists will be skeptical about the natives using it consciously "for the purpose of avoiding impregnation." The "passivity" is sometimes a kind of self-hypnosis or a mental preoccupation by turning the mind to

[77] Alfred Cort Haddon, "Birth and Childhood Customs, and Limitation of Children," in Cambridge Anthropological Expedition to Torres Straits, Reports of, pp. 105–111, vol. VI on *Sociology, Magic and Religion of the Eastern Islanders* (Cambridge, University Press, 1908), p. 107.

[78] George Brown, *Melanesians and Polynesians* (London, 1910), p. 38.

[79] Kisch, *Sexual Life of Woman*, p. 403.

subjects other than the event in hand.   My theory is that it proceeds from
a sense of guilt in coitus; if it is not enjoyed, the consequences will not be
so unfortunate.   The notion is very old and very widespread that "holding
back" prevents impregnation by preventing an orgasm.   Of course, the
orgasm is not so completely under control as many assume.   The idea that
"holding back" an orgasm prevents impregnation is also related to the
sucking-in theory of the cervix.   If the uterus actually did suck in semen
during orgasm, as it probably does not, it might facilitate conception; but
there is scant evidence on this matter.

More effective than the means just described were those reported by
Walter Knoche[80] as in use among the native women of Easter Island.   Before they had sexual relations with foreigners, usually sailors, these women
would sometimes place just in front of the os uteri a piece of algae or seaweed.
The women considered this method effective.   Knoche tells us that it was
unfortunately not possible to determine whether the measure was generally
applied in past times, or whether it was applied solely for the object of
keeping the stock free from dilution by foreign blood.   In opposition to
the latter view is the circumstance "that the women of Easter Island have
children by 'foreigners' who have lived for some time on the island, but
that today the women use contraceptives, when they have coitus with such
foreigners as come and disappear quickly.   The ostensible reason seems to
be," avows Knoche, "that in the latter case there is no man to support the
child when it is born.   It is indeed, highly probable," he adds, "that the
application of contraceptives originally had its origin in Malthusian principles.   The small island, whose population, according to reports of various
eighteenth and nineteenth century travellers, oscillated a few thousands,
had by this time reached its maximum of numbers, and hence it became
necessary to keep births and deaths at an equilibrium."[81]   Knoche considers the presence of anti-conceptional methods among these people quite
as much evidence of a relatively high culture as the famous stone idols, a
system of writing, etc.   Knoche is, however, in error in thinking that the
inhabitants of Easter Island are the only preliterate people in the Oceanic-
Island region to have knowledge of prevention;[82] and Fehlinger, who quotes
Knoche, falls into the same error.[83]

[80] Walter Knoche, "Einige Beobachtungen über Geschlechtsleben und Niederkunft auf
der Osterinsel," *Zeitschr. f. Ethnol.*, xliv (1912), 659–661.   Cited by H. Fehlinger in "Das
Geschlechtsleben der Naturvölker," Nr. 1 in *Monographien zur Frauenkunde und Eugenetik, Sexual-biologie und Vererbungslehre* (Ed. by Max Hirsch. Lpz: Curt Kabitsch, 1921,
pp. 93), p. 62.

[81] Knoche, p. 660.

[82] *Ibid.*, p. 661.

[83] Fehlinger, *Geschlechtsleben*, pp. 62–63.

Margaret Mead reports that the Samoans practice *coitus interruptus*. This, their only method, is not in Dr. Mead's opinion, a consequence of contact with whites.[84]

A rather unusual practice, that of the male sucking the semen from the vagina, is reported as in vogue among the Marquesans of Oceania:

I am under the impression that the Marquesans used no mechanical or chemical contraceptives [writes Dr. Ralph Linton in a letter]. Children were rarely born to unmarried mothers, but I think that the chances of conception were cut down mainly by the use of perversions instead of [by the use of artificial devices during] actual intercourse. The natives were extremely expert in the arts of love. However, the perversions were always practiced in private. When a group of men went out with one woman, and had intercourse with her in rapid succession, publicly, which was a common amusement, the last man had to suck semen from her vagina. This was sometimes practiced in individual intercourse as well. I believe that this is true, although it sounds improbable; for excitement of women with the tongue [cunnilingus] was a regular part of love play.[85]

I append Dr. Linton's observations on abortion as practised by the same natives, because of the unusual nature of his interpretative remarks:

Abortion was fairly common even after marriage. Due to the universal practice of adoption, many women objected to bearing children which they knew would be taken from them, and reared by some one else. Herb remedies were used, although I did not learn their nature; and also mechanical abortion by means of a sliver of bamboo inserted into the uterus. I do not know at what stage this was used. There seem to have been few casualties from this method, for the people were expert anatomists, due to the knowledge gained by cutting up bodies to eat.[86]

The Maori of New Zealand have an odd ritual designed to cause a woman's fruitfulness to cease. It is referred to by the natives as *Taupa* or *kokoti-uru*. Elsdon Best, the observer of this rite, was not able to learn the particulars of it. He was able only to say that "a piece of stone was employed therein, and [that] the woman was supposed to be made as sterile as the stone."[87] Of the same magical nature is the procedure of Maori

[84] Letter to W. Lloyd Warner. Used by permission. Miss Mead writes: "I did not find any knowledge of contraception among the Samoans except a knowledge of *coitus interruptus*. . . . They practiced abortions by pressure, either by rather skillful manipulation by the old masseurs, or roughly by the boy placing the sole of his foot against the girl's side. Kava was also believed to be an abortifacient, if chewed in large enough quantities."

[85] Letter of Dr. Ralph Linton, anthropologist, University of Wisconsin to Mr. W. Lloyd Warner, University of Chicago anthropologist. Used by permission of both parties.

[86] *Ibid.*

[87] *Jour. Anthrop. Inst.*, xliv (1914), 132. The ritual was doubtless as ineffective as that which Best describes as prevalent to cause a *pukupa* (sterile) woman to bear.

medicine men who are believed by the natives able to prevent conception by throwing a little blood into the fire as they murmur incantations. A woman arranges to have her confinement in the presence of a medicine man, who carries out the above during the expulsion of the placenta. Henceforth the woman will not conceive.[87a]

Fiji Island women, who live just east of New Zealand, take local flora internally in an effort to prevent conception. Says Blyth, reporting in 1887:

> Just as the Fijian midwife undertakes to rectify sterility, so, on the other hand, amusing expedients are resorted to with the object of preventing conception, and these methods are believed to be sometimes successful and sometimes not. The medicine employed for this purpose is obtained from the leaves and root of the Roqa tree, and from the leaves and root of the Samalo in conjunction. The roots are first denuded of bark and then scraped. The scrapings and the leaves bruised are made into an infusion with cold water, and this, when strained, is ready for use. This herbal medicine is taken sometimes once, and sometimes twice, in order to produce the desired effect. If coitus take place, say in the evening, the decoction is given on the following day, and this without any reference to the relation in point of time which the coitus may bear to the menstrual period. This remedy, besides being given to prevent a first conception, is also administered in the case of a woman who has had one or more children, in order to prevent future pregnancies.[88]

Such methods are undoubtedly ineffective. Similar medicines are taken to induce fertility. The women have small families as a rule, but sterile marriages are reported as not infrequent. "If a woman is sterile, she is at once believed to have drunk at some time or other 'the waters of barrenness,' that is to say, sterility is looked upon as a self-induced condition."[89]

The reasons for limitation are very interesting. "Fijian women have a decided aversion to large families, and have a feeling of shame if they become pregnant too often, believing that those women who bear a large number of children are laughing-stocks to the community.... If a woman believes that her present pregnancy has too quickly succeeded her previous one, she deems it necessary to bring about abortion."[90]

In New Ireland, not far from the Fiji Islands, similar methods for preventing conception have been tried. Pfeil was the first reporter in 1899.[91] A more recent investigator, however, is of the opinion which the writer shares, that while the natives think they have a contraceptive that works,

---

[87a] Edward Tregear, *The Maori Race.* (Wanganui, N. Z.: Willis, 1904), p. 38.

[88] *Glasgow Med. Jour.*, xxviii (1887), p. 180. Blyth was for some years on the British Government Medical Staff in Fiji.

[89] *Ibid.*, p. 179.

[90] *Ibid.*, p. 181.

[91] J. G. Pfeil, *Studien und Beobachtungen aus der Südsee* (Braunschweig, 1899), pp. 30–31.

in reality they have none. Dr. Hortense Powdermaker of the Yale Institute of Human Relations has recently done field work among these natives, and reports in *Life in Lesu*[92] the contraceptive and abortifacient herbs used by the natives. Prior to publication of the report, the author wrote me that the natives "think they have a method of birth control. Certain leaves are supposed to have the power of making a woman sterile, and others are said to have an abortive value. The leaves are chewed, the juice swallowed, and the pulp spit out. Natives swear by the efficacy of these leaves. But so also do they swear by the ability of the rain magician to bring rain. The knowledge of the sterilizing and abortive leaves is usually owned by men who have received it from the maternal uncle or some other relative. It is zealously guarded, for, like all medical and magical knowledge, it is a source of income. When a man is requested to procure the necessary leaves, he is paid for his services." Dr. Powdermaker brought back seven varieties of leaves supposed by the natives to have abortifacient properties. These she has since had identified. One of these, *Rubus miluccanus*, has the same function in India; while four are used in India, but with different functions. Two have constituents that might make them useful as emmenagogues: *Acanthacae*, which contains a bitter alkaloid, and *Curcuma*,[93] which contains a volatile oil. These are undoubtedly ineffective since no drug taken by the mouth is known to Western science that will prevent conception or abort.

Testimony very similar to Dr. Powdermaker's comes from Professor Radcliffe-Brown who declares that "a very large proportion of the tribes of New Guinea and the adjacent islands (Bismarck Archipelago, etc.) believe in the possibility of producing sterility in women by means of vegetable substances taken orally. The actual species of tree or plant which supply the berries, bark, or roots so used differ in various districts. I tried," he continues, "to get some of them subjected to pharmacological analysis. There is evidence that at least one of these medicines does produce in a few days a shrinking of the female breast. One may, however, be fairly certain that the native belief that the taking of these substances orally for a period will produce sterility is unfounded in fact." He adds: "Similar beliefs and practices have not been found in Australia, though they might possibly exist in the North of Cape York Peninsula, where there is considerable influence from New Guinea."[94]

Regarding the effect of the self-administration orally of drugs supposedly

[92] Hortense Powdermaker, *Life in Lesu. The Study of a Melanesian Society in New Ireland* (New York: W. W. Norton, 1933), pp. 242–244; 293–297.

[93] *Cf.*, *infra* p. 38.

[94] Letter to author dated Nov. 6, 1932.

abortifacient, an observation by von Oefele is relevant. He has contended that if certain abortifacient drugs, namely ergot and *Aristolochia*, are taken regularly by women, as has been the case since antiquity, and in other forms probably since prehistory, a certain under-development of the uterus takes place; and that this in itself either causes sterility or acts as a hindrance to conception.[95] Many dangerous drugs, he holds, also cause inflammation and catarrh of the cervix, which interfere with conception. If such is the case, this practice may have brought about some diminution of births.

From drugs we turn temporarily to a method of expelling the semen used by a South Sea Island tribe reported by Pfeil:

Rarely are the women confined in the first year after their marriage. Usually two or three years pass before the birth of their first child. The women fear children since they increase their working load. To be sure the girls help their mothers, but years must pass before they are able to be really serviceable. Accordingly, abortion is frequently resorted to intentionally. The women jump from a height, or permit themselves to be massaged by another in order to expel the foetus. Moreover, they possess the noteworthy ability, up to a certain degree, to make pregnancy dependent upon their will, since they are in a position after cohabitation to emit immediately from themselves all that they have received (alles Empfangene sofort wieder von sich zu geben).[96]

Here reference is made to a method of expelling the semen, possibly by bodily movements or even by a downward straining while squatting.

Erdweg reports that the inhabitants of Tumleo, an island in Dutch New Guinea, "know how to prevent the birth of children" when they do not want them.

Four obviously harmless plants are already known to us, the drinking of which produces sterility. One of these called *kakaú*, grows by the thousands hereabout.

---

[95] Felix Freiherr von Oefele, "Anticonceptionelle Arzneistoffe. Ein Beitrag zur Frage des Malthusianismus in alter und neuer Zeit," *Heilkunde* (Wien), ii (1898), 206; 273; 409; 486. For this reference see the second article in the series, pp. 273–284. This scholarly and able series is the best single source on contraceptive practices since Greek times. If one may judge by the absence of citations, this work is, to American and English writers, quite unknown. The articles have usefully been collected and published in Dutch under the following title: *Over het Gebruik van Kruiden en dranken ter Voorkoming van Zwangerschap.* (On the Custom of Drinking Drugs for the Prevention of Pregnancy) Amsterdam: Graauw, ed. 3, 1899, pp. 159 (trans. from German into Dutch by the late Dutch Neo-Malthusian, Dr. J. Rutgers). I have collated this page by page with the German articles and have established that they are virtually identical. Since no copy of this work (the collected series in Dutch) was known to be on deposit in any American Library it was necessary to import a copy from Holland. Thanks are due the eminent medical historian, Dr. R. de Waard, of Groningen, Holland, for calling my attention to this Dutch edition.

[96] Pfeil, *Studien*, pp. 30–31.

The women eat the leaves of that with sago bread. Both the leaves and fruit of another plant *natunmum* (making one incapable of conceiving) are eaten with sago bread. Another plant, the name of which is unknown to us, is dried on the fire like tobacco, ground, made into a cigarette and smoked. The women swallow the smoke which makes them sterile. The worst plant of this kind is the last, called *lapalet*. This plant has a root which is peeled, cut into little disks, and then eaten alternately with cocoanut kernels. One does not dare to chew the stuff, for its taste is too bitter; it must be swallowed whole. The poison of this plant is so destructive that it not only produces sterility [?], but can also kill a three or four months old foetus. Why the people wish to produce sterility and even abortion is still quite unknown to us. Even the men do not know what to say about it. They know neither the secret means of the women, nor the art by which this childlessness is made possible. Only the fact that the women do this is known to them, and also the fact that they take plant poisons for that purpose. On the more intimate circumstances the married women, who alone are initiated into the secrets, observe an unbreakable silence.[97]

Natives of the Eddystone Islands, a mere speck of land in the southern part of the Solomon Islands, have, according to the report of Rivers,[98] a magico-religious rite called *egoro* (meaning "barrenness") which they believe not only prevents conception temporarily, but produces permanent sterility. Rivers, like many other anthropologists who have followed him, noted that, although the natives freely indulged in sexual relations prior to marriage, premarital births were, in fact, so "extremely rare" that "in the whole of the pedigrees collected by us only one such case was given, and that many generations ago." No such birth was reported during his visit; and so far as he could learn "there was no one on the island who was the child of premarital intercourse." Such births had occurred, but no actual instances could be cited.

Two causes were given to account for this: abortion, and the *egoro* rite.

Several examples of *egoro* rites were obtained [by Rivers]. One came from Ruviana, in which bark is scraped with a *rikerike* from the two nut-trees called *ngari* and *vino* and from *petepete* tree. The bark is mixed with scrapings from a special reddish stone procured from the island of Gizo, and the mixture put inside a betel-leaf and given to the woman to be eaten with a nut of *anggavapiru* and lime, to the accompaniment of the following formula:

"Ngge va pialia na rekoreko pini; mi patu to pa na soloso; mi ke pondu komburu; mi egoro tu."

"I make this woman here eat betel; let her be as the stone on the mountain; let her not make a child; let her be barren."

A girdle is put on of *molu* taken where it crosses the path. This is done for four months, once in each month.

[97] P. M. J. Erdweg, "Die Bewohner der Insel Tumleo, Berlinhafen, Deutsch-Neu-Guinea," *Mitt. d. Anthrop. Ges. in Wien*, xxxii (1902), 383.
[98] W. H. R. Rivers, *Psychology and Ethnology*, p. 76ff.

Another method, elicited from a very old woman, was the scraping of bark from the *nggema* and *vino* trees. The bark was eaten with betel-leaf, together with *anggavapiri*, but without any formula. In the case of a married couple the mixture was eaten by both sexes, and it was said that, even if eaten by the man only, his wife would not bear any children. This rite was carried out for four months, four times in each month, . . . A case was mentioned in which this *egoro* had been given to a girl before puberty, who, though now a grown woman, had had no children.

This egoro bears so close a resemblance to the process already described that there are very probably two versions of the same rite. A third example is very different. In it, part of the nest of the bee or hornet called *mbumbu* and the flower of the *undundalo* plant are put inside betel-leaf and eaten with areca-nut, which is the *imburu* of the usual kind, while the betel-leaf is that called *uala igigisi*. No formula is used. This is eaten by men and women, and is said to be efficacious if eaten only by the man. The place of origin of this *egoro* is not known, and it may possibly have come from Ruviana like the first.[99]

Rivers goes on to state that the significance of this rite is essentially magico-religious. Indeed the use of a girdle made of a creeper where it crosses the path supports such a view. But Rivers adds that something may be used in the *egoro* rite which has "genuine pharmocological action." This is improbable. More likely the almost total lack of premarital children is to be explained rather by the circumstance that girls have a sterile period, or at least a quasi-sterile period, for three or four years following the onset of menstruation (see p. 35).

A Melbourne anthropologist, D. F. Thomson, has lately shown[100] that the natives of several tribes constituting the Kawadji on the Cape York peninsula are aware that pregnancy results from sexual intercourse and that they recognize a *physical* as well as a *social* bond between father and child. These views are quite contrary to Malinowski's.

The Koko Ya'o, Kanju, Yänkonyu, Ompelä and Yintjingga tribes of the Kawadji group have a firm belief in the contraceptive, as distinct from abortifacient, properties of certain plants. Thomson was informed of this by both men and women in widely separated localities while collecting genealogies. The two plants used were called *tjarri* or *ka'atä* (*Dioscorea sativa var. rotunda*) and *pi'alä* (*Entada scandens*).[101] The natives replied that certain childless women had no offspring because they "had shut themselves up" by eating medicine. The men, though usually pleading ignorance of women's matters, admit that women use such a medicine and

---

[99] *Ibid.*, pp. 77–78.

[100] *J. Roy. Anthrop. Inst. Gr. Brit. & Ire.*, lxiii, 519.   See sec. 12, pp. 505–510.

[101] Both are used for foods, the root of the former and the bean of the latter, but only after a tedious cooking process and frequent changes of water. The latter is called the Queensland matchbox bean. The former is a tuber.

declare they would be angry if they found their women using it. The reason given by the women for the use of contraceptives was that they could not carry their children about. One woman said: "I have only one child, not a great number. I have no canoe to carry them about the country. My belly is no good, nor my shoulder [to carry children]."

When taken as contraceptives these medicines are generally eaten raw, sometimes roasted, but always without the prolonged washing employed when the same are taken as food. It is administered to the young women by older women credited with special knowledge of such matters. The medicine "is taken in the early morning on an empty stomach, after which the woman lies down, refraining from drinking throughout the day, until sundown. The old women declared that once a woman had taken this medicine [*tjarra*] she would never have a child. One explanation of its action was that it 'dried them up,' another that it closed the genital passages so that the *täll'äll* [seminal fluid] could not enter. These are, of course merely the speculations of my informants," says Thomson, "for in such matters, which are not freely discussed, there is probably nothing that could be called an orthodox belief."

Thomson has no evidence on the reliability and effectiveness of these. Many native medicines are magical (e.g., love charms), but some (e.g., fish poisons) are very potent. But the native has as much faith in one as in the other. Thomson is convinced of the sincerity of the native beliefs in the contraceptive medicines.

§6   THE PUZZLE OF INFERTILE PREMARITAL PROMISCUITY

A similar problem, infertile premarital promiscuity, is raised regarding the natives of the Trobriand Islands (North-West Melanesia, British New Guinea). Professor Malinowski, the anthropological authority on the sex life of the aborigines of this area, not only denies that the natives have any knowledge of methods to prevent, or to reduce the likelihood of, conception;[102] but he asserts, and presents evidence tending to prove, that they are ignorant of the physiology of paternity.[103]   He says:

[102] Bronislaw Malinowski, *The Sexual Life of Savages in North-Western Melanesia.* London: Routledge, 1929. So far as can be determined, none of Dr. Malinowski's other numerous works present any evidence on the subject of conception control.

[103] See especially Ch. vii, §3. Dr. Malinowski argues that the Trobriand natives believe that in order for a woman to become pregnant only perforation or dilation of the vagina is necessary. Other groups have been known to hold this view. Physiological insemination by sexual congress is not required (pp. 154–155). "They do not know the generative power of the male discharge." P. 155. Elsewhere Dr. Malinowski says, "physical fatherhood is unknown." P. 171. *Cf.*, p. 172.

Since there is so much sexual freedom [among the Trobriand Islanders], must there not be a great number of children born out of wedlock? If this is not so, what means of prevention do the natives possess? . . .

As to the first question, it is very remarkable to note that illegitimate children are rare. The girls seem to remain sterile throughout their period of licence, which begins when they are small children and continues until they marry; when they are married they conceive and breed, sometimes quite prolifically.[104]

Since giving birth to prenuptial children is considered by the natives "reprehensible," and hence leads to concealment, Dr. Malinowski could not speak with complete confidence regarding the number of illegitimate children. But he believes such births to be approximately one per cent of the total.[105]

In attempting to explain the small number of illegitimate children, Dr. Malinowski speaks with a curious combination of diffidence and self-assurance:

On this subject I can only speak tentatively, and I feel that my information is perhaps not quite as full as it might have been, had I concentrated more attention upon it. [But] *One thing I can say with complete confidence: no preventive means of any description are known, nor [is] the slightest idea of them entertained* (italics mine). This, of course, is quite natural [since the natives do not understand the physiology of parenthood]. . . . Indeed, any suggestion of neo-Malthusian appliances makes them shudder or laugh according to their mood or temperament. They never practise *coitus interruptus*, and still less have [they] any notion about chemical or mechanical preventives.[106]

This statement seems all the more clear as Dr. Malinowski says

that the natives, when discussing these matters, feel neither fear nor constraint, so there can be no question of any difficulties in finding out the state of affairs because of reticence or concealment.[107]

The situation is puzzling. There is general promiscuity before marriage but almost no illegitimacy. When the same girls marry and "settle down," they bear children sometimes prolifically. Dr. Malinowski's query is to the point:

Can there be any physiological law which makes conception less likely when women begin their sexual life young, lead it indefatigably, and mix their lovers freely? This . . . cannot be answered here, as it is a purely biological question; but some such solution of the difficulty seems to me the only one, unless I have missed some very important ethnological clue.[108]

[104] *Ibid.*, 166–7.
[105] *Ibid.*, p. 167.
[106] *Ibid.*, pp. 167–168.
[107] *Ibid.*
[108] *Ibid.*, p. 168.

A. C. Rentoul, a Resident Magistrate,[109] believes Malinowski did miss a "very important ethnological clue:" expulsion of the male seed.[110] As proof that the natives understand the physiology of conception he cites this alleged practice:

> Dr. Malinowski has asserted that no contraceptives are known to the natives of the Trobriands. Be that as it may, I have been informed by many independent and intelligent natives that the female of the species is specially endowed or gifted with ejaculatory powers, which may be called upon after an act of coition *to expel the male seed*. It is understandable that such powers might be increased by use and practice, and I am satisfied that such a method does exist.
>
> It would appear from evidence that I have been able to collate on the spot that the precaution referred to is taken by single girls to prevent conception, and also by married women who do not wish to become pregnant.[111]

Malinowski scoffs at this idea. Back in 1929, in his *Sexual Life of Savages*, he had admitted that "there is a belief prevalent among the white citizens of Eastern New Guinea that the Trobrianders are in possession of some mysterious and powerful means of prevention or abortion."[112] But he was even then firm in the conviction that this belief, which he described as "incorrect and fantastic," could arise only from an inability to explain away the infertile premarital promiscuity, from the "insufficient knowledge" of the local white residents,[113] and from "a tendency towards exaggeration and sensationalism so characteristic of the crude European mind." Even the residents who held the conviction could cite no evidence to Dr. Malinowski.

In reply to Rentoul's implication that he missed significant ethnological evidence—which implication, incidentally, has led to an acrimonious but entertaining debate in *Man*—Malinowski, in an article on "Pigs, Papuans, and Police Court Perspective,"[114] has in 1932 presented much the same point of view as in 1929. He described the expulsion story as "one of the typical myths which circulate among the semi-educated white residents,

[109] Rentoul has been connected with the Court of Native Matters, and, as a District Officer, has come into contact with the domestic problems of the natives. At present he is Resident Magistrate in charge of the South-Eastern Division of Papua, embracing a large portion of Western Melanesia and the Trobriand group.

[110] Alex. C. Rentoul, "Physiological Paternity and the Trobrianders," *Man*, xxxi (1931), Art. No. 162.

[111] *Ibid.*, p. 153.

[112] Pp. 168–9.

[113] As partial proof of the inaccurate information of local whites regarding native affairs Malinowski says the whites dogmatically assert that unmarried native girls never have children save those who live with white traders, whereas the fact is that native girls sometimes do have prenuptial children. Malinowski thinks Rentoul had such an informant.

[114] *Man*, 1932, Art. (not p.) 44.

ascribing to the members of the inferior culture all sorts of preternatural powers." He lampoons its effectiveness, is astonished that Rentoul accepted the story, and calls for real evidence on the existence of the practice.

Malinowski quotes R. F. Fortune's, *The Sorcerers of Dobu* (p. 239) as coming to essentially the same conclusions with regard to the Trobriand belief that procreation is by reincarnation of dead spirits rather than by activity of the biological father.[115] He adds that Dr. Sarasin and Professor Nieuwenhuis have also come to the conclusion that the unphysiological theory of conception held in the Trobriands extends generally to Australia and Oceania. In fact Malinowski goes so far as to assert[116] that "not one assertion" in Rentoul's article is "scientifically substantiated." Moreover, Malinowski denies that in his former writings his thesis was to prove that the Trobrianders know nothing about paternity. More exactly his view is that, though the natives have "a vague idea as to some nexus between sexual connection and pregnancy," they have "no idea whatever concerning the man's contribution towards the new life. . . ." They believe that the *Baloma* is the real cause of later birth but that cohabitation is *also* a cause. It is in this sense evidently that "physical fatherhood is unknown." If Malinowski's later statements do not mean this, then the statements made by him on various occasions hardly check.

Rentoul's rejoinder under the title of "Papuans, Professors, and Platitudes" has little to add regarding the specific contraceptive practice originally reported. The author merely adds that he had learned from a friend,

---

[115] W. J. Perry interprets in just the opposite manner from Malinowski the passage in Fortune. This passage reads:

> The Dobuans know the Trobriand belief that procreation is from the reincarnation of spirits of the dead, not from the biological father. . . . The Trobrianders asserted the spiritual belief, just as Dr. Malinowski has published it. . . . With the exception of the part played by the seminal fluid, Dr. Malinowski's rendering of the Trobriand ideas on the physiology of sex applies also to the Dobuan state of knowledge. (Fortune, *Sorcerers*, p. 239.)

Concerning the above Perry writes:

> This quotation surely implies that the Trobrianders are *not* ignorant of the physiological doctrine of paternity. They obviously have heard of it many times from their Dobuan friends. The friction engendered by discussions about it shows quite clearly that in their minds there is a conflict between common sense and tradition. The rational is struggling with the non-rational, but the non-rational triumphs because of the prestige of its association. They deny the doctrine of physiological paternity because they have been taught a fantastic alternative theory which they accept because of the authority that so often even amongst ourselves causes sophisticated nonsense to be accepted in preference to patent truth. (*Man*, 1932, Art. No. 218.)

Thus do the same observations lead to opposite conclusions. This shows in what an unfortunate state modern anthropological knowledge is on this subject.

[116] *Man*, 1932, p. 37.

Dr. Cecil Cook of North Australia, that such a method was unreliable contraceptively. An additional case is cited to support his view that the natives realize the rôle of the father in paternity. In concluding that the natives probably hold two beliefs: first, that the offspring is the gift of God, or of the *Baloma*; second, that it is given to the mother through the agency of the male seed,[117] Rentoul does not seem to differ very widely from Malinowski. But as to the reality of the practice in this particular region of expelling the semen there is still a clash of opinion.

Additional light can, however, be thrown on this problem. What is undoubtedly the same technique, seminal expulsion by violent bodily movements, is reported below as used by Australian natives. Therefore, its occasional use by some Trobriand women is a possibility. Other circumstances being equal, a positive declaration of use seems more credible than a denial by natives in conversation with an anthropologist.

As we have seen, the question whether primitive peoples understand the rôle of the father in paternity is still unanswerable so far as all groups are concerned. But the conclusion is justified that it seems highly probable that some groups have only a magico-religious theory of conception, others a quasi-rational explanation to *supplement* some magico-religious theory. Almost without exception the half-informed, rational explanation is only a *supplement*. The natives believe that conception can take place by either method. This is probably the situation among the Trobriands.

But it seems like *non sequitur* reasoning for Dr. Malinowski to contend that because the Trobriands do not *completely* understand the physiology of conception it is "quite natural" that they should make no attempts to prevent conception. My survey of the contraceptive knowledge of preliterates shows that some tribes have knowledge of techniques fairly reliable from a theoretical standpoint. And the presumption is that such groups

---

[117] F. W. Williams, government anthropologist in Papua, has recently pointed out that in the Morehead District of Papua two discordant theories of conception are held at the same time: the woman is impregnated by an eel copulating with her while bathing; the semen impregnates her. Williams describes the second theory as "generally accepted" and as overlying the first. Despite the inconsistency of the two theories, the native has sincere belief in each at different times. (*Man*, xxxiii (1933), Art. No. 128.) Williams concludes that these natives well knew that the father played his part in the procreation of the child. It was generally held that pregnancy resulted from repeated intercourse, and the actual body of the child was said to be formed by the accumulation of *jengere* (semen). . . . Some natives, seeking to explain the barrenness of certain women, suggested that they were in the habit of ejecting the semen after intercourse. It was also claimed that the woman's refusal to cohabit again until her last child was walking accounted for the smallness of families. . . . The males of this district are without exception sodomists . . . and they hold the belief that the practice may lead to pregnancy in the male." (p. 123) They eat lime to prevent pregnancy.

have no more knowledge (and no less) of the physiology of conception than have the Trobrianders.[118]   We have seen that seminal expulsion is reported elsewhere in the region.   So great have been the variations in sexual conduct in various early groups throughout the whole period of cultural evolution that it would seem highly probable that some groups hit upon reliable or quasi-reliable contraceptive methods even though their knowledge of the mechanism of conception was meagre indeed.   Such historical accidents, if they may be so described, are explicable upon the theory of variation, trial and failure, trial and eventual success.   No other sociological theory seems adequate to explain the facts.   Clear it is that anthropology alone has never solved the riddle.

Following Malinowski's reasoning we would have to conclude that man would never have used a condom or sheath to prevent venereal infection until the gonococcus or spirochaete had been identified under a microscope as the cause of the disease; whereas all that is required is that men should observe an association between sexual contact and a disease subsequently arising.   Some primitive people have doubtless made a similar association. They have observed a connection between coitus and a later birth.   When Professor Warner asked some Australian native men what semen was for they replied: "That makes babies."

Similarly, one of Dr. Malinowski's students, Dr. Hortense Powdermaker, observes of certain New Ireland natives that "These Lesu people are fully aware of the causal connection between intercourse and birth, although they do not know the exact physiological process by which the embryo is formed."[119]

---

[118] It would be interesting, and perhaps worth while, for someone to correlate the extent of contraceptive knowledge and the extent   of physiological understanding of different primitive groups.   I have not done so.   The data might not be available in many instances.   It might be charged by some anthropologists, especially by the modern functionalist school, that I have committed a serious methodological error in extracting one element from different cultures, that is, knowledge of contraceptive technique, without making allowance for its relation to the totality.   Neither of the anthropologists who read the manuscript of this chapter criticized it on that ground.   But if such a methodological criticism were made, the reply would be that the selection of one cultural element for comparative study is fully justified.   Furthermore, I have tried to take into account other cultural circumstances in extracting this one element for comparison, as I think this chapter shows.   There is such a thing as making a fetish of the principle: "Study each cultural element in relation to the total situation, in relation to the whole culture."   This is a sensible rule of methodology, but when carried to extremes it becomes *prima facie* absurd for the reason that we never can know all the modifying circumstances any more than we can ever know much about first causes.   Furthermore, many who preach this doctrine, never live up to it in their own studies.

[119] Hortense Powdermaker, *Life in Lesu*, p. 242.

It is highly important to realize, however, that even if expulsion of the semen were generally prevalent among the Trobrianders (as it evidently is not), it could not be sufficiently effective to explain, under conditions of general promiscuity prior to marriage, an illegitimacy rate as low as one per cent. We are not told in any report of the method that the fingers are used to wipe out the vagina; and even had this been the case, not all the semen would be removed from the folds and fornices. Bodily movements alone could not be effective particularly if delayed; nor would they result in complete removal of sperms.

The infertile promiscuity is probably to be explained on Hartman's theory[120] that girls have an infecund period for three or four years after the onset of menstruation. They have no children because they are biologically immature, not because of any generally diffused contraceptive technique. Puberty and sexual maturity are not identical as commonly supposed. The births begin shortly after physiological maturity, which probably arrives in most instances shortly after the early marriages of the girls. Whether the Trobrianders or any other group have a full knowledge of the physiology of conception or biological fatherhood is immaterial for our problem since the sterility of the promiscuous period is to be explained on biological not contraceptive grounds.

The evidence on these points pro and con has been presented in some detail because infertile promiscuity among primitives has been a great problem. And it has not been sufficiently probed. The Trobrianders are merely a case in point. The generalization is probably sound that wherever we find this phenomenon among natives the explanation is to be found not in contraceptive practices (as a rule)[121] but in biological immaturity of the young girls.

In an effort to render the account of contraceptive practices among the natives of the Indian Archipelago as complete as possible the assistance of Professor J. P. Kleiweg de Zwaan of the Colonial Institute, Amsterdam, was enlisted. This outstanding authority on the ethnography of that region reports as follows:

I have found little mention in the literature concerning methods of preventing pregnancy employed by the natives of the Indian Archipelago—strikingly little

---

[120] *Science*, lxxiv (1931), 226–227. I have referred to this distinction between puberty and maturity as Hartman's theory. It may be that F. A. E. Crew deserves credit for it, since in 1930 he made the importance of this distinction the subject of his presidential address before the Second International Congress for Sex Research. *Proceedings* (London: Oliver & Boyd, 1931, edited by A. W. Greenwood), p. 18.

[121] African instances of *coitus interruptus* may be in a somewhat different category. If the girls were fecund, this technique would be partially effective.

mention in comparison with what one finds therein concerning the induction of abortion. May one conclude from this paucity of reports in the literature that the natives attempt to prevent conception on a small scale only? This need not necessarily be the case. In the first place, it is possible that no one has attempted to gather from the natives with sufficient thoroughness data in regard to these practices. It may be observed, however, that it is certainly true that the natives in general do not care to discuss such intimately personal matters. Among many tribes in the Indian Archipelago premarital coitus is quite frequent. If the girl becomes pregnant, marriage follows shortly afterwards as a rule; or the girl resorts to abortion, for which a variety of methods are known. Many motives are reported in the literature. That attempts to prevent conception among many tribes in the Indian Archipelago, both by single as well as by married women, are not rare appears to be quite certain.

Stratz pointed out[122] some time ago (1897) that the native women of Java quite frequently induce a retroflexed uterus with the object of preventing pregnancy.[123] In more than 50 per cent. of all women examined by him Stratz found the uterus tipped backwards. He is, moreover, of the opinion that this retroflexion, in most cases, is produced artificially, and, moreover, for the specific purpose of preventing conception. It was from a native woman that he learned of this method: "First the abdomen of the woman, closely above the symphisis, was pushed downwards by the *Dukun* [midwife] with stiff, spread fingers. Then, with both hands close above the *Ligamentum Pouparti* the midwife rubs upwards very forcefully, caus-

[122] C. H. Stratz, *Die Frauen auf Java. Eine gynäkologische Studie*. Stuttgart, 1897.

[123] It may be here pointed out that a decade prior to Stratz's observations on retroversion induced by the *Dukun*, van der Burg published the following regarding the same practice in the Dutch East Indies:

> In the girls the sexual impulse develops very early, and is gratified, even though they have regular sexual intercourse with men, without fear of consequences, when the services of certain skilled elderly women (*doekoen*) have been requisitioned. . . . These women appear, in fact, to understand, by means of pressure, rubbing, and kneading, through the abdominal walls (not by the vaginal route), how to induce anteversion or retroversion of the uterus, to such an extent as to prevent the occurrence of conception. It is said that the only inconvenient consequences of this procedure are trifling pains in the lumbo-sacral and inguinal regions, and some trouble in passing water during the first few days after the manipulations have been effected. Later, when a girl who has been treated in this way wishes to marry and become a mother, by a reversal of the manipulations, the uterus is restored to its natural position.

> It is said that these skilled women have been called in by European women in the Dutch Indies, who did not wish to have many children; but it appears that in a woman who has once given birth to a child, the result of the manipulations is less to be depended upon than in the case of a virgin.

[Cornelius Leendert van der Burg, *De Geneesheer in Nederlandsch-Indië* (Batavia, 1884–1887. 3 vols.), i, 71–72. Van der Burg also observes that while the half-breeds are very fertile, in many cases producing a child every year, and menstruating one month after childbirth even though they suckle their children, "many women belonging to the better class [of hybrids] use after coitus cold water douches." But among the half-breeds in general, van der Burg says that "means to prevent pregnancy are not general or are ineffective." Abortion is frequent. *Op. cit.*, i, 104.]

ing the abdominal muscles to relax.   Then both hands grasp the uterus from the side, pulling this forward; while the thumbs, with a forceful pressure, push the uterus downward.   This latter movement, as well as the first pressure above the symphisis, causes extraordinarily severe pain."[124]

This procedure is known to the natives as *ankatproet* (German = Ankat-prut) and is usually executed shortly after an abortion or delivery.   Stratz also discusses the effect of the operation upon health and its reliability in preventing conception.   He finds that it is only suitable in less than half the women, and moreover, it is likely to have injurious results.   It is by no means a certain preventive, since women with retroflexed uteri can and do conceive.[125]   Dr. R. L. Dickinson is likewise of the opinion that such manipulations are not likely to be generally effective since the elastic supports of the uterus draw back the organ into position.   The *Dukun* (German for *doekoen*) are also supposed to be able to return the uterus to its normal position by a corresponding massage, but Stratz rightly doubts to what extent this is responsible for future pregnancies.[126]   Schmidt reports this uterus-displacing procedure as existing also in the East Indies.[127]
Kleiweg de Zwaan continues his report:

Eerland, who has made a study of the position of the uterus in Javanese women,[128] is, however, of the opinion that Stratz has over-emphasized his particular interpretation of the etiology of the frequent incidence of retroflexed uteri.   Of 1120 Javanese women, Eerland found only 4.2 per cent having an ante-flexed uterus.   In the cases of all the other women the uterus was tipped backwards.   [Can it be that none of them had a uterus in normal position?]   Eerland ascribes this to a general weakness of the muscles[129] and to a diminishing tone of the uterus among Javanese women, but also, in some measure, to an artificial tipping of the uterus in order to prevent conception.

I found [continues Professor de Zwaan] that the Minangkabau, Malayans of middle Sumatra, have methods available whereby, according to their opinion, pregnancy can be prevented.   I was told, for instance, about the *toemanang* fruit, which has to be chewed with a *sirih* "plug," and the juice of which is swallowed by the woman.   These chewed-out plugs must be saved; they are deposited on a board above the fire of the fireplace in the room of the woman.   The women believe that this procedure will prevent them from becoming pregnant.   [I take it that the natives hold that it is the chewing of the plug, and not the ritual of placing the chewed-out plug above the fireplace which is the really effective portion of the procedure.]

[124] Stratz, *op. cit.*, p. 45.
[125] Ibid., p. 47.
[126] *Ibid.*
[127] R. Schmidt, *Liebe und Ehe im alten und modernen Indien.*   Berlin: Barsdorf, 1922.
[128] *Geneeskundig Tydschrift voor Nederlandsch Indië*, vol. xi, 1930.
[129] Dr. Robert L. Dickinson thinks it may be due to the fact that the women get up and go about soon after delivery, when the uterus is large and heavy.

Another method employed by these Malayans of Sumatra to prevent conception, again reported to me by Professor Kleiweg de Zwaan, is the following: A piece of *ingoe* (*asa foetida*) is put into a *pisang* (banana). Thrice monthly a woman who desires to remain free from pregnancy must eat such a fruit. She is also obliged to use an extract made from *daun doekoeng anak* (*Phyllanthus urinaria*), *oerat doekoeng anak, tjapo mali* (*Blumea sp.*) and *oerat kadoedoek* (*Pteroloma trignetrum*). These Malayan women also practice a massage of the abdomen in order to prevent conception. Professor de Zwaan reports that he could not, however, find out whether it was the intention of the natives to cause, by this process, a retroflexion of the uterus.

On the island of Nias, near Sumatra, Professor de Zwaan was informed that a woman who does not wish to become pregnant is obliged to rub a knife on a grindstone; then to pour some water on the knife and grindstone, and subsequently to drink this water while pronouncing a magical incantation. This is obviously one of many superstitious practices found among the natives of the Indian Archipelago, the exact procedure and intent of which are not always clear. Several tribes of the region ascribe a strong magical influence to iron and steel, and this contraceptive ritual is probably an example.

The Karo-Bataks, natives of Sumatra, employ several contraceptive techniques essentially magical and ineffective. Joustra says that these people introduce a small ball of opium into the vagina;[129a] and he is under the impression that they also use *coitus interruptus*.

Single girls, as well as married women, try to prevent conception.[130] For that purpose the female takes *koelit tangah* (a kind of tree bark), *curcuma*[131] and old *pinang* (areca or betel nut). These ingredients are rubbed until they are fine; and the mixture must be taken internally by the woman for three days every morning upon awakening. In order that it may be effective, she should pronounce certain words beforehand! Massage of the abdomen is also practised in this district to prevent pregnancy.

According to J. Kreemer [132] the methods used by the people of Acheh in Sumatra to prevent pregnancy are imported, as a rule, by people from Klingal.

[129a] M. Joustra, *Hygienische Misstanden in het Karoland* [*Hygienic Abuses in the Karo-Country*] (Published by the Batak Institute, No. 1, 1909), p. 287.

[130] "Ethnographische bijzonderheden betreffende de onderafdeeling VIII Kota en VII Loerah. Godsdienst en bijgeloof." [Ethnographic peculiarities regarding subincision VIII Kota and VIII Loerah], *Indische Gids* (*Indian Guide*), 18th annual publication I, 1896, pp. 585–598. See also p. 831 and p. 963.

[131] For an earlier report on the use of *Curcuma* see p. 25.

[132] *Atjeh*, ii (1922), 410.

Professor Snouck Hurgronje writes[133] of the Achehnese that they "are far from being afraid of over-population." The Achehnese "themselves assert that married couples with a number of children are very much in the minority; by their own confession they make much use both in and out of wedlock of expedients for preventing pregnancy or causing miscarriage."

He adds that

Recipes for this purpose are to be found in all the books of memoranda of literate Achehnese. These recipes sometimes consist merely in *tangkays* (formulas) to be recited on certain occasions, but more material methods are also recommended in great variety. The following is one of the commonest: choose a ripe pineapple, and cut off a piece from the top, letting the fruit still remain attached to the stalk. Then take out a little of the inside and fill up the space so made with yeast. Close the fruit up again by replacing the piece cut off; fasten it up tight and let it hang for another day or two. The fruit is then plucked and it is said that the woman who eats it will find it a sure preventive of pregnancy.[134]

Jacobs[135] distinguishes two techniques in use by the Achehnese for the prevention of pregnancy: (1) those which prevent a fruitful coitus (*oebat tjawat*); (2) methods to induce abortion (*oebat bĕh anèk*). Jacobs could not, however, determine their exact nature. He also states that several techniques do not originate with the Achehnese, being prepared and sold by the Klings (Klingalese) living in Acheh. In the course of his study among the Achehnese, Jacobs was given by one of the natives a black mass in the form of a pill, which the natives were accustomed to introduce into the vagina before coitus, and which was supposed to prevent impregnation. Upon examination, this black mass was found to contain a large quantity of tannic acid. Quite possibly these natives had, by trial and error, hit upon a vaginal suppository sound in principle.

Recent laboratory tests by Baker and Voge have shown that tannic acid ranks very high as a spermicide—much higher than lactic acid, which is the supposed active agent[136] in jellies applied to vaginal diaphragms in the modern birth-control clinics. Tannic acid immobilizes sperms immediately in a 1000 solution, while lactic acid, according to Günther, requires 107 minutes at this strength.[137] The use of a tannic acid suppository by the Achehnese women is thus an excellent illustration of one of the minor theses of this book, namely, that some sound principles of contraception were

---

[133] Christian Snouck Hurgronje, *De Ajehers*, i, 73. English translation by A. W. S. O'Sullivan as *The Achehnese*, i, 70, note.

[134] *Ibid.*

[135] Julius Jacobs, *Het Familie-en Kampongleven op Groot-Atjeh. Eene Bijdrage tot de Ethnographie van Noord Sumatra.* Leiden: Brill, 1894.

[136] I say "the supposed active agent" advisedly. Probably the physical impediment is more important than the presence of lactic acid.

[137] R. L. Dickinson and L. S. Bryant, *The Control of Conception*, p. 41.

accidentally hit upon early in man's history as a result of trial, rejection, re-trial, and success. Nor is this the only instance in which a study of primitive society is likely to teach us something about sexual life.

The natives of Australia have several practices which need to be considered in detail in relation to the question whether they are effective in preventing conception. They are: (1) expelling the semen by violent abdominal movements. This is reported as practised by the native women of Vincent Gulf near Adelaide to avoid impregnation by white men. (2) Ovariotomy practised by the natives on the Parapitshuri Sea, Cape York, and on the Condamine River;[138] (3) Subincision. Each of these will be considered in turn.

The native women of Port Darwin, Australia, who evidently have some contact with white men, are accustomed after coitus to make violent movements of the abdomen backward and forward in order to expel the semen. Mr. Albert Morton, a collector for the Australian Museum in Sydney, who observed coitus among the natives in that locality, which observations have been reported by N. von Miklucho-Maclay,[139] an ethnographer writing in the eighteen eighties, states that this practice is executed by the native women, according to the views of white settlers of North Australia, for the purpose of avoiding impregnation after coitus with white men. It is not known whether the native women follow the same practice after connection with native men.

Roth, who knew the natives of Queensland from personal experience, reports through N. von Miklucho-Maclay,[140] that the natives on the Parapitshuri Sea (33° lat. and about 139° long.) practise ovariotomy in order to produce for the young men of the tribe a special class of prostitutes, who could never become pregnant.[141] Roth noticed among these natives, who also practise the *mica* or subincision operation described below, "an odd appearing girl who avoided the company of women, and kept company only

---

[138] According to Ploss-Bartels ovariotomy is practised with contraceptive intent in Malay. For modern usage, see Spengler in *Marriage Hygiene*, Nov. 1935.

[139] N. von Miklucho-Maclay, "The position of the couple in coitus and the hurling forth of the sperm from the woman after the same." *Zeitschr. f. Ethnol.* [*Verhandl.*] xii (1880) 87–88. This article is noteworthy in other respects. It describes in detail, by the use of drawings, positions in coitus among the Australian natives at Port Darwin. The article contains the only sketches I have seen of positions in coitus among primitive peoples. However, one will find in Malinowski's *The Sexual Life of Savages* (ch. x, §12) an excellent set of descriptions of coitus as practised by the Trobriand Islanders. See also W. E. Roth, *Ethnological Studies among the North-West Central Queensland Aborigines.* 1897. Also H. Basedow, "Subincision and Kindred Rites of the Australian Aboriginal," *Jour. Royal Anthrop. Instit.*, 1927, pp. 151–156.

[140] Observer Roth; reporter N. von-Miklucho-Maclay in an Address before the Berlin Anthrop. Soc. on Nov. 12, 1881 in *Zeitschr. f. Ethnol.*, xiv (1882), 27.

[141] According to Hovorka (*op. cit.*, ii, 525) ovariotomy is also practised in Malay.

with the young men of the tribe, with whom she shared their duties and hardships. He reports that the girl showed a very poor development of the breasts and especially of buttocks; the thin buttocks, and hair growing on the chin, giving her the appearance of a boy. She not only avoided the women, but showed no special inclination to the young men to whose sexual satisfaction she was appointed. One of the natives, interpreting the two long scars on the abdomen, and who, as a result of a residence on various stock farms could speak some English, observed that the girl was like a "spayed cow." The native also stated that the girl indicated was "not the only case of her kind, and that the operation was undertaken from time to time on girls in order to produce for the young men a special kind of prostitute, who could never become a mother."[142]

Another report of the same operation among the natives of a tribe at Cape York, Australia is available in the same account, the observer being Mr. John MacGillivray.[143] MacGillivray had himself seen the ovariotomized woman and had noted the scars on the abdomen. He had no doubt that the job had been done by the natives themselves. The same operation seems to have been performed, at least at one time, on certain native women living on the Condamine River.[144] Here again the custom is to turn the sterilized women over to all the men for their sexual satisfaction. Miklucho-Maclay has full confidence in the authenticity of these reports. He believes, moreover, that ovariotomy can scarcely be more difficult or complicated than subincision; but this view overlooks the fact that ovariotomy involves an abdominal incision which is likely to be more serious in its consequences. Regarding Miklucho-Maclay's confidence in the authenticity of these reports, it is only fair to say that Buschan, writing in Moll's *Handbuch der Sexualwissenschaft*,[145] flatly denies that any Australian natives ever removed the ovaries as an anti-conceptional technique. I gather that Buschan thinks this unlikely because, in his judgment, Australian natives have no knowledge of the physiology of conception. But, as we have seen before, this is not an adequate basis for a denial.

§7 SUBINCISION (MICA[146] OR KOOLPI OPERATION)

One of the most interesting practices allegedly related to the early history of contraception is the subincision rite of Australian natives. The Dieri call it *mica*; the natives of Cooper's Creek call it *koolpi*.

---

[142] *Zeitschr. f. Ethnol.* xiv, 26–27.

[143] *Ibid.*, p. 27.

[144] *Ibid.*

[145] Albert Moll, Ed., *Handbuch der Sexualwissenschaften* (Leipzig: F. C. W. Vogel, 1912), p. 307. See incidentally pp. 449–456 for Moll's discussion of techniques and indications for Präventivverkehr.

[146] Pronounced with a short "i" as in pin.

The exact nature of the operation varies in different groups.   The urethra may be slit open for its entire length from the glans to the scrotum.   In other instances the length of the incision varies with the operator.   Portions only of the urethra may be dissected out.   During ejaculation the semen then dribbles over the testicles.   The men have to urinate with widely separated legs.   Among the natives the rite is widely distributed geographically throughout Australia.   It is a sort of extension of the circumcision rite, and all young males in the tribes employing the rite are operated upon before marriage.

Statements have so frequently appeared in the literature citing this rite as a population check that it seems desirable to review the literature in some detail on two points: (1) the nature of the operation, (2) the motives behind it and its purpose.   The literature will then be evaluated in the light of modern anthropological thought.   We turn first to early reports of the nature of subincision.

As early as 1845 Edward J. Eyre reported[147] the subincision rite of the natives of the Port Lincoln Peninsula and along the coast of Australia to the westward.   Eyre avowed that he examined many of the men in the group he studied, and that all had been operated upon.   Thirty-four years after Eyre's observation, that is, in 1879, the Rev. G. Taplin described the operation as follows: A suitably-fashioned kangaroo bone is introduced into the urethra at the beginning of the scrotum, and then is pressed forward until it comes through the end near the glans.   Then the operator takes a stone knife and strips open the urethra lengthwise.[148]   C. W. Schürmann, a missionary, reporting on Port Lincoln natives said that a chip of quartz was the instrument used.[149]

Describing subincision among the Dieri—they call it *koolpi*—Gason says, "So soon as the hair on the face of the young man is sufficiently grown to admit the end of the beard being tied, the ceremony of the Koolpi decided on. . . .   The operation is then commenced by first laying his penis on a piece of bark, when one of the party, provided with a sharp flint, makes an incision underneath into its passage, from the foreskin to its base.   This done, a piece of bark is then placed over the wound and tied so as to prevent its closing up. . . ."[150]

---

[147] Edward J. Eyre, *Journals of Expeditions of Discovery into Central Australia, and Overland from Adelaide to King George's Sound, in the years 1840–41.*   London: Boone, 1845.

[148] Report in *The Native Tribes of South Australia.*   Adelaide, 1879.

[149] C. W. Schürmann, in a paper on "The Aboriginal Tribes of Port Lincoln and South Australia" in *The Native Tribes of South Australia.*

[150] S. Gason, in a paper on "Manners and Customs of the Dieyerie Tribe" in *The Native Tribes of South Australia*, p. 273.   An early report states that after the rite described, and

The Nasims on Carpenter Gulf use for the operation, besides splinters of quartz, a sharpened shell. Though N. von Miklucho-Maclay describes a knife which he alleges is used for subincision by the natives of Herbert River, Queensland, Professor A. R. Radcliffe-Brown, a careful scientific observer and an authority on the Australian natives, avows in a letter that the Herbert River natives do not practice it. Perhaps they formerly did; or else Miklucho-Maclay must have reference to a knife used by another group. At all events, the instrument described is a quartz splinter with a handle made of the hardened juice of Australian "grass tree" (Xanthor-

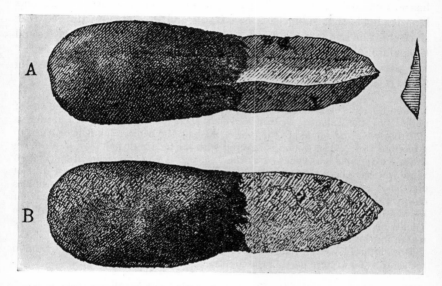

FIG. I. Flint Knife Used in Subincision (Mica) Operation by Australian Natives (Herbert River). A, B. Views of Both Sides. C. Quartz Splinter. Source: *Zeitschr. f. Ethnol.*, xiv (1882), 28.

rhoea) [See Figure I]. Just as the Dieri fasten a piece of bark on the wound to keep it from closing, so the Nasims employ a little stick or a thin bone for the same purpose.

Semon, a much later reporter (1899), declared that the youths were "decoyed away from the camp by a conspiracy of the old men, and then thrown down and mutilated."[151] This hardly suggests that the operation was willingly and voluntarily entered upon. If the operation, however, is a

---

when the wound is healed, the male organ takes on the appearance, during detumescence, of a large button or knob. On erection it is very broad and flat.

[151] Richard Semon, *In the Australian Bush* (London, 1899), p. 234.

status giving ceremony, as modern authorities believe, all the young men must expect to submit to the ordeal, in which case Semon's suggestion is erroneous. The same observer adds that "In some tribes we find it a custom that every man submits to this operation [hypospadia] after the birth of his second or third child."[152] According to Radcliffe-Brown it is erroneous to suggest that the operation is performed after the birth of a certain number of children. Where subincision is customary, it is always performed before a man is permitted to marry. It is in fact a status-giving ceremony. To be sure, the incision may be lengthened after the man is married, but it has nothing to do with the children he may or may not have had.[153] Porteus likewise holds that subincision is a status-giving ceremony; further, that since abortion and infanticide are much more certain population checks and less painful to adults, subincision is not adopted for contraceptive reasons.[154]

A pseudonymous writer, Dr. Jacobus X, declares[155] that the natives of Santo (Oceania) use the *mica* operation:

I found a native of Santo with an artificial hypospadia, performed at the age of puberty by the Takata. With a well-sharpened piece of quartz, the urethra is slit from the gland [glans] to the root of the bag, the penis being first fastened to a piece of bark. The wound is covered with a bandage of fine bark, after being dressed with some herbs chewed by the Takata. This curious operation compels those who have been thus mutilated to stoop down to make water. In a state of erection, the member becomes large and flat, and when emitting, the sperm dribbles out over the bag. The native, who exhibited this curious mutilation, told me that he was not the only one, and that it was not unfrequently performed by the Takata on persons specially named by the Chief. He could not explain to me the reason for this singular custom.

It is certain, however, that it comes from Australia . . . where it is practised in the central and western parts of the country.[156]

Figure II shows the operation being carried out by the Warramunga.

According to Radcliffe-Brown the operation is carried on with varied degrees of completeness. "In some tribes the urethra is laid open to the scrotum. In others the extent of the incision varies with the operator.

[152] *Ibid.*

[153] Letter to the author, Nov. 6, 1932.

[154] Stanley D. Porteus, *The Psychology of a Primitive People. A Study of the Australian Aborigine* (New York: Longmans Green. London: Arnold, 1931), pp. 279–282. For a discussion of the knowledge of conception held by primitives see pp. 217–223.

[155] A French Army Surgeon, *Untrodden Fields of Anthropology*. Paris, 1898, 2 vols. There is some doubt whether the observation is original. It may be from a secondary source. Though *Untrodden Fields* is hardly a first-class scientific source, the evidence of this anonymous French Army Surgeon is presented for whatever interest it may have for us in completing the picture of the geographical distribution of this operation.

[156] *Ibid.*, ii, 363–364.

The first operation may merely be an incision of an inch or so. In some tribes an individual may undergo a series of operations each extending a little further down the urethra."[157]   After the operation the underside of the penis now has a shallow hollow (see Figure III) representing the slit or partially extirpated urethra.   Hirschfeld's monumental *Geschlechtskunde* and Garson in the *Medical Press*[158] furnish illustrations of it, but the clearest is in Dickinson's *Atlas*.   This figure is reproduced on the next page.

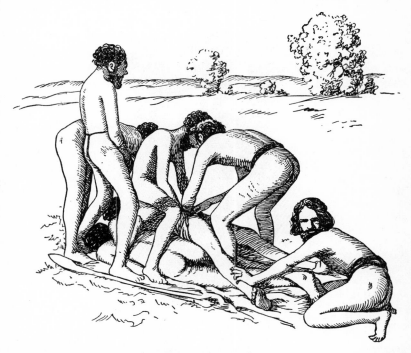

FIG. II. Warramunga Natives Performing a Subincision Operation.   Source: Hirschfeld, *Geschlechtskunde*, Figure 95.   Redrawn by Alfred Feinberg.

Concerning the effectiveness of subincision (*mica, koolpi*) in preventing conception there are two schools of thought.   Generally speaking the German literature, especially the works of Ploss and Bartels and the secondary accounts based thereon, holds that the operation is more or less effective in preventing conception; holds even that in some instances the operation is so intended by the natives.   Such statements have also been repeated in

[157] Letter to author, dated Nov. 6, 1932.

[158] London, lvii (1894), 189–190.

the less scientific, quasi-erotic sexological books of which Jacobus X's *Untrodden Fields of Anthropology* is typical.   Other observers whose judgments carry greater weight (e.g., Roth, Spencer, Gillen, Radcliffe-Brown, Warner) insist that the operation is ineffective in preventing conception and hence has nothing to do with birth control.   Though Spencer and Gillen[159] thought subincision might have an injurious effect upon fecundity, Roth[160] and

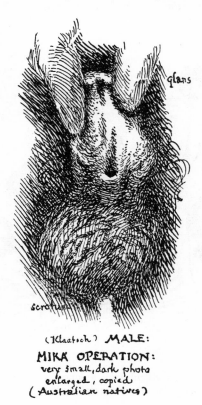

(Klaatsch) MALE:
MIKA OPERATION:
very small, dark photo
enlarged, copied
(Australian natives)

FIG. III. Male Organ after Subincision.   Source: Dickinson, *Human Sex Anatomy*, Fig. 117.

Mathews[161] have denied this.   Carr-Saunders, after reviewing the literature on mutilation of the sex organs by primitives, concludes that "there is apparently no reason to believe that this mutilation has any effect upon

[159] Spencer and Gillen, *Native Tribes of Central Australia*, p. 52.
[160] W. E. Roth, *Ethnological Studies*, p. 179.
[161] R. H. Mathews, *Ethnological Notes*, p. 177.

fecundity, except possibly among the Australians."[162] He then expresses doubt that subincision was effective; and thinks it still more certain that it was not practised with the intention of producing sterility or partial sterility.[163]

These views fit in well with the conclusions of modern anthropologists. They argue that if all males were operated upon, and if the operation were effective in preventing conception, the groups would die out, an argument logical enough. They contend that practically all males are operated upon in those tribes using the ceremony at all; second, that subincision is not effective in preventing conception. Radcliffe-Brown, for instance declares[164]

All available evidence tends to show that the operation of subincision does not interfere with conception. In most of the tribes in which subincision is carried out on males an operation of introcision is performed on females. A very common attitude adopted in coitus is one which allows the sperm from even the completely subincised penis to flow into the artificially enlarged vulva. Since in many tribes every adult male is subincised, if it were really an effective contraceptive method, there would be no children at all or very few. Yet these tribes formerly had to practise infanticide to keep down their numbers. In West Australia my genealogies show no differences in the number of children in a family in the Kariera tribe where there is no subincision and in the Nyamal tribe where every male is subincised.

This statement is probably authoritative. Many will be skeptical though, about semen dribbling on an artificially enlarged vulva being as effective in promoting conception as when the semen is expelled, during coitus, through the glans. Probably it is only recently that there has been any realization even among many physicians of how small a deviation from optimum conditions may prevent fertilization. It is my view, eminent anthropologists notwithstanding, that it is highly probable that subincision constitutes such a deviation from optimum conditions. This is not to say that it is an infallible preventive, like the excision of a portion of the vas deferens in the male; it is merely argued that subincision probably reduces the likelihood of fertilization.

What are the subsidiary effects of subincision? Miklucho-Maclay declares that, judging by the frequency of coitus, it does not reduce sexual desire. One writer has even stated that the natives perform the operation because it enhances pleasure. But this may be rejected until better evidence is forthcoming. Miklucho-Maclay guesses that coitus is of shorter

---

[162] A. M. Carr-Saunders, *The Population Problem*, p. 138.

[163] *Ibid.*, p. 139.

[164] In a letter to the author.

duration among subincised men, the ejaculation coming sooner than with those non-subincised.

Several theories have been proposed to account for the existence of a mutilating operation which seems so odd to Westerners. The various theories are: (1) That the act is purely ceremonial and has no contraceptive significance whatsoever. (2) That it proceeds originally from eugenic motives, whether such reasons are now held consciously or not. (3) That the practice is purely traditional, done because the natives' forefathers did it. (4) That it serves the function of a population check whether consciously adopted for that purpose or not.

The ceremonial view is more or less emphasized by Roth, Spencer and Gillen, von Reitzenstein, Strehlow, Buschan; more recently by Warner, Radcliffe-Brown, and Porteus. According to this view subincision is merely a portion of the religious, initiatory, status-giving rites. It is symbolical of the fact that the boy has now become a man. An individual who had not been subjected to the rites of which subincision is often a part would be treated as a boy or woman. "He could take no part in the sacred ceremonial life of the tribe, could not be admitted to the men's camp, would not be permitted to marry, and if he ran away with a woman, would be killed unless he was under white protection." Radcliffe-Brown says:

As part of the initiation ceremonies, nearly every Australian tribe practices some deformation which differentiates the man from the boy. Some tribes content themselves with raising scars on the shoulders, back and breast, some knock out one or two incisor teeth. A few tribes content themselves with circumcision. When subincision occurs, it follows circumcision, and is a sort of continuation of the circumcision rite. It is so regarded by the tribes of Western Australia that I know personally. Circumcision is the first step towards making a man, subincision is a second step of the same general kind.

I do not think there is any fundamental difference between tooth-avulsion as practised in Eastern Australia and circumsion plus subincision as practised in the western two-thirds of the Continent except in the two social activities to which the rites have symbolic reference—the eating of food in the one case and copulation in the other.[165]

Warner says, "This operation is found throughout the greater part of Australia. Spencer and Gillen rightly point out that it has nothing to do with birth control practices."[166]

The second explanation is that the operation proceeds originally from

[165] Letter to author dated Nov. 6, 1932.
[166] W. Lloyd Warner, "Birth Control in Primitive Society." *Birth Control Review*, xv, 107 (April, 1931). *Cf.*, Buschan in Moll's *Handbuch*, pp. 306–307.

eugenic motives, whether such reasons are now held consciously or not. Some writers (e.g., Garson,[167] Stopes,[168] and Aptekar[169]) declare that only the weaker men are selected; others say the stronger.[170] Professor Radcliffe-Brown, an authority on Australian native life, says there is absolutely no conscious eugenic selection; that, as early writers have declared, among those tribes where subincision is customary, all males are subincised. Nor is there any evidence even for unconscious selection, for there is no selection at all. This point is clear; and the earlier writers, including Stopes and Aptekar in our time, are in error.

The theory that subincision is customary or traditional explains nothing, if true. It arose no doubt from statements made by natives to some of the early reporters. Customs, to remain intact over very long periods of time, must serve some need. Does subincision serve merely a ceremonial need? Is its function solely that of giving status to the adolescent boy? Can it be that it has maintained itself because it supports and fits in with the maintenance mores of the group?

Several early observers held that subincision proceeded from Malthusian motives. But few have argued, though some[171] have implied, that the motives were consciously held by the natives. As a matter of historical record, let us review some of the older judgments before presenting our own. Eyre declared in 1845 that

This extraordinary and inexplicable custom must have a great tendency to prevent the rapid increase of the population; and its adoption may perhaps be a wise ordination of Providence, for that purpose in a country of so desert and arid a character as that which these people occupy.[172]

J. M. Davis likewise speculated that the

[167] J. G. Garson, "Notes on Deformations of the Genital Organs, practised by the Natives of Australia," *Med. Press* (London), lvii (1894), 189–190. After describing in detail three variations of subincision, Garson says incorrectly: "These operations are performed on youths at the age of 18 years, and only upon a certain number of them, namely, those who prove themselves indolent and the least useful members of their tribes." This is probably the origin of the view held by Stopes and Aptekar that the motive is eugenic.

[168] Marie C. Stopes, *Contraception* (London, 1931), p. 252.

[169] H. Aptekar, *Anjea*, p. 124.

[170] M. Bartels, *Die Medicin der Naturvölker* (Leipzig, 1893), §125, pp. 296–298. Bartels says the stronger men are selected, except among the Nazims, who operate on the weaker.

[171] Garson (*op. cit.*), however, says that the "operation . . . has been practised for the purpose of preventing him [the male] from having any family." Garson is unreliable on this point as on the eugenic purpose previously discussed within.

[172] *Op. cit.*, i, 212.

practice was perhaps introduced by some Aboriginal Solomon to prevent the too rapid propagation and thereby starvation of the race; and it is certainly surprising [he adds] how, under the circumstances, there are any children at all.[173]

Semon, another early observer, agrees with Eyre and Davis that the ultimate purpose is population control:

If the hordes of a tribe are to live near each other in peace and amity, it is necessary that the number of the population remain stationary. Provided the hordes increase, it would grow impossible for all to exist upon the yields of hunting and fishing and upon the produce of the wild-growing plants. As things are, the land is able to nourish only a scanty populace, so that we must regard it as a fitting accommodation if the Australian tries by artificial means to prevent the growth of the tribe, and thus render the population stationary. Some tribes attain this by exposing or killing a certain number of new-born infants. Others castrate [sic] a number of the youths as soon as they are grown up and before they enter the class of adults, or render them infertile by slitting the urethra (Hypospadie).[174]

Lasch,[175] interpreting the statement by Lumholtz[176] that among many groups the operation is performed after a man has become the father of one or two children,[177] thinks the motive Malthusian.

Probably the conclusion of Eyre, Davis, Semon, Lasch, Garson and Bartels needs discounting in the light of more recent investigation. Of course, if subincision is completely ineffective even in reducing the likelihood of conception, it would be fruitless to argue that whatever the conscious ceremonial purpose of the rite may be, its unconscious, ultimate function is to control population. We have, however, suggested the view that while it is a very inefficient contraceptive practice, it may cause deviations from the optimum conditions conducive to impregnation. However, until it is clearly shown by further investigation that subincision is more contraceptive in its effect than any report has yet demonstrated, it would seem most in accord with recent anthropological investigation to accept the view of Professor Radcliffe-Brown and others that its significance is ceremonial. He maintains that "it can be stated quite definitely that in no tribe known to us is subincision practised with the conscious purpose of limiting conception."[178] If it is mainly ineffective in preventing the birth of children,

---

[173] John Moore Davis, "Notes Relating to the Aborigines of Australia," being Appendix A in Brough Smith, *The Aborigines of Victoria*, (1878), ii, 312.

[174] Semon, *op. cit.*, pp. 233–234.

[175] *Zeitschr. f. Sozialwissensch.*, v (1902), 85–86.

[176] *Unter Menschenfressern*, p. 66.

[177] We have seen that this is not always the case. The mutilation sometimes takes place before the boy reaches puberty.

[178] Letter to the author dated November 6, 1932.

as modern testimony seems to bear out, limitation could not be its unconscious, ultimate purpose.

Has subincision been employed by any groups above the preliterate level? There seems to be little evidence on this subject. Tentatively it may be concluded that, if it has been employed, instances are rare. Dr. Solomon Gandz, however, thinks that there are veiled references to it, hitherto misunderstood, in the Bible and Talmud. He expects to prepare a paper on this subject.

§8 PRE-PUBERTAL COITUS AND DEVIATIONS

These are not, properly speaking, birth-control measures, yet they had the effect of limiting births, whatever the conscious intentions of the agents. Professor H. G. Duncan cites a number of references in anthropological literature to pre-pubertal coition among primitive peoples.[179] He declares that "Copulation before puberty appears to have been common among the American Indians, Eskimos, and the tribes of Africa, India, Australia, and New Zealand."[180] Duncan also suggests, but does not explicitly state, that pre-pubertal coitus was consciously practised as a means of birth limitation. This one may deduce from the fact that Duncan treats the subject under the general heading of "The Control of Population by Preventive Methods." Perhaps Professor Duncan does not mean to imply that the practice is consciously adopted as a population expedient. This seems the most tenable position; for usually such early coitus is merely sex play common enough among primitive peoples. This is not to gainsay that pre-pubertal coitus would have the effect of limitation especially if, as Hartman contends, women have a sterile period for three or four years after the onset of menstruation. The practice would limit fertility in so far as mature men substituted infecund girls for mature women.

What has been said of pre-pubertal coitus applies also to those deviations from normal coitus commonly known as the perversions. Any divergent mode of performing the sexual act, any method of providing a substitute outlet would necessarily have the effect of reducing births. The surviving pottery of some of the ancient races of Peru shows that they practised oral and anal coitus.[181] Vorberg's illustrations of Greek vases show that the Greeks knew the same sexual deviations as the Peruvians.[182] Almost every

---

[179] *Op. cit.*, p. 295 *et seq.*

[180] *Ibid.* See also the works of Carr-Saunders, Briffault, Malinowski, and numerous others.

[181] See the various volumes of *Anthropophyteia*, edited by F. S. Krauss.

[182] Gaston Vorberg, *Glossarium eroticum* (Stuttgart: Püttman, 1928–1932); *Antique Erotik in Kleinkunst und Keramik* (München: Müller, 1921). About one in six of the

large museum possesses vases showing these forms of sexual life.   Kisch, who also points out the prevalence of homosexuality among the Greeks, adds that its purpose was the prevention of overpopulation.[183]   One wonders whether this is a modern rationalization after the fact.   Dr. Solomon Gandz informs me that anal coitus and *coitus reservatus* are mentioned in the Talmud.[184]   But they are treated from the legal side; they are not suggested as preventives.   However, it is probable that the early Hebrews employed such practices as did other groups. •

Probably these practices were not adopted consciously as a means of population limitation.   Though variety of experience and the enhancement of sexual pleasure were more likely motives, they had the effect of limiting births by creating substitutes.

Why was contraception not more frequently resorted to by preliterate peoples?   The widespread adoption of abortion and more especially of infanticide filled the need.   These checks are immediate, practicable and certainly effective.   In most uncivilized groups life is not held sacred until the child has gone through a formal ceremony of tribal recognition, usually marriage.   Until such a time the child is not considered a member of society, hence, properly speaking, not a human.   Accordingly, it could be killed without compunction, and the parents had full authority to determine whether it would be done away with or not.

Professor Ralph Linton argues in a letter to me that in a sense infanticide more effectively met the needs of primitive *groups* than contraception, however well the prevention of conception might more effectively serve the needs of individuals, more especially unmarried women.   Contraception, he argues, results in an uncontrolled, uncertain, hit-or-miss limitation of the population.   But infanticide not only makes limitation in relation to food supply certain, but also makes possible a conscious control of the sex ratio—important where there is a division of labor on sex lines.   Thus a hunting culture could elect a surplus of men, an agricultural tribe a surplus of women.   There can be no doubt but that infanticide has contributed to group survival in a certain state of cultural evolution.   This is not to say that we need it now.   We do not, for we have a reliable substitute.

Another circumstance limiting resort to contraception in primitive socie-

---

pictures of coitus in Hans Licht's *Sexual Life in Ancient Greece* (London: Routledge, 1932), in A. Feuchtwanger's and A. Reichold's *Griechische Vasen Malereien* (Munich: Bruchman, 1904) and in Vorberg's *Glossarium* suggest anal coitus.   *Cf.*, Aretino's women, about one-third of whom ask for it.

[183] *Sexual Life of Woman*, p. 414.

[184] Many writers seem to think that the first report of *coitus reservatus* is its use in the Oneida Community led by John Humphrey Noyes in the U. S. in the eighteen seventies.

ties is the fact that natives have such a rudimentary knowledge of the nature of conception. Though it is a disputable point of ethnology, it seems quite clear that most primitive people had little or no such knowledge. I am aware that a few anthropologists are of a contrary opinion; but the judgment I have expressed seems supported by the weight of authority.[185] Furthermore, when we realize how little even the most learned Greek and Islamic physicians knew of the mechanisms involved, we will not impute too much knowledge to savages. Even Leeuwenhoek's great discovery of human spermatozoa had to await the invention of the microscope. Only since Swammerdam, who died in 1685, have we known that a contact between the sperm and the egg has been necessary for fertilization. Only since Barry (1850) have we known that the spermatozoa must penetrate the egg. *It cannot be too strongly emphasized, therefore, that whatever primitive peoples may have known about contraception, they hit upon by trial and error, by trial-success-and-survival processes, not as a consequence of a thorough understanding of the physiology of conception.*

§9 SUMMARY

The first point made in this chapter was that contraceptive practices were rare among preliterate peoples when compared with abortion and infanticide, the chief primitive substitutes for conception control. The anti-conceptional techniques, both rational and magical, were then reviewed taking the tribes by geographical location on various continents. Among

[185] Among the anthropologists or other observers who have minimized the knowledge of conception of primitives are Frazer, Spencer and Gillen, Malinowski, von Reitzenstein, Fehlinger, Strehlow, Buschan and numerous others. See Frazer's *Golden Bough* for many unphysiological ideas of the nature of conception held by preliterates. *Cf.*, also Durkheim's *Primitive Religion*, the works of Westermarck, Robert Briffault (especially *The Mothers*, ii, 443 ff.) and the literature cited by these authors. There are literally scores of theories of conception not in any way connected with coitus. Some of the younger students of anthropology incline to the view that the naïveté of primitive peoples has been exaggerated. These students credit early man with a knowledge of the connection between coitus and subsequent birth [e.g., see W. Lloyd Warner, in *Birth Control Review*, xv (1931), 107; Herbert Aptekar, in *Birth Control Review*, xv (1931), 112–114; 127; xiv (1930), 202–203; 218; xiv, 233–235. *Anjea*, New York: William Godwin, 1931. H. Powdermaker, *Life in Lesu*, New York, 1933.] It is easy to ascribe too much knowledge to primitive peoples, to react too strongly from the assumptions of the man on the street that primitives are usually ignorant. My view is that while some natives probably realize that "coitus makes babies," this is about as far as their "knowledge" goes. Most natives hold a magical theory, for example, a spirit entering the woman's body. It is only necessary for natives to see a connection between coitus and a later birth, for them to desire to take steps aimed at prevention. Thus I hold that a preventive technique can exist even though knowledge of the physiology of conception is very crude or even absent. Accidental variation in conduct is the answer.

the Thonga, Masai, Nandi, Swahili, Amhara and several other tribes in Africa *coitus interruptus* is reported. Doubtless it is quite general in Africa. The Samoans and the Karo-Bataks in Sumatra also resort to it. In German East Africa *coitus inter femora* is reported.

Numerous are the magical rites, formulae, and potions given by medicine men, in whom the women often have supreme faith. Potions are nearly as frequently mentioned as the hocus-pocus, magical procedures. A considerable variety of leaves, herbs, and roots, as well as all manner of odd and obnoxious substances are pulverized, liquified, swallowed. It almost seems that the less palatable the substance the greater the faith in its effectiveness. It would be a dubious service to essay a summary of these recipes here. Note, though, that they show a desire for prevention.

More worthy of attention are certain ingenious, quasi-rational techniques. Among these are the use of the female condom made of an okra-like seed-pod by the Djukas in South America, douching with a solution of lemon juice by the negro women of Guiana and Martinique, *coitus interruptus* which is widely diffused among, though probably not frequently used by, primitive peoples; the use of tampons of roots (Dahomey in Africa), of algae or seaweed (Eastern Islanders), of chopped grass or rags (Bapindas and Bambundas in Africa). Kiwai Papuan women do more than tie a rope around the waist; they wash the genitals. Remarkable, too, is the use by Achehnese women of a "pill" or tampon employing the very effectively spermicidal tannic acid. Perhaps the small ball of opium placed before the *os uteri* by Karo-Batak women (Sumatra) is at least a partial impediment physically. They also use *coitus interruptus* and potions with a rite. This case well illustrates the principle that groups that have a rational method will also often have magical, ineffective techniques. The sensible and the nonsensical go along together—just as they do in our age, as yet unsifted by time, experience and accumulated knowledge.

Perversions are more or less widespread. Prolonged suckling is present, though one cannot always be sure that the purpose is prevention.

The only genuine case records of attempts at contraception by primitives are those reported by Masters. Probably these practices never would have been discovered had not the practices (stoppage of vagina) landed the natives in a white man's hospital.

Quite remarkable, it seems to me, are the occasional reports on medical and economic indications given by primitive women. These reports show how old are the reasons given for attempts at prevention. Among them are, in modern phraseology, high infant mortality, suffering during parturition, a previous history of several dead babies, difficulty in providing for children economically, the fact that having children or additional children might endanger the mother's life. All these indications have a very modern ring. Sometimes these reasons are not given by native mothers themselves; sometimes they are mentioned by other natives or by observers of aboriginal life. Primitive women are sensitive about such matters, as are modern women. There is reason to believe that many of them realized that it was easier on them, more economical of their energy, to prevent pregnancy than repeatedly to abort themselves at great cost of pain and discomfort. Such women are, moreover, anxious to do justice to their children according to the mores of their particular group. One guesses that they are more sensitive to medical than economic conditions. But this is only a guess. Modern men and women are sensitive to other forces in greater degree: desire for personal independence, for a higher standard of living, etc. But so far as the most common indications for contraception are concerned, we find them not only in modern societies but in primitive. *The desire for control is neither time nor space bound. It is a universal characteristic of social life.*

Perhaps midway between genuinely clever techniques, on the one hand, and magical rites and potions, on the other, stands the attempt to prevent conception by expulsion of the semen by abdominal movements. There are several reports on this in the region of Australasia. In the same category, no doubt, belongs artificial retroflexion of the uterus. The reports on ovariotomy are few; and one writer (Buschan) denies the authenticity of them. I share his skepticism. The germ of "modern" sterile-period theory—accidentally hit upon, of course, without any comprehension of the theory involved—may perhaps be seen in the practice of the Isleta Indians (New Mexico) in omitting intercourse for nine days after the cessation of menstruation. This was evidently a part of their tabu period. Siegel's curve seems to show the first nine days relatively infertile. If this is not to be considered a genuine case of use of the "safe period," the first report appears in the *Gynecology* of Soranos, a Greek physician of the second century A.D. (see Chap. IV).

Subincision was then described in detail, and the earlier literature reviewed critically. Various theories of motivation were considered. The eugenic theory was held to be clearly false. Though it was concluded that subincision would reduce optimum conditions for impregnation, it was held to be, in general, ineffective in preventing conception. It is a status-giving ceremony rather than a consciously-intended population check.

It would seem that contraception played a minor rôle in primitive societies chiefly because the more common expedients, abortion, infanticide and sexual tabus, were more certainly effective. A minor factor may have been, in most instances, an absence of any real comprehension of the physiology of conception.

However, it is clear that the *desire* to control conception is very old and quite universal. Its sphere is wide. Narrower is the sphere of *practice*. Narrowest of all is the sphere of effective contraception. This is, indeed, small. But modern clinical theory suggests that primitive man did hit upon some expedients workable at least in theory. Probably these were sheer luck—practices hit upon by trial, failure, re-trial, and finally success. It is a widely debatable point whether the more rational methods had any better chance of survival during social evolution than the potions and magical formulae.

From primitive societies it may seem a long jump to such early civilizations as those of the Egyptians, early Christians, Hebrews, and the Greek and Roman medical writers. Yet the continuity in desire for prevention, even in some of the practices, is striking. Especially noteworthy was the advancement made in contraceptive techniques by certain Greek physicians, notably Soranos and Aëtios. The practices of the civilizations mentioned will be the subject of the various chapters in Part Two. Eastern cultures, China, India, Japan, are considered in Part Three.

PART TWO

CONTRACEPTIVE TECHNIQUE IN ANTIQUITY
(WESTERN WORLD)

CHAPTER II

THE EGYPTIANS

IF OUR prehistoric ancestors knew something of contraceptive technique, we shall not be surprised to learn that in the civilizations of antiquity such knowledge was greater in extent than heretofore supposed. The antique peoples studied in this Part are the Egyptians, ancient Hebrews and early Christians, as well as certain writers representing the thought of Greece and Rome. Attention will first be directed to contraceptive technique as reported in Egyptian papyri.

§1 PETRI OR KAHUN PAPYRUS (1850 B.C.)

The oldest medical prescriptions for the prevention of conception still extant in writing are to be found in certain Egyptian papyri. The Petri Papyrus, found at Kahun in April 1889, and dating from the reign of Amenemhat III of the Twelfth Dynasty (c. 1850 B.C.), is a medical papyrus consisting of gynecological instructions and prescriptions without title or introduction. The papyrus consists of three pages about $39\frac{1}{2}$ inches long and $12\frac{3}{4}$ inches wide. The first page is in a fair state of preservation; but the third, which alone concerns us (see page 61), was reconstructed from no less than forty-six separate pieces, the small stiff hand in which it was written always ensuring their identification from amongst the vast heap which composed the so-called find No. VI. Griffith,[1] the editor of the papyrus, goes so far as to say that most of the prescriptions are "obvious quackery" since they relate to ascertaining sterility, the sex of unborn children, and so on. He notes that it is in one of these prescriptions that there occurs the only incantation in the papyrus. But it is by no means certain that the contraceptive practices recommended were sheer quackery. Before attempting to determine this, let us turn to the text of the original prescriptions numbered XXI, XXII, and XXIII:

Prescription No. XXI
> *To prevent* [conception] . . . Crocodile's dung cut up (?) on *auyt*-paste, sprinkled . . .

---

[1] F. Ll. Griffith, *The Petri Papyri-Hieratic Papyri from Kahun and Gurob* (*Principally of the Middle Kingdom*). London: Bernard Quaritch, 1898.

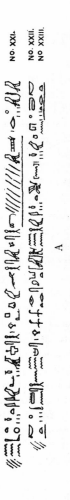

A

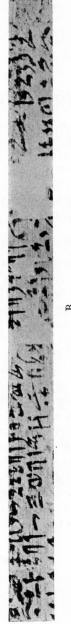

B

FIGS. IV A AND B. First Contraceptive Texts Still Extant in Writing. Kahun or Petri Papyrus. *c.* 1850 B.C. Above: Hieratic form. Below: Demotic form. Source: F. L. Griffith, *The Petri Papyri*

Prescription No. XXII

    (7) *Another medicine:* 1 pint (henu) of honey, consperge in vulvam ejus; [sprinkle on her uterus] this is to be done upon *sehem* (?) of natron.

Prescription No. XXIII

    Another ... (8) upon *auyt*-gum, consperge in vulvam ejus [sprinkle on her uterus]

Dawson[2] has well summarized the purport of these prescriptions in saying that "The first consists of crocodile's dung mixed with a paste-like vehicle,

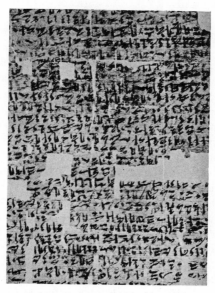

FIG. IV C. Page 3 of Kahun or Petri Medical Papyrus reduced.   Source: F. Ll. Griffith, *The Petri Papyri.*

and is probably a pessary for insertion in the vagina; the second consists of irrigating [or plugging?] the vagina with honey and natron [native sodium carbonate], and the third mentions a gum-like substance for insertion in the vagina."[3]

We may now consider whether the use of these substances was exclusively magical or whether perchance their use, empirically determined in the first instance, was not also based upon some appreciation of their physiological

[2] Warren Dawson, "Early Ideas Concerning Conception and Contraception," in *Medical Help on Birth Control* (London: Putnam, 1928), pp. 189–200.   Internal evidence leads me to believe that *Medical Help* was edited by Dr. Marie Stopes.

[3] Dawson, *op. cit.*, p. 193.

properties. Dawson[4] accepts the former view; but goes on to note that honey, like oil, has a physical clogging capacity; and that greasy substances form the base of many modern contraceptive suppositories. He observes further that the use of crocodile's dung inserted as a pessary in the vagina "is not essentially unlike a sponge soaked in some weak acid,"[5] a contraceptive more or less effectively employed in our time. As a matter of fact Egyptian crocodile dung may be alkaline. Tests[6] on the dung of the Cuban variety (*Crocodilus rhombifer*) showed alkalinity (pH of 7.9. A neutral solution like water has a pH of 7.0. A figure above 7.0 indicates alkalinity; below 7.0, acidity.)

Later in this volume we shall trace this prescription through the antique literature in which elephant's dung was substituted for crocodile's dung. But here it may be mentioned that the faeces of Indian elephant (*Elephas indicus*) had a pH of 5.6, while that of the African elephant (*Elephas africanus*) had a pH of 5.9. Since the vagina generally has a pH range of 3.86 to 4.45, running somewhat higher in the presence of cocci,[7] the use of crocodile (as distinct from elephant) dung (pH 7.9) in a suppository would tend to increase alkalinity in most cases; but not sufficiently to create optimum conditions for spermatozoa (pH 8.5 to 9.5). It would, however, tend to neutralize vaginal acidity. Hence, except for its mechanical effect, such a suppository would tend to promote, rather than to restrict fertilization.

These deductions are based upon the pH of Cuban crocodile not Egyptian which was not available. Furthermore, it makes no allowance for the pH of the substances with which the dung is mixed (e.g., buffers). This is rather a serious hiatus in the basis of our interpretation; but the task of filling it will have to fall, I fear, to some Egyptologist and bio-chemist rolled into one. Before closing this discussion, it may, however, be remarked that the substitution in much later recipes of elephant's for crocodile's dung was probably an accidental improvement from the standpoint of effective contraception, since the faeces of the Indian elephant has a pH of 5.6, that of the African elephant a pH of 5.9. The motility of spermatozoa is arrested at a pH of 6.0 or below.[8] At 4.0 revival is unlikely. In a word, crocodile dung, in most instances, would increase alkalinity and pro-

[4] *Ibid.*, p. 194.

[5] *Ibid.*

[6] Thanks are due to the director and staff of the Food Research Laboratories, New York City, who made the following determinations from samples sent from the New York Zoological Park through the courtesy of Dr. C. V. Novack, director. The determinations were made by the quinhydrone potentiometric method.

[7] R. L. Dickinson and L. S. Bryant, *The Control of Conception* (Baltimore: Williams & Wilkins, 1931), p. 41.

[8] *Ibid.*

mote conception; the use of elephant dung would hardly have a serious spermicidal effect by chemical means, though both might exercise some mechanical effect.

The second prescription (No. XXII) in the Petri papyrus mentions honey and natron (native sodium carbonate). This employs quite a universal principle, the use of a sticky substance, honey. The third prescription mentions a gum. A gum appears in another Egyptian medical papyrus. As we shall see in later chapters, oily and gummy substances are mentioned quite frequently in the contraceptive recipes of antiquity.

The use of dung in a contraceptive pessary can be traced in the literature for over 3000 years. After the Kahun papyrus (1850 B.C.) it reappeared in various works produced in the ninth, eleventh, and thirteenth centuries. Of course, the prescriptions varied somewhat; but their continuity is the significant feature. From the Egyptians, the prescription passed into the Arabic literature. Originally it may have had an Oriental source. It is unknown in the Greek literature. Quṣṭā ibn Lūqā [of Baalbek or Heliopus, Syria] the Arabian physician, philosopher, and mathematician, of the ninth century, citing an unknown ancient Indian text, substitutes elephant for crocodile dung, avowing that "Elephant dung mixed with honey and placed in the vagina of a woman prevents conception."[9] The same prescription, in identically the same Latin words, reappears in the eleventh century in the *Book on Surgery* by Constantine the African[10] [Constantinus Africanus (c. 1015–1080)]. Finally it appears in the *Canon* of Ibn Sīnā (XI century) and in Ibn al-Baiṭār's *Treatise on Simples* (XIII century). This is a remarkable continuity. No trace of it has been found since the thirteenth century. It does not seem to have passed into the oral tradition of folk medicine as did an early Greek potion. One of the few magical prescriptions cited by Soranos was drinking a potion of the water in which smiths quench their forceps and other hot metals. That has been found recently among a few European peasants. But even this span (1800 years) hardly compares with the persistence of the Egyptian prescription (3000 years).

§2   EBERS PAPYRUS (1550 B.C.)

The Ebers papyrus, a compendium of medical writings dating at the latest from 1550 B.C., and which Bryan[11] describes as "The Most Ancient

---

[9] "Stercum elephantinum cum melle mixtum et in vulva mulieris positum nunquam permittit concipere." Quoted by Lynn Thorndike, *History of Magic and Experimental Science* (London, 1923), i, 656. *Cf., infra* p. 154.

[10] *De Chirurgia*, p. 320. Cited by George F. Fort, *Medical Economy During the Middle Ages* (New York: Bouton; London: Quaritch, 1883), p. 47, note.

[11] Cyril P. Bryan, *The Papyrus Ebers* (London: Bles, 1930), p. xl. This is a popular account.

Book in the World," contains perhaps the first reference in writing to a medicated lint tampon designed to prevent conception.

The original prescription reads as follows:

Beginning of the recipes made for women in order to cause that a woman should cease to conceive for one year, two years, or three years:

Tips (?) of acacia

D' r. t

Triturate with a measure of honey, moisten lint therewith and place in her vulva.[12]

The tips of the shrub acacia contain gum arabic, which under fermentation liberates lactic acid anhydride ($C_6H_{10}O_5$). This dissolves readily in water forming lactic acid ($C_6 H_{10} O_5 + H_2 O \rightarrow 2 C_3 H_6 O_3$). The remarkable nature of this recipe, dating from 1550 B.C., is apparent when it is recalled that jellies in which lactic acid is the active agent are used by most of the birth-control clinics in England and the U. S. A.,[13] sometimes alone (being smeared on the cervix and into the fornices by turning a key on a tube which expels the jelly or paste through a nozzle previously inserted), sometimes as a smear on cervical rubber caps or vaginal diaphragms to prevent spermatozoa from swimming around the edge. Gum arabic, or gum acacia, is also generally used in the production of modern contraceptive jellies as a vehicle or medium.[14]

§3 BERLIN PAPYRUS (1300 B.C.)

Another early Egyptian source is the Berlin Medical Papyrus dating from the Nineteenth Dynasty (c. 1300 B.C.). Textual evidence leads one to believe that it was copied from an older manuscript. Although in a

[12] Georg Moritz Ebers, *Papyros Ebers* (Leipzig: W. Engelmann, 1875), Plate 93, Lines 6–8. Joachim's edition of the papyrus omits the passage. The German translation given in Ebers's translation (i, 35) is an incorrect translation of the Egyptian text. Ebers's German translation considers the means described abortifacients, when they are, in fact, contraceptives, and intended as such by the ancient Egyptians. So I am assured by Dr. James H. Breasted, the eminent egyptologist, and Director of the Oriental Institute, University of Chicago, and by Dr. Robert J. Barr, Assistant to the Director. Bryan's English account of the papyrus makes no mention of the birth-control passage. Bryan used Joachim's inaccurate German edition.

[13] As a matter of fact, despite its wide adoption, lactic acid is less effective in immobilizing sperms than acetic or tannic acids. The latter immobilizes immediately in a 1,000 solution, while Günther affirms that lactic requires 107 minutes at this strength. Baker, the English investigator of the chemistry of contraception, found lactic one-half as effective as acetic (1:1600 vs. 1:3200). The clinic jellies rarely contain more than 2.0 per cent. A 3.0 per cent. solution is effective immediately and completely (Voge), but has been rejected by the clinics in this strength as smarting about one woman in five. (Dickinson & Bryant, *op. cit.*, p. 41.)

[14] Dickinson and Bryant, *Control of Conception* p. 47.

better state of preservation than the Kahun Papyrus, the text is so corrupt that it is impossible to interpret certain details with certainty. But the general purport is clear. Eight sections deal with contraception and the ascertainment of pregnancy, sterility, and the sex of unborn children.

The following fragmentary, quasi-magical prescriptions are of some interest:

(1) Fumigate her in her vulva with *mimi* [a drug]: then she will not receive her seed. Afterwards give her a prescription to get rid of it; grease, *m'atet* herb, sweet ale. Cook them. To be swallowed for four mornings.

(2) To know a woman who will bear from a woman who will not bear. Watermelon, pounded and bottled with the milk of a woman who has borne a male child; make it into a dose. To be swallowed by the woman. If she vomits, she will bear. If she has eructations she will never bear.

Regarding the first prescription, Dawson remarks that "presumably the fumigation is a preparatory measure before coition, and the administration of the dose is made after."[15]

The second prescription is of special interest inasmuch as a passage in the pseudo-Hippocratic writings (Ch. 6 on *Concerning the Sterile*) seems to have been based upon it:

If you wish to know if a woman will become pregnant, give her to swallow butyron (βούτυρον) and the milk of a woman who has borne a male child. If she has eructations, she will conceive, but if not, then she will not.

This passage was translated by Dawson from the Greek text of the Van der Linden edition of Hippocrates (Leiden, 1665). Dawson goes on to say: "In Littré's great edition of Hippocrates (*Oeuvres*, Paris, 1839–61, viii, 415) a similar, but not quite identical text is given. In Kühn's edition (Leipzig, 1825, viii, 6) a variant text is to be found, where, instead of βούτυρον simply we have σικύην ἤ βούτυρον 'cucumber or butyron.' This is of great importance because it shows that butyron is not butter, as most editors have translated it, but a fruit in parallelism with the cucumber. Theophrastus does not mention βούτυρον, but we know from Hesychius, Athanæus, and others that there was a plant so called; and as it is given as an alternative to the cucumber, it is evidently a large, juicy fruit of the same kind. The Egyptian word for melon, which occurs in the passage of the Berlin papyrus quoted above, is *bdd* (the consonants only are written in Egyptian, the vowels being omitted); and it seems quite evident that when the prescription was borrowed by the Greeks they adopted their similarly sounding word βούτυρον as a translation of the Egyptian *bdd*, which represents the same or a similar fruit."[16]

[15] *Op. cit.*, p. 196.
[16] *Op. cit.*, p. 197.

It should be noted that the diagnosis in the second prescription as to whether or not a woman will prove fertile upon taking the concoction prescribed, is just reversed by the pseudo-Hippocratic writer. Among two irrational diagnoses, one choice is as good as another. Indeed it may be said that the prescriptions in the Berlin papyrus are less rational in theory and less effective in practice than those found in the earlier Kahun papyrus. The use of grease mixed with an herb, recommended in the first prescription, was evidently intended not for use in the vagina, but was to be taken by the mouth.

How do the prescriptions in the three different papyri rank in terms of presumed rationality? The Berlin (1300 B.C.) prescriptions are magical and worthless, those in the Petri papyrus (1850 B.C.), in so far as they may be partially effective, depend more upon physical than chemical features. The use of honey and possibly also lactic acid on lint as a tampon (Ebers) is pretty good procedure, combining chemical and physical features.

§4 MISCELLANEOUS SOURCES AND METHODS

It seems altogether strange that the Egyptian women, who used quantities of olive oil (often perfumed) in beautification, did not hit upon it as a contraceptive, as did the Greeks. The Greeks used olives for many purposes, one being contraceptive (see Chapter IV).

The survival in modern Egypt of a method of contraception hardly less magical than some found in Egyptian papyri has been shown by Miss W. S. Blackman's *The Fellahin of Upper Egypt*:

> If an expectant mother wishes to have no more children for a certain period, she will take the seeds of a castor-oil plant, and, on the day after the child is born, she will eat one of the seeds, if she wishes to be without another child for one year, two if for two years, and so on. This is believed to be invariably effective.[17]

We have already noted (see p. 9) that the women of modern Fez believe themselves protected from pregnancy when they eat one castor bean for each year that they desire to be free from conception. This type of symbolic magic has existed for hundreds of years in the folk beliefs of modern Europe (see Chapter VII). An instance is the belief that sitting upon a certain number of fingers will render one sterile for a number of years—one year for each finger. It may be noted, however, that the Greeks believed that castor would induce sterility.

There is reason to believe that the ancient Egyptians used prolonged lactation to reduce fertility. One writer has declared that primitive Egyp-

---

[17] W. S. Blackman, *The Fellahin of Upper Egypt* (London, 1927), p. 107. Cited by Dawson, *op. cit.*, p. 198. Punctuation mine.

tian women were not expected to bear children more frequently than once every three years; and that accordingly they nursed their children for a corresponding period.

Equally interesting is the account of Athenæus of Naucrates (Egypt, second century) who, in describing the profligacy of the ancient Lydians, observed that Adramyttes, their king, "was the first man who ever castrated women, and used female eunuchs instead of male eunuchs."[18] Whether or not he was the first is immaterial. Though the motive for castrating is not clear, it is a reasonable inference that it was to avoid offspring as a consequence of the sexual orgies of the people. At least Francis Adams, editor of the works of, and authority on, Paul of Aegenita, thinks it was practised to prevent conception.[19]

Probably the method was ovariotomy, for Strabo says the ancient Egyptians and Lydians were acquainted with the art of removing the ovaries of women and girls.[20] The kings of Lydia, Adramyttes and Gyges, castrated the women of their harems in order that they might continually be used with the full bloom of youth and beauty.[21] Though eunuchism in China seems to have had motives other than contraception, in the present instance sterilization seems to have been the purpose.

Sir Ernest Wallis Budge, an authority on Egyptian magic and on amulets, reports "I never saw an amulet to *prevent* conception, but I have seen thousands to produce it."[22] Presumably, therefore, the Egyptians, so far as present knowledge goes, did not rely upon amulets for this purpose.

Striking is the fact that all the Egyptian recipes mentioned above seem to have been dependent upon the female rather than on the male.[23] This is in accordance with the best modern theoretical thought on the subject. Inasmuch as the woman experiences the travail of child-bearing, it is preferable that control should be in her hands. This is especially important when women have unusually aggressive husbands disposed to alcoholic intoxication.

To what extent were the methods known to the Egyptians in general use?

[18] Athenæus, *Deipnosophists*. Bk. XII, Ch. 11. Yonge ed., iii, 826. Athenæus cites Xanthus as a source.

[19] *Seven Books of Paulus Aegenita*, i, 612.

[20] The fact (on the authority of Strabo and the editor of Paul of Aegenita) that the Egyptians knew this technique lends credence to the scattered anthropological reports that some primitive groups also practised ovariotomy. The death rate must have been high in the days before aseptic control.

[21] Cited by E. H. Kisch, *Sexual Life of Woman*, p. 415.

[22] Communication to the author dated November 4, 1931.

[23] We shall see that the same tendency is exhibited in the Greek and Roman prescriptions; though Aristotle mentioned anointing the male organ with cedar gum. Perhaps it is less true of Arabic recipes.

Here we are in a fog; we can only speculate. It seems reasonable to suppose that prolonged lactation may have been resorted to somewhat. We know that some preliterate groups used it. It is, however, unreliable and insufficient protection;[24] and it seems doubtful if it could have appreciably restricted population. Drugs taken by the mouth may have been resorted to by a few women. Must not operative procedures have been rare? What of the frequency of use of methods recommended in the papyri? Was knowledge of them limited chiefly to physicians? There seems to be no way of determining the extent of diffusion among individuals of such knowledge. It may be remarked, however, that when compared with modern agencies of communication those of the ancient Egyptians were restricted. Nor were the motives for practising contraception so general or so intense as in Western societies of our time. Our mores are quite different. Such circumstances suggest that while contraceptive techniques were recognized in Egyptian medicine, they were not diffused, not democratized. In fact, it is one of the major generalizations of this book that contraceptive knowledge, at least of a quasi-reliable, harmless sort, did not begin to become a mass phenomenon until late modern times (early nineteenth century). The incomplete process is still continuing.

It is reasonable to suppose that the Egyptian tradition was handed on to the Greeks, who, in turn, after contributing to it notably, handed it on to the Arabian or Islamic school of medicine. To these groups we turn after an examination of contraception in the Bible and Talmud.

[24] *Cf.*, Dickinson and Bryant, *op. cit.*, p. 54.

CHAPTER III

THE BIBLE AND THE TALMUD[1]

§1 HISTORICAL AND LEGAL ASPECTS

(1a) The Blessing of Fertility and the Jewish Law

THE precept "Be fruitful, and multiply, and replenish the earth"[2] was pronounced in the Bible as a blessing. Proliferousness was promised as a reward for a good life.[3] Barrenness was threatened as a punishment and curse for a wicked life.[4] In later times the blessing, interpreted as a commandment and duty, became formulated as a law. The *Mishna*[5] teaches: "A man must not stop from propagation of the race unless he already has children." The Shammaites (c. 30 B.C.) say: "Have two boys." The Hillelites (c. 30 B.C.) say: "Have one boy and one girl." For it is written:[6] "Male and female created He them." The commandment of propagation of the race is encumbent only upon the man, not upon the woman. Rabbi Yohanan ben Boroqa (c. 100–150 A.D.) says: "In reference to both of them the Bible declares: 'And God blessed them, and said unto them: Be fruitful and multiply.'"

(1b) The Old Law and its Modification

A change in conditions brought about modification of the older law. After the Babylonian exile (536 B.C.), the Jews settled down to a peaceful life. But, by the time of Alexander the Great (330 B.C.), Palestine could no longer support all its agricultural population. When the Jewish emigra-

---

[1] Most of what is valuable in this chapter is the work of Dr. Solomon Gandz, distinguished American Talmudic scholar, until lately librarian at Yeshiva College, New York City. Save for changes of an editorial nature (in collaboration with Dr. Gandz) and except for a few paragraphs from my own pen and assistance in calling his attention to one or two references, Dr. Gandz deserves sole credit for this interesting and able account.

[2] *Genesis*, i, 28; ix, 1.

[3] *Leviticus*, xxvi, 9; *Deuteronomy*, xxviii, 4: "Blessed shall be the fruit of thy body."

[4] *Deuteronomy*, xxviii, 18: "Cursed shall be the fruit of thy body." *Hosea*, iv, 10: "And they shall eat, and not have enough, they shall commit harlotry, and not increase."

[5] *Yebamot*, vi, 6, 61b and 65b; *Tosephta*, *ibid*., ed. Zuckermandel, viii, 4, p. 249. Final edition of the *Mishna* c. 200 A.D., that of the *Tosephta* one generation later. Both, however, contain very old traditions.

[6] *Genesis*, v, 2.

tion and dispersion set in, large families were no longer regarded as a blessing. Polygamy, though legal, was practically abandoned in favor of monogamy. Hence, the race, adapting itself to the changed conditions, adopted new views and new practices. The old views and practices were protected and fortified by law and statute. The wording of the *Mishna* suggests that there was an old, rigid law enjoining marriage and procreation under all circumstances and without any restrictions. The later stage of the law is satisfied with preservation of the race. After the birth of two children the duty is fulfilled.[7] Similarly, the divergent minority opinion of R. Yohanan seems to represent the old rigid law; while the accepted majority opinion, restricting the validity of the law to men only, appears to be a later interpretation making allowance for new needs that justify an exemption from the strict rule.[8] Thus the law, as formulated in the *Mishna*, reflects a compromise between the requirements of old and new conditions.

§2 TECHNIQUES

(2a) *Interruption of Pregnancy: Embryotomy*

The general rule is that, in cases of dangerous deliveries, the life of the mother may be saved by the sacrifice of her unborn child. "When a woman giving birth to a child is in danger, the unborn child may be cut to pieces and removed, for her life takes precedence over the life of the unborn child."[9] In such cases, however, where pregnancy would constitute a menace to the woman, or to her suckling child, prevention of conception is recommended by certain Rabbis.

(2b) *Coitus Interruptus*

One of the most ancient and primitive methods of family limitation is *coitus interruptus*. The Bible mentions it in the following story:[10]

---

[7] We now know that not two but three or four children are, as an average, required for survival. Not all children live until the marriageable age; of those that do, not all marry; of those that marry, some are involuntarily sterile. In any given population at any given time, the number required for replacement depends upon many conditions such as the above. Hence, the number varies as conditions vary. In early Hebrew times, infant mortality must have been high. Probably the marriage rate was high. In the absence of specific knowledge we may guess that the percentage of involuntary sterility was about that found in our time—ten per cent.

[8] See section *infra* on "The Sponge."

[9] *Mishna Oholot*, vii, 6. *Cf.*, also Julius Preuss, *Biblisch-Talmudische Medizin* (Berlin, 1923), p. 169. Modern Catholic doctrine, it may be noted, does not permit craniotomy to save the life of the mother in childbed. It prefers to let both die rather than enable the mother to survive. The ethical grounds are that evil may never be done for a presumably good purpose.

[10] *Genesis*, xxxviii, 7–10. Moffat translation, New York: Doran, 1924.

And Er, Judah's first-born, was wicked in the sight of the Lord; and the Lord slew him.   And Judah said unto Onan: "Go in unto thy brother's wife, and perform the duty of a husband's brother unto her, and raise up seed to thy brother!"   And Onan knew that the seed would not be his; and it came to pass, whenever he went in unto his brothers wife, that he used to spill it on the ground, lest he should give seed to his brother.   And the thing which he did was evil in the sight of the Lord; and He slew him also.

Hence, according to the Bible, Onan's sin did not consist in the use of *coitus interruptus* itself, but in the fact that he refused to perform the levirate marriage,[11] and to give seed to his brother's wife.   Onan was not lacking in appreciation of children.   On the contrary, he appreciated them so much, that he would create none under his brother's name.   Besides, he acted wrongly by concealing his disinclination to give seed to his brother and his brother's wife.   He deceived Judah and Tamar.   Had he frankly confessed his intention, Tamar could have married another.   Apparently, this act of selfishness and cheating of a poor widow constituted his sin.   The rabbis, however, laid more stress upon the act of *coitus interruptus* itself; they proclaimed it a mortal sin.   They said[12] that not only Onan but also Er practised *coitus interruptus*; and that Er, too, died on account of this sin. They must have felt that laxity and indulgence in such practices would constitute a menace to the good morals and preservation of the race.

In cases, however, when it seemed indicated medically, some Rabbis recommended *coitus interruptus*.   R. Eliezer, for example, who flourished about 80–100 A.D. writes: "During the twenty-four months[13] [that the mother nurses her child], he must thresh inside and winnow outside."[14] Other Rabbis, however, have protested that to do so is to act as Er and Onan did.   Yet Professor Lauterbach[15] justly remarks that the later teachers did not expressly say that it was forbidden to do so; they merely refused to recommend the practice.   The inference, therefore, is that the sponge was later suggested to meet this objection.   We shall return to this point presently.

[11] The levirate, not to mention marriage customs very similar, is quite widely diffused among primitive peoples.   For the evidence, see Sumner and Keller, *The Science of Society*.

[12] *Genesis Rabbah, ad locum*, lxxxv, 4, 5.   They are using two euphemistic terms for *coitus interruptus*.   Onan "was threshing inside and winnowing outside," and Er was "ploughing in the garden and emptying upon the dunghill."   *Cf.*, below the section on "The Removal of the Semen from the Vagina."   Note 42 this chapter and Preuss, *loc. cit.*, p. 534–5.

[13] *Yebamot*, 34b.   The Talmud regards twenty-four months as the proper period of lactation.   See also Preuss, *loc. cit.*, p. 471.

[14] Compare also the opinion of R. Meir as quoted in the *Tosephta*,   §2(c).

[15] Jacob Z. Lauterbach, "Talmudic-Rabbinic View on Birth Control," *Yearbook* of the Central Conference of American Rabbis, xxxvii, (1927), p. 373, *seq.*

The view that Onan was slain because he refused to follow the law of the levirate is not commonly followed by Catholic theologians, who seem to prefer, regardless of the nature of the text, to interpret the severe punishment of Onan as a consequence of practising *coitus interruptus*. Since Thomas Aquinas produced the *Summa Theologica*, Catholic theologians have whole-heartedly condemned the prevention of conception by artificial means, even when medically indicated in the most severe cases, and have regularly used, in contemporary controversial discussions, this text from *Genesis* (xxxviii, 9–10) as one of the main authorities.[16]

That Onan was slain for refusing to follow the levirate law is avowed not only by the text itself and by such writers on population problems as Harold Cox,[17] but by the Catholic author, Canon A. de Smet, in his recent book *Betrothment and Marriage:*

From the text and context, however, it would seem that the blame of the sacred writer applies directly and formally to the wrongful frustration of the law of the levirate, intended by Onan, rather than to the spilling of his seed.[18]

Canon de Smet cites as authority St. Augustine, *De nuptiis et concupiscentia*, cap. xv, n. 17 (*Migne*, cxliv, col. 423 s.)

(2c)   The Sponge (Spongy Substances?)

Until recently the writer was under the impression that the first mention in literature of the use of the moistened sponge as a contraceptive occurred in the handbills disseminated in England by Francis Place and his assistants in 1823 (see accompanying pages for reproduction of these handbills). Now it seems that this method was known to the authors of the Talmud. Moreover, the conditions under which it might legitimately be used were also laid down. One wonders whether the use of *mokh* (a spongy substance) is in any way related to the use of lint by the Egyptians, and whether the suggestion of an occlusive agent was passed on to the Hebrews during the captivity.

[16] The Catholic literature on the subject is enormous; but most of it is of little scientific value. Probably the most intelligent modern critic of birth control from the Catholic point of view is Father John A. Ryan of the Department of Social Action, National Catholic Welfare Conference, Washington, D. C. See the listings in the bibliography of the volume to follow on the economic and social history of birth control. Consult the following names: John A. Ryan, Father John Cooper, Bishop Charles Gore, Vermeersch, Frederick J. McCann, Edward Roberts Moore, Raoul De Guchteneere, and Rev. C. H. Sharp[e]. The League of National Life in London and the [American] National Catholic Welfare Conference publishes pamphlets on the subject. See also such standard Catholic periodicals in the U. S. as the *Pilot, Commonweal,* and *America*; and the English *G. K's Weekly, Pilot,* and other British Catholic periodicals.

[17] *The Population Problem* (London: Putnam, 1923), p. 208 ff.

[18] i, 165, note.

The inference that the sponge was later suggested by the early Rabbis to overcome logical difficulties associated with *coitus interruptus* is supported by the following tradition.[19] "There are three women that must[20] cohabit with a sponge:[21] a minor,[22] a pregnant woman, and one that nurses her child—a minor, because she might become pregnant and die; a pregnant woman, because the foetus might become a *foetus compressus* (or *papyraceus*);[23] one that nurses her child, because she might kill her child."[24] For R. Meir (150 A.D.) used to say: "During all the twenty-four months [that a mother nurses her child], he must thresh inside and winnow outside." And the other Rabbis said: "He may cohabit as usual, and the Lord will protect him; for it is written that 'The Lord preserveth the simple.' "[25] The text of this *Tosephta* (230 A.D.) admits only the following natural explanation. The obligation or the permissibility of the sponge is the *consensus omnium*. The controversy between R. Meir and the Rabbis, like the controversy between R. Eliezer and the other teachers, refers only to *coitus interruptus*. This controversy is quoted in the *Tosephta* only to explain why the sponge was generally recommended. *Coitus interruptus*, the practice of Er and Onan, was very objectionable. Besides, the act of prevention of conception was performed by the man, upon whom the commandment of the propagation of the race lay; hence it constituted a viola-

[19] *Tosephta Niddah*, ii, 6, p. 642. Edition c. 230 A.D. The tradition itself is older.

[20] This is Dr. Solomon Gandz's conception. Among the Rabbinic commentaries the question of whether cohabitation with a sponge is permitted or compulsory is controversial; cf., especially *Yam shel Shelomoh* on *Yebamot*, i, 8, and Jacob Z. Lauterbach, *op. cit.*, pp. 377–379.

[21] Hebrew *mokh* is a soft spongy substance, an absorbent material like cotton or hackled wool. This is the same material that Theilhaber refers to when he says that "An Hebraic law-book of a later date, Eben Haeser, recommended to very sick women, who should have no children, a suitable method of birth prevention in the introduction [presumably into the vagina] of 'much,' a kind of wadding." (Felix A. Theilhaber, *Das Sterile Berlin*, Berlin, 1913, p. 10.) Theilhaber here refers to a sixteenth century code authoritative for the Jews. Dr. Gandz has, however, given the original source of the *Eben ha 'Ezer* which, in this instance, is the *Tosephta* (c. 230 A.D.).

[22] A minor is defined as one aged from eleven years and one day to twelve years and one day. If she is either older or younger, a man may cohabit with her without apprehension. The Orient, especially at that time, did not object to marriages with minors.

[23] According to the Talmud, superfoetation is possible, but it causes the former foetus to become an abortion in the shape of a flat fish like the sole or turbot. Even when superfoetation does not occur, the Rabbis believe that cohabitation during the first three months after conception is harmful to the woman and to the child. See *Niddah*, 31a and Preuss, *op. cit.*, pp. 445–48, 486–87.

[24] By losing her milk and being compelled prematurely to wean her child. *Cf.*, *Yebamot*, 42a.

[25] *Psalms*, cxvi, 6.

tion of this commandment. This was the reason for the dissension of the Rabbis. *By the use of the sponge it was the woman, free from the duty of propagation, that committed the act of the prevention of conception; hence, especially in instances where contraception was medically indicated, there was no reason for anybody to forbid it.*

The Babylonian Talmud,[26] which appeared later than the *Tosephta*,[27] quotes, however, the same tradition with a minor but significant variation. There[28] one reads: "There are three women that must cohabit with a sponge: a minor, a pregnant woman, and one that nurses her child—a minor, because she might become pregnant and die; a pregnant woman, because the foetus might become a *foetus compressus*; one that nurses her child, *because she might wean her child, which would cause its death*." The earlier phrase had been "because she might kill her child." A minor is defined as one aged from eleven years and one day to twelve years and one day. If the girl is younger or older, she may cohabit as usual. Such is the opinion of R. Meir. The other Rabbis say: "This one and that one may cohabit as usual, and the Lord will have pity on them, for it is written that 'The Lord preserveth the simple.' " According to this reading the legality of the use of the sponge would be controversial, and, since the majority is against it, forbidden. This interpretation is generally accepted by the rabbinic authorities.[29] Professor Lauterbach[30] thinks that the controversy refers only to the case of a minor. Furthermore, he points out that even if we should understand from the passage that the Rabbis differ with R. Meir in all three cases, it would only follow that they do not make the use of the sponge obligatory, which interpretation was early suggested by R. Solomon Lurya (1510–1573).[31]

The meaning of the term "to cohabit with a sponge" is plain and unequivocal. It is this: to put the sponge into the vagina before cohabitation, in order to cover the *os uteri*, absorb the semen, and prevent direct insemination. Such is the explanation of Rashi (d. 1105) in *Yebamot* 12b and 100b. Rabbi Jacob Tam, the grandson of Rashi, explains the term to mean that the woman uses the sponge to remove the sperms from the vagina after cohabitation. Philologically R. Tam's interpretation is without foundation, and the plain sense of the text, especially in *Niddah 3a*, contra-

---

[26] Final edition c. 500 A.D.

[27] Edited in Palestine c. 230 A.D.

[28] *Yebamot*, 12b, 100b; *Ketubbot*, 39a; *Nedarim*, 35b; *Niddah*, 45a.

[29] Apparently they did not see fit that a woman should form a habit of using such devices.

[30] *Op. cit.*, p. 379 *seq.*

[31] See n. 20.

dicts it.[32] Strangely enough, Rashi himself, in *Ketubbot 37a*, changes his opinion, and accepts R. Tam's explanation.[33] Dr. Reissner[34] follows Rashi, and does not notice that he contradicts himself by using one and the same term in two different meanings. Upon one occasion[35] he understands it to mean removal of the sperms after cohabitation; at another time,[36] he considers it to imply actual use of the sponge as an occlusive agent. Reissner is again mistaken when he says that the removal of the sperms after cohabitation is unconditionally forbidden because it is the usage of prostitutes. The fact that prostitutes use a means is no reason for its prohibition. On the contrary, according to R. Tam and his followers, the removal of the sperms after coitus is less objectionable than the use of the sponge, which is the very reason why they adopted this forced interpretation.[37]

(2d) Violent Movements. The Practice of Prostitutes

According to Hebrew law, a divorced woman or widow must wait three months before remarrying in order to ascertain whether the paternity belongs to the first or to the second husband. But if a woman is unmarried, and there is a suspicion, or even the certainty, of illegal intercourse, then she must not wait before marrying, because the legal assumption is that she used the sponge to prevent conception. In this connection another contraceptive method is mentioned, namely twisting oneself and making violent movements after cohabitation.[38] This practice was well known in antiquity, and is still known and used in modern times.[39] For the use of this method among primitive peoples, see the section on Australia in Chapter I. Rabbi Meir Adalbi[40] (c. 1360) quotes Galen's opinion that violent movements after coitus prevent conception.

[32] *Cf., Yam shel Shelomoh* on *Yebamot*, i, 8, and Lauterbach, *op. cit.*, p. 378.

[33] In *Ketubbot*, 37a, the Talmud says that a prostitute usually cohabits with a sponge. Rashi might have learned from some source that the custom of prostitutes was to remove the semen after cohabitation. Hence the different explanation of this special passage.

[34] Dr. Hans Reissner, "Die Stellung des Judentums zur Frage der Geburtenkontrolle," *Die Neue Generation*, xxvi (1930), 295–299.

[35] On p. 297, referring to *Ketubbot*, 37a.

[36] On p. 298, referring to *Yebamot*, 12b.

[37] On the other side, Hans Reissner, *op. cit.*, 295–299 fails to mention this source which expressly speaks of the removal of the semen after coitus; see below, the section on "Removal of the Sperms from the Vagina." Also he does not notice the legal difference between man and woman.

[38] *Babli, ibid.*, and *Niddah*, 42a.

[39] Preuss, *op. cit.*, p. 530.

[40] In his book *Shebilè Emùnah*, v, §1 (Warsaw, 1887), p. 112. Rabbi Adalbi gives no reference to Galen. Dr. Moïssidès of Athens informs me that he has searched the works of Galen, and has been able to find no discussion of contraception. If the subject is mentioned by him, perhaps it is only a passing comment. Dr. Gandz says that Rabbi Adalbi's source was probably a Hebrew or Arabic translation and that Adalbi hardly knew Greek.

(2e)   The Removal of Semen from the Vagina

Removal of the semen from the vagina was a well known technique. The Talmud teaches:[41] "If somebody enjoins his wife by a vow to fill up and empty out upon the dunghill, the court compels him to divorce her, and to pay her stipulated widowhood." Now "to fill up and empty out upon the dunghill" is a euphemism meaning to receive the semen but remove it after intercourse.[42] Nothing is said about the method and procedure of the removal. Rashi,[43] and after him Preuss,[44] think that it was brought about by quick, violent movements. What the Talmud says is only that, if the woman complains, she is supported by the court, and entitled to divorce and payment of her widowhood. No mention is made of whether or not the practice in itself, in the case of mutual agreement or medical indication, is forbidden.[45]

(2f)   Potions: The Cup of Roots

The plain teaching of the Talmud is that there are no legal objections to a woman's taking internally a medicine which would make her barren. So we read:[46] "A man is not allowed to drink a cup of roots in order to become sterile, but a woman is allowed to drink a cup of roots in order to become sterile." The following story is characteristic:[47] "Judith, the wife of R. Hiyya (c. 200 A.D.), suffered from great pains during childbirth.[48] Disguised, with changed clothes, she appeared before R. Hiyya and asked him: 'Does the commandment of propagation include the woman?' He said, 'No.'[49] Accordingly, she took the root medicine that made her sterile. Eventually it became known, and R. Hiyya said to her: 'I wish you had given me at least one birth more.' "

The *Midrash*[50] says that in the time of the great flood a man used to marry two women, one to bear him children, and another for sexual intercourse only. The latter took the "cup of roots" to render herself sterile, and was accustomed to keep company with him dressed like a mistress.

---

[41] *Mishna Ketubbot*, vii, 5; *Tosephta, ibid.*, vii, 6, p.269; *Babli, ibid.*, 72a; *Yerushalmi, ibid.*, 31b.

[42] *Cf.*, this chapter n. 2 and the remark of the *Yerushalmi* that it is like the practice of Er. See also Preuss, *op. cit.*, p. 530.

[43] *Ketubbot*, 72a.

[44] *Op. cit.*, p. 530.

[45] *Cf.*, §2c.

[46] *Tosephta Yebamot*, viii, 4, p. 249.

[47] *Yebamot*, 65 b.

[48] She gave birth to twin sons and twin daughters; *Yebamot, ibid.*

[49] In accordance with the teaching of the *Mishna*, in §1(a), and the *Tosephta*, here. R. Hiyya is regarded as the editor of the *Tosephta*.

[50] *Genesis Rabbah*, xxiii, 2.

R. Yohanan (d. 279 A.D.), regarded also as a skilled physician,[51] has the following to say regarding the preparation of this medicine:[52] "Alexandrian gum [of the *Spina Aegyptia*], liquid alum, and garden crocus, each in the weight of a denar, are mixed together. Three cups of wine with this medicine are good for gonorrhea, and do not sterilize. Two cups of beer with this medicine cure jaundice and sterilize."[53] Isaak Lampronti (1679–1756), an Italian Rabbi and physician, testified[54] that, in cases where prevention was medically indicated, the Jewish physicians of his time used to administer the *trifera*,[55] or other medicines, to Jewish women to sterilize them, or to prevent them from conceiving.

(2g) Professor Lauterbach's Summary on the Attitude of Talmudic-Rabbinic Law

Dr. Jacob Z. Lauterbach, Professor of Talmud at the Hebrew Union College, Cincinnati, a distinguished authority on rabbinic literature, sums up his studies of the subject as follows: ". . . While there may be some differences of opinion about one detail or another, or about the exact meaning of one talmudic passage or another, we can formulate the following principles in regard to the question of birth control as based upon a correct understanding of the halakic teachings of the Talmud, as accepted by the medieval rabbinic authorities, and especially upon the sound interpretation given by R. Solomon Lurya to some of these talmudic passages:

"(1) The Talmudic-Rabbinic law does not consider the use of contraceptives, as such, immoral or against the law. It does not forbid birth control, but it forbids birth suppression.

"(2) The Talmudic-Rabbinic law requires that every Jew have at least two children in fulfillment of the biblical command to propagate the race, which is incumbent upon every man.

"(3) There are, however, conditions under which a man may be exempt from this prime duty: (a) when a man is engaged in religious work, like the study of the Torah, and fears that he may be hindered in his work by taking on the responsibilities of a family; (b) when a man, because of love or other considerations, marries a woman who is incapable of having children, as an old or sterile woman; (c) when a man is married to a woman

---

[51] *'Adodah Zarah*, 28a; *The Jewish Encyclopedia*, vii, 211.

[52] *Shabbat*, 110a.

[53] This is the explanation of Maimonides in his commentary to *Shabbat*, xiv, 3. The explanation of Rashi is that three species mixed with wine are good for gonorrhea and do not sterilize, while two species mixed with beer do sterilize, etc. He does not say, however, which two species are meant. *Cf.*, also Preuss, *op. cit.*, p. 439.

[54] In his *Pahad Yishaq* (Venice-Reggio, 1813), part 4, f. 52b. under *Kōs 'iqqarīn*.

[55] Fanfani, *Italian Dictionary*, explains it as *Lattovaro inventato dagli Arabi*.

whose health is in such a condition as to make it dangerous for her to bear children.

"Of course, in any case," Professor Lauterbach continues, "the use of contraceptives, or any device to prevent conception, is allowed only when both parties, i.e., husband and wife, consent."[56] This attitude certainly has many enlightened and modern elements. Later on we shall see that the religions of the Islamic peoples were likewise not opposed to contraception. But we shall first summarize what has preceded in this chapter.

§3 SUMMARY

It is clear from this account that the ancient Hebrews knew and practised to some extent such contraceptive techniques as *coitus interruptus*, the intravaginal use of spongy substances, violent movements, removal of the sperms from the vagina, such potions as the cup of roots. They also practised embryotomy. Further, Jewish law permitted prevention under certain circumstances.[57] Though the old law was gradually modified as circumstances changed, we have no means of knowing to what extent anti-conceptional measures may have been used. Probably, as in the instance of primitive tribes, and the peoples of antiquity, they were not greatly resorted to. It would seem a safe inference that custom and religious law as well as the absence of strong incentives to limitation, prevented wide-spread use. But this is only a guess. At all events, it is clear that the ancient Hebrews manifested a desire to avoid both excessive sterility and excessive fertility. This we shall find characteristic of every civilization we study. It is one of the major generalizations of this book.

It is as well exemplified in Greek and Roman society as in any others. To these writers we now turn.

[56] *Op. cit.*, as quoted by *Amer. Hebrew*, March 27, 1931, p. 495. *Punctuation mine.*

[57] For a contrary view see Rabbi J. Horowitz, "Prevention of Conception According to the Jews's Religious Law," an article in Hebrew contributed to the *Festschrift für Jacob Rosenheim* (Frankfort a. Main, 1931), pp. 87–119.

CHAPTER IV

GREEK AND ROMAN WRITERS

THE elementary knowledge of contraceptive technique possessed by the Egyptians and early Hebrews was notably advanced by several Greek and Roman writers. Chief among them were Aristotle, the Hippocratic writers, Lucretius, Pliny, Dioscorides, Soranos, Aëtios and Oribasios. It was in Soranos that Greek gynaecological thought and contraceptive medicine found its culmination.

Aristotle, Plato, Hesiod, Polybius and many other writers of antiquity discussed various general aspects of the population problem, including limitation, as is well-known to anyone familiar with the standard histories of economic and social thought.[1] Hesiod, Xenocrates, Lycurgus, for example, were partisans of the one-child family. Plato and Aristotle favored a stationary population for the Greek city state. Abortion and infanticide were commonly condoned and even recommended under certain circumstances as a matter of public policy. Certain writers, of whom Plato was one, believed that the age of procreation should be regulated by law (30–35 years for the male and 20–40 years for the woman). Procreation beyond these limits was to be condemned. Aristotle would regulate by law the number of children one might have, and approved abortion and the exposure of deformed infants. We know how Polybius complained eloquently of depopulation in his time. All this is common knowledge, and has been treated in the histories of social and economic thought of the period. But that Aristotle was acquainted with a more or less rational anti-conceptional technique has not, to my knowledge, been mentioned by any of these historians; nor has it been noted by the medical historians. It has been overlooked even by the Greek medical historian and editor, Moïssidès, in an excellent article[2] recently published on Neo-Malthusian expedients known to the Greeks.

[1] See, for example, Lewis H. Haney, *History of Economic Thought*. New York: Macmillan, 1923. Joseph Rambaud, *Histoire des Doctrines Économiques*. Paris, 1909. René Gonnard, *Histoire des Doctrines Économiques*. Paris, 1924, 3 vols., especially vol. i.

[2] M. Moïssidès, "Le Malthusianisme dans l'Antiquité Grecque," *Janus*, xxxvi (1932), 169–179.

§1   ARISTOTLE (IV-2 B.C.)[3]

Aristotle's *Historia Animalium* seems to contain the first mention of a contraceptive in the writings of the Greeks. This great philosopher and keen observer there notes that some of his contemporaries prevent conception "by anoint[ing] that part of the womb on which the seed falls with oil of cedar, or with ointment of lead or with frankincense, commingled with olive oil."[4] There is no reason to believe, however, that Aristotle understood the principle upon which this practice operated.[5] It is clear from the context that he regarded the quality of smoothness as the *modus operandi* of prevention; whereas we now know that oil has a contraceptive effect by reducing the motility of spermatozoa and by gumming up the external os.

[3] This dating system is used frequently below. The Roman numeral refers to the century, the Arabic numeral to the first or second half. All are A.D. unless otherwise specified.

[4] *Works*, iv, 583a.   Smith and Ross ed., Oxford, 1910.   It is interesting to note in this connection that Dr. Marie C. Stopes, the leading lay advocate of contraception in England, in the course of urging the necessity of developing some ultra-simple contraceptive for poor and uneducated women, recommends the use of olive oil on a rubber sponge.   In a recent paper she states that "one of the best and most effective things is simple olive oil. We [at the Mother's Clinic for Constructive Birth Control in London] have approaching 2,000 cases in which we have given as the sole instruction the use of olive oil. . . . Some of these cases go back about two years, and house to house visits of some hundreds of them show a percentage of failure of *zero*."   [Marie C. Stopes, "Positive and Negative Control of Conception in its Various Technical Aspects," *Jour. State Medicine*, xxxix (1931), 359; reprint p. 6.]   While the declaration that this method is infallible is not likely to be accepted by the scientifically-minded, it is quite possible that a carefully-controlled case series composed of sufficient numbers of cases might well show that olive oil was reasonably effective as a contraceptive.   Recent research by Dr. John R. Baker (see Bibliography) has shown that, in the case of many suppositories, the physical impediment to fertilization frequently proves more effective than the chemical ingredients used.   He has conclusively demonstrated that chinosol has, for example, been much over-rated as a spermicide.

[5] There is nothing unusual in this circumstance.   There is every reason to believe that most variations in conduct and in the mores are discovered by a hit and miss, trial and error method.   When an individual finds this effective, he communicates the fact to others. Gradually there is a diffusion of the practice.   When such practices become institutionalized, and are elevated to doctrines of welfare, they become mores as distinct from folkways.   It is not necessary that an individual or a group should understand the theoretical basis for a given useful practice in order to discover, adopt and spread it.   Those practices the beneficial results of which are clear and not too remote are, other things being equal, more likely to be readily adopted and diffused than practices the beneficial results of which are remote, intangible, or questionable.   For an excellent theoretical discussion of some of these points see A. G. Keller, *Societal Evolution.   A Study of the Evolutionary Basis of the Science of Society*.   New York: Macmillan, 1915.

§2 PSEUDO-HIPPOCRATIC WRITERS: (IV & V B.C.)

Certain sections of the Hippocratic writings, which, like the writings of Aristotle, ante-date by some centuries the birth of Christ, make mention of a potion supposed to prevent conception. Assuredly the following passage excerpted from the section "On the Nature of Woman" was written not by Hippocrates himself but by a disciple:

If a woman does not wish to become pregnant, dissolve in water misy as large as a bean and give it to her to drink, and for a year she will not become pregnant.[6]

Virtually the same passage appears in the section on the "Diseases of Women."[7] Various authorities have tried, as Oliver notes,[8] to identify misy. The following are the various guesses: Sulphur, sulphate of copper, iron sulphate, iron vitriol, the salts of sulphuric acid with copper and alum. Dierbach[9] concludes that the substance is "undeterminable."

The following prescription of the Hippocratic writer would seem, upon superficial examination, to be recommending a contraceptive for the cure of sterility. It will be noted, however, that the application is for a specific period only, seven days, and that thereafter the woman is to withdraw the tampon and lie with her husband. Dr. R. L. Dickinson informs me that the prescription (which follows) is good treatment for the most common cause of sterility, catarrh of the cervix.

If a woman does not conceive over a long period in spite of the fact that her periods appear, take on the third or fourth day some alum, crush it fine, dissolve it in perfume, apply it on wool as a pessary; the woman will wear it for three days; on the fourth day boil the dried bile of beef in oil, moisten lint with it, and apply this pessary; she will wear it for three days; the next day she will withdraw it, and will go to her husband.[10]

---

[6] E. Littré, *Oeuvres complètes d'Hippocrate*, vii, 415, §98. *Cf.*, Robert Fuchs's German edition of Hippocrates, iii, 382, §98. The passage has been noted by H. Fasbender, *Entwicklungslehre*, p. 240, and by Klotz-Forest, "Contraceptive Prophylaxis at the Time of Hippocrates," in *Chronique Médicale*, xii (1905), 142. Haeser (*Lehrbuch*, 1875 ed., i, 202) states that "Hippocrates also recommended as a preventive method the production of corpulence." Doubtless this would have been as ineffective as the misy. It is now known that corpulence is not a cause of sterility, but only associated with it. The fat woman sometimes has organic defects interfering with fertility.

Since these passages have been written, Dr. M. Moïssidès writes (*op. cit.*) as if this passage were by Hippocrates himself. But this is doubtful. Incidentally, Moïssidès believes "misy" to be "very probably sulphate of iron or copper." (p. 173).

[7] Littré, *Oeuvres*, viii, 171, §76. *Cf.*, Fuchs's edition, iii, 465, §76.

[8] Dr. John Rathbone Oliver, in a letter to the author.

[9] J. H. Dierbach, *Die Arzneimittel des Hippokrates*. Heidelberg, 1824.

[10] Littré, *Oeuvres*, viii, 59.

In another passage[11] goose fat applied in a pessary was prescribed to aid conception.   But here again we must distinguish between immediate and long run effects of the treatment.

In the Hippocratic chapter "On the Nature of Woman" it is stated that "After coitus, if a woman ought not to conceive, she makes it a custom for the semen to fall outside when she wishes this."[12]   This is probably a factual report rather than a contraceptive recommendation by Hippocrates.   He clearly understood that both the male and female elements had to unite to cause conception.   The passage is so euphemistic that one cannot be certain whether *coitus interruptus* is the technique used or whether the women expel the semen by bodily movements (see earlier discussion of this among primitives in Chapter I) or the use of fingers to wipe out the vagina.   Women have been known to use the finger or fingers to direct urine to flush out the vagina.   Whatever the technique the Hippocratic writer had in mind, it is probably very old and persists to some extent even in our day.

§3   LUCRETIUS (I-1 B.C.)

Lucretius (99 B.C. –55 B.C.), the great Latin poet, who combined with his poetic ability a scientific and rationalist viewpoint, made some interesting observations on human fertility and sterility, and on the prevention of conception.   He observed that it was not a consequence of the wrath of the gods that humans were sterile; in vain did his male contemporaries raise offerings to the gods to make their wives pregnant.[13]   Sterility is caused by "too great thickness," or by undue "fluidity and thinness" of the semen.[14] Lucretius observed that

some males impregnate some females more readily than others, and other females conceive and become pregnant more readily from other males.   And many women

---

[11] *Ibid.*, viii, 53.

[12] Elsewhere in the same chapter the Hippocratic writer tells of a certain musician who, having coitus with many men, came to the conclusion, after hearing oral reports to that effect, that she would be less likely to conceive if the semen were thrown off.   "When she one day noticed that the semen had not flowed out, she told her husband about it.   The report even got to me."   Hippokrates, *Sämmt. Werke* (Fuchs ed., München, 1895), i, 219.

[13] "Nor do the divine powers debar anybody from the power of begetting, forbidding him ever to receive the name of father from sweet children, and forcing him to pass his life in a barren wedlock; as men commonly fancy when in sorrow they drench the altars with much blood, and pile the raised altars with offerings, to make their wives pregnant with abundant seed.   In vain they weary the divinity of the gods and the sacred lots."   Lucretius *On the Nature of Things*.   Bk. iv, pp. 165–6 in translation by H. A. J. Munro.   London: Bell, 1913.   The passages below occur all at the end of Book iv.   Punctuation mine. Munro had a passion for omitting it.

[14] *Ibid.*, p. 166.

have hitherto been barren during several marriages, and have yet in the end found mates from whom they could conceive children and be enriched with a sweet offspring.[15]

These were shrewd observations for the time. Both "diet" and the "modes of intercourse" are important in promoting or restraining fertility. "By some foods seed is thickened . . . and by others again [it] is thinned and wasted." Intercourse in the quadruped position promotes fertility;[16] the semen is more likely to enter the os. But effeminate motions during intercourse reduce the chances of fertility.[16] Hence harlots execute these motions (not detailed) to prevent conception and heighten pleasure for their men.

And in what modes the intercourse goes on is likewise of very great moment; for women are commonly thought to conceive more readily [when they have intercourse] after the manner of wild beasts and quadrupeds, because the seeds in this way can find the proper spots [os] in consequence of the position of the body. Nor have wives the least use for effeminate motions [during intercourse]; a woman hinders and stands in the way of her own conceiving, when thus she acts; for she drives the furrow [vagina] out of the direct course and path of the share, and turns away from the proper spots [os] the stroke of the seed. And thus for their own ends harlots are wont to move, in order not to conceive and lie in child-bed frequently, and at the same time to render Venus more attractive to men. This [mode of intercourse to prevent conception and give the men especial pleasure, avows Lucretius] our wives have surely no need of.[17]

§4 PLINY THE ELDER (1-2)

The *Natural History*[18] by Pliny the Elder (23–79 A.D.)[19] is an uncritical, largely unorganized, gossipy, dilettante encyclopedia, on the medical side

[15] *Ibid.*

[16] This idea is questioned by modern science.

[17] *Ibid.*, p. 167. One wonders whether the reference to "effeminate motions" is a euphemism for violent movements calculated to expel the semen. The reference to this practice as that of prostitutes might make one suspect that this is the case; on the other hand, by another interpretation, Lucretius seems to be speaking of effeminate motions during, rather than after, coitus.

[18] I have used the Bostock and Riley 6 vol. ed. in the Bohn Classical Library series. This includes notes by the latest commentators.

[19] Gaius Plinius Secundus, the elder, author of the *Historia Naturalis*, was born at Como in 23 A.D., and died at Stabiae during the great outbreak of Vesuvius of the 22nd of August, 79 A.D. The facts of his life we know through the reports of his namesake and nephew, Pliny, the younger, (*Epst.* iii, 5): That he was a soldier in the campaigns with Germany, later lived in Spain as Proconsul, held in Rome an appointment at the court, was active as a legal adviser, and later commanded the fleet at Misenum. Pliny was unusually active in a literary way, despite his public responsibilities. Except the *Historia Naturalis*, we possess none of his numerous works. Irreplaceable above all is the loss of his twenty books on the German wars.

based largely on folk medicine. Pliny's occasional statements on contraception are merely incidental, unsystematized; but they deserve to be winnowed from the chaff of a quarter of a million words simply as a matter of record. Moreover, the influence of the *Natural History* throughout the Middle Ages was great.

First, as to anaphrodisiacs one finds: "Mouse-dung . . . applied in the form of a liniment;"[20] the broth of scincus taken with honey;[21] clymenus;[22] nasturtium;[23] the ashes of dill;[24] purslane;[25] the softer orchis taken in goat's milk;[26] hemlock applied to the testes at puberty;[27] two species of "vitex;"[28] the ashes of a tree called brya;[29] willow leaves, crushed and taken as a potion—all these "check libidinous tendencies, and effectually put an end to them, if habitually employed."[30] Rue, boiled with rose-oil, with the addition of an ounce of aloes, has the effect of impeding the generative function.[31] "According to Osthanes, if a woman's loins are rubbed with blood taken from the ticks upon a black wild bull, she will be inspired with an aversion to sexual intercourse."[32] "The skin of the left side of the forehead [of the hippopotamus], attached to the groin, acts as an antaphrodisiac."[33] Hempseed[34] and condrion[35] render males impotent. A plant called "nymphea," when taken as a drink, renders an individual impotent for twelve days.[36] Nor should this bizarre prescription be overlooked:

A most powerful medicament is obtained by reducing to ashes the nails of the lynx, together with the hide; . . . these ashes, taken in drink, have the effect of checking abominable desires in men; and, . . . if they are sprinkled upon women, all libidinous thoughts will be restrained.[37]

Among the sterilizing plant or animal products taken as a potion or eaten, Pliny mentions these: Epimedion,[38] esplenon,[39] (he warns women against using these), parsley,[40] *Pteris* or *Thelypteris*.[41] Mint taken internally, since it curdles (?) milk, will impede generation, "by preventing the seminal fluids from obtaining the requisite consistency."[42]

Nor are purely magical recipes absent: From a spider called phalangium, described as having a hairy body and enormous head, are to be extracted two small worms. These, according to Pliny, attached in a piece of deer's skin, before sunrise, to a woman's body will prevent conception.[43] Clearly,

[20] Bk. 28, ch. 80. *Cf.*, use of elephant and crocodile dung in other prescriptions within.
[21] Bk. 28, ch. 30.   [22] Bk. 25, ch. 33.   [23] Bk. 20, ch. 50.   [24] Bk. 20, ch. 74.
[25] Bk. 20, ch. 81.   [26] Bk. 26, ch. 62.   [27] Bk. 25, ch. 95.   [28] Bk. 24, ch. 38.
[29] Bk. 24, ch. 42.   [30] Bk. 24, ch. 37.   [31] Bk. 20, ch. 51.   [32] Bk. 28, ch. 77.
[33] Bk. 28, ch. 31.   [34] Bk. 20, ch. 97.   [35] Bk. 22, ch. 45.   [36] Bk. 25, ch. 37.
[37] Bk. 28, ch. 32. There may be still other prescriptions in Pliny of a similar nature.
[38] Bk. 27, ch. 53.   [39] Bk. 27, ch. 17.   [40] Bk. 20, ch. 44.
[41] Bk. 27, ch. 55.   [42] Bk. 20, ch. 53.   [43] Bk. 29, ch. 27.

the following passage might be classed either with the anaphrodisiacs above
or under the magical prescriptions:

A lizard drowned in a man's urine has the effect of an antaphrodisiac upon the
person whose urine it is. . . . The same property is attributed to the excrements of
snails, and to pigeon's dung, taken with oil and wine. . . . the testes of a game-
cock . . . rubbed with goose-grease and attached to the body in a ram's skin, have
all the effect of an antaphrodisiac; the same, too, with the testes of any kind of
dunghill cock, placed, together with the blood of a cock, beneath the bed. . . . If a
man makes water upon a dog's urine, he will become disinclined to copulation. . . .[44]

After all these digressions—albeit, lost in perhaps a quarter of a million
words—Pliny's modesty impresses one when he says:

It [phalangium] is the only one of all the anti-conceptives that I feel myself at
liberty to mention, in favour of some women whose fecundity, quite teeming with
children, stands in need of some such respite.[45]

Worthy restraint for a Roman soldier! But Pliny does not live up to his
promise. For he repeats Aristotle's more or less effective technique: rubbing the male organ with cedar [oil or gum?] just before coitus. This, we
are assured, "will effectually prevent impregnation."[46] Aristotle, however,
had recommended application of the cedar oil to the cervix, not to the penis.
Cervical application is clearly preferable, though use by the male would be
better than nothing at all. Thus did Pliny venture to improve on Aristotle!

To summarize: Pliny's account is diffuse, the techniques mainly ineffective and sometimes purely magical. Potions and amulets find a central
place. When he follows Aristotle he writes more sense.

§5 DIOSCORIDES (1–2)

Pandanios Dioscorides of Anazarbos in Cilicia has been selected as representative of the early works on materia medica because his work by that
title, *De materia medica*, "ought," in the words of Daremberg, "to be considered as the primary source of everything on simple medicaments to be
found in the work of his successors."[47] To Haeser[48] it was the most important pharmacological and botanical treatise in antiquity. Up to the sixteenth century Dioscorides' works were consulted as if they were an oracle.
Before the invention of printing, they were frequently reproduced by copying the manuscript. Subsequently, more than seventy editions appeared
in practically all the languages of Europe, except, remarkably enough, in

---

[44] Bk. 30, ch. 49.   [45] Bk. 29, ch. 27.   [46] Bk. 24, ch. 11.
[47] *Oeuvres d'Oribase*, i, xxii.
[48] H. Haeser, *Lehrbuch* (1875 ed.), i, 303.

English.[49] Not until the discovery of the original manuscript of Dioscorides, rather late in modern times, was it possible to compare this with the
somewhat truncated copies used by the Arabs and the medieval scholastics.
The manuscript was discovered in Constantinople by a Belgian, and later
brought to Europe. I understand that it is a beautifully decorated manuscript, and that it now reposes in the library of the palace at Vienna. Its
Greek author flourished during the time of Nero, and accompanied the
Roman armies as a physician, collecting a store of information on plants.
The treatise is divided into five books, details the properties of about 1600
medicinal plants, and describes animal products of dietetic and medicinal
value. For fifteen centuries Dioscorides, who greatly influenced Islamic
physicians,[50] maintained undisputed authority in botany. His work
became "the oracle of physicians throughout the entire Middle Ages."[51]

Dioscorides gives us four types of recommendations for the prevention
of conception: Magical prescriptions (e.g., wearing of amulets); ineffective
potions; medicated pessaries; anointing the genitals with sticky substances.

Among Dioscorides' magical prescriptions are the following: "The menstrual blood of women appears to prevent conception when they [the women]
spread themselves with it, or when they step over it."[52] Asparagus, tied up
as an amulet or drunk as a decoction, will prevent conception and render one
sterile.[53] The roots of large heliotropes tied up, presumably as a charm, are
also reported as used to prevent conception.[54]

The potions are: The finely ground leaves of willow taken with water,[55]
iron rust (*ferrum oxydatum*),[56] iron slag (less effective).[57] The root of barrenwort or bishop's hat, *Epimedium alpinum* L. or *Botrychium Lunaria*—the
plant has not with certainty been identified—causes sterility; when the
finely ground leaves of this plant are taken to the amount of five drachms in
wine after menstruation, they prevent conception for the duration of five

[49] Carolus, "Sur un manuscrit du Vme Siècle de Dioscoride," *Annales d'académie
d'archéologie de Belgique* [Anvers, xiii (1856), 295–299], xiii, 296–7.

[50] See ch. vi *infra*.

[51] H. Haeser, *Lehrbuch* (1875 ed.), i, 303.

[52] *De materia medica*, edition by J. Berendes (see Bibliography for full title). Bk. ii,
ch. 98, p. 191. All succeeding references are to the same edition. Stepping over the
menstrual blood is reminiscent of the practice of the Aiţ Sáddĕn in North Africa. See
p. 9.

[53] *Ibid.*, Bk. ii, ch. 151, p. 220. It is quite a matter of indifference whether Dioscorides
has reference to *Asparagus acutifolius* or *Asparagus officinalis*.

[54] *Ibid.*, Bk. iv, ch. 190 (193), p. 475.

[55] *Ibid.*, Bk. i, ch. 135, p. 121. It is not known whether Dioscorides here refers to white
or black willow; and it is quite a matter of indifference.

[56] *Ibid.*, Bk. v, ch. 93, p. 513. Applied in a pessary, it stops the menstrual flow.

[57] *Ibid.*, Bk. v, ch. 94, p. 514.

days.[58] The roots of the brake or fern are given to women to prevent conception; if taken by pregnant women they cause a miscarriage.[59] Two drachms of Ostracite [a kind of potters clay][60] drunk [for each of ?] four days after menstruation will prevent conception.[61] Sprengel thinks the stone a fossil, Berendes, cuttle-fish skin.

Medicated pessaries are reported by Dioscorides as follows: Pepper "appears to prevent conception if it is introduced as a pessary after coitus."[62] Note that the medication takes place after coitus. The juice of peppermint (?) [Gebauteminze] mixed with honey (in German, Honigmeth) prevents pregnancy as a suppository prior to coitus.[63] A sword-shaped sickle-wort (*Coronilla securidaca*) "mixed with honey as a pessary introduced before coitus appears to prevent conception."[64]

Approaching perhaps in effectiveness the use of honey in a vaginal pessary are the following: anointing the genitals with cedar-gum prior to coitus;[65] applying alum in various forms to the uterus prior to coitus.[66]

Dioscorides also makes vague allusions to certain substances causing sterility (as contrasted with methods preventing conception). It is not quite clear whether in these instances Dioscorides believes the materials to produce the effect physiologically, or whether he thinks they operate directly by preventing conception on mechanical or chemical principles. Perhaps the former is the proper implication. When he says, however, that "The bark of the white poplar [*Populus alba*] taken with the kidney of the mule causes sterility,"[67] he is probably reiterating a popular superstition. The superstition that poplar could produce sterility persisted into the Middle Ages; and may even be accepted in some portions of Europe today. Nor was Dioscorides alone in thinking that a portion of the anatomy of the mule would cause sterility. In another passage he says that "the rennet of the hare drunk for three days after menstruation should cause sterility."[68] He notes that the finely pulverized berries of ivy drunk after purification

[58] *Ibid.*, Bk. iv, ch. 19, p. 376.

[59] *Ibid.*, Bk. iv, ch. 184 (187), p. 472.

[60] See ch. vi, n. 41, p. 151.

[61] *Ibid.*, Bk. v, ch. 164 (165), p. 553.

[62] *Ibid.*, Bk. ii, ch. 188, p. 238.

[63] *Ibid.*, Bk. iii, ch. 36 (41), p. 287.

[64] *Ibid.*, Bk. iii, ch. 136 (146) p. 349.

[65] *Ibid.*, Bk. i, ch. 105, p. 99.

[66] *Ibid.*, Bk. v, ch. 122, (123) p. 533. The form of the alum recommended is not clear. Probably it was raw alum formed by the decomposition of a kind of lava to be found in volcanic regions; or else an alum schist as a crystalline deposit of alum-bearing water. Alum entered very considerably into the trade of antiquity.

[67] *Ibid.*, Bk. i, ch. 109, p. 101.

[68] *Ibid.*, Bk. ii, ch. 21, p. 159.

in the dose of one drachm causes sterility.[69]   In the same passage our author notes that the young rundles of ivy leaves spread with honey, and introduced into the uterus, provoke menstruation and evacuate the embryo. The leaves of spleenwort, picked on a moonless night, cooked in wine and drunk for four days appear to be able to cause sterility.[70]   If taken by themselves or bound up with the spleen of a mule [as an amulet?] they produce the same result.[71]   The roots of barrenwort cause sterility.[72] Though the upper roots of the gladiola (*Gladiolus segetum*, a variety of *Gladiolus communis*) applied with wine as a pessary increase sexual desire, the lower ones, used presumably in the same manner, cause sterility.[73]

To promote fertility Dioscorides recommended placing against the uterus after menstruation a pessary made of the rennet of the hare mixed with butter.   Likewise fawn rennet, introduced three days after menstruation, is mentioned.   Hare rennet, when swallowed, caused the death of the embryo; after menstruation, sterility.   He mentions the rennet of approximately ten different animals, not all of which have been certainly identified.

Whether rennet pessaries acted as a contraceptive or as a cure for sterility would depend on how they were used.   If continually used, they might act as a contraceptive.   If used only to clear up cervical inflammation—its thick muco-pus is the most frequent cause of sterility—they might well promote conception.   It is quite possible that rennet pessaries digest or dissolve the excessive cervical mucus.   Digestants are used today in caroid or pawpaw preparations to clear the cervix.   If such pessaries as those mentioned by Dioscorides and, previously herein, by Hippocratic writers, were solely controlled by the medical profession, their rôle was doubtless limited to the cure of sterility; if they became a part of oral tradition, it is perhaps a safe inference that some people applied them for long periods; hence they would have acted, in such instances, as contraceptives.

§6   SORANOS OF EPHESUS (II-1)

The most brilliant and original account of contraceptive technique written prior to the nineteenth century is undoubtedly that in the *Gynaecology* of Soranos of Ephesus (98–138).   He was not only the most illustrious member of the Methodist sect but the greatest gynaecologist of antiquity.   After studying at the school in Alexandria, Soranos went to Rome, where he practised medicine during the reigns of Trajan and Hadrian (91–117).

Though his book dates from the first half of the second century, the origi-

[69] *Ibid.*, Bk. ii, ch. 210, p. 255.
[70] *Ibid.*, Bk. iii, ch. 141 (151), p. 351.
[71] *Ibid.*
[72] *Ibid.*, Bk. iv, ch. 19, p. 376.   *Cf.*, reference above to the finely ground leaves.
[73] *Ibid.*, Bk. iv, ch. 20, p. 377.

nal text was lost for many centuries, in fact not published until 1838. Consequently Soranos's originality has been under-estimated; he was known to the Middle Ages largely through Moschion,[74] who received much of the credit due Soranos. His literary productivity was prodigious. According to Emerins, the Dutch savant, he was the author of no less than forty treatises. In one or another of these he wrote on nearly all the subjects then known to the healing art, though his main interest was in gynaecology, obstetrics, and pediatrics. In view of the encyclopedic nature of his efforts we are the more impressed with the rationality and originality of his discussion of contraception. Though Soranos's medical writings are noted for their rationality, nowhere does this emerge more clearly than in his discussion of contraceptive technique.

The full text reads as follows:

On the Use of Abortifacients and of Measures to Prevent Conception

§60. Atokion differs from phthorion in this, that the first designates a remedy which prevents conception, while the second, on the contrary, designates a remedy which kills the foetus. Some think of ekbolion as a synonym for phthorion; others however say that in contrast to phthorion, ekbolion does not designate a medicine but on the contrary a violent convulsion of the body, as for example in jumping. Thus Hippocrates in his[75] book ON THE NATURE OF THE CHILD has rejected abortifacients, and has advised a method to procure abortion by jumping so that the buttocks are touched with the feet. Opinion, however, on the use of abortifacients differs. Many reject them, referring to the words of Hippocrates, "I shall never prescribe a phthorion" and further declaring it to be the task of medical art to preserve and save the works of nature. Others permit the use of phthoria in exceptional cases, but never in cases where the killing of the foetus is desired as a consequence of adultery or as the consequence of the desire to maintain beauty; but, on the contrary, always when birth threatens to become dangerous, or when the uterus is too small so that delivery is impossible, or when rips and new formations have formed themselves in the mouth of the womb, or when any other hindrance to birth exists. To these views correspond also the opinions on the use of means for the prevention of conception. In agreement with these, we think it surer, to prevent conception than to kill the foetus.

§61. In cases where it is more advantageous to prevent conception [than to

---

[74] Quite possibly Moschion's popular treatise on *Gynaecology* (*Gynaecia*: *De mulieribus passionibus*) also discusses contraceptive technique for it was based on Soranos. Moschion was a Latin gynecologist living in North Africa in the sixth century. Until recently he was given greater credit for originality than Soranos, for the latter's work had become lost and forgotten. So much was this the case that in the fifteenth century Moschion's book was translated into Greek; later retranslated back into Latin. In fact the original text of Soranos was not published until 1838. Moschion's text should be searched for anti-conceptional techniques. If they exist, they are probably much like Soranos's. The only edition of Moschion (probably a poor one) readily available to me contained nothing on contraception.

[75] Actually it is pseudo-Hippocratic.

induce abortion], people should abstain from coitus at the times when we have indicated as especially dangerous, that is, the time directly before and after menstruation.[76] Further, the woman ought, in the moment during coitus when the man ejaculates his sperm, to hold her breath,[77] draw her body back a little so that the semen cannot penetrate into the os uteri, then immediately get up and sit down with bent knees, and, in this position, provoke sneezes.[78] She should then wipe out the vagina carefully or drink cold water in addition. Further, conception is prevented by smearing the mouth of the womb with old [sour] oil or honey or cedar gum or opobalsam, either alone or mixed with ceruse (white lead), or with ointment which is prepared with myrtle oil and ceruse, or with alum, which is likewise to be watered before coitus, or galbanum in wine. Soft wool introduced into the mouth of the womb, or the use of astringent or occlusive pessaries before coitus are also effective. For, if such means operate astringently and coolingly, they close the mouth of the womb before the moment of coitus and prevent the entrance of the sperm into the os uteri; if they have this stimulating effect, then they not only prevent the sperm from remaining in the os uteri, but they extract even another fluid from it.

§62. I mention still other means of that kind: Pine bark, rhus coriaria, both to equal parts: Pulverize it with wine, and use it shortly before coitus with the help of wool. Withdraw it after two or three hours, and then coitus may take place.

Another method: Cimolus soil [a chalky soil] and panaseroot to equal parts alone or mixed with water as an ointment. Application as before.

Or: Use pulp of fresh granate pulverized with water.

Or: Two parts of pomegranate rind, one part of gallnut; reduce by pulverization to small balls, and lay them just below the os uteri after the cessation of menstruation.

Or: Dissolved alum and the pulp of the granate pulverized with water. The application is carried out by means of wool.

Or: Unripe gallnut, pomegranate pith, ginger. Take of each two drachms, make into little balls of pea size, dry in the shade, and use as pessaries before coitus.

Or: Pulverize the pulp of dry figs with natron [native sodium carbonate] and use it in the same way.

Or: Pomegranate skins with gum and rose oil to equal parts.

The same effect is produced by drinking honey mixtures. All methods which cause burning must, however, be avoided, because they have a caustic effect. All the methods mentioned are to be used after the cessation of menstruation.

§63. Many also recommend the use once a month of a quantity of cyrenaic sap [juice ?] to the size of a chick pea, with two cyathi of water, for menstruation is promoted by it. Or also: Two obols of opopanax, of cyrenaic sap [juice ?] and the juice of rue formed into pills with wax and swallowed. Watered wine is then drunk after this, or this medicine is drunk in watered wine. Or drink for three days in wine a potion made of three obols of gilly flower seeds and of myrtle seeds, one drachm of myrrh and two kernels of white pepper. Or drink one obol of hedge-mustard seeds and one-half obol of sphondylium mixed with sour honey.

---

[76] Is this the beginning of confidence in the sterile-period superstition?

[77] This notion is still prevalent among the ignorant. Holding the breath, by tightening the levator muscle, increases abdominal and vaginal tension and may act to retard or prevent an orgasm; but it could hardly be very effective in preventing sperms from reaching the os.

[78] Sneezing has a tendency to expel semen.

These medicines not only prevent conception, but also destroy its product. According to our opinion the damage caused by them is, however, very considerable, for they cause indigestion, and vomiting; also they cause a heavy head. Many use amulets in a firm belief in their antipathetic effect. These amulets contain the womb of a mule or the ear-dirt of the same and such things. But the usefulness of this amulet is delusive.[79]

Note that Soranos distinguished between contraceptives and abortifacients; mentioned indications for abortion (dangerous births) as well as contra-indications. Abortion should not be resorted to in order to conceal the consequences of adultery, nor simply to maintain the chaste female form. He observed further that, wherever repeated abortions are indicated, efforts to prevent conception are advisable.

Though Soranos included ineffective potions, his main reliance was upon more rational techniques: an elaborate array of occlusive pessaries of various types, vaginal plugs, using wool as a base, and those impregnated with gummy substances such as sour oil, honey, cedar-gum, opobalsam, and galbanum.[80] Astringent solutions (e.g., alum[81] and natron) contract the os, and thus make impregnation less likely. The use of native fruit acids is not without interest. Pomegranate pulp or rind is acid, of course, while gallnut contains gallotanic acid. Fig pulp is also mentioned.

Theoretically any gum-like or oily substance will not only tend to occlude the os, but reduce the motility of spermatozoa. Moreover, any strongly alkaline or acid condition will likewise tend to provide a hostile environment for sperms.

Soranos thinks the "damage" done by drinking potions with the intention of preventing conception is "very considerable,"—a modern view. Consequently he warns against this. Notable also is his discouragement of the use of amulets, doubtless prevalent in his time, as they were during the Middle Ages. One finds cropping up in the latter period the superstition that the ear-wax of a mule, worn as an amulet, will prevent pregnancy. Haeser, in an undocumented statement, reports that Soranos also states somewhere that some of his contemporaries believed that eating the uterus

[79] The text used in this translation is that by H. Lüneburg, *Die Gynäkologie des Soranus von Ephesus* (München: Lehmann, 1894), bk. i, ch. xix, pp. 43–45.

[80] Galbanum is a yellow or brown gum resin of objectionable odor derived from an Asiatic plant. Besides its medicinal use, it is employed in our time in the manufacture of varnish, galbanum being a base.

[81] It is interesting to note that Charles Knowlton, the first American physician to publish a treatise on contraception in 1832 (see Bibliography), thought the use of alum as a contraceptive original with him; and he was very much incensed that he was not accorded due credit. Alum is rather commonly mentioned in the early literature. *Cf.*, Dioscorides, Aëtios, and the Islamic writers who mentioned it. See chapter vi *infra*.

of a she mule would prevent conception.   If so, this shows that some of the ancient Greeks accepted a primitive magical belief.   It suggests the fundamental continuity of a concept connected with reproduction.   Haeser likewise reports that Soranos mentions the following: "the water from the firebucket of the smith, when drunk continuously after every menstrual period, causes sterility."[82]   This prescription has come down through the centuries and is now, or has been until very lately, accepted by some peasants in remote sections of Europe—another illustration of cultural persistence even when the prescription, in all probability, is relatively useless.   Little is known of the physiological effect of such a potion; but it is supposed to contain iron sulphate.   As for the more rationally-founded prescriptions mentioned by Soranos, many of these, too, have come down to us: Douching with astringent solutions, and vaginal pessaries of more modern form being perhaps the most commonly persistent.   And as for the pseudo-Hippocratic *coitus interruptus*, that is by all odds still the most common method.

§7   ORIBASIOS (IV-2) AND ST. JEROME (HIERONYMOUS) (IV-2)

Though the fourth century was not a period of great scientific advance, medicine saw reasonable development.   It is interesting to note that the eminent Greek medical encyclopedist, Oribasios,[83] the greatest physician of the century, included in his vast compendium ('Ιατρικαὶ συναγωγαί) a short chapter (116) on contraception.   Oribasios's greatness lies not only in his vast medical encyclopedia, only one-third of which is now extant, but in his paving the way for Galen's popularity, whom he often quoted with commendation.   Noteworthy also is the fact that Oribasios courageously fought the rising superstitions of his day.

[82] H. Haeser, *Lehrbuch* (1875 ed.), i, 309.   On the same page Haeser gives us a summary of Soranos's abortifacients.

[83] Born at Pergamus about 325, Oribasios studied medicine under Zenon of Chypre, becoming learned not only in the technique, but in the history of his art.   This latter knowledge is well revealed in his *Medical Collection*, written at the request of Julius Caesar, his intimate friend and patron.   Oribasios accompanied Caesar on many of his expeditions, and was at his side when he perished in combat with the Persians in 363.   Exiled by the Christian Emperors as a retaliation against his religious activities, Oribasios developed such an enviable reputation professionally that he was recalled about 367, married a woman of high station and some wealth, by whom he had four children; and devoted the remainder of his life to medical practice and literary activity.

The *Medical Collection* may perhaps be best described as an encyclopedia.   His *Synopsis*, an elementary treatise on hygiene and therapeutics, draws largely on Galen.   The *Euphorists* is a lay manual.   Oribasios's works, especially the *Synopsis* and *Euphorists* enjoyed a great vogue during the Middle Ages, possibly owing to their brevity.   Manuscripts of translations abound.

We translate literally, chapter 116 of the *Medical Collection* dealing with anti-conception:

In order to prevent conception, drink male or female fern root in sweet tasting wine, blossoms and leaves of the willow, and cabbage blossoms in wine, after coitus; but when one wants to prevent conception before copulation one anoints the virile part of the man with "hédysome" [Fr.] juice. The application in a pessary after coitus of ground-up cabbage blossoms prevents the semen from congealing; before coitus, one injects a decoction of coronilla seed into the vagina.[84]

Unlike Oribasios, St. Jerome (Hieronymous), the Latin Church Father, and Christian contemporary of Oribasios, strongly condemned potion-drinking to induce sterility approximately nine centuries before Thomas Aquinas. Methods intended to be preventive of impregnation are condemned in the same breath with deliberate abortion, a confusion still cleverly promoted by the sophistry of many Catholic leaders.

In a letter dating from 384 addressed to an aristocratic girl, Eustochium, St. Hieronymous complains to the Holy One about the free and immoral life of many girls and widows, and notes that some women—what proportion we have no means of knowing—drink before coitus a potion in order to remain sterile. Presumably the practice had some currency or he would not have condemned it. We are not told what the decoction is. The translated passage runs as follows:

Others, however, drink before [coitus] a potion in order to remain sterile, and go on even to practice abortion. Many, when they become aware of the results of their immorality, mediate on how they may deliver themselves by means of poisonous expedients, and, often dying themselves for that reason, go to hell as threefold murderesses: as suicides, as adulteresses to their heavenly bridegroom Christ, and as murderesses of their still unborn child.[85]

Other potions and means than those mentioned above were evidently also resorted to by Roman women for the prevention of conception, for Aigremont avows, though upon what authority is not clear, that Roman women drank during menstruation myrtle tea not only for its evacuating effect, but "as a means against conception."[86] And Juvenal reports[87] that Roman women were accustomed to have intercourse with eunuchs in order that they might enjoy themselves without becoming pregnant. It is

[84] Bussemaker and Daremberg, *Oeuvres d'Oribase* (Paris, 1851–1876), v, 777–8. See Bibliography for full title.

[85] *De custodia virginitatis* in P. Leipelts, *Bibl. der Kirchenväter*, liv, 211 f. Cited by Rudolf Huber, "Tränklein gegen Empfängnis in altem Rom," *Archiv f. Kriminal-Anthropologie u. Kriminalistik*, lviii (1914), 161.

[86] Aigremont, *Volkserotik und Pflanzenwelt* (2nd ed.), i, 109. No source is cited.

[87] Juvenal, vi, 367, commencing *Sunt quas eunuchi imbelles . . . tantum rapit Heliodorus.*

possible, too, that goat bladders were used in ancient Rome for preventing conception.[88]

§8 AËTIOS OF AMIDA (VI-1)

Almost as brilliant as Soranos's account is that of Aëtios, Greek physician of the sixth century (first half). Born in Amida, Mesopotamia, Aëtios flourished under Justinian I, Emperor of the East, 527–565. He was a physician at the Byzantine Court, and is known chiefly as the author of a medical encyclopedia, *On Medicine in Sixteen Books or Discourses* (βιβλία ιατρικα εκκαιδεκα), an eclectic compilation of great historical value, inasmuch as it quotes many medical works of antiquity. Book XVI contains two chapters (XVI and XVII) on contraceptive technique, the full text[89] of which reads as follows. The indebtedness to Soranos is striking.

Chapter XVI

Diseases of the Womb

Certain women, when they have become pregnant, run a danger during parturition. Either on account of a small uterine neck, or on account of a small uterus, they are not able to function up to the end, either on account of a condyloma or something similar in the neck of the uterus, which is an obstacle to delivery. For these women it is preferable that they should not become pregnant.

On Contraceptives and Abortifacients

Contraception differs from abortion. The first prevents conception, the second destroys the product of conception and drives it out of the uterus. In order to avoid conception it is necessary to abstain from coitus during the days favorable to conception, for example, at the beginning or end of menstruation. During coitus, when the man is about to ejaculate, the woman ought to hold her breath and withdraw a little in order that the sperm might not penetrate the uterine cavity; she ought to get up immediately and squat down on her haunches, provoke a sneeze, and carefully clean the vagina.

Smearing the cervix before coitus with honey or opobalsam or cedar rosin alone or in combination with lead or liquid ointment with myrtle and lead or liquid alum or galbanum with wine aids contraception. These medicaments, when they are astringent, unctuous and refrigerant, close the orifice of the womb before coitus and prevent the sperm of the man from entering the uterus. When they are cold they irritate; and they not only prevent the sperm of the man from remaining in the uterine cavity but they draw a liquid from the uterus. All these medicaments belong to the anti-conceptional class.

[88] For an account of the use in ancient Rome of the goat bladder to prevent conception, see ch. viii, § 2a *infra*.

[89] This is the edition used: Aëtios, *Des Affections de la Matrice, ou Discours seizième*. Édition Skevos Zervos, Leipzig, 1901. Since this text was not available in the U. S. A., I am grateful to Dr. M. Moïssidès of Athens, able student of Malthusianism in antiquity, for copying for me the French text. There is no edition of the entire Greek text of Aëtios. There are only partial texts.

Chapter XVII

Anti-Conceptional Pessaries

Pine bark, *rhus cotinus* in equal quantities: triturate with wine and make a pessary of wool. Place it [before the os] prior to coitus, withdraw it after two hours, and then have coitus.

Or else: The inside of young pomegranates: mix with water and prepare pessaries to introduce into the vagina.

Or else: Pomegranates, 2 parts, gallnut, 1 part: triturate and make into small suppositories. Introduce into the vagina after the end of menstruation.

Or else: 3 drachms gallnut, 2 drachms myrrh: prepare some pessaries with wine of the size of peas. Dry in the shade and introduce into the vagina before coitus.

Or else: Make pessaries with the pulp of dried figs and mix with niter and put into the vagina.

Or else: 2 drachms pomegranate, 2 drachms gallnut, 1 drachm absinth: after having pulverized these, mix with cedar rosin, and prepare barley-sized pessaries, and put on the cervix for two days immediately after the end of menstruation. The woman ought to remain quite tranquil for a day, and then have sexual congress, not before. This contraceptive is infallible.

Anti-conceptional potion: Cyrenaic sap, of the size of a pea in two glasses of winy water: to be drunk once a month. This also causes onset of menstruation.

Or else: Cyrenaic sap, opopanax, rue leaves to equal parts: triturate, mix with some sap. Take an amount the size of a bean and drink with winy water. This potion is also an emmenagogue.

Or else: 1 drachm aloes, 3 obols of stock seed, 3 drachms ginger, 2 grains of pepper, and saffron: give it to the woman to drink with wine in three doses immediately after the end of menstruation. Copper water in which one extinguishes [hot] iron, drunk continually, and above all immediately after the end of menstruation, is anti-conceptional. One drachm of root of poplar, with a seventh of a small glass of water; give it to the woman to drink once a month during menstruation.

Anti-conceptional: Wear cat liver in a tube on the left foot, or wear the testicles of a cat in a tube around the umbilicus.

Or else: Wear part of the womb of a lioness in a tube of ivory. This is very effective. Or lead with oil in a pessary; put in the vagina before coitus or sooner. Pomegranate and gallnut and 2 drachms sour fruit juice [usually grape ?], 1 drachm absinth: mix with cedar rosin and prepare pessaries of the size of barley, and put into the vagina for two days after menstruation.

Another contraceptive: As long as a woman desires to remain sterile, she ought to drink during this time a quantity of black ivy berries in winy water after menstruation; or the seeds of henbane gathered from the plant before they have fallen to the ground. Mix with the milk of a she ass, a little myrtle and a berry of black ivy or some corymb: to be worn after having been wrapped in the skin of the hare or the mule or the stag. The amulet ought not to touch the ground at all. Or give the woman cold copper water[90] to drink on an empty stomach after menstruation.

Or else: Give the woman a decoction of willow bark with honey to temper its bitterness. To be drunk continually.

Or else: The woman should carry as an amulet around the anus the tooth of a child or a glass from a marble quarry.

---

[90] Is this the Hippocratic "misy?"

Another experiment: Wrap in stag skin the seed of henbane diluted in the milk of a mare nourishing a mule. Carry that as an amulet on the left arm, and take care that it does not fall to the ground. And give the woman the seed of artemisia to drink. [These] prevent conception for a year.

Or else: The man ought to smear his penis with astringents, as for example, with alum or pomegranate or gallnut triturated with vinegar; or wash the genital organs with brine, and he will not impregnate. The burned testicles of castrated mules drunk with a decoction of willow constitute contraceptives for men.

Aëtios is here following Soranos especially in discussing the more reasonable remedies. Significantly enough Aëtios added amulets in which Soranos avowedly had no faith whatever. The more we learn of the history of contraceptive techniques from antiquity down the more brilliant does Soranos's genius tower above that of his contemporaries and most of his successors. Note that Aëtios mentions washing the male genitals with vinegar or brine. This is a very early mention of these substances, the first I can recall. So far as our limited knowledge at present goes, vinegar was not again mentioned in the literature until Charles Knowlton (1832). He seems to have been first in suggesting douching with vinegar solutions, a technique more effective than Aëtios's method of applying it to the phallus.

Both brine and vinegar are highly spermicidal. Acetic acid immobilizes human sperms in 10–15 seconds at a 1 to 2,000 solution. Ordinary vinegar ranges about 4–5 per cent acetic, wine vinegar running to 6 per cent. Two tablespoonfuls of vinegar to a quart of water is stronger than 1 to 1,000. Vinegar is one of the most effective of "modern" douching spermicides. How much more effective Aëtios's prescription would have been had diluted vinegar been applied to the vagina instead of to the penis! But douching, so far as one can now judge, was completely unknown to the ancients. Similarly, contraceptive jellies, properly defined, are also ultra-modern.

§9 RESTRICTED DIFFUSION OF CONTRACEPTIVE KNOWLEDGE IN ANTIQUITY

To what extent were anti-conceptional measures employed in ancient Greece and Rome? Our tentative answer is: probably to some extent but hardly extensively. The question is not capable of definitive answer in the present state of our knowledge. It is likely that we shall never know. Antique accounts are lacking. Nor should we make the mistake of inferring too much from the lamentations regarding depopulation with which the pages of history are strewn.

For it remains to be shown that when the populations in certain areas declined, it was due to widespread use of anti-conceptional measures and not to a low marriage rate, increased abortions, infanticide, frequent divorce, etc. These circumstances are overlooked by those who allude to the fall of Rome when discussing the awful future of any country that allows birth-control knowledge to become diffused.

There are at least a score of theories why Rome fell. One is that there was a dearth of native soldiers; that consequently it was necessary to hire mercenaries. The implication is that soldiers were lacking because the birth rate was low. And why was the birth rate low? Because birth control was used. This reasoning is fallacious and contrary to fact; fallacious because the conclusion does not logically follow; false, or contrary to fact, because birth-control knowledge was never sufficiently diffused materially to alter the picture.

Birth control had little or nothing to do with the decline of Roman hegemony. The view of most economic historians is more acceptable. In a word, Rome declined because its economic life was parasitic; it did not earn what it consumed; it stamped the iron heel of militarism on the necks of other producing groups and extracted from them by military force all it could. When the springs that fed it dried up, Roman imperialism withered. The "bread and circus" regime at home also promoted decay. Whether this brief account is accepted or not, we should remember that no one has ever demonstrated that effective contraceptive knowledge was sufficiently diffused in either Greece or Rome to cause population to decrease. Hence the decline could not have been due to a situation which never existed.

The lamentations of depopulators mean nothing for another reason. I have never met in all history with a depopulationist (by which I mean a bewailer of declining population) nor with a population booster (one who is never satisfied with the present rate of increase) who ever understood the economic and sociological theory of demographic movements. Never do such writers really understand the phenomena they mouth about. Never do they see demographic phenomena as adjustment or equilibrium phenomena. In a word, this is because the depopulators or optimists start with preconceived notions about what the people, under the circumstances of the time, *ought* to do. The masses know more about these matters than do statesmen, physicians and pamphleteers. The reason is briefly that it is the masses and not the advisers, who feel the pressures set up by economic and social situations. It is a fact of history that population has consistently grown since the first colonies or settlements along the Mediterranean, a fact which suggests that the bewailers have, up to this time at least, wasted their efforts.

One is quite safe in predicting that once effective contraceptive knowledge is diffused, no longer will we see whole nations spawning irresponsibly. The reason it has happened in the past is that contraceptive ignorance has been general, whatever the writers of medical encyclopedias may have known.

The general subject of the decline of civilizations is too big to be entered upon in this place. But it may be suggested that a cycle of cultural rise, flowering and senescence is normal, usual. And so long as that which is valuable is preserved, what difference does it make? The abnormal view is precisely the assumption that a given cultural configuration should always remain intact. History proves the subjectivity and falsity of such an assumption. Cultural syntheses are constantly dissolving, disintegrating, re-integrating. What most historians and would-be historians call decline is simply the creation of new cultural complexes. And the reasons why new ones form are as numerous as philosophies of history. This being so it is time to stop talking nonsense about cultures declining and becoming decadent because of birth control. This is not to say that such an event cannot occur; it is only to say that proof of its occurrence in the past has never been made.

§10 SUMMARY

It is not suggested that the texts presented in this chapter are the only ones of the period available. They are not. But it is probably a safe guess that they are representative. An effort has been made to study contraceptive medicine as taught by those leaders of thought who influenced others.

It is clear from the above that Greek and Roman writers, more especially two Greek physicians, Soranos and Aëtios, carried rational contraceptive medicine to a much higher degree of development than any of their predecessors.

Moreover, those Greek physicians who treated the subject were among the greatest physicians of all time, men who have a permanent place in the history of medicine for other reasons. Many people nowadays frown upon a physician who supports contraception as a "radical;" whereas the simple fact is that the awakening interest in contraception on the part of contemporary doctors is merely a return to the classical attitude. In antiquity anti-conceptional technique had a definite place in preventive medicine.

The early texts published in this chapter gave much less space to indications than to technique. This is invariably the case until late modern times, and indeed may even be true of our day. As early as the fifth century B.C. we find Aristotle mentioning smearing the cervix with cedar oil, or lead with olive oil. The pseudo-Hippocratic writings are of small importance in the history of contraceptive medicine. There we find only potions (of "misy") and the time-honored *coitus interruptus*. Lucretius (first century B.C.), a poet rather than a physician, has likewise little to add that is specific. None the less, his analysis of certain factors promoting and restraining fertility anticipate a certain modern school of thought which holds that certain positions in coitus sometimes check or encourage conception. Though Pliny the Elder (first century A.D.) mentions in his diffuse *Natural History* a great array of botanical plants used for potions; and though charms and amulets in considerable number likewise find a central place, Pliny's treatment of contraceptive medicine is indeed shabby. Only when he essays to modify Aristotle's advice does he furnish a rational contraceptive technique. Pliny feigned modesty, diffidence. He affected to think the subject a little obscene; and made no contribution to our knowledge.

Dioscorides, contemporary of Pliny, who had great influence for centuries upon medicine, discussed magical prescriptions (amulets), potions, medicated pessaries, and anointing the genitals with sticky substances. He mentions about a score of "prescriptions" only three being medicated pessaries, two quasi-rational preventives in the form of sticky substances smeared on the genitals. There are three charms, six potions, and seven "sterilizing" drugs. The emphasis throughout is on materia medica. In view of the large irrational element, Dioscorides's place in contraceptive medicine is a modest one.

With Soranos, the case is otherwise: his treatment of contraceptive technique is the most brilliant until very late in modern times. True, his discussion is tinged with ineffective recommendations; there is mention of holding the breath—a notion which has persisted to our day; but attention is focussed on medicated suppositories of many varieties using wool as a base and oily substances as the medication. Old oil, honey, cedar gum, opobalsam, myrtle oil, and alum are mentioned. Probably thirty or forty different combinations are suggested. Astringents and fruit acids have a prominent place. We are cautioned against the use of burning substances. The use of amulets is "delusive;" the damage of potions is considerable. Wherever repeated abortions are necessary prevention is indicated.

Oribasios, greatest medical encyclopedist of the fourth century, was another supporter of contraception, but his *Medical Collection* contains only a brief passage and that not very distinguished. Besides three potions (willow, fernroot, cabbage blossoms), anointing the penis with *Hedysarum* juice is advised, as well as cabbage-blossom and coronilla-seed pessaries (i.e., suppositories). Manifestly this is a great step backward after the account by Soranos. There seems to have been a decline between the second and sixth centuries, that is, between Soranos and Aëtios. The passage from St. Jerome, the Church Father, is of interest chiefly in showing by its protest that potion-drinking in an effort to prevent conception was actually in practice by the people. Of its real extent we know little, for the lamentations of the contemporary depopulators need discounting.

Though Aëtios holds an important place in Greek contraceptive medicine, it is a rank definitely below that of Soranos, from whom he copied a great deal. Yet one must admit that it takes a certain level of intelligence to choose wisely models for copying. Was it merely an accident that Aëtios chose so good an one? Despite his able model, Aëtios's treatment lacks the originality and rationality of Soranos's account. That he possessed much less scientific caution than Soranos is shown by his recommendation of the use of the womb of an animal as an amulet. Aëtios thought this "very effective," though Soranos had specifically rejected it about four centuries before. It is probably true to say, however, that amulets and potions are subordinated to substances for anointing the male genitals and a wide array of medicated pessaries. Notable is the use of vinegar and brine.

It is much to be doubted whether the goat-bladder sheath, for male or female use, was ever used in Imperial Rome to any extent. Quite probably the mention of it is a mere historical curiosity (see Chapter VIII on the Condom).

The question was next discussed whether there was sufficient diffusion of contraceptive knowledge among the populace of antiquity to explain causally declining populations at various periods; further, whether it was the cause of the "fall" of Rome. It was suggested that the answer to both questions was in the negative. The disintegration and re-integration of new cultural syntheses on a large scale (e.g., "nations") cannot be explained by an analysis so naïve, narrow and simple.

Some use of contraceptives was doubtless made by the Greeks and Romans; but it was on a scale in no way comparable to modern usage. That had to await a democratizing revolution, such changes as industrialization, the loosening of old religious bonds, urbanization, the Industrial and Agricultural Revolutions, the rise of preventive medicine, and their consequent effect on the growth of population, the vulcanization of rubber (and hence the cheap manufacture of condoms, cervical caps and vaginal diaphragms of the Mensinga type)—all changes of a fundamental nature but not operative in the antique world.

The scanty evidence available suggests that the contraceptive knowledge of antiquity was confined largely to the heads of medical encyclopedists, to a few physicians and scholars. The average citizen was probably quite ignorant of the subject—even, indeed, as he is today. Ten to fifteen centuries had still to elapse before the invention of movable type caused a technological revolution in printing, in the published communication of ideas; still several more centuries before printing was really cheapened. The manuscripts of antiquity were, of course, laboriously copied at considerable expense.   In a word, all the social circumstances of the time conspired to prevent the communication of contraceptive knowledge as we understand communication and democratization in our time.   But this in no wise dims the torch of knowledge that a few gifted, independent minds of antiquity handed down to the modern world through Islam.   That heritage is indeed a noble one.   Before we consider the development of contraceptive medicine in Islam, it will be convenient to explore another taproot that has nourished the whole tree.   I refer to the great Eastern cultures—China, India, and Japan—commonly supposed never to have given thought to this subject, owing to the nature of Oriental religion and other forces.   But as in the instance of the early West, we shall find that in the East, even when knowledge of effective remedies was lacking, the *desire* to prevent conception was a characteristic feature of the civilizations.

PART THREE

CONTRACEPTIVE TECHNIQUE
IN EASTERN CULTURES

CHAPTER V

CHINA, INDIA, AND JAPAN

THE history of contraception in the three great Oriental civilizations—China, India, and Japan—will be treated as a unit since, from a Western point of view, they have been subject to somewhat similar cultural influences. Specific conditions of mental outlook, of social organization, of cultural tradition combine to present a special cultural configuration. This has, in turn, profoundly affected the development of contraceptive medicine. This is not to suggest that conditions have been identical in the three countries; they are at best only similar.

§1 CHINA

(1a) Influence of the Social Organization and Mores of the Chinese on the Development of Contraceptive Medicine

Perhaps the chief reason that evidence on the early anti-conceptional techniques employed in China, India and Japan are difficult to secure lies in the circumstance that they were, on the whole, little resorted to in Oriental cultures owing to the dominance, especially in China, of the doctrine of filial piety and the presence of family communism. Let us examine briefly the social significance of these factors.

Filial piety has been so entrenched in China and Japan that large families, to provide ancestor worshippers and to serve as the ancient equivalent of old age insurance, have generally been preferred to small ones. Accordingly, the Orient is the classic instance of proliferation and its results—mass poverty and misery. Ever since Confucius said, "There are three things which are unfilial, but the most unfilial of these is to have no sons," the Chinese people have had more than adequate reproduction. In fact, as is generally known, the rate of reproduction is so high, the arts of production so retarded (as compared with Western standards), and preventive medicine so ill-developed that a high death rate has generally prevailed. The mortality-inducing dangers being great, the birth rate tended to be high. Since labor is cheap and capital scarce, it is next to impossible to introduce an essential ameliorative agent, machinery. Over-supplied coolies working as stevedores to unload boats, for example, get such low wages that in some instances it does not pay to introduce hoisting machinery and motor trucks.

It is cheaper to hire coolies than to import an American motor truck, make the initial outlay for the investment, pay the interest on it, and take care of the minimum operating and repair charges.   Thus we have the vicious circle: People are too poor to get out of poverty.

Such is the drama of excessive reproduction in China.   Recently, a beginning has been made in breaking the vicious circle; for mechanization and capital accumulation are proceeding, albeit slowly.   In the meantime, there will be much suffering during the readjustment period.

Even the distant industrial future is not bright for China.[1]   It lacks the necessary mineral resources.   Its coal supplies have been greatly exaggerated until recently; and the supply of high grade iron ore is not great.   It might be rather inconvenient for China to be obliged to import great quantities of iron and steel, one of the essential bases of modern industrialization. For these reasons there are definite limits, though they will not operate for several decades probably, to the extent to which China can relieve her population pressure by industrialization.   Japan has somewhat similar limitations though she is already in a more advanced stage and has, in addition, seized Manchukuo.   Of such stuff is the struggle for national survival made.

The other great cause of a high birth rate in China—to a lesser extent in Japan—has been the communistic form of family organization.   Wherever those who produce offspring are not responsible for the support of them, but gain their sustenance from a "family" which includes not only the parents themselves but all their blood relatives, friends and business associates, few checks on spawning can operate.   This system of familism has been perhaps the chief force in retarding the growth of capitalism in China, and though capitalism has never succeeded in eliminating poverty completely—it can hardly be expected to do so since there will always be people to squander or unwisely invest even an adequate income—it has done more to raise the standard of living than any other single institutional change in man's history.   Now a Chinese who, by superior intelligence, ability, or wise expenditure, grows prosperous, is likely to be called upon to support not only his own offspring but those of his impecunious relatives, friends, and even business (i.e., occupational) associates.   Thus the prosperous man can save but little; if he still has wealth, he is quite likely to hide the fact from those likely to make familial claims upon him.   Thus is the accumulation of capital, a prerequisite to industrial and agricultural development retarded.   The market for inventions is likewise restricted.   To be sure, other factors such as unstable government and insecurity of investment

<hr/>

[1] George B. Cressey, *China's Geographic Foundations.   A Survey of the Land and its People.*   New York & London: McGraw-Hill, 1934, pp. xvii, 436.

have slowed up the adoption of more efficient methods of production; but family communism has been no small factor. Thus does poverty, the scratch line from which the human race starts, persist. Poverty is associated with a high death rate and a high birth rate. Many factors play their parts in these correlations; but it would seem that in the instance of China and Japan, and to a considerable extent in the case also of India, family communism has slowed up the evolution away from poverty by increasing the number of consumers without due consideration for the other end of the equation: productivity.

Doubtless there is much of value for Western society in Chinese family solidarity, but this should not blind us to the awful consequences it has, in other respects, visited upon the Chinese people. Many great thinkers from Aristotle to James Mill, John Stuart Mill and Malthus have repeatedly warned that where there is little responsibility for bringing children into the world, there must necessarily, unless it is counteracted by other forces, be mass poverty. This is true regardless of the form of social organization prevalent. China, Japan and India have yet to learn and act upon this principle. So, too, have those who see no defects in Oriental family solidarity.

Other essential factors associated with high reproductive rates in the Orient are: the low status of women, early marriage, the ease of elimination (abortion and infanticide), a lack of mass education, especially higher education for females, the low standard of living and the tendency to be contented with the satisfaction of the simpler economic wants (e.g., Hindu doctrine of "desirelessness"). Caste barriers and the uncritical worship of custom and tradition have also played some part. The operation of these forces and their results in the Orient have been graphically pictured by Professor E. A. Ross with a thoroughness of sound economic reasoning, and with a finish of literary presentation not surpassed in the whole range of sociological literature on population.[2]

(1b) Scarcity of Sources

Since contraceptive practices have played a minor rôle in the life of the Chinese and Japanese, compared with Western peoples, it has been difficult to secure evidence on them. Dr. George H. Danton of Union College assures me that "the ancient Chinese classics would, as a matter of principle,

[2] Edward A. Ross, *Standing Room Only?* New York: Century, 1927, pp. xiv, 3–368. Despite the somewhat sensational title of this book and the fact that its general point of view—the danger of overpopulation in the Western world—is already out of date, its reasoning is, on the major points, sound. Sociologists have probably underestimated its importance.

contain no information on, or discussion of, contraceptive methods, since the first principle of the Chinese social system was, according to Mencius, that the greatest of sins was to have no son."[3]

If the canonical works contain any medical or social observations on this subject, they are yet to be discovered. Two of the world's great sinologists, Dr. Paul Pelliot of Paris and Dr. Berthold Laufer of the Field Museum, Chicago, were unable to direct the writer to likely sources.

Dr. Laufer personally searched several books on Chinese medicine, but could find no mention of contraceptives.[4] He stated further that he had "never heard or read of contraceptive practices among the Chinese."[5] Unwilling to accept this negative evidence as final proof that the ancient Chinese medical writers had given no thought to the subject, I enlisted the coöperation of Dr. Arthur W. Hummel, Chief of the Division of Chinese Literature, Library of Congress. He put me in touch with Mr. Michael J. Hagerty of the U. S. Dept. of Agriculture now stationed at the University of California. Mr. Hagerty has searched some of the old Chinese medical texts in the original, and through his diligence and courtesy it is now possible to offer some tentative information on the subject.

(1c) *Examples of Early Contraceptive Texts*

In the ancient Chinese texts it is sometimes difficult to distinguish contraceptives from abortifacients; and at the risk of introducing some irrelevant passages, those on abortion will be added, inasmuch as these have not been treated even by the specialists on the history of Chinese medicine,[6] much less by the historians of Chinese social customs.[7]

[3] Letter to the author dated December 13, 1930.

[4] This is not strange in view of the fact that histories of medicine in the English language commonly made no mention of the subject. It is as if this practice, of no inconsiderable medical interest and importance, were non-existent! Garrison, however, devotes a few superficial and inaccurate lines to the situation in the U. S. A., but mention is much more frequent in German works.

[5] Letter to the author dated December 13, 1930.

[6] See, for example, Franz Huebotter, "Die Chinesische Medizin zu Beginn des xx Jahrhunderts und ihr historischer Entwicklungsgang." *China Bibliothek der Asia Major.* Bd. I, 1929. Leipzig.

[7] Note the absence of data in, for instance, Léon Wieger, *Moral Tenets and Customs in China* (trans. by L. Davrout, S. J.). Ho-Kien-fu: Catholic Mission Press, 1913; and even in Marcel Granet, *Chinese Civilization* (as trans. by Chavannes). London: Kegan Paul, 1930, pp. 435. Granet touches upon the subject, but hardly in an illuminating manner. He says (p. 147), referring to the *Historical Annals of Sse-ma Ch'ien* (Bk. ii, 188, note 1) that an early Chinese potentate, Kou-chien, "adopted a policy of birth control little in conformity with healthy conditions." The rest he leaves to one's imagination. It may be that Granet uses the term without care. The word is commonly misused to cover conditions other than the control of conception.

The earliest mention of contraceptive recipes we have found in Chinese medical texts appears in the form of prescriptions quoted from the *Ch'ien chin fang* 千金方 "Thousand of Gold Prescriptions" by Sun Ssu-mo 孫思邈 who died A.D. 695. However, it is clear from the quotation referring originally to the text of the *Shên Nung pên ts'ao ching* 神農本草經, that the Chinese were practicing abortion in the pre-Christian era. This latter may be one of the oldest abortifacient prescriptions in existence, excepting, of course, those found among preliterate peoples. The *Shên Nung pên ts'ao ching* is the most ancient medical work in the Chinese language, and is supposed to have been written by the Emperor Shên Nung, who, according to Chinese chronology, reigned in 2737–2696 B.C.

To return to the contraceptive recipes. In a work entitled *Fu jên liang fang ta ch'üan*[8] 婦人良方大全 "Complete Collection of Valuable Prescriptions for Women," in 24 books, the following interesting formulae are found under the heading, *Tuan ch'an fang lun* 斷產方論 "Contraceptive Prescriptions":

[Ch'ên Tzu-ming's text, Bk. 13:7] "The *I ching* 易經 or Book of Changes, one of the Chinese canonical works, states: 'The great virtue of heaven and earth is called *shêng* 生 "produce." But married women have difficulties at the time of childbirth. Some bear offspring unceasingly but desire to stop this, therefore prescriptions are written so that they may be prepared for use. If one takes a dose of substance such as *shui yin* 水銀 or quicksilver, *mêng ch'ung* 蝱蟲 or gadfly [*Tabanus trigonus*, Coq.] and *shui chih* 水蛭 or medicinal leeches [*Hirudo nipponica*, Whitman], not only will pregnancy not again occur but disaster will ensue as quickly as the turning of the hand.'"

[Comment on the preceding by Hsieh Chi]: "Take a square foot or more sheet of paper on which silkworm eggs have been hatched, burn to an ash and pulverize. After childbirth mix this in liquor and take. Those with impoverished blood will not again become pregnant for the rest of their lives. As a rule, in contraceptive prescriptions, many use dangerous and violent ones, so that we constantly have cases wherein they do not recover. Really then the injury from childbirth is not as great as the injury from preventing childbirth. I have heard that the wives of Chang Lo-fêng 張羅峯 the Grand Secretary and Li Hêng-chai 李恆齋 the Director of the Court of Sacrificial Worship both took contraceptive prescriptions.

[8] This work was written by Ch'ên Tzu-ming 陳子明, and was first published in 1237. The text we are quoting is that which has been edited and incorporated into the collection of medical works entitled *Hsieh shih i an* 薛氏醫案, some of which were written by Hsieh Chi 薛巳, *tzu* Li-chai 立齋, who flourished about 1506–21, while others he merely commented upon.

They personally explained that they were weak in physique and vitality and that excessive exertion was certain to bring on illness.   There are cases such as these."

This statement on indications and the one contained in the second sentence of the paragraph above are undoubtedly among the earliest medical indications for contraception so far discovered in the ancient Chinese sources.   Credit for the discovery belongs to Mr. Hagerty, whose finds are all the more noteworthy in view of the negative reports of the most distinguished sinologists.   It may be remarked that indications for contraception appear much less frequently in the early literature than prescriptions.   *Cf.*, however, the evidence reported by Hrdlička and Olbrechts on American Indians, and the evidence on indications reported in the Talmud, the last to be found in Chapter III.

Next Ch'ên Tzu-ming quotes the following three prescriptions from the *Ch'ien chin fang* by Sun Ssu-mo, who, as we have stated, died A.D. 695: (1) *Ch'ien chin tuan fang* 千金斷方 "Thousand of Gold Contraceptive Prescription."   Take some oil and quicksilver and fry a whole day without stopping.   Take one pill as large as a jujube seed on an empty stomach and it will forever prevent one from becoming pregnant.   Furthermore, it will not injure the person.   (2) *Ch'ien chin ch'ü t'ai* 千金去胎, "Thousand of Gold Prescription for Abortion."   Take five pints of *ta ch'ü* 大麴 [barley leaven],[9] one *tou* 斗 [Chinese peck measure] of clear liquor, bring to a boil twice and strain off to remove the sediment.   Divide the liquid into five doses.   Do not take any food during the night and in the morning repeatedly take.   The foetus will become like rice gruel and the mother will be without any suffering.   One should not part with this prescription for a thousand of gold.   (3) *Yu fang* 又方 "Another Prescription."   Take the *Ssu wu t'ang* 四物湯 "Four ingredients broth."[10]   Each dose is five mace.

[9] Barley or wheat leaven is made as follows: Take some un-hulled grain, wash clean, sun-dry, grind into grits, mix with water which was used in scouring the grain, knead into a lump, wrap it in leaves of the paper-mulberry tree, hang it up in a place exposed to the wind for seven to ten days and then it may be used.   See *Cyclopedia of Chinese Medicine*, p. 317.

[10] Formula:

Shu ti huang 熟地黃 or cooked *Rehmannia glutinosa*.   (If the blood is hot substitute raw *Rehmannia glutinosa*).   3 mace.

Tang kuei shên 當歸身 or *Angelica polymorpha*, var. *sinensis* root.   (If the bowel movements are not firm fry it with earth).   3 mace.

Pai shao yao 白芍藥 or white *Paeonia albiflora* root.   (If there is dysentery and bowel trouble fry with *Cassia* liquor; if the patient has hemorrhage fry with vinegar).   2 mace.

Ch'üan hsiung 川芎 or *Conioselinum univittatum* from Szechwan.   (If the blood is poor soak in the urine of a child).   1½ mace.

These ingredients are ground into a coarse powder and boiled in pure water.   At bed

Add two pinches of *yün t'ai tzu* 蕓薹子 or rape [*Brassica rapa*] seeds. After menstruation take warm on an empty stomach.

Some additional formulae are given in the *Chi yin kang mu* 濟陰綱目 or *Treatise on Gynecology and Obstetrics*,[11] under the heading, *Fu tuan tzu fa* 附斷子法 or Supplement on Methods of Contraception, from which we have extracted the following:

Formula No. 1

Take 1 *shêng* 升 [Chinese pint] of a leaven called *mien ch'ü*[12] 麵麴 and 5 pints of liquor without dregs. Knead this into a paste and boil until there are but 2½ pints left. Use a silken cloth to strain and throw away the dregs. Divide the liquid into three doses. Wait until the menstruation is about to come and in the evening take one dose; on the following morning take another dose. The menstruation will then flow and for the rest of her life she will be without children.

The *I chien chih*[13] 夷堅志 states: "A woman of Tonking named Mu Tan 牡丹 sold a drug preparation to cause abortion and this brought an awful retribution upon her. Now, although the above prescriptions are set forth, they may only be used in one out of ten-thousand cases; therefore those who use them should do so with caution."

(1d)   Early Prescription for abortion (2737–2696 B.C.)

We turn now from these contraceptive recipes to a most interesting one for abortion. Hagerty has discovered in the *Chung hsiu Chêng Ho chêng lei pên ts'ao* 重修政和證類本草, a famous Chinese herbal written by T'ang Shên-wei 唐慎微 about 1108 A.D., the following (in Bk. 4:16) under the heading *Shui yin* 水銀 or mercury:

---

time heat and take a dose. Eat before and after taking but do not eat excessively. If prepared in the spring season add *fang fêng* 防風 or *Peucedanum rigidum* and double the quantity of *ch'üan hsiung*. If prepared in the summer add *huang ch'in* 黃岑 or skullcap (*Scutellaria macrantha*) and add double the quantity of *shao yao*. If prepared in the autumn add *t'ien men tung* 天門冬 or *Asparagus lucidus* and double the quantity of *ti huang*. If prepared in the winter add *kuei chih* 桂枝 or *Cassia* twigs and double the quantity of *tang kuei*. See *Cyclopedia of Chinese Medicine*, p. 724.

[11] This work was written by Wu Chih-wang 武之望, a native of Shênsi Province, whose *tzu* is Shu-ch'ing 叔卿, and others of the Manchu dynasty period and was published in 1728. The author is also indebted to Mr. Li Chi-fan 李其璠 of San Francisco who lent this work and called Mr. Hagerty's attention to these additional references.

[12] This leaven is made with wheat flour mixed with kidney beans, the juice of *shui liao* 水蓼 [*Polygonum flaccidum*], and apricot kernels. It is made during the dog-days (July 15th to August 15th). The peptic, nutritive and abortifacient properties of these ingredients are well recognized in the Chinese herbals. See Stuart's *Chinese Materia Medica*, p. 233.

[13] A work by Hung Mai 洪邁 of the Sung period. It is a collection of miscellaneous notes concerning matters of a fabulous nature. See *Tz'u yüan*, Pt. Ch'ou 丑, p. 240.

"*Shui yin* tastes bitter, is of cold nature, and contains poison. It is a specific for ulcers, white itching sores on the scalp, will kill parasitical worms in the skin and flesh, cause abortion, and cure fevers. . . . "[14]

(1e) Eunuchism

Eunuchism is a very ancient practice in China, dating from 1100 B.C. (Chou Dynasty). This we know from a code of the Emperor Chou-Koung which mentions it as a punitive measure. Readers interested in the history of castration in China should refer to the account by Matignon.[15] These interesting data do not properly concern us here, since there is no reason to believe that the intent is a genuinely contraceptive one. Most of the Chinese eunuchs are, and have been, in the Imperial service. The motive for castration seems to have been to prevent the palace attendants from having sexual relations with the imperial concubines. Outside of China the religious motive for castration is also prominent throughout history. The male castrates of the Catholic church were desired up to the eighteenth century for their soprano voices. The practice was condemned by the Council of Nice; and later, Pope Clement XIV prohibited castrates from singing in the churches. Matignon, however, reported in 1896 that they were still employed in the Sistine Chapel.[16]

Are we to conclude then that castration has never been used in China for contraceptive purposes? Probably not; for Professor Danton writes: "I know from my own conversations with the Chinese that contraceptive methods were used in the palaces without reference to Western science or contraceptive instruments of Western origin. In this case, the Emperor determined whether or not the chief eunuch should prevent the conception of any particular concubine through manipulative measures. How successful these were is, of course, very problematical, and I have no information as to whether such methods were also used on the Empress. My informant," adds Professor Danton, "was one who was closely associated with palace affairs during the time of the Empire, and I regard the information as fairly authentic."[17]

Several other ancient Chinese works refer to contraceptive technique. But their search will have to await a special inquiry. Enough has been

---

[14] It is of great significance that the above statement has been quoted by T'ang Shên-wei from the *Shên Nung pên ts'ao ching*, which is, as we have said above, the most ancient medical work in the Chinese language and attributed to Emperor Shên Nung, who, according to Chinese chronology, reigned 2737–2696 B.C.

[15] Matignon, J. J., "Les Eunuques du Palais Impérial à Pékin," *Bulletins de la Société d'Anthropologie de Paris*, 4s. vii (1896): 325–336.

[16] *Ibid.*, p. 326.

[17] Letter to the author dated December 13, 1930. (Punctuation and unimportant phraseology slightly altered.)

said, however, to suggest that the story is not so blank as some sinologists have assumed.

(1f) Miscellaneous Magical Contraceptive Recipes

Passing reference may be made to certain Chinese magical procedures of unknown age reported by Ersch and Gruber,[18] through Wilde,[19] German gynecologist and first-known reporter of what seems to be the modern cervical cap (see pp. 319–320 *infra*). Some Chinese women, when they desired to be free from pregnancy, have burned on the navel three *moxa* balls (Ger. = Moxakegel). On the other hand, a woman who wishes to become pregnant puts eleven such balls on both sides of the twelfth dorsal vertabrae. Girls who serve Venus pandemos also drink every month a certain amount of white lead to suppress menstruation and to prevent impregnation.[20] Lead has a sterilizing effect; the other prescriptions are worthless.

Before closing this section a word may be said about the changing situation in China in our time.

(1g) The Democratization of Birth Control Begins

There is reason to believe that a start has already been made in adopting more modern and effective contraceptive measures. "Already," says Peffer, who knows the country and the people, "the Chinese are conscious of the advantage of smaller families and are resorting to means for limiting their size, as may be seen by looking in at the windows of modern drug stores, where devices are openly displayed with that matter-of-factness about such things that is so natural to an Oriental and so shocking to the Occidental."[21] Birth control clinics have been opened in Shanghai and Peiping, and medical missionaries have furthered modern birth control. Peffer goes on to express the judgment that, though the Chinese have always proliferated to glorify the family, successful industrialization implies urbanization and education. The combination, he thinks, "always has one result—birth control."[22] As they become more industrialized, democratize education, gain access to medical knowledge, "they will inevitably limit reproduction." Since the old family system is breaking down, one of the chief motives to spawning will have been taken away.

[18] Ersch und Gruber, *Allgemeine Encyclopädie der Wissenschaften und Künste*, ii, 385.
[19] Friedrich Adolph Wilde, *Das weibliche Gebär-unvermögen* (Berlin, 1838, pp. xvi, 413), p. 315.
[20] *Ibid.*
[21] Nathaniel Peffer, *China: The Collapse of a Civilization* (New York: John Day, 1930), p. 285.
[22] *Ibid.*

§2 INDIA

(2a) Sanskrit Sources

That the literature of ancient India richly reports the sexual life of the people is evident to anyone who has perused the standard histories of Indian literature.[23] The Indian people had a balanced outlook on life, though they are not usually credited with this by uninformed Westerners.[24] Indian literature stressed a three-fold way of life: the *artha-çāstras* stressed the ways and means by which man could secure and maintain material welfare, while the *dharma-çāstras* dealt with religious duties and obligations. The *kāma-çāstras* concerned themselves with maximizing sexual enjoyment. They elevated love to a fine art, developed an *ars amoris*.

Devotion to *kāma*, or to desire, is presented in Indian literature as a very serious business—as one worthy of study.[25] The man of taste, known as the nagaraka, or man about town, was particularly indebted to this literature, much of which is, from the ordinary Western point of view, obscene. The East Indians as a people were never as ascetic as commonly supposed.

It has not been possible for this study to search all this literature.[26] It is

---

[23] Moritz Winternitz, *Geschichte der indischen Literatur*. Leipzig, 1908–[22], 3 vols. (The first volume has been translated into English.) A. Berriedale Keith, *A History of Sanskrit Literature*. Oxford, 1928. See chap. xxiv on "The Science of Love." Herbert H. Gowen, *A History of Indian Literature*. New York & London: Appleton, 1931. Arthur A. Macdonnell, *A History of Sanskrit Literature*. New York, 1900. Albrecht Weber, *The History of Indian Literature*. London, 1878. Max Müller, *History of Ancient Sanscrit Literature*. London, 1860.

[24] Gowen declares: "Thus it happens that the literature which contained some of the profoundest speculation the world has ever known contains also, through devotion to *artha*, some of the most cold-bloodedly practical and, in the case of *kāma*, some of the most licentious." (*op. cit.*, p. 172.)

The *artha cāstras* dealt realistically with government and administration. They discussed agriculture, the arts, the census, and such topics as arts and crafts, foresting, mining, irrigation, famine, etc. In the *Dharma-sūtras* one finds much on taxes, judicial procedure and military preparation, while the 12th book of that famous poem, the *Mahābhārata*, deals with the science of kingship. The *artha-cāstra* of Kautilya has been recently translated and published in German (1926) by Johann Jacob Meyer.

[25] In this sense these works are forerunners of all the modern scientific investigators of sex life—and of some not so scientific. Much of what they taught—not the details so much as the point of view—is only recently coming to find acceptance in the Western world among physicians, psychiatrists, mental hygienists, social hygienists, etc. *Cf.*, the well-known works of Robie, Van de Velde, Helena Wright, M. J. Exner, I. E. Hutton, etc. See Sir Bhagvat Sinh Jee, *A Short History of Aryan Medical Science* (London: MacMillan, 1896), p. 75.

[26] There is an immense Arabic as well as Indian literature on *ars amoris*. See Ahlwardt, catalogue of the Arabic MSS. in Berlin. *Cf.*, Sarton *Introduction to the History of Science* for a few titles scattered throughout the volumes.

a subject for a monograph in itself.   Most of it is inaccessible in the U. S. A., or has never been translated.   Moreover, reports on anti-conceptional technique are invariably lost in a mass of irrelevant details.   But that techniques are reported in this literature is not to be doubted.   Some are presented below, though not all are from the *kāma-çāstras*.   The entire range of *Āyur-veda* literature, dealing with Sanskrit medicine, needs also to be searched from this point of view.   To my knowledge it has not been done by anyone to date.   Here again is a monumental task in itself.   The fact is mentioned here so the reader may understand the limits of this investigation.

A word may be said about the antiquity of the *Kāma çāstras*.   Though these great erotic lyrics go back to Vedic times, the first great treatise of the kind which has come down to us is the *Kāma-Sūtra* of Vatsyāyana Mallanāga (early fourth century A.D.).[27]   He has been called by Keith and Gowen "the Machiavelli of erotics."   Familiar with Kautilya's *Artha-çāstra*, the author of the *Kāma-Sūtra*, a physician, built upon Kautilya's work.   As Kautilya had taught that everything was fair in war and statecraft, so Vatsyāyana held that everything was fair in love.   And the seduction of women is here reduced to a fine art.

The seven parts of the work follow:

1. The statement of generalities in praise of the *trivarga*.
2. The various ways of enjoying love.
3. Hints for courtship.
4. Relations with married women.
5. Relations with other people's mistresses.
6. Relations with courtesans.
7. On love potions and aphrodisiacs.

The Indian poets and dramatists studied carefully, and were much influenced by, the *Kāma-Sūtra*.[28]   Through them knowledge of erotics, and probably also some crude knowledge of contraception, was spread.

The publication and influence of the *Kāma-Sūtra* naturally led to the publication of imitative works.   About 1200 there appeared the *Ratirahasya*, or "Secret of Love," sometimes called the *Koka-çāstra*, written by Kokkoka.   A contraceptive recipe from this source is reproduced below.   Then in the thirteenth century came the *Jayamangala* by Yaçodhara Indrapada.

The techniques,[29] probably representative, having their origin in this

[27] Gowen, *op. cit.*, p. 192.
[28] Gowen, *op. cit.*   For an account of the *Kāma-Sūtra*, see also Keith, *op. cit.*, pp. 467–471; Winternitz, *op. cit.*, iii, 536–541.
[29] It is worthy of interest from the standpoint of population control that there was,

literature, are more frequently magical than rational. At present it is impossible to date the origin of these techniques; and the following account is not chronological.

(2b) The Anàngaranga by Kalyànamalla (XVI)

The *Anàngaranga*, or *The Stage of the God of Love*, a volume of erotic poetry by Kalyànamalla dating probably from the sixteenth century, says:[30]

The woman who drinks daily for half a month a pala [measure = $2\frac{2}{15}$ ounces] of three year old molasses will remain without doubt barren for the duration of her life. [1] The woman who, at the end of her period, drinks daily for three days the roots of the agni tree (*Semecarpus anacardium, Plumbago zeylanica* or *Citrus acida*) cooked in sour rice water will be barren. [2] The fruit of *kadamba* (*Nauclea cadamba*) and the feet of flies, drunk with hot water for three days, will cause

---

among the ancient Indians, much emphasis upon ceremonial abstention from coitus. Jee avows (*op. cit.*) that the Hindu principles of hygiene require the restriction of intercourse to certain periods. Cohabitation is not to be indulged in during sunset (p. 73). He adds:

Sexual intercourse is prohibited for the first four days after the appearance of the menstrual flow, as well as on the 8th, 14th, and 15th days of both the fortnights—light and dark; on the anniversary days of dead parents, nights previous to the anniversaries; on Vyatipta (the seventeenth of the astrological Yogas), Vaidhrata (the twenty-seventh astrological Yoga), Sanskranti (the passage of the sun or planetary bodies from one sign of the zodiac to another); in the daytime, at midnight, and during an eclipse. (p. 76)

The Hindoos are, however, enjoined, as are the Chinese, to beget progeny,—a *putra* (son) or a *putri* (daughter). Childlessness, being a frustration of the chief object of marriage, is anathema; and one dying without a son is offered no salvation.

In addition to ceremonial abstention, mention may be made of the fact—though it is not a birth-control measure as herein defined—that in India widows are not allowed to re-marry. When Masters says (*op. cit.*, p. 90) that the prevention of conception "is very common in India" he clearly exaggerates. For abstention from re-marriage is not a birth-control measure at all, even though it may have some effect in limiting procreation.

[30] From the translation into German from the Sanskrit made by Richard Schmidt *Beiträge zur Indischen Erotik. Das Liebesleben des Sanskritvolkes....* Berlin: Barsdorf, 1922. Ed. 3rd, pp. 691. *Cf.*, Stopes, *Contraception*, 2nd ed., p. 280 for a somewhat different rendering taken from the English translation: *Ananga-Ranga (Stage of the Bodiless One), or, the Hindu Art of Love. Translated from the Sanskrit, and annotated by A. F. F. & B. F. R. Reprint: Cosmopoli*, 1885 *for the Kama Shastra Society of London and Benàres and for private circulation only.* Schmidt says that the translator avows that only four copies of the original edition are known to exist; while the translator of the *Kàma-Sùtra* states—whether referring to the original or the reprint, I do not know—that "only six copies were printed for private circulation." A translation from the French into English by Isidore Liseaux was published in Paris, 1886 (pp. xvii + 196) under the title: *Anàngaranga, traité hindou de l'amour conjugal....* Neither the English nor the French edition seem to be available in America.

It is by no means certain when the *Anàngaranga* was written. Schmidt (*op. cit.*, p. 28) thinks it was during the reign in Gujarat of Làd Chàn (1450–1526).

unfruitfulness. [3] A half pala of the seeds of red lotus, drunk with rice water for the seven days duration of the period, will make those with gazelle eyes unfruitful. [4][31]

(2c) The Pañcasāyaka by Kaviśekhara (XI–XIII)

The *Pañcasāyaka*, or *The Five Arrows* [of the God of Love], by Jyotirīśvara Kaviśekhara, dating from the eleventh to thirteenth centuries says:

The woman who drinks on a lucky day palasa (*Butea frondosa*) and . . . fruits as well as flowers of the śālmali tree (*Salmalia malabarica*) together with melted butter, will certainly become unfruitful. (1) If she drinks regularly of the decoction of the root of the pāvaka tree (*Semecarpus anacardium* ?) and sour rice water, and keeps it up for three days after the end of the menstrual period, she will remain unfruitful until death. (2) If she drinks regularly the kadamba fruit (*Nauclea cadamba*) and honey together with sour rice water for three days or even only once after the end of the (cleansing) bath she will surely render herself unfruitful thereby. (3) If a woman eats or drinks continuously for half a month a large pala of three year old molasses, the greatest of the poets (Kaviśekhara) says that she will surely be unfruitful to the end of her life. (4) Two large karsa of the seeds of the rākṣasa tree (?) drunk with white rice water for seven days after the end of the menstrual period, causes certain unfruitfulness for those with gazelle eyes.[32]

[31] The original Sanskrit passage as published by Schmidt (p. 646) reads:
gudaṃ traihāyaṇaṃ yātti palamātraṃ tu nityaśaḥ
māsārdhaṃ sā bhaved vandhyā yāvad āyur na saṃśayaḥ || 1 ||
tuṣatoyena saṃkvāthya mūlam agnitarūdbhavam
puṣpāvasāne tridinaṃ pītvā vandhyābhijāyate || 2 ||
kadambasya phalaṃ pādaṃ makṣikāyā dinatrayam
pītam uṣṇodakenaiva vandhyātvaṃ pratipādayet || 3 ||
raktāmbhoruhabījānāṃ palārdhaṃ taṇḍulābhasā
ṛtau pītaṃ tu saptāhaṃ vandhyāṃ kuryān mṛgīdṛśam || 4 ||

[32] Translated from Schmidt, *op. cit.*, pp. 647–48. The original Sanskrit passage (fol 13a) in *The Five Arrows* reads:
palāśa . . . yoḥ phalāni
puṣpāṇy atho śālmalipādapasya
ghṛtena sārdhaṃ sudine pibantī
vandhyā bhaven niścitam eva nārī
tuṣāmbunā pāvakavṛkṣamūlaṃ
niḥkvāthya pītvā niyamaṃ carantī
ṛtvantakāle tridinaṃ pibantī
vandhyā bhaved ā maraṇāntam eva
phalaṃ kadambasya samākṣikaṃ ca
tuṣodanena tridinaṃ sakṛd vā
snānāvasāne niyamena pītvā
vandhyām avaśyam kurute haṭhena
traihāyanaṃ yā gudam atti nityaṃ
palapramāṇaṃ vanitārdhamāsam
jīvāntakaṃ niścitam eva tasyā

It seems highly improbable that any of these receipts could have been effective in preventing conception.   They are essentially magical.   Others reported below are more effective.

(2d)   The Ratirahasya by Kokkoka (Before XIV)

Not only the Anangaranga and the Pancasayaka, but Kokkoka's Ratirahasya, or The Secret of Sexual Desire, antedating the fourteenth century, furnish us, collectively considered, with a score or more of recipes for forestalling the emission of the male semen.   While many of these are weirdly magical, one at least possesses a rational basis:

> If one, at the time of sexual enjoyment [orgasm] presses firmly with the finger on the fore part of the testicle [base of the urethra], turns his mind to other things, and holds his breath while doing so, a too rapid ejaculation of the sperm will be prevented.[33]

This is nothing other than *coitus obstructus*, still unfortunately practised in our day.   It functions in this manner: Since the urethra is occluded by pressure of the finger, the ejaculate is forced into the bladder whence it later passes with the urine.   It is interesting to find it mentioned in a fourteenth century Sanskrit text.   The presumption is that it antedates[34] that period; al-Razi seems to refer to it.   (See p. 137.)

---

vandhyatvam uktam kavipumgavena
karsadvayam raksasavrksabijam
saptahamatram sitasalivara
rtau nipitam mrgasavakaksya
vandhyatvam etan niyatam karoti

[33] *Ratirahasya*, fol. 20b.   Schmidt, *op. cit.*, p. 622, 623.   Turning one's mind "to other things" is the same as the Chinese method of *cong-fou* (see *infra*).   The belief that holding the breath will assist one in preventing impregnation is, I believe, still widely prevalent in various parts of the world.   The notion may have its source in some of these ancient Sanskrit texts.

[34] For a questionable report of passiveness during coitus by natives of Buro (Malay Archipelago) with the supposed intent of preventing conception, see page 21.   Riedel may be in error both regarding the natives' intent and the actual performance.   If not, we may be sure that passiveness is rare among primitives.   In sex matters they have a philosophy of maximizing pleasure save for stringent taboos and other controls.   It seems reasonable to suppose that the practice of remaining passive proceeds from a feeling, conscious or unconscious, of guilt about intercourse.   The notion may be current that the act is less reprehensible if the woman only half enjoys it.   In India, no doubt, passiveness in coitus partook of a "purifying" self-discipline.   It is ceremonial discipline, a phase of Hindu "desirelessness" in general.   A branch from the same root seems to me to flower in Puritanism and Christian asceticism.   By this tradition of asceticism the Western as well as the Eastern world has been influenced.   But unless I am mistaken, sexual asceticism never particularly characterized preliterate societies.   Savages left such foolishness for civilized peoples.

The fact that it existed as one of a score of magical receipts designed primarily to slow up the male orgasm and to avoid premature ejaculation, rather than as a recipe to prevent conception, leads one to infer that it was not widely adopted by the populace for the latter purpose.   Moreover, the initiated alone probably had access to such information.   The magical recipes for retarding ejaculation ranged from rubbing the navel or the soles of the feet with various salves made from native flora, to taking potions. But the recommendation to practise *coitus obstructus* would have been at least partially effective.   The birth rate in India suggests the extent to which this custom was effectively employed.

(2e)   The Bridhadyôgatarangiṇî (VIII)

This work contains some interesting contraceptive recipes.   Though belonging approximately to the eighth century, the book is a collection of extracts from various older works to which references are not given.   For instance, some are probably from the well-known medical work by Charaka (first century B.C.).   I am indebted to a Bombay correspondent, Mr. R. D. Karvé, for searching out and translating the following recipes:

1. One tôlâ [2½ tolas = 1 ounce] of powdered palm leaf and red chalk taken with cold water on the fourth day [of the menstrual period] makes a woman sterile with certainty.

2. The seed of the *Palâsha* tree being mixed with honey and ghee, and smeared inside the vagina during the menses.   By the power of this application, the woman will never conceive.

3. The woman who has intercourse after menstruation, after treating the vaginal passage with the smoke of the *Neem* wood [by the method explained below], does not conceive.

4. The prostitute who has intercourse with a man, after having inserted into her vagina a piece of rock salt[35] dipped into oil, never conceives.

5. The root of the *Datura* plant [yielding *Hyoscyamine*] gathered in the month of Powsha [the tenth month of the Hindu lunar calendar, corresponding normally to January, the calendar being adjusted to the solar calendar every three years by the addition of an extra month] and tied round the waist, prevents conception in prostitutes and others.

6. The roots of the *Tandûlîyaka* tree, ground with rice-water [water in which rice has been washed before cooking], and taken for three days at the end of the menstrual period, make women sterile.

7. Mustard seeds ground in sesame oil, and taken [by the mouth ?] for three days during menses, prevents all chance of pregnancy.

8. If a woman drinks, at the time of delivery, flowers of the *Japâ* [China Rose]

It may be pointed out that sexual asceticism may be expected to diminish in the future, for there is less need for it functionally.   There are better population controls.   Doubtless religious asceticism will always persist to some extent.

[35] See n. 39.

tree in gruel, even if she conceives again, the foetus will disappear, and she will never carry to delivery.

9. A woman who has lost her husband, or whose husband has abandoned her, may, at her ease, have intercourse with anyone, [but] she should afterwards insert into her vagina a foetus-preventing tampon of *Ajowan* seeds and rock salt ground in oil.[36]

(2f) Miscellaneous Sanskrit Sources

Similar passages are to be found in other Sanskrit sources of considerable antiquity:

1. Libidinous men, who do not want their wives to bear children, produce sterility in women for their pleasure.

2. She who drinks during menses a mixture of equal parts of long pepper (*Pippali*), *widanga* [used as a vermifuge], and borax, in milk never conceives.

3. The woman who eats the flowers of the *Japâ* tree ground in gruel [made by the fermentation of boiled rice], or who eats four tolas of raw sugar, never conceives.

4. She who eats *Japâ* flowers with gruel every day does not menstruate, or even if there is a suspicion of menstruation, does not conceive.

5. She who has intercourse after skilfully treating the vagina with smoke from the *Neem* wood after menstruation, can do so without fear of pregnancy.

[The method is to put live coals into a vessel with a spout, to put some powdered *Neem* wood on it, to cover the opening of the vessel and insert the spout into the vagina. This explanation is recorded in the original Sanskrit.]

6. A woman who eats every day for a fortnight, three-year-old raw sugar, [a lump] the size of a nutmeg fruit, will become sterile for life.

7. A woman will become sterile by drinking a decoction of the roots of the *Chitraka* tree in rice-bran-water for three days after menstruation.

8. Sandal-wood, mustard, and sugar, drunk in rice-water in equal parts, make a woman sterile.

9. The woman will never conceive again who drinks during the menses the flowers of the *Jambûla* tree ground in the urine of a cow.

10. The woman will certainly become sterile who drinks in wine the fruits of the *Kutaja* and *Kadamba* trees with *wâlaka* and sandal-wood. [The roots of *wâlaka* are used for their fragrance.]

(2g) Summary and Evaluation of the Practices Recommended

The recipes from these sources may be classified as follows:

Magical and Ritualistic
Swallowing:
1 Three year old molasses
2 Roots of *agni* tree cooked in sour rice water
3 Fruit of *kadamba* with feet of flies
4 Seeds of red lotus with rice water

[36] *Bridhadyôgatarangiṇṭ.* Adhyara, ch. 143, verses 53–61 inclusive. *Anandâshram Sanscrit Series.*

5 *palasa*
6 Fruits and flowers of *śālmali*
7 Root of *pāvaka* tree and sour rice water
8 *Kadamba* fruit with honey and sour rice water
9 Seeds of *rākṣasa* tree with rice water
10 Palm leaf and red chalk
11 Roots of *tandûlîyaka* tree
12 Flowers of the Japâ tree
13 Pepper, *widanga* and borax in milk
14 Ground mustard seed in sesame oil
15 Raw sugar, three year old sugar
16 Roots of the *chitraka* tree
17 Sandal wood, mustard and sugar
18 Flowers of the *jambûla* tree
19 Fruits of the *kutaja* and *kadamba* trees with *wâlaka* and sandal wood

Vaginal fumigations with the smoke of *neem* wood
Passiveness in coitus
Holding the breath
Amulet
Root of the *Datura* plant tied around the waist

Quasi-rational or Rational
Coitus obstructus
Smearing the vagina with honey and ghee (oil)[37]
Vaginal medication of rock salt dipped in oil
Tampons of ground *ajowan* seed and rock salt with oil.[38]

This summary shows that nineteen recipes consist of concoctions to be taken by the mouth, and which are therefore ineffective. Vaginal fumigations, passiveness in coitus, holding the breath, and amulets each receive mention once. Of twenty-six different recipes, quasi-rational or rational methods are mentioned only three times.

Smearing the vagina with honey and ghee would seem quite reasonable. Tampons and plugs of rock salt with oil might also be more or less effective. Ordinary modern table salt is an excellent spermicide. An 8% solution kills sperms rapidly.[39] As used in our time five tablespoonsful are dissolved in a quart of water; or, half a teaspoonful to a vaginal bulbful.

Viewing the matter in broad perspective the chief difficulty with these prescriptions as a group is this: Even the most experimentally-minded Indian physician would be unable, upon reading such accounts, to sort out the ineffective from the (theoretically) partially effective means. He would be as likely to recommend the internal use of decoctions as to apply the

[37] Ghee is clarified butter; or butter converted into a kind of oil by boiling.
[38] The use of the word "afterwards" in the original text is confusing. Probably it means not after intercourse but after menstruation.
[39] Dickinson and Bryant, *Control of Conception*, p. 44.

quasi-rational methods.   If lay women read such accounts—probably they were not accessible to them—they would be even more confused than the physicians.   Hence the whole possibility of conception control would come to be doubted, and brought into contempt.   Failing to achieve results, women would come to believe no method possible; and this feeling would no doubt be communicated to others.   In fact the persistence for centuries of magical along with rational methods of preventing conception may account for the superstition—for such it is—of some modern physicians that there are no reliable methods for preventing conception.

(2h)   The Contemporary Situation and the Future

A few words may be said about the modern situation in India, and especially about the prospects of the general diffusion of contraceptive knowledge in India in the future.

The Sanitary Commissioner for Assam, commenting on the slow increase in numbers of the tea-garden coolies, reports that

An important factor in producing the defective birth-rate appears to be due to voluntary limitation of births, a practice which is not confined to highly civilized and sophisticated communities.[40]

The Commissioner avows that a birth rate higher than that actually reported might reasonably be expected "owing to the amount of care and thought which is devoted by the tea industry towards maintaining the health of the labour force at as high a level as is economically possible."[41] Whether this is a white viewpoint toward a colored increase that needs discounting it is impossible to say.   It is relevant to observe, however, that government health officers the world round have been too prone, at least until very recently, when there has been a marked face-about, to enter upon a chorus of disapproval of the declining birth rate.   Rarely do such officers view the declining birth rate as a vital adjustment to social and economic conditions.

Exactly what form the "voluntary limitation of births" takes, the Commissioner does not venture to suggest.   The phenomenon among the coolies is corroborated also by the Indian Census Report, which states that "It is a matter of common belief that among the tea-garden coolies of Assam means are frequently taken to prevent conception, or to procure abortion."[42] Techniques are not reported.   Perhaps something is swallowed.

The latest census report for India (1931) not only makes passing reference

---

[40] Report, 1913.   Quoted by P. K. Wattal, *The Population Problem in India*, p. 29.
[41] Wattal, *op. cit.*, p. 28.
[42] *Ibid.*, citing Indian Census Report, 1901.

to contraception, but seems optimistic about the future prospects of its general adoption:

[Until recently] Artificial modes of keeping down the population have not been consciously adopted [on any considerable scale] . . . but there is a tendency for men certainly to marry later, and the beginnings of a like tendency in the other sex will probably appear ere long. The effects of this should be seen ultimately in a lower birthrate and slower increase in population. Birth control, though advocated by among others a Judge of the High Court, and extensively advertised in the press, and not unknown in the higher social circles, cannot be said to have as yet taken any marked place in the social system. *When it will, however, is merely deferred, and ten years should show a marked growth in its popularity.* Books on the subject are to be found in any bookstall or publisher's list and . . . it is unlikely that they can fail to exert some influence.

Contraception of a crude kind has been observed among Goundans of Salem apparently in order to prevent the undue growth of families, and consequent fragmentation of holdings and weakening of the joint family system and influence. The portent is of great interest.[43]

Anstey's recent able survey of economic and social conditions in India[44] concludes, as did Orchard's comparable analysis of Japanese conditions, that no enduring economic improvement will be possible in India until certain obstacles, such as the high birth rate and the uneconomic (at least, non-capitalistic) outlook of the people, are overcome. That the more informed native leaders in India are themselves beginning to realize this needs no proof.

Though the diffusion of contraceptive information, so necessary to bring reproduction under control, will be hampered by cultural traditions, by the Oriental outlook toward the family and toward reproduction, by a slow levelling upward of the standard of living, and hence by widespread illiteracy and poverty, it is only a matter of decades—say a century at most—before contraceptive practices, after the modern Western manner, will become general.

The Madras Neo-Malthusian League (founded July, 1929) publishes a propaganda journal of rather high merit, all circumstances considered. It is the *Madras Birth Control Bulletin.* To the March and April 1931 numbers Sherwood Eddy contributed an article on "Birth Control in India," which gives a brief summary of contraceptive methods. The League has

[43] *Census of India,* 1931, xiv, 46. Madras. Part I. Report by M. W. Yeats of the Indian Civil Service. Supt. of Census Operations, Madras. Punctuation and italics mine.

[44] Vera Anstey, *The Economic Development of India.* London, 1931. Miss Anstey, now of the London School of Economics, is not only a competent economic theorist, but she was for seven years a resident of Bombay. Her conclusions merit, therefore, more weight than those of the casual observer or traveller.

reprinted this as a pamphlet for sale at a low price (As. 2). The League also issued in 1930 a pamphlet entitled "Dr. Sherwood Eddy on Family Limitation" (pp. 14). This does not discuss technique, is merely an argument for birth control; but a League notice at the end informs the reader that "the following appliances are available for sale at the League:

1. Artificial rubber sponges
2. Jelly made of vaseline and boric acid
3. Jelly made of glycerine, starch and chinosol.

In addition to English and American pamphlets on technique, which it sells, this active League issues a pamphlet on technique of its own.[45] A number of other pamphlets of an educational nature have been issued. These will be considered in a subsequent volume devoted to the economic and social phases of the history of birth control. Here our concern is chiefly medical.

Several treatises on technique, some popular, have been published in India within recent years. These are by Karvé, Phadke, and Ayyur (also Aiyer.)[46] There are native (Marathi) as well as English editions of at least one of these. In addition, a goodly number of works on the subject with English imprints are being sold in India. There are several commercial firms handling modern devices. A few contraceptive clinics are operating. Dr. A. P. Pillay pioneered in opening one in Bombay. In the near future the clinic movement will doubtless expand considerably.

Bombay is also the place of publication of the only scientific journal in the world devoted to advancing our knowledge of conjugal hygiene. The title of the new quarterly is *Marriage Hygiene*, and the first number appeared in August, 1934. Dr. A. P. Pillay is the editor-in-chief, the present author, editor for the U. S. A. An international board of editors is gradually being set up. Another object of the journal is to unite the interests of those connected with contraceptive clinics and marriage advice bureaux. To some it will seem strange that such a journal should be started in India; but in the light of its traditionally natural attitude toward sexual phenomena it is really not strange.

I know of no quantitative data on the extent of sale of contraceptive

[45] Anon. [Aiyer], "Select Methods of Family Limitation compiled by a Committee of the Madras Neo-Malthusian League." Second ed. Madras: Madras Neo-Malthusian League, 1929, pp. 16. The title of the first edition was "Approved Methods of Family Limitation compiled by a Committee of the Madras Neo-Malthusian League with the assistance of Dr. M. S. Krishnamurthi Aiyer, M. B. & C. M.," 1928, pp. 8.

[46] R. D. Karvé, *Birth Control. Theory and Practice.* Fourth edition. Bombay: Right Agency, 1931, pp. 123; and N. S. Phadke, *Birth Control. Theory and Practice.* Poona: Vijaya-Sāhitya, 1925, pp. 107. See note above for Aiyer's pamphlet.

devices in India, and we have none on the percolation downward to the lower social groups of modern knowledge and practice. These matters are certainly worthy of local investigation.

§3 JAPAN

(3a) The Kabutogata (Hard Condom)

Little information is available at present on the early history of contraception in Japan. Schedel, however, reports the use of a " 'kabuto-gata' or helmet [for the glans] made of tortoise shell or horn which not only gives the woman much satisfaction but also prevents conception at the same time."[47] This instrument might be described as a hard condom. The age or extent of its use is unknown to me. One would infer, in the absence of contrary evidence, that its use must have been restricted. Probably it was used as a device for the impotent. Both Schedel and Krauss have given us photographs of it.[48] The former also notes that the *kabutogata* was sometimes used by women on a plain or fluted stick as an instrument of self-gratification.

In a recent, remarkable treatise on Japanese sexual life by Krauss, Satow, and Ihm we have a report of a *Kabutogata* made not of shell or horn but of leather, and which Krauss considers tolerably effective as a contraceptive. A Japanese erotic book of the 10th Bunsei year (*c.* 1827) gives the following description of such a hard condom:

Kawagata; it is also called Kyōtai. Such a Kyōtai is made of thin leather, and foreigners call it Ryūrusakku. This is an object which prevents the male semen from entering the vagina thus preventing conception.[49]

Probably the word *Ryūrusakka* is a corruption of a foreign word. Satow thinks it derived from Rüde-Sack; Krauss from the Dutch roede-zak. Krauss says "it is supposed" that the Dutch first introduced such leather condoms into Japan. The word *Ryūru* appears to have been known in the form *Ryoru* much before this; for, in the book *Naemara Initsuden* (*Life History of an Important Person*) by Hiraga Gennai (Yedo Period, year unknown) one reads:

"Komo nite wa Ryoru to ii."

"The foreigners call it (the penis) Ryoru." The word *Kyōtai* in the passage quoted above means "root-sack" or "penis-sack." The people also use

[47] J. Schedel, "Reizmittel im Geschlechtleben der Japaner," *Anthropophyteia*, vi (1909), 93–95. See p. 94.

[48] Schedel, *ibid.* Photographs at end of volume. Schedel also states that the picture in the earlier edition of Krauss's *Geschlechtsleben der Japaner* is mistakenly understood by Krauss to be a pessary instead of a *kabutogata*.

[49] F. S. Krauss, Tamio Satow, and Hermann Ihm, *Japanisches Geschlechtsleben*, ii, 439.

the term *Marabukuro* for penis-sack.   Since the end of the Yedo Period both words have gradually fallen into disuse.[50]

Krauss is of the opinion that the rubber condom was first introduced into Japan in perhaps the 4th or 5th Meiji year (1871–2); and he states that in the 19th Meiji year (1886) a dozen cost three yen (about $1.50).[51]   Writing in 1922, G. Teruoka, says that it was only about forty years ago that the [rubber] condom was introduced into Japan.[52]   That would place the date at say 1880 or 1882.   Hence the dates of Krauss and Teruoka roughly agree.

(3b) *Misugami (Bamboo Tissue-paper Tampon)*

It is reported[53] that the prostitutes of Japan and China have applied disks of oiled paper to the cervix to prevent conception.   Kurella[54] states, without producing the evidence, that these methods date from ancient times.   This is evidently the use of *Misugami* reported more recently by Krauss, Satow and Ihm who, one gathers, do not agree among themselves as to the intent of those employing it.   *Misugami* is a thin transparent paper, much like toilet paper, made of bamboo tissue.   According to some reports it is used mainly *after* coitus to prevent the clothing from being soiled by semen.   (It seems that coitus often takes place in Japan with the clothing on, perhaps owing to the difficulty of securing privacy, perhaps owing to an absence of the winter heating of rooms.)   Satow thinks that it was used as a tampon prior to coitus, but that its purpose was the prevention of venereal infection; and that it was well-adapted for that purpose. Krauss seems correct in rejecting this view.[55]   For it would afford only a very limited protection to the cervix.   A Japanese erotic book, *Kōgō Zatsuwa (Vermischte Abhandlungen über den Coitus)*, by Insai Hakasui says:

Make a ball of Misugami and put it into the vagina in order to prevent the penis from touching the uterus; that is called Agezoko.[56]

Evidently the purpose here was the prevention of conception.

(3c) *Miscellaneous Techniques*

Less effective than the *Kabutogata* or *Misugami* must have been the resort to internal means.   An anti-conceptional means recommended and

---

[50] *Ibid.*, ii, 439.

[51] *Ibid.*, ii, 440.

[52] *Arch. f. Frauenk. u. Eugenetik*, viii (1922), 217.

[53] Artur Streich in Sudhoff's *Arch. f. Gesch. d. Med.*, xxii (1929), 210.

[54] Hans Kurella, *Geschlecht und Gesellschaft* (Würzburg, 1911), p. 381.

[55] I gather that Krauss rejects this view because he speaks [*op. cit.*, ii, 438–439] of the use of the soft paper, *Misugami*, as one of the simplest means used in Japan for the prevention of conception.   He adds (ii, 438) that cotton is sometimes used in place of paper.

[56] Krauss, Satow, and Ihm, *op. cit.*, ii, 361–2.

sold by the women doctors of the Chūjō school was a decoction called *Tsuitachigwan* to be drunk on the first day of the month.[57] It was supposed to prevent conception, even if a women had frequent intercourse. The basis of this superstition is now unknown.

We are also told that a means of prevention widespread among Japanese women was the use of the *Mogusa*, or burning ball, which was burned on the mons veneris (Venusberg). It is apparently so ineffective that the Japanese folk-poets have poked fun at it in their satirical verse. And though it maintains a quiet existence here and there among superstitious women, the *Mogusa* has today almost completely fallen into oblivion.[58] Note that this practice seems virtually identical with the burning on the navel by Chinese women of *moxa* balls (see p. 113), a custom reported by the German gynecologist, Wilde, as early as 1838.

A popular Japanese educator of the seventeenth century, Yokiken Kaibara[59] (1630–1714), advocated the suppression of ejaculation on the part of old men in the interests of longevity. Though it was not a birth control measure, being prompted rather by a mistaken physiological notion doubtless very old, the practice, at least if the old men had young wives, would have a birth-limiting effect. Kaibara was thus a forerunner of those in America (e.g., J. H. Noyes, Alice Stockham) who counselled so-called "Karezza," "Male Continence" or *coitus reservatus*.

Elsewhere within (Chap. I, §5) there is an extensive discussion of the artificially-induced retroflexion of the uterus as practised in southeastern Asia (Java, Sumatra, etc.) for the purpose of preventing conception. Here we must note that Helbig reports the same practices employed by Japanese women, presumably in Japan. Though this is quite possible, Helbig cites no first-hand observer or authority. Perhaps he had personal knowledge of the practice in Japan; but this may be doubted. Helbig's accounts have been found somewhat inaccurate in other respects. He says the Japanese call it *ankatprut* [German for the Dutch *angkat proet*]. In support of the likelihood of the practice in Japan is the fact that, especially in recent decades, there has been a certain amount of inter-migration between Japan and southeastern Asia, a circumstance calculated to diffuse such a custom. It would be a service to the history of medical science and social customs if some of the Japanese physicians, such as Drs. Majima and Tsutsumi, now

[57] *Ibid.*, ii, 440.

[58] *Ibid.*, ii, 439.

[59] Kaibara is described by Tsurumi as Japan's "first popular educator"; as one who "expounded the difficult Confucian teachings with the plainest of words and wrote over a hundred books that went into the hands of the poor." Jusuki Tsurumi, *Present Day Japan* (New York: Columbia Univ. Press, 1926), p. 41.

concerned with modern contraception in that developing country of the East, would investigate the history of anti-conceptional practices there in order that some of the disputed points might be cleared up and our knowledge deepened.

(3d)   Recent Developments in Japan

Though the birth-control movement is in its initial stages in present-day Japan, there will be a lag of several decades before it can materially influence the demographic situation.   In getting off to a slow start the Japanese movement is no different from that in England, Germany, or the United States.   In fact the peculiar circumstances cited earlier in this chapter, chief among which are the religious system, ancestor worship, and the still-extant rural mores, will only gradually be overcome by the loosening of religious bonds, by industrialization and urbanization.   All these movements are, however, proceeding more rapidly in Japan than in China and India.

Popular education in modern contraceptive methods has only recently begun.   Margaret Sanger's visit in 1920 gave stimulation and encouragement to it.   Though her visit was more than frowned upon at first, her determination, as usual, won out.   Local leaders have gradually arisen, chief among them being Baroness Ishimoto.   Lately a few birth-control clinics have been set up under municipal toleration if not encouragement. A propaganda movement is started, and representatives have attended recent international conferences.   Two tolerably good medical handbooks on technique have recently appeared in the Japanese language.[60]

A few high governmental officials, seeing in birth control a way out for Japan's over-population problem, have begun to interest themselves in the subject.   And though the government has set up an official commission to study and report on the population problem, more especially as it relates to food supply, emigration, etc., evidently the military group now in control has deemed it inexpedient to adopt even the somewhat timid recommendations of the official commission.   Even the Commission did not face squarely the economic and health issues implied in Japan's extraordinary rate of natural increase.   This increase for 1932 was 1,007,868.   The birth rate was 32.92 and the death rate 17.72.   As in the instance of large natural increase of population in Western countries during the nineteenth century, the Japanese differential is mainly caused by a declining death rate: de-

[60] Kau Majima, *Be Wise Mothers!   The Practical Guide to Contraception.* [Introduction by Roswell H. Johnson] Kyobashi, Tokyo: Jitsugyo-no Nippon Sha, 1931.   The author is a Japanese Assemblyman.   Tatsuo Tsutsumi, *Medical Knowledge for the Control of Conception.*   Tokyo: Jitsugyo-no Nippon Sha, 1930, pp. 21.

creased infant mortality and the absence of epidemics.   When one realizes, however, that only about one-fifth of the area of Japan is tillable, that the hillsides are already "sculptured" to secure every possible foot of ground for cultivation; that as long ago as 1920 the density per square kilometer was 969 as compared with 226 for England and 394 for Belgium (among the highest densities in Europe); and when we realize that Japan is only in the initial stages of industrialization and the exportation of manufactures, we see how difficult it is for her to meet the economic problems implied in the demographic situation.   The situation is so glaringly obvious to students of population that it may be said that almost no writer of standing on the Japanese population problem who has published in recent years has failed to note that this situation cannot long endure without dire consequences. And many of them grant, though some reluctantly, that birth control is the only way out.   But even when such writers do not recognize contraception as the solution, it is no exaggeration to say that the considerable body of literature prepared in recent years on the Japanese population problem forms a significant ideational background for the development of a birth-control movement there.[61]   In substantiation of the point of view

[61] A few of the more useful general titles may be cited here: Keikai Hayashi, *Theories of Population*, Tokyo: Tokyo Publishing Co., 1930, pp. 281 (in Japanese); H. G. Moulton, *Japan: An Economic and Financial Appraisal*, Washington: Brookings Institution, 1931; Étienne Dennery, *Foules d'Asie. Surpopulation Japonaise, Expansion Chinoise, Émigration Indienne*, Paris: A. Colin, 1931, pp. 247; Translated from the French by John Peile, with a Foreword by Harold Cox, as *Asia's Teeming Millions and its Problems for the West*. London: J. Cape [1931]; Walter Russell Crocker, *The Japanese Population Problem. The Coming Crisis*, London: Allen & Unwin, 1931, pp. 240, New York: Macmillan; E. Honjo, "Population Problems in the Tokugawa Era," *Kyoto Economic Review*, December, 1927, pp. 42–63; City of Tokyo, *A Study of the Birth Rate of the Low Classes*, Tokyo, 1927 (in Japanese); I. Takano, *The Present and Future of Japanese Population*, Tokyo, 1916; John Orchard, *Japan's Economic Position; The Progress of Industrialization*, New York: McGraw-Hill, 1930, pp. 504; E. F. Penrose, *Food Supply and Raw Materials in Japan*, Chicago: Univ. Chicago Press, [1930], pp. 75.

Certain master of arts theses at Columbia University contain valuable information: Teruye Otsuki, *Japanese Population Problems*, (1931); Ai Sasaki, *The Population Problem in Japan*, (1930) pp. 66; Toshio Fujie, *Over Population in Japan and Proposed Remedies*, (1928) pp. 35; R. M. Kamida, *An Interpretation of Population Statistics in Japan to the Year 1913*, (1925) pp. 57; Yano Tsurki, *On the Food Supply of Japan*, (1917) pp. 68.   Note also the bibliographies in these sources.

See also Shuichi Harada, *Labor Conditions in Japan* (New York: Columbia Univ. Press, 1928), pp. 5–8, 75–106, 138–163; Fuminori Okazaki, *Study of Population Statistics*, (in Japanese).   Tokyo: Huhikaku Book Co., 1922, pp. 266; Naomasa Yamasaki, "A Note on the Geographical Distribution of the Density of Population, Birth- and Death Rates of Japan," in *Problems of the Pacific, Institute of Pacific Relations* (1928), pp. 361–364; John E. Orchard, "The Pressure of Population in Japan," *Geog. Rev.*, xviii (1928), 374–401.

The annual reports of the Sanitary Bureau and of the Bureau of Statistics are a source

here represented I shall be content with citing a few paragraphs from a recent book by Professor Warren S. Thompson.

There is a well-conducted movement for the propagation of birth control already in existence in Japan, and, judging from what has happened in the Western world, this movement will grow and will be recognized in time as the only satisfactory method of offsetting the effects of the saving of life by modern sanitation and medicine. This seems inevitable. Not for long can we have both uncontrolled births and controlled deaths. The two things cannot exist together for many decades in any particular country or in the world at large. This proposition is axiomatic.

But even if birth control is the ultimate solution of the problem of population pressure in Japan, it does not follow that it will become sufficiently general to relieve this pressure in time to prevent an expansive movement on the part of Japan. [These are prophetic words at a time when Japan is seeking expansion through force of arms in Asia.] There is a very strong traditional opposition to birth control in Japan. We are not speaking here of authoritarian opposition; this exists also, as in many other countries, but in Japan the whole social organization centres in the family to a degree that is difficult for us in the West to realize. Consequently such a movement meets a passive resistance in the attitude of mind of the people at large which it has never encountered in the West. Among us the development of industrialism has led to the breaking down of family ties to a very great extent. Each individual has come to be looked upon as a separate unit in the social organization, responsible, not to the family, but only to the nation or state. Almost inevitably this produces a state of mind in which the pleasure and welfare of the individual become the chief concern of each. There is now with us but little feeling of belonging so intimately to a family group that our first and paramount duty is to this group. This strong feeling of family allegiance had been thoroughly dissipated among us before birth control became generally known or before there was any urgent need of its practice. Hence its practice among us never involved any feeling of disloyalty to the welfare of the family or of the nation.

In Japan, on the other hand, the practice of birth control cannot be expected to make rapid headway. There is no doubt that this movement is under way now, but it will not attain the development it has among us for some decades, perhaps several generations.[62]

---

quite untapped by Westerners. See also the Reports of the Commission on Population, Tokyo, 1930, (Japanese).

In view of recent events in the political relations between Japan and China the following, written in 1927, is of interest: S. Washio, "Imperialism or Birth Control?" *Trans-Pacific*, April 4, 1927.

[62] Warren S. Thompson, *Danger Spots of World Population* (1929), pp. 33–35. *Cf.*, the papers and book of John Orchard, and É. Dennery on "La Surpopulation Japonaise," *Ann. de Géog.*, xxxviii (1929), 148–168.

For further information on recent developments on birth control in Japan, which it is no object of this volume to consider in detail, see *Jour. Amer. Med. Asso.*, lxxxi (1923), 588; xcv (1930), 877. Edgar and Sanger in *Medical Times*, li (1923), 73–74; 77. Harold G. Moulton, with collaboration of Junichi Ko, *Japan. An Economic and Financial Appraisal*. Washington: Brookings Institution, 1931. John Orchard, *Japan's Economic*

§4 SUMMARY

The history of anti-conceptional technique in the Oriental countries has been considered as a unit because of certain cultural similarities which bind India, China and Japan. On account of the fragmentary nature of the reports available it has been necessary to present the evidence on various practices without full consideration of their time sequence. The antiquity of some of the Chinese and Sanskrit texts and the age of certain practices are often obscure. None the less, it is clear that even in Oriental cultures, which have stressed family solidarity and ancestor worship rather than scrambling, self-maximizing individualism, the *desire* for prevention is old. So likewise are some of the techniques.

As might have been expected in the early period of our era, magical procedures hold the center of the stage. Only the most rational of the Oriental practices will be reviewed here.

The early Chinese prescriptions consisted largely of potions. But here again the universality and antiquity of the desire for prevention is demonstrated. The Chinese potions are too technical usefully to recapitulate them here; so we shall merely recall the existence of eunuchism (intent other than contraceptive) and the influence of the Oriental mental outlook, institutional set-up and social organization in retarding the development of contraceptive medicine. The future is not bright for rapid development inasmuch as China's industrial future has probably been overestimated in many quarters.

The techniques culled from Sanskrit sources are summarized in the text. Omitting the potions and rites mentioned, it is interesting to note the antiquity of certain superstitions still held by ignorant European women: that passiveness in coitus or holding the breath will prevent conception.

More rational East Indian techniques are smearing the vagina with honey and oil, or vaginal medication with rock salt and oil. Tampons are also impregnated with these. Recall that salt is very highly spermicidal. Ghee (butter clarified by boiling) is also mentioned. This is cheap, available, and probably quite reliable. Here, in short, were good measures. But for every such technique, many magical recipes[63] were in circulation.

Position. New York: McGraw-Hill, 1930. One of the best recent works is E. F. Penrose, *Population Theories and their Application with Special Reference to Japan.* Stanford University, Calif.: Food Research Inst., 1934, pp. xiv, 347. The Japanese newspapers and magazines have lately devoted considerable space to birth control.

For a brief account on China see Agnes Smedley, "Birth Control Work in China" in Sanger & Stone, *Practice of Contraception*, pp. 283–284.

[63] Six out of twenty-six of the Sanskrit recipes, to be exact.

Thus the ineffective nullified the effective.　For who was there to guide an ignorant populace in such matters?

In Japan rational procedures are, according to our fragmentary reports, more common than in China.　The hard glans condom (tortoise shell or horn) is mentioned, as is one of leather.　The rubber sheath seems to have been introduced about 1880.　More sensible than potions is the practice of some prostitutes who place before the os a disk of oiled tissue paper made of bamboo.　This is one of the few Oriental tampons reported.　We have noted a few from the Sanskrit literature.　*Coitus reservatus* again appears, as does artificial retroflexion of the uterus (*cf.*, Chapter I).　As in all other cultures, decoctions and rites are not absent.

It is evident from this account that advance in contraceptive medicine has been less rapid in the East than in the West, especially among Greek writers.　Perhaps an intermediate position was occupied in the Middle Ages by the Islamic writers.　To them attention will be directed in the next chapter.

PART FOUR

TECHNIQUE IN THE WEST DURING THE MIDDLE AGES AND EARLY MODERN TIMES

CHAPTER VI

THE ISLAMIC WORLD AND EUROPE DURING THE MIDDLE AGES

§1 INTRODUCTION

THE influence of Greek culture upon Islamic civilization is well known. This is no less true of medicine, and of that branch of it known as contraception. While the work of Islamic physicians on conception control is not as brilliant as that of Soranos or Aëtios, it is, none the less, work of distinction. Their techniques were, considering the small accumulation of medical knowledge in those days, often reasonable and more or less workable. To be sure, one finds mention of amulets and medicines to be taken by the mouth. And it is doubtless true that Islamic techniques were inferior to ours, but that is hardly a fair basis of comparison. Viewing them as a whole, they were sounder in theory than most of the notions current in the Christian world of the time. One needs only to compare the recipes of 'Ali ibn 'Abbās or Ibn Sīnā (Avicenna), or even the recipes of Ibn al-Baiṭār with those in the apocryphal works of Albert the Great, Arnold of Villanova and Constantine the African to see a marked deterioration.

One cannot understand the development of contraceptive medicine in the Middle Ages without devoting at least passing attention to the views of the Catholic Church. Though St. Thomas contributed nothing to contraceptive technique, his philosophical views became incorporated in the general body of Catholic theology and doctrine; and they have profoundly influenced the position of religious writers, Catholic and Protestant, from that day to this.

On the contrary, the attention which the greatest medical writers of the Islamic world gave to contraceptive technique and indications seems extraordinary—extraordinary, that is, in comparison with the conception frequently met with even in informed circles regarding the knowledge of these peoples of contraception. It is not extraordinary in the sense that the amount of material on contraception is not great in the old *scientific* Arabic literature.[1] In bygone ages such instruction was largely, and still is, in the hands of midwives. But, on the other hand, medical treatises are not

---

[1] This is the opinion of Dr. Max Meyerhof, the great Arabic scholar of Cairo, expressed in a personal letter dated December 13, 1932.

without fairly elaborate accounts of technique.   Meyerhof is authority for the statement that *popular* contraceptive remedies are innumerable in the lands of Islam.   They are so numerous according to him that it would be quite impossible to furnish even a superficial survey of such methods without several years of research in many lands, and moreover, on many hundreds of Arabic medical manuscripts dispersed in libraries throughout the world.   Since no such undertaking is at present possible, attention in §2 is confined to five works: (1) A tenth century treatise by Al-Rāzī, *Quintessence of Experience*, (2) another tenth century Persian treatise in Arabic, *The Royal Book* of 'Ali ibn 'Abbās, (3) the *Canon* of Ibn Sīnā (980–1037), (4) *The Treasure of the King of Khwārazm* by Ismā 'īl al-Jurjānī (d. 1135–36), a Persian physician; (5) *The Book of Right Conduct* of Ibn al-Jamī.́ In §3 under the decline of Islamic medicine we take up the *Treatise on Simples* of Ibn al-Baiṭār (1197?–1248), and Dāwūd al- Antākī's, *The Memorial*.

Thus the practice of contraception was a cultural element present in Arabian or Islamic civilization just as it was characteristic of many primitive cultures, and the civilizations of the Egyptians, the ancient Hebrews, Greeks, Romans, the ancient Chinese, Indians, etc.

Islamic religious law differs fundamentally from Christianity in its attitude toward the employment of anti-conceptional measures.   In Islam the foetus is not considered a human being until it has reached a distinctly human form; hence abortion is not forbidden.   Still less forbidden are anti-conceptional measures of which the most frequent, mentioned even in the earliest traditions of the Prophet, is *coitus interruptus* (*'azl*).   The reason Islam does not consider such conduct sinful lies in the fatalism which characterizes the religious outlook.   For Allah creates children against the will of the parents.

In an article in the *Encyclopedia of Islam* (iv, 1014) by Professor Joseph Schacht on *Umm al-Walad* (literally: "the mother of the child," a technical term in Islamic law meaning "a slave-girl who has borne her master a child") we read the following:

> In order to prevent the birth of a child the practice of *'azl* was frequent in intercourse with slave-girls, and it is therefore often discussed in connection with the *Umm al-Walad*.   The most important of the references in tradition on this subject have been collected by Wensinck, *Handbook of Early Muhammadan Tradition*, s.v. *intercourse*; here it is sufficient to say that *'azl* was considered to be permitted with slave-girls.

From the above we see that *coitus interruptus* is very old in Islamic lands and that anti-conceptional measures were not in any sense condemned by Islamic religious law as they were by Christianity until very recent times.

The texts of various treatises show that the physicians of Islam did not neglect, even in the Middle Ages, anti-conceptional preventive medicine.

§2 THE RISE AND FLOWERING OF ISLAMIC CONTRACEPTIVE MEDICINE

(2a) Al-Rāzī (Rhazes), Quintessence of Experience (X-2)

I shall begin the chronological presentation of Islamic texts on contraceptive medicine with the account in al-Rāzī (Latin: Rhazes), *Khulāsat-al-Tajārib* or *Quintessence of Experience*. The Persian physician Abū Bakr Muḥammed ibn Zakarīyā al-Rāzī, born in Ray, near Teheran, Persia, about the middle of the ninth century, and who flourished in Ray and Bagdad (d. 923–924), was the greatest clinician of Islam, in fact the greatest physician of the Middle Ages.[2] Sarton says that Rhazes "combined with his immense learning true Hippocratic wisdom." He made many contributions to gynecology, obstetrics, and opthalmic surgery, compiled several encyclopedic works, the best known being his *Kitāb al-Ḥāwī (Continens)*.[3] He was the author of a famous treatise on measles and smallpox, and applied chemistry to medicine more than many of his contemporaries. Al-Rāzī illustrates well a principle that constantly impresses itself on the investigator as he studies the history of contraceptive medicine: It was the great physicians of all time who thought contraception worthy of discussion and analysis; who held it to be a legitimate part of medical practice; who left for the modern small-fry the idea that it was obscene.

We now turn to Rhazes' text in the *Quintessence of Experience*:

Chapter 24. On the Organs of Generation and the Breasts, Their Anatomy and Uses: On the Various Temperaments of the Uterus: On Diseases Peculiar to Women, Their Symptoms, Signs, and Treatment: On the Diagnosis of Pregnancy and its Management: And on the Means of Preventing Conception.

Occasionally it is very important that the semen should not enter the womb, as for instance when there is danger to the woman in pregnancy, or, if it has entered, that it should come out again. There are several ways of preventing its entrance. The first is that at the time of ejaculation the man withdraw from the woman so that the semen does not approach the os uteri. The second way is to prevent ejaculation, a method practiced by some. A third method is to apply to the os uteri before introgression some drug which blocks the uterine aperture or which expels the semen and prevents conception, such as pills or pessaries [we would now say, more accurately, suppositories] of cabbage, colocynth pulp, bryony, ?, iron scoria, ?, tamarisk dew [gum?], pitch, ox gall, inner skin of a pomegranate, animals' ear wax, the ? of a mulberry bush, elephant's dung, scammony, and whitewash. These may be used alone or in combination.

---

[2] George Sarton, *Introduction to the History of Science* (Baltimore: Williams & Wilkins, 1927–31. 2 vols. Pub. for the Carnegie Inst. of Wash.), i, 609. William C. D. Dampier-Whetham, *A History of Science and its Relations with Philosophy and Religion* (New York: Macmillan, 1930), p. 81.

[3] This has never been published. There is not even a complete MS. text in existence; but there are partial Latin translations.

Again, the expulsion of semen from the uterus may be effected in several ways. Firstly, immediately after ejaculation, let the two come apart and let the woman arise roughly, sneeze and blow her nose several times, and call out in a loud voice. She should jump violently backwards 7 to 9 paces. Secondly, there are drugs which can be applied to the womb for this purpose, such as sal ammoniac, sugar candy, potash (reading qulya, though my ms. has qulyab = amulets), bamboo concretions, ?, and other similar drugs which bring on the menses. In some cases pills of the above drugs have the same property. Thirdly, the woman may sit upon the tips of her toes and squeeze and rub her navel with her thumb. She may smell foul odors or fumigate her under parts, as has been described in the section on "Hurrying on Labour."[3a] Or she may take by the mouth some labefacient drug.

If these methods do not succeed and the semen has become lodged, there is no help for it but that she insert into her womb a probe or a stick cut into the shape of a probe, especially good being the root of the mallow. One end of the probe should be made fast to the thigh with a thread that it may go in no further. Leave it there all night, often all day as well. Use no force: do not hurry: and do not repeat the operation or you will cause pain. Wait thus for one or two weeks until gradually the menses appear and the whole thing will slowly become open and clean. Some people screw paper up tight in the shape of a probe and after binding it securely with silk smear over it ginger dissolved in water. They leave this to dry and then insert it into the uterus. If one is unsuccessful, they take it out and insert another, until the menses do appear and the woman is cleansed. This procedure causes no harm. But if the paper is passed too high up, the woman is not cleansed because it rapidly grows soft and comes out again. There is no better operation than this.

The use of drugs both internally and externally is often successful. While the uterus is being watched, the patient should guard herself against cold and should not eat any dishes containing things which are astringent and bitter nor cold things, cold water, melons, peaches, wind-causing foods, and ?. She should go to the hot bath every other day. She should massage the abdomen and uterus with soft infusions and oils and eat soft dishes which are aperient and solvent, such as soups containing eggs and broth of onions, leeks, mallows, and saffron, and animals' tails with fat of fowls, oil of almonds, and so forth, and the flesh of young fowls and their feet. She should indulge in violent movements and vigorous sexual intercourse. Joking too is useful.[4]

[3a] See page 119 for reference in an eighth century Sanskrit source to fumigations as a contraceptive. The patient was instructed to sit over the spout of a kettle in which *Neem* wood is burned. I am very reliably informed that to this very day a similar pattern of conduct exists for the same purposes among certain Jews of the lower East Side of New York City. A midwife prescribes that the women sit over a pot of hot stewed onions, believing that the fumes will be effective in inducing an early abortion or return of the menstrual flow. Here we find the persistence of a cultural pattern over eleven centuries. The span is not to be compared, however, with that existing for suppositories of animal's dung, elephant and crocodile especially; nor with the persistence of potions made of smithy's fire-bucket water, and certainly not with the continuity and antiquity of *coitus interruptus*.

[4] I am indebted to Dr. Cyril Elgood of Wareham, Dorset, England, for this translation.

All told, there are approximately twenty-four different prescriptions in the above text, omitting, of course, abortion. On the whole, the numerical emphasis is upon suppositories of which there are fifteen. But magical numbers (jumping backwards seven or nine times) and drugs to be taken by the mouth appear. The prevention of ejaculation doubtless refers to finger pressure at the base of the phallus. Fumigations and squeezing and rubbing the navel while squatting seem primitive and savor of the Oriental influence. Considered as a unit, however, Rhazes' text is a good account for the tenth century; but inferior to the texts of Soranos and Aëtios in my judgment.

(2b) ʻAlī ibn ʻAbbās, The Royal Book (X-2)

During the second half of the tenth century the Persian physician ʻAlī ibn ʻAbbās al-Majūsī (d. about 994 A.D.) produced a treatise called Kāmil aṣ-Ṣināʻa⁵ (The Perfection of the Art) or The Royal Book (Liber regius). ʻAlī ibn ʻAbbās was born in Ahwāz in southwestern Persia, flourished under the Buwayhid ʻAḍud al-Dawla and died in 994. He is considered "one of the three greatest physicians of the Eastern Caliphate."⁶ His medical encyclopedia is more systematic and concise than Rāzī's Ḥāwī, but more practical than Avicenna's Qānūn (Canon) quoted below, by which it was superseded. The work is divided into twenty discourses, one of the best portions being on materia medica.

In an Arabic text of The Royal Book one finds the following passage on contraception:

Chapter 28. On That Which Prevents Conception

As to the remedies which prevent conception, although it ought to be a duty not to mention them [in this treatise] in order that they might not be used by certain ill-famed women, it is nevertheless indispensable to administer them to those women who have a small uterus, or to those suffering from a disease which would render gravidity so dangerous that the patient might die during parturition. Except for women in such predicaments the physician should never impart contraceptive information to women, nor should he ever prescribe remedies calculated to suppress the menses, nor remedies for causing abortion, except to trustworthy women [sic], inasmuch as all these remedies kill the embryo and expel it.

Conception will be prevented if women insert rock salt⁷ (milḥ andarānī) [in the vagina] during coitus, or induce the man to anoint his penis with the same material,

---

⁵ Sarton, op. cit., i, 677. Sarton gives other versions of the title as (1) Kitāb al-Malikī (2) Kāmil al-Ṣanāʻa al-Ṭibbīya.

⁶ Ibid., i, 677.

⁷ Ordinary modern table salt is an excellent spermicide. An 8 per cent solution kills sperms rapidly. As used in our time five tablespoonfuls are dissolved in a quart of water; or half a teaspoonful to a vaginal bulbful.

or with tar; or if a woman inserts the flowers and seeds of cabbage (*kurunb*) and the juice of rue (*sadhāb*) during or after coitus; or carries [in her vagina] the rennet of rabbit or the leaves or fruits of the weeping-willow (*gharab*).[8]

Noteworthy in the above passage is the sensitivity of 'Alī ibn 'Abbās to the possibility of misuse of contraceptive knowledge by those of promiscuous habits or intent and more especially by midwives, who are always the advisers of Oriental women.   He would have the physician exercise prudence in disseminating such information; and there is here something of the implication that imparting such skill should be in the hands of the medical profession.   These views would undoubtedly be approved by the over-

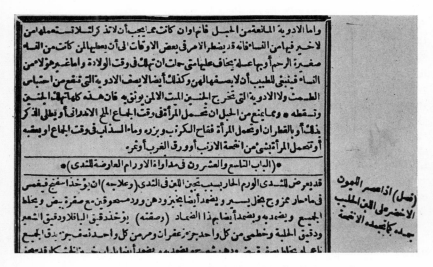

FIG. V. 'Ali ibn 'Abbās, Kitāb al-Malikī (Vol. ii, p. 440)

whelming proportion of American physicians in our time and quite probably by most of their European colleagues.

The passage is noteworthy also not only for the rather high level of recipes, —they are less complete than those of Ibn Sīnā (mentioned below)—but for the emphasis on medical indications.   These are conservative—for health only.   It may be observed parenthetically, that the discussion of indications is rare in the early literature on contraception; and I cannot remember hav-

---

[8] Ed. of Arabic text: Cairo-Būlāq, 1294, Hedjrae, ii, 439 ff.   For the translation of this text and that of the following one I am indebted to Dr. Max Meyerhof, M.D., Ph.D. of Cairo who searched them out.   Dr. Meyerhof requested that I smooth the English of his clear translation; and this has been done.

ing met with an *economic* indication prior to J. Bentham's advocacy (1797) of the sponge to reduce the English poor rates (see *Economic Jour. Hist. Supp.*, January, 1936) and the Mill-Place propaganda (1823–25). Techniques far outnumber indications in all the early literature.

There is an emphasis in *The Royal Book* upon the preventive point of view which is altogether admirable: imparting contraceptive information is indispensable if gravidity is likely to endanger the life of the woman during parturition. It seems reasonable to infer that this Persian physician would not have thought highly of those among his modern followers who repeatedly abort women without instructing them in contraceptive technique even in the presence of weighty indications. Would 'Ali ibn 'Abbās have considered such conduct malpractice?

Regarding the effectiveness of the methods mentioned, the rock salt and tar seem most likely to succeed; the seeds or flowers of cabbage with rue juice would seem less likely to achieve their purpose; while the amulet is, of course, worthless, save in promoting peace of mind.

Even more elaborate and complete than these recipes are those of Ibn Sīnā (Avicenna).

(2c) Ibn Sīnā, Qānūn (Canon of Avicenna) (XI-1)

Abū 'Alī al-Ḥusain ibn 'Abdallah ibn Sīnā, more briefly known as Ibn Sīnā (Hebrew, Aven Sina; Latin, Avicenna) was born near Bukhārā in 980 and died in Hamadhān in West Africa in 1037 where his tomb is still held in veneration. Ibn Sīnā was not only an encyclopedist, philosopher, physician, mathematician and astronomer; he was "the most famous scientist of Islām and one of the most famous of all races, places and times; one may say that his thought represents the climax of mediaeval philosophy."[9] There can be no doubt about Ibn Sīnā's erudition, wisdom, versatility, originality and insight in many fields of knowledge—fields now sharply demarcated. The work which interests us most is the *Qānūn fi'ṭ-Tibb*, or *Canon*, well known under the Latin title *Canon Avicennae*. This enormous medical encyclopedia, containing about a million words, is "a codification of the whole of ancient and Muslim knowledge."[10] "Because of its formal perfection as well as its intrinsic value, the *Qānūn* superseded Rāzī's *Ḥāwi*, 'Ali ibn 'Abbās's *Malikī* [i.e., *The Royal Book*], and even the works of Galen, and remained supreme for six centuries."[11] So great were Ibn Sīnā's encyclopedic efforts in reporting facts in diverse fields of learning and theorizing about them that his very originality was dwarfed. So thorough was the

[9] Sarton, *op. cit.*, i, 709.

[10] *Ibid.*, i, 710.

[11] *Ibid.* Some italics mine.

acceptance of the work that it stifled original investigation and sterilized intellectual life.   It is not too much to say that his authority approached that of Aristotle; he was at once oracle and magician.

This great scholar, like many notable figures before him, considered the prevention of conception a legitimate part of medical practice.   This is well demonstrated in the first paragraph quoted below.

Ibn Sīnā's account of contraceptive technique is excellent for the period, perhaps second only to that of Soranos and Aëtios before him, to either or both of whom he was evidently indebted.   Clearly his techniques exceed in rationality those of many later writers.   The following passages from the *Qānūn* are of considerable historical importance:

[Chapter] On the Prevention of Conception[12]

The physician is sometimes obliged to prevent pregnancy in a small woman to whom childbirth would be dangerous, or in women who are suffering from a disease of the uterus or from a weakness of the bladder; . . .

Among the prescriptions for the prevention of conception are the following: [1] Avoid the form [time?] of coition which favors conception, and which we have already mentioned.   Moreover, [2] the partners should avoid simultaneous ejaculations [orgasms].   [3] Quick separation of the two individuals [that is withdrawal just before the male orgasm].   [4] The woman should rise at the end of coitus and jump backward seven or nine times [magical numbers].   In this way the sperm may conceivably come out.   Jumping and leaping forward causes the sperm to remain [in the female genital tract].   [5] Another way to void the sperm is to provoke sneezing.   [6] The woman must also be careful to smear tar in the vagina [both] before and after coitus and [7] to anoint the penis [of the man] with it, or else [8] anoint it with balm oil and white lead (*isfīdāj*).   Another recipe is [9] for a woman to insert [intravaginally] before and after [coitus] the pulp of pomegranates with alum, or [10] she can insert the flowers and seeds of cabbage[13] during the period of purity[14] [i.e., after menstruation].   The use of the latter before and after coitus is also an efficacious means for the same purpose, especially if [11] mixed with tar, or dipped into a decoction of the juice of pennyroyal (*fūtanaj*).   [12] Inserting intravaginally the leaves of the weeping-willow after the purity in a flock of wool [will make an effective contraceptive], especially [13] if dipped in the juice of weeping-willow.   The same [objective] is obtained by [14]

[12] This chapter is not in the Hebrew translation.

[13] Oribasios mentioned cabbage in the fourth century.

[14] It is interesting to observe that Ibn Sīnā points out that many of these pessaries or plugs are to be inserted *after* the purity begins.   Presumably coitus was relatively rare during menstruation inasmuch as it was, and still is, strictly forbidden by the Islamic and Jewish religions.   Perhaps the women went about with these pessaries for days at a time. If this was not cleanly, the women were at least always prepared for preventive coitus.   In a partial sense there is an implication in the instructions here similar to those of some modern physicians who advise a woman to insert a rubber vaginal diaphragm or cervical cap *each* evening as a regular part of her toilet.   She is then more likely, perhaps, to become psychologically adjusted to the procedure.

[a pessary composed of] equal parts of pulp of colocynth (*ḥanẓal*), mandrake (*hazārjushān*[15]), iron-dross, sulphur, scammony, and cabbage-seeds, collected, mixed with tar, and inserted [literally "worn"]. [15] Inserting pepper after coitus likewise prevents conception, and so does [16] [insertion of] elephant's dung alone, or [17] in fumigations at the times mentioned previously. It is also useful [18] to drink three *okas* [pints] of an infusion of sweet-basil (*bādrūj*)[16] [for] it prevents

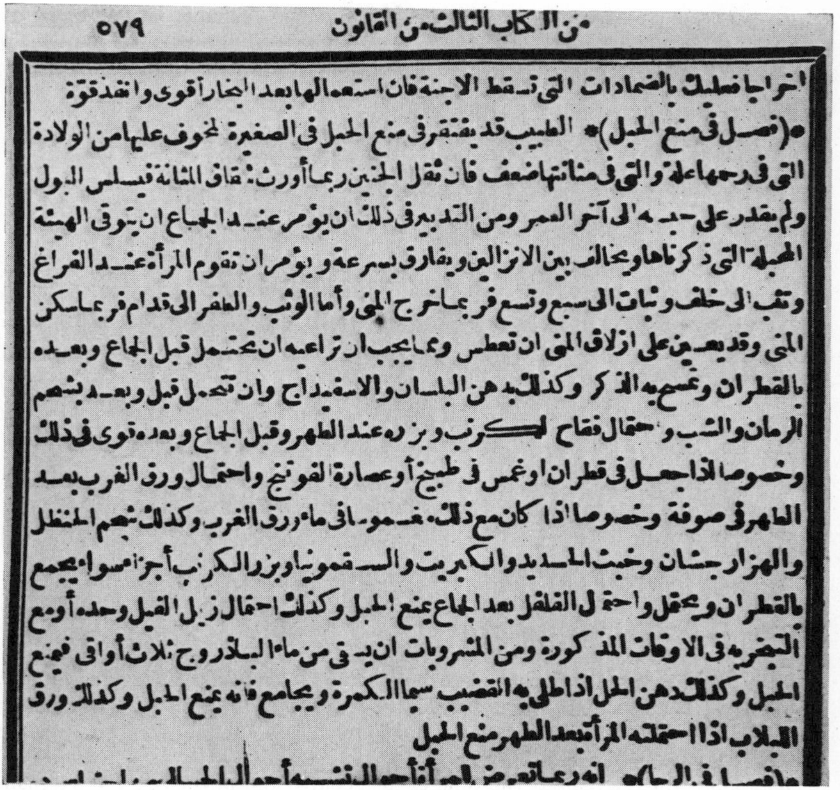

٥٧٩ من الكتاب الثالث من القانون

اخراجا فعليك بالضمادات التي تسقط الاجنة فان استعمالها بعد ايجار اقوى وانفذ قوة

(فصل في منع الحبل) الطبيب قد يفتقر في منع الحبل في الصغيرة يخوف عليها من الولادة

التي في رحمها علة والتي في مثانتها ضعف فان ثقل الجنين ربما أورث انشقاق المثانة فيسلس البول

ولم يقدر على حبسه الى آخر العمر ومن التدبير في ذلك ان يؤمر عند الجماع ان يتوقى الهيئة

المحبلة التي ذكرناها ويخالف بين الانزالين ويفارق بسرعة ويؤمر ان تقوم المرأة عند الفراغ

وتثب الى خلف وثبات الى سبع وتسع فربما خرج المني وأما الوثب والطفر الى قدام فربما سكن

المني وقد يعين على ازلاق المني ان تعطس ومما يجب ان تراعيه ان تحتمل قبل الجماع وبعده

بالقطران وتمسح به الذكر وكذلك بدهن البلسان والاسفيداج وان تحتمل قبل وبعد بشحم

الرمان والشب واحتمال فقاح الكرنب وبزره عند الطهر وقبل الجماع وبعده قوي في ذلك

وخصوصا اذا جعل في قطران او غمس في طبيخ أو عصارة الفوتنج واحتمال ورق الغرب بعد

الطهر في صوفة وخصوصا اذا كان مع ذلك مغموسا في ماء ورق الغرب وكذلك شحم الحنظل

والهزارجشان وخبث الحديد والكبريت والسقمونيا وبزر الكرنب أجزاء سواء يجمع

بالقطران ويحمل واحتمال الفلفل بعد الجماع يمنع الحبل وكذلك احتمال زبل الفيل وحده أو مع

التبخر به في الاوقات المذكورة ومن المشروبات ان يسقى من ماء البادروج ثلاث أواقي فيمنع

الحبل وكذلك دهن الحل اذا طلي به القضيب سيما الكمرة ويجامع فانه يمنع الحبل وكذلك ورق

اللبلاب اذا احتملته المرأة بعد الطهر منع الحبل

FIG. VI. Ibn Sīnā, *Qānūn* (Būlāq edition) (Vol. ii, p. 579)

conception. [19] If the penis, particularly the glans, is anointed with sweet oil before coitus, conception is prevented. [20] Likewise the leaves of bindweed (*lablāb*) prevents conception if women insert them after their purity [begins].[17]

[15] This Persian word appears in the Arabic text. Other equally Persian drug names which appear frequently in Arabic forms are *isfîdaj* and *fūtanaj* as mentioned above.

[16] This Persian word appears in the Arabic text; *vide supra*.

[17] *Qānūn fi'ṭ-Ṭibb* (*Canon Avicennae*). Translated especially for this work by Dr. Max Meyerhof from the Arabic text: Cairo-Būlāq, 1924; 1877, ii, 579.

Here again we find one of the greatest figures in Arabic medicine devoting attention to contraceptive technique and its medical indications. Twenty recipes may be distinguished. If the indications seem fragmentary, it may be pointed out that they have not been, even in our day, completely worked out. Ibn Sīnā was in advance of many modern physicians in recognizing the legitimacy of any medical indications whatsoever. The other marked features of the passage are the evident influence of either Soranos or Aëtios or both, the inherent reasonableness and workability of the recipes and the relative absence of magical procedures.

Approximately a century after 'Alī ibn 'Abbās and Ibn Sīnā there appeared a Persian physician of great importance in the history of contraceptive medicine.

(2d) Ismā'īl al-Jurjānī, Treasure of Medicine (XII-1)

Zain al-dīn Abu-l-Fadā'il Ismā'īl ibn al-Husain al-Jurjānī, more briefly Ismā'īl al-Jurjānī (i.e., of Jurjan),[18] sometimes referred to as Sayyid Ismā'īl, was a great Persian physician of the first half of the twelfth century (d. 1135–36). He lived at the court of Khwārazm,[19] and wrote in Persian and Arabic. His *Dhakhīra-i-Khwārazmshāhī*, or *Treasure of Medicine Dedicated to the King of Khwārazm*, was probably the first medical encyclopedia written in Persian instead of Arabic, and was completed shortly after 1110. It is, like Avicenna's *Canon*, a work of enormous bulk containing nearly a quarter million words, being divided into nine books (75 discourses, 1107 chapters).[20] The work is still unpublished. Accordingly, I am indebted to Dr. Cyril Elgood of Wareham, Dorset, England, for the following translation into English of the contraceptive passages. Dr. Elgood's manuscript is in Persian.[21]

Whenever a woman is of tender years, or suffers from weakness of the bladder; or whenever there is a fear that pregnancy will bring on some ailment such as incontinence of urine, uterine erosions, and so forth, it is thought good to use some plan to prevent pregnancy.

One plan is for the man at the time of intercourse and of the seminal emission to abstain from holding the woman close to himself, to raise her thighs, and rapidly to come apart from her. They should try to avoid the orgasm being simultaneous. When the male does come apart from her, he should order her to have a good shake

---

[18] Jurjan is the ancient Hyrcania on the southeast coast of the Caspian Sea.

[19] Now Khiva (Turkestan, Russian territory).

[20] For an analysis of the contents see E. G. Browne, *Arabian Medicine* (1921), pp. 110–112.

[21] Sarton says (*op. cit.*, ii, 235) that the *Dhakhīra* was translated in abbreviated form into Hebrew by an anonymous author. Sarton adds that this is remarkable inasmuch as there are practically no other translations of medical writings from Persian into Hebrew.

seven times.[22]   When they get up, he should again try to make her expel the semen. For this he should cause her to sneeze.

If the man at the time of intercourse moistens his glans penis with oil of sesame, his semen will not stick within the vulva, but will slip out again.   If he anoints himself with oil of balsam or with tar or with ceruse, conception will not take place. Let the woman eat flower of cabbage and its seeds mixed together after purity and before sexual intercourse.   If after this she elevates her thighs, conception will not ensue, above all if these are mixed with tar.[23]   To drink three ounces of the infusion of sweet basil will also prevent pregnancy.

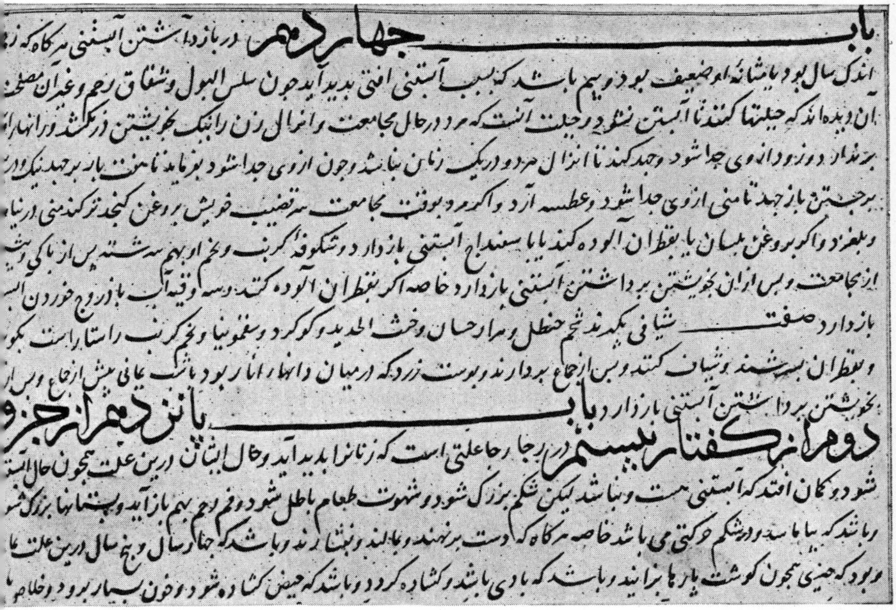

FIG. VII. Isma 'īl al-Jurjani, *Treasure of Medicine*, (c. 1110 A.D.)

A Prescription for a Pessary.

Take colocynth pulp, bryony, iron scoria, sulphur, scammony, and cabbage seed; grind these up thoroughly and mix with tar.   Make into a vaginal pessary. Insert one after intercourse.

Mix, too, the yellow pulp which lies between the pips of a pomegranate, with

[22] "This would appear to be the meaning," says Elgood.   "Literally translated the sentence runs: 'Let him command seven times to a good exertion.'   Possibly the MS. is corrupt."   Seven is a magical number.

[23] In these two sentences the text may be corrupt.   I believe the intention is not that the leaves of cabbage should be eaten, but rather ground and mixed with tar; then used as suppositories.   So reads the corresponding passage in the *Canon*.   Since this is my interpretation of the meaning, the prescription is classified accordingly below.

alum, and insert this before intercourse.   If after these measures a woman raises her thighs,[24] pregnancy will not follow.[25]

It will be seen that many of these prescriptions date back to Soranos. Seven are like those of Ibn Sīnā; six are not mentioned by Ibn Sīnā.   Oribasios had mentioned cabbage leaves; but they were to be taken by the mouth. 'Ali ibn 'Abbās mentioned cabbage flowers and seeds; but they were to be used in his prescription with the juice of rue presumably as a vaginal plug.

(2e)   Ibn al-Jamī', The Book of Right Conduct (XII-2)

This work, if not as distinguished in the history of contraceptive medicine as some of its predecessors, nevertheless deserves a definite place in the history of contraception.   But the account is shorter than that in the *Canon*. Ibn al-Jamī' was a Jewish, Egyptian physician, at one time physician in ordinary to Sultan Saladin (1171–1193).   His work, *The Book of Right Conduct Regarding the Supervision of the Soul and Body*[26] exists only in Arabic manuscript.   From this medical encyclopedia, the following contraceptive recipes are extracted:

Anti-conceptional means: Anointing the penis before copulation with the expressed juice of onion will prevent conception.   Likewise conception will be prevented if a woman inserts after purification a tampon impregnated with peppermint-juice (*na' nā'*), pennyroyal (*fūtanaj*), or the seeds of leek (*kurrāth*); for this [impregnated tampon] has a particular anti-conceptional effect.   Moreover, a woman may insert pessaries (*farāzikh*) made from myrrh (*murr*), opopanax (*jāwshīr*), rue (*sadhāb*) and hellebore (*kharbaq*) kneaded with ox-gall.   It is said that if a woman will eat beans on an empty stomach, she will not become pregnant; and that the same result will be obtained if the man anoints his penis with any kind of oil.[27]

Though this account is brief, the recipes are, judged as a whole, on a high level of rationality and effectiveness; yet the eating of beans on an empty

[24] On the contrary, raising the thighs or buttocks on a pillow is the best possible position for the retention of semen, and is therefore conducive to impregnation.   For the anatomy of conception and contraception see Robert L. Dickinson, *Human Sex Anatomy: A Topographical Hand Atlas* (Baltimore: Williams & Wilkins, 1933), pp. 97, 98, and Figures 9 and 152.

[25] MS. of *Dhakhīra* in possession of Dr. Cyril Elgood.   Bk. vi, Section 20.2.14 (p. 917 of MS.).

[26] Sarton (*op. cit.*, ii, 86) translates the title as *Direction for the Improvement of Souls and Bodies*.   The title I have used is that translated by Dr. Max Meyerhof.   The *Irshād* was a general treatise on medicine.   Ibn al-Jamī' was the author also of a commentary on the fifth book of Ibn Sīnā's *Qānūn*, and of two essays reproduced by Ibn al-Baiṭār.

[27] Ibn al Jamī', Kitāb al-irshād li-maṣāliḥ al-anfās wa'l ajsād (*The Book of Right Conduct Regarding the Supervision of the Soul and Body*).   Translated by Dr. Max Meyerhof from the manuscript in the Egyptian Library in Cairo (No: Medicine 345).   This is a free but accurate translation.

stomach is worthy of no confidence. Had the recipe any validity, the population of Boston would have died out long ago!

(2f) Summary of Recipes and Indications

In the following summary and classification of the anti-conceptional techniques of four early Islamic physicians—I omit Rhazes' text since it

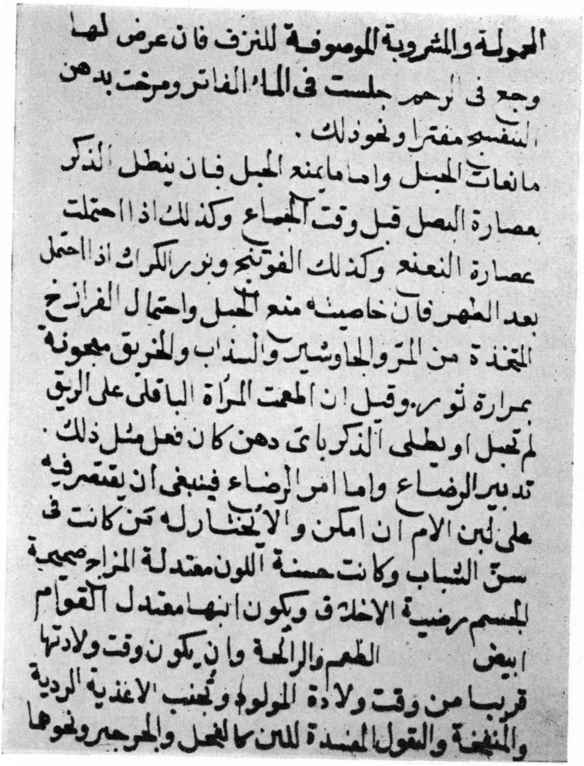

Fig. VIII. Ibn al-Jamiʻ, *Irshād* (Cairo MS., second copy, modern)

has some gaps—which classification is based upon the presumed rationality of the techniques, each technique is followed by a number indicating its source according to the following plan:

ʻAli ibn ʻAbbās (1)
Ibn Sīnā (2)
Ismāʻīl al-Jurjānī (3)
Ibn al-Jamiʻ (4)

This enables one to trace repetitions, similarities, and differences. It proved helpful to the writer also in indicating a probable corruption in the text of Ismā'īl al-Jurjānī's *Dhakhīra* or *Treasure*. The summary of the recipes of the four Islamic writers preceding Ibn al-Baiṭār, who represents the beginning of decline, is as follows:

(A) *Means to be taken by the mouth:*

An infusion of sweet basil [three pints (2); three ounces (3)]
Eating beans on an empty stomach (4)

(B) *Magical means:*

Rennet of rabbit or weeping-willow leaves or fruits worn as an amulet (1)

(C) *Suppositories and tampons:*

Rock salt (1)
Flowers and seeds of cabbage with rue juice (1)
Same without rue juice (2)
Suppository of cabbage leaves with tar or with pennyroyal juice (2, 3)
Pulp of pomegranates with alum (2)
Leaves of weeping-willow in flock of wool (2)
Equal parts of pulp of colocynth, mandrake [bryony], iron dross [or iron scoria], sulphur, scammony, and cabbage leaves, mixed with tar to form suppositories (2, 3)
Pepper (2)
Elephant's dung (alone or with fumigations) (2)
Leaves of bindweed (2)
Yellow pulp of pomegranate with alum as suppositories (3)
A tampon impregnated with peppermint-juice, pennyroyal, or the seeds of leek (4)
Suppositories made of myrrh, opopanax, rue and hellebore kneaded with ox-gall (4)

(D) *Techniques used by the man:*

Anointing the penis with
(a) Rock salt (1)
(b) Tar (1, 2, 3)
(c) Balm oil and white lead (2, 3?)
(d) Sweet oil (2)
(e) Any kind of oil (4)
(f) Expressed juice of onion (4)
(g) Oil of balsam (3)
(h) Oil of sesame (3)
Withdrawal (2, 3)

(E) *Miscellaneous techniques:*

Safe period ? (2)
Avoiding simultaneous orgasms (2, 3)
Bodily movements to void semen [e.g., jumping backward (2) or "shaking" (3)]
Provoking sneezing (2, 3)

Smearing tar in vagina (2)
Raising the thighs (3) [This is used after suppositories.]

This collection of techniques seems rather remarkable for so early a period. The rational element bulks large in them. Note, however, that in many instances the pessaries are to be inserted after coitus rather than before. This is contrary to modern practice. Still, they probably would have been effective in many instances even though used after coitus, especially in instances of frequent coitus.

Summarizing the fragmentary discussion of indications we may recall that they were confined to the medical; so far as present knowledge goes, economic and social indications did not appear until the writings of Bentham, Mill and Place. Regarding medical reasons 'Ali ibn 'Abbās (X cent.) mentioned a "small uterus" and any "disease which would render gravidity so dangerous that the patient might die during parturition." Ibn Sīnā (XI cent.) mentions "a small woman to whom childbirth would be dangerous, or . . . women who are suffering from a disease of the uterus or from a weakness of the bladder." Ismā'īl al-Jurjānī (XII cent.) mentions a woman of "tender years," also anyone suffering from "weakness of the bladder;" any case in which "there is fear that pregnancy will bring on some ailment such as incontinence of urine, uterine erosions, and so forth." The passage from Ibn al-Jamī' (XII cent.) contains no discussion of indications. If the indications cited are, from a modern standpoint, narrow, the authors deserve credit for emphasis upon the preventive point of view. In this respect the medieval writers mentioned are more in advance of some of their modern successors who permit theological biases to interfere with their proper functions as preservers and promoters of the public health.

Note also that the discussion of techniques occupies much more space than indications.

We now turn to a thirteenth century Arabic writer, Ibn al-Baiṭār, who, great as he was, represents the beginning of the decline of Islamic contraceptive medicine.

§3 THE DECLINE OF ISLAMIC CONTRACEPTIVE MEDICINE

(3a) Ibn al-Baiṭār, Treatise on Simples (XIII-1)

Diyā' al-dīn Abū Muḥammad 'Abdallāh ibn Aḥmad ibn al-Baiṭār al-Mālaqī, the great Arabic pharmacologist, the son of a veterinary—the name Ibn al-Baiṭār means son of a veterinary—was born toward the end of the twelfth century (1197?), and died in Damascus in 1248. He travelled widely throughout the Mediterranean basin on his botanical tours, was occasionally in the royal service, and made notable contributions to the botanical and pharmacological knowledge of his time.[28]   Sarton considers him the greatest botanist and herbalist that western Muslim produced; to Meyerhof he is essentially a compiler.   The latter is probably right.

Ibn al-Baiṭār's chief work is a *Treatise on Simples*, the Kitāb al-jāmi' fi-l-adwiya al mufrada;[29] it is hereinafter referred to either as the *Treatise* or the *Jāmi'*.   Sarton considers it "the foremost Arabic and mediaeval treatise of its kind, the greatest from the time of Dioscorides to the middle of the sixteenth century."[30]   However, Ibn al-Baiṭār's originality has been greatly exaggerated.   He is primarily a compiler,[31] and judging by his account of contraception, a compiler none too critical.[32]   The *Treatise* deals not only with simples but with various species of food.   Omitting duplications, some 1400 different items are considered; about 300, including some 200 plants, are novelties.   All these are methodically arranged, and some new observations added.   Virtually all of Dioscorides' and Galen's knowledge on materia medica and botany was incorporated in the *Jāmi'*; but many other authors were quoted, some 150 in all, among whom were twenty Greeks.   Since the middle of the tenth century Dioscorides had been diligently studied in Muslim Spain.[33]

The *Treatise* is available in a French translation by Lucien Leclerc[34] (used below) and in an inaccurate German translation by Sontheimer.[35]   A second great work by Ibn al-Baiṭār on simples, the *Mughnī*, arranged this time not alphabetically but therapeutically, is still unpublished.   It seems highly probable that, like the *Jāmi'*, it devoted attention to anti-conceptional techniques.   It has not been searched for this study.   Both the

---

[28] For an excellent biographical account, see George Sarton, *op. cit.*, ii, 663–4.

[29] Literally: *The Book of Collection about Simple Drugs*.

[30] Sarton, ii, 663.

[31] See the Introduction to M. Meyerhof & G. Sobhy, the abridged version of *The Book of Simple Drugs* of Aḥmad ibn Muhammad al-Ghāfiqī by Gregorius Abu'l-Faraj (Barhebraeus) (Faculty of Medicine Publ. No. 4), Cairo, 1932.

[32] Dr. Meyerhof is convinced that Ibn al-Baiṭār's reputation has been exaggerated, that he was, in fact, a scholar of mediocrity.   Dr. Meyerhof writes me that he is now translating a treatise on drug names by Maimonides copied by the very hand of Ibn al-Baiṭār, who was often unable to read correctly the names recorded by Maimonides.   Consequently he mutilated the text in an extraordinary manner.   Dr. Meyerhof adds that many Hispano-Arabic scholars of the XI and XII centuries were superior to Ibn al-Baiṭār.

[33] M. Meyerhof, *Die Materia Medica des Dioskurides bei den Arabern*.   In Wellman Festschrift.   Berlin, 1933.   *Cf.*, also Sarton, ii, 663.

[34] *Traité des Simples*, in *Notices et Extraits de la Bibliothèque Nationale et autres Bibliothèques*, published by l'Institut National de France, Part I = vol. 23 (1877); Part II = vol. 25 (1881); Part III = vol. 26 (1883).   Paris.

[35] Abu Mohammed Abdullah ben Ahmed, *Grosse Zusammenstellung über die Kräfte der bekannten einfachen Heil- und Nahrungsmittel.   Bekannt unter dem Namen Ebn Baithar.   Aus den Arabischen übersetzt von Joseph v. Sontheimer*.   Stuttgart, 1840–42, 2 vols.

Jāmi' and the *Mughnī* were completed in that order in the fifth decade of the thirteenth century.

Sarton believes that the influence of Ibn al-Baiṭār's *Treatise* "was not at all commensurate with its real importance" because it "appeared too late."[36] But such a statement doubtless under-estimates the value of the work of Ibn al-Baiṭār's predecessors. The *Jāmi'* was practically untranslated until the nineteenth century.

The Leclerc edition of the *Treatise*, from which the anti-conceptional techniques below have been extracted and translated, comprises three large tomes of approximately fifteen hundred printed pages. Among a mass of recipes for the cure of all sorts of illnesses, for the procuring of abortion, for increasing sexual pleasure both in the male and the female, are to be found a score or more recipes. The six which immediately follow have come down from Dioscorides:

It is said that the rennet of earthly hare, taken for the three days which follow the period, will cause a woman to become sterile.[37]

The root of barrenwort taken internally will prevent conception. Its leaves pulverized and administered in a dose of two drachms with wine after the appearance of the menses will prevent a woman from conceiving.[38]

It is said that Hedysarum, a plant which has a small bitter fruit, if used with honey as a suppository before coitus, will prevent conception.[39]

The rennet of a stag will prevent conception, if used by a woman for three days after the period.[40]

If a woman takes Ostracite to the value of two drachms after the period for four days consecutively, she will not conceive.[41]

It is said that white poplar taken with the kidney or testicle of a he-mule will prevent conception. It is said that the leaves of this tree act in the same way, if a woman takes them after her period.[42]

---

[36] *Op. cit.*, ii, 664.

[37] *Traité des Simples*, Part I, p. 51 (No. 53).

[38] *Ibid.*, Part I, p. 109 (No. 117).

[39] *Ibid.*, Part I, p. 150 (No. 163).

[40] *Ibid.*, Part I, p. 181 (No. 219). This recipe does not specify how the rennet is to be used, whether applied in a suppository or carried as a charm. One might guess the former.

[41] *Ibid.*, Part I, p. 411 (No. 612). This is a stone that is very plentiful in Egypt. It resembles potter's clay, breaks easily, and is scaly. If it is pulverized, and given in a dose of two drachms, and drunk with milk, it will, according to Dioscorides, cause the menses to flow.

[42] *Ibid.*, Part I, p. 472 (No. 724).

Besides the above, a recipe is given for the *promotion* of conception:

Rennet used as a suppository with butter after the period will aid conception.[43]

The interpretation of the effectiveness or rationality of such a recipe offers difficulties. The immediate effect of such use would be to lessen, at least in a highly fertile woman, the likelihood of conception; for any greasy substance such as butter interferes with the motility of spermatozoa.[44] On the other hand, such a recipe, if applied for a rather long period to a woman relatively sterile as a result of the presence of profuse cervical pus or mucus, would be good treatment. In judging the rationality of the recipe much depends upon the circumstances of use. These are not made clear in the account.

When Ibn al-Baiṭār quotes others—and he is primarily a compiler—he often abridges. Hence the method of application of a given contraceptive technique is frequently left obscure. For instance, Rufus is quoted to the effect that rue will prevent conception;[45] that Ibn Sīnā mentioned scoria is also recalled.[46] The reader is left in the dark by Ibn al-Baiṭār regarding the exact method of application.

We should not overlook magical techniques:

If a woman urinates on the urine of a wolf, she will never be with child. If she takes the right testicle of a wolf, rubs it with oil, puts it on wool and uses it as a suppository, she will lose all venereal desire.[47]

It seems difficult for us to believe that such a method was ever used. Yet oily wool, inserted before coitus, would have helped, not to reduce desire, but to prevent conception.

From this same *Properties* by Ibn Zuhr another formula equally fantastic is quoted:

If one takes, before it falls, the tooth of a child who is losing his teeth, and puts it in a silver leaf, and [if] a woman carries it, it will prevent her from conceiving.[48]

[43] *Ibid.*, Part I, p. 157 (No. 172). Quoted by Dioscorides.

[44] Dr. Marie C. Stopes, and more latterly, R. L. Dickinson and Cecil Voge, have given some attention to the problem of devising a cheap, easily applied, readily accessible contraceptive, one peculiarly adapted to the poor. In an oral conversation in 1927 Dr. Stopes suggested butter. Hence, it is interesting to find this mentioned in the thirteenth century by Ibn al-Baiṭār. So far as known, the effectiveness of butter has never been tested either in laboratory trials or in case series.

[45] *Traité des Simples*, Part II, pp. 240–241 (No. 1166).

[46] *Ibid.*, Part II, p. 9 (No. 754). Scoria is slag from the reduction of metallic ore.

[47] *Ibid.*, Part II, p. 163 (No. 1016). Quoted from *The Properties* (al-Khawāṣṣ) [*of Drugs and Ailments*] by Ibn Zuhr.

[48] *Ibid.*, Part II, p. 455 (No. 1560).

From Costus's book on *Agriculture* another magical recipe is quoted:

The seed of patience or sorrel enclosed in a linen cloth and carried on the left arm of a woman will prevent her from conceiving as long as she carries it.[49]

There are several recipes for substances to be taken internally:

It is said that, if a woman, after having had her period, takes for seven days [note magical numbers] seven seeds of solanum, she will not conceive. It is a fact proved by experience.[50]

From the same author [al-Idrīsī] another recipe is quoted:

If *kermes* [a scale insect allied to the cochineal insects, and which lives on trees and vegetables] is taken with vinegar, a woman will lose the faculty of conceiving.[51]

From an important ninth century translator, Ibn al-Baiṭār extracts the following:

Ḥunain says, apropos the male hare, that his rennet taken for three days internally after a woman's period prevents her from conceiving.[52]

Cloves taken daily is a recipe extracted from a work by Isḥāq ibn 'Amrân:

If a woman does not wish to conceive, she should take every day a grain of male clove.[53]

Four recipes more rational and effective are given:

The rennet of doe in particular will prevent conception, if used by a woman as a suppository for three days after her period.[54]

[49] *Ibid.*, Part I, p. 453 (No. 698). Dr. Meyerhof informs me that in reality the passage comes from Cassianos Bassos. It seems that the name Costus is, in fact, a corruption of the name Bassos. Bassos was a great Byzantine writer on husbandry who compiled a collection of Greek writings on that subject. He flourished probably in the second half of the VI century in the time of Alexander of Tralles. His treatise became the basis of the compilation made c. 950 A. D. by order of Emperor Constantine VII.

[50] *Ibid.*, Part II, p. 473 (No. 1589). Ibn al-Baiṭār quoting Le Chérif, i.e., al-Sharīf al-Idrīsī, one of the greatest geographers and cartographers of the Middle Ages. A MS. recently discovered in Constantinople contains a treatise on botany and materia medica ascribed to al-Idrīsī. See M. Meyerhof, "Über die Pharmakologie u. Botanik des arabischen Geographen Edrisi," *Arch. f. Gesch. d. Math., Naturwiss. u. d. Technik*, xii (1930), 45–53, 225–236.

[51] *Ibid.*, Part III, p. 75 (No. 1756).

[52] *Ibid.*, Part I, p. 157 (No. 172).

[53] *Ibid.*, Part III, p. 64 (No. 1748). Ibn al-Baiṭār quoting Isḥaq ibn 'Amrân.

[54] *Ibid.*, Part I, p. 158 (No. 172). Ibn al-Baiṭār quoting Isaac Israeli (Isḥāq al-Isrā'īlī), the Elder, noted Jewish physician and philosopher of the tenth century. Probably Ibn al-Baiṭār is quoting from Israeli's book on simple drugs and nutriments (Kitāb al-adwiya

Darnel,[55] a bitter plant with a bitter fruit, if used in a suppository, has the property of preventing conception.[56]

The root of woodbine[57] (European honeysuckle) inserted by a woman will prevent conception.[58]

The dung of elephant, used with honey in a suppository, will render a woman sterile forever.[59]

The last recipe is interesting as reminiscent of one appearing in the Petri or Kahun papyrus[60] (Egyptian).

Throughout folk medicine a significant rôle has been played by dung. To it many healing properties have been ascribed. In Ibn al-Baiṭār's treatise the faeces of many different animals are mentioned as used for plasters, suppositories, or pessaries. He follows Al-Baṣrī in recommending it for the prevention of conception.

Summarizing and classifying ibn al-Baiṭār's prescriptions we get the following:

> (A) *Means to be taken by the mouth:*
>> Rennet of the hare
>> Rennet of stag
>> Ostracite
>> White poplar leaves alone or with the kidney or testicle of a "he-mule"
>> Rue
>> Scoria
>> Barrenwort roots or leaves with wine
>> Solanum
>> Kermes with vinegar
>> Rennet of male hare for three days
>> Clove

---

al mufrada wal-aghdhiya). Israeli composed many medical works in Arabic, and was one of the first to direct the attention of Jews to Greek science and philosophy. See Sarton, i, 639–640; Leclerc, *Histoire*, i, 409–412; Wüstenfeld, *Geschichte*, 51–52.

[55] The Arabic word given by Leclerc, the editor, is *kotītna* but he fails to identify it. Meyerhof says it is undoubtedly darnel [*Cf.*, Issa, *Dictionnaire des Noms des Plantes*. Le Caire, 1930, p. 1116. Lit. *Kathīb = Lolium temulentum* (darnel)]. Darnel is an annual grass, a common weed in grain fields.

[56] *Ibid.*, Part III, p. 145 (No. 1887). Ibn al-Baiṭār quoting Abu 'l-Abbās an Nabātī.

[57] The term given by Leclerc is *bokhour mariem akhar*. Meyerhof's erudition again assists me by pointing out that the above mentioned term is probably a translation of Dioscorides' κυαλάμινος ἔτερα i.e., woodbine (*Lonicera periclymenon*).

[58] *Ibid.*, Part I, p. 203 (No. 248). Ibn al-Baiṭār quoting Ibn al-Haitham.

[59] *Ibid.*, Part III, p. 52 (No. 1714). See *supra*, Ibn Sīnā. *Cf.*, Constantinus Africanus, *De chirurgia* (1536) p. 320, for the same prescription.

[60] See *infra*, p. 62.

(B) *Magical Means:*

    Urinating on the urine of a wolf

    Wolf's testicle wrapped in oiled wool as a suppository [If really used, this might have been partially effective through the oiled wool.]

    Carrying a child's tooth

    Seed of patience wrapped in linen cloth and worn on the left arm

(C) *Suppositories:*

    Hedysarum with honey

    Doe rennet

    Darnel

    Root of woodbine

    Elephant dung with honey

(3b) Dāwūd al-Anṭākī, The Memorial (XVI) and Al-Ispahani, Mirat-al-Sahhat. (XV-2)

Islamic contraceptive techniques reached their lowest point in the magical formulae of Dāwūd al-Anṭākī (sixteenth century). In place of the tampons and pessaries of the earlier writers, this author relies on magical words, letters, and numbers. If Ibn al-Baiṭār's *Treatise* represents decline in its initial stage, the *Kitāb at-Tadkhira (The Memorial)* exhibits Islamic contraceptive medicine at its lowest ebb.

Dāwūd al-Anṭākī was a Syrian physician and traditionist from Antioch who lived in Cairo and died in Mecca in 1599. Though he belongs to a later period, his name is included here in order to complete the story of Islamic decline.

The *Kitāb at-Tadkhira*[61] is a record of drugs, and it contains in the third volume a long record of magical proceedings including methods for writing amulets. It is in this section of the treatise that one finds a discussion of the prevention of conception. There are two pages of magical anti-conceptional formulae, here reproduced, which begin as follows: "In order to prevent conception one writes and suspends on the woman [a paper on which have been written the following magical formulae]. Then she will not conceive." Then follow two full pages of magical words, letters, and numbers.[62]

---

[61] Dr. Meyerhof who has examined this often printed treatise describes this sixteenth century *Kitāb* as containing in the first half an alphabetical list of simple drugs following much the procedure found in Ibn al-Baiṭār's *Treatise*; as containing in the second half an alphabetical record of diseases and their treatment. Among the latter are long chapters on astrological and magical methods which are missing from older treatises. It is not, as Sarton says, the book on drugs next best to Ibn al-Baiṭār's, but is distributed even in this day mostly by bazaar druggists and quacks. It was printed as early as 1838, and eight or nine times since, the most recent being Cairo, 1906.

[62] Vol. iii, pp. 294–295 of the best printed edition (Cairo: 1281).

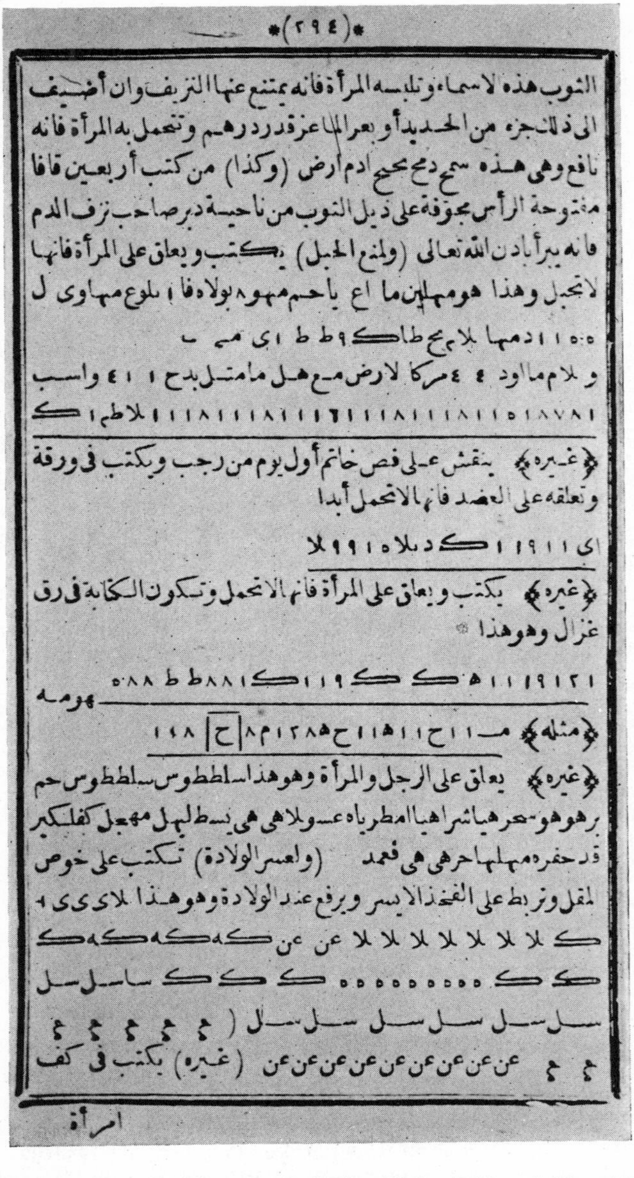

(٢٩٤)

الثوب هذه لاسمائه وتلبسه المرأة فانه يمتنع عنها النزف وان أضيف
الى ذلك الجزء من الحديد أو بعر الماعز قدر درهم وتعمل به المرأة فانه
نافع وهى هذه سمع دع محج محج ادم أرض (وكذا) من كتب أربعين فاذا
منتوحة الرأس بجوزفة على ذبل النوب من ناحية دبر صاحب زف الدم
فانه يرأ بادن الله تعالى (ولمنع الحبل) يكتب ويعلق على المرأة فانها
لا تحبل وهذا هو مهلين ما اع با حمم مهو ٨ بولاد ٨ فا لموع مهاوى ل
ا ١٥٥ ادمها بلا يع طاك ٩ ط ط اى مى ٮ
ولام ما ود ٤ ٤ مرك لارض مع هل ما متـل بدح ٤٤١ واسب
للاطى ١ ك ١ ١٨ ١ ١٨ ١ ١٢ ١ ١ ١ ١٨ ١ ١٨ ١ ٥ ١٨ ٧ ٨ ١

{غيره} ينقش على فص خاتم أول يوم من رجب ويكتب فى ورقة
وتعلقه على العضد فانه لا تحمل أبدا
اى ١٩١١ ك د بلاه ١٩١١ لا

{غيره} يكتب ويعلق على المرأة فانه لا تحمل وتكون الكتابة فى رق
غزال وهو هذا

١٢١٩١١ ك ك ١١٩ ك ك ١ ٨٨١ ط ٨٨٨ ٥
مومه
{مثله} مـ ١١ ١ ح ١١ ١ ح ١١ ١ ح ١١ ١ ٨٢١٢٨٨ ١١٨

{غيره} يعلق على الرجل والمرأة وهو هذا اسطططوس سلطططوس حم
رهوهو عرهياشراهبا مطرباه عسولاهى هى بسطلهل مهجل كفلكبر
قدحفره ممهلها حرهى هى فعمد (ولعسر الولادة) تكتب على خوص
لقل وتربط على الفخذ الايسر وبرفع عند الولادة وهو هذا لاى ى ى ١
ك لا لا لا لا لا لا لا عن عن ك ك ه ك ه ك ه ك
ك ك ٥٠٥٠٥٥٥ ك ك ك ك سا سل سل
سل سل سل سل سل سل (٢ ٢ ٢ ٢ ٢
٢ عن عن عن عن عن عن عن عن (غيره) بكتب فى كف
امرأة

FIG. IX. Dāwūd al-Anṭākī, *Tadhkira* (Cairo 1281, vol. iii, p. 294)

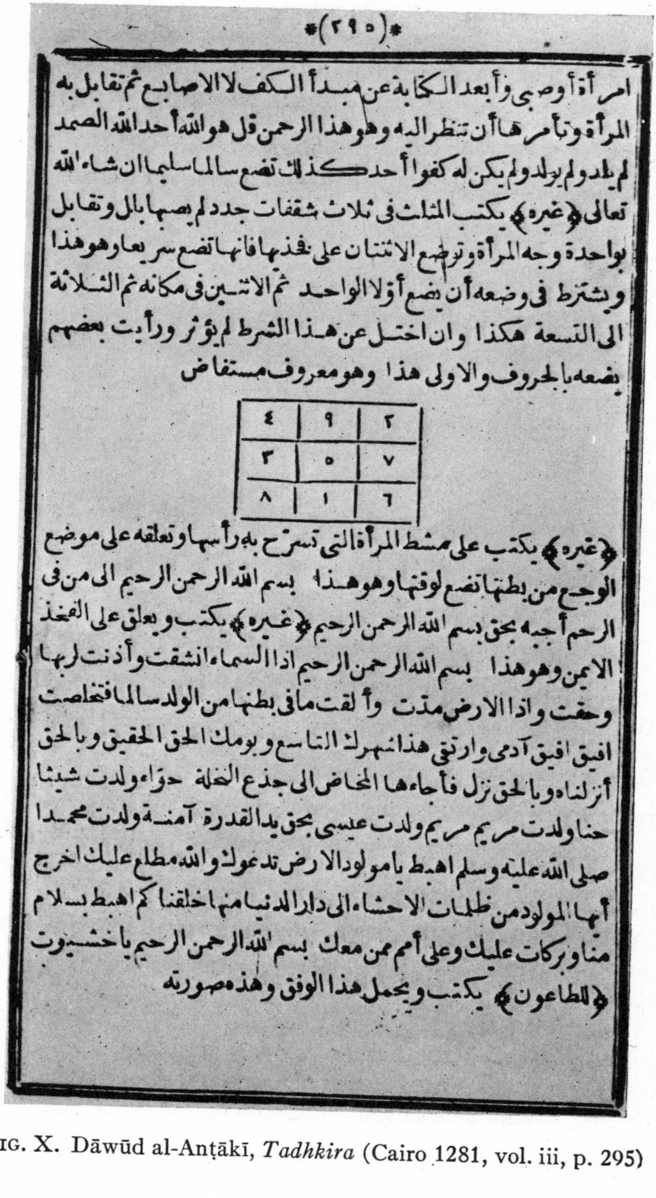

(٢٩٥)

امر أذا وصى وأبعد الكتابة عن مبدأ الكف لا الاصابع ثم تقابل به
المرأة وتأمرها أن تنظر اليه وهو هذا الرحمن قل هو الله أحد الله الصمد
لم يلد ولم يولد ولم يكن له كفوا أحد كذلك تضع سالما سليما ان شاء الله
تعالى ﴿غيره﴾ يكتب المثلث في ثلاث شققات جدد لم يصبها بلل وتقابل
بواحدة وجه المرأة وترضع الاثنتان على نهذها فانها تضع سريعا وهو هذا
ويشترط فى وضعه أن يضع أولا الواحد ثم الاثنين فى مكانه ثم الثلاثة
الى التسعة هكذا وان اختل عن هذا الشرط لم يؤثر ورأيت بعضهم
يضعه بالحروف والاولى هذا وهو معروف مستفاض

٤	٩	٢
٣	٥	٧
٨	١	٦

﴿غيره﴾ يكتب على مشط المرأة التي تسرح به رأسها وتعلقه على موضع
الوجع من بطنها تضع لوثها وهو هذا بسم الله الرحمن الرحيم الى من فى
الرحم أجبه بحق بسم الله الرحمن الرحيم ﴿غيره﴾ يكتب ويعلق على الفخذ
الايمن وهو هذا بسم الله الرحمن الرحيم اذا السماء انشقت وأذنت لربها
وحقت واذا الارض مدت وألقت ما فى بطنها من الولد سالما فتقاصت
افق افى آدمى وارتقى هذا نهرك التاسع وبومك الحق الحقيق وبالحق
أنزلناه وبالحق نزل فأجاءها المخاض الى جذع النخلة حوّا وولدت شيئا
حنا وولدت مريم مريم ولدت عيسى بحق بذا القدرة آمنة وولدت محمدا
صلى الله عليه وسلم اهبط يا مولودا الارض تدعونك والله مطلع عليك اخرج
أيها المولود من ظلمات الاحشاء الى دار الدنيا منها اخلقنا كم اهبط بسلام
منا وبركات عليك وعلى أمم ممن معك بسم الله الرحمن الرحيم يا خشيوت
﴿الطاعون﴾ يكتب ويحمل هذا الوفق وهذا مصورته

FIG. X. Dāwūd al-Anṭākī, *Tadhkira* (Cairo 1281, vol. iii, p. 295)

A late fifteenth century Persian medical manuscript, *Mirat-al-Sahhat*,[63] by one Ghiyas ibn Muhammad al-Mutatabib al-Ispahani, mentions several drugs to prevent conception which we have met with in earlier sources, and some of which still persist in European folk medicine. They are rennet, mule's hoof, iron scoria, iron rust, elephant's dung, pepper—all to be taken by the mouth.

§4 A CLASSIFICATION AND COMPARISON OF ISLAMIC CONTRACEPTIVE
TECHNIQUES

If the recipes we treated in §2 (those of 'Ali ibn 'Abbas, Ibn Sīnā, Ismā 'īl al-Jurjānī, and Ibn al-Jamī') are placed in Group I and those of Ibn al-Baiṭār in Group II, we may observe at a glance the superiority of the former.

	Group I	Group II
Total	41*	20
(A) Means to be taken by the mouth	3	11
(B) Magical means	1	4
(C) Suppositories and tampons	15	5
(D) Techniques used by the man	13	0
(E) Miscellaneous techniques	9	0

* Counted each time that a given recipe appears, even though copied. If an author selected the more rational techniques of his predecessors, he should receive credit for this.

Of Ibn al-Baiṭār's twenty recipes, three-quarters (fifteen) were clearly ineffective. On the other hand, the four early writers (Group I) mentioned severally forty-one techniques of which only four were magical or recipes to be taken by the mouth.

The prescriptions here reported constitute, no doubt, only a portion of those known to various Islamic writers. Undoubtedly many physicians, other than those here considered, treated anti-conceptional measures. There are at least forty treatises in Arabic similar to Ibn al-Baiṭār's *Treatise on Simples*. Many are still untranslated and unpublished. It is certain that Ibn Serapion and Mesuë discussed contraceptive technique; but there has been no opportunity as yet to search these sources. I have no doubt that Ibn al-Baiṭār's unpublished *Mughnī* discusses it; and the formidable output of Rāzī (Rhazes), the greatest clinician and medical observer of the Islamic world, is still unpublished. However, I have presented one text from Rhazes. There are several thousand unpublished and mostly un-

[63] Dedicated to Sultan Bayazeed II (1481–1512). In the concluding paragraph the author states that he finished the work in 869 A.H. (c. 1490 A.D.). My attention was called to this by Dr. C. Elgood of England.

translated Arabian medical manuscripts. Constantinople alone has eighty-three libraries full of such unpublished medical manuscripts. Dr. Meyerhof ventures the opinion that it will be two hundred years before a real history of Islamic medicine can be written. I am well aware of the sketchy nature of this account and under no illusions regarding its completeness. It is useful mainly in pointing the way, and in suggesting rich sources for future investigation.

The extent to which contraceptive practices were actually used by the Islamic peoples in the period of their cultural hegemony is not known. It is known, however, that they were not forbidden by religion. It is probable that medical writers gave more attention to the subject than legal, religious, and ethical authors. There probably exist Arabic codes discussing the legal and religious side of contraception, but no one unfortunately seems to have searched them for our purpose.

A recent report[64] on modern Mecca shows that certain contraceptive folk practices have persisted into very late modern times. Speaking of that city in the middle of the nineteenth century, Professor C. Snouck Hurgronje declares that since half the unions are pure concubinage, and are expected to be dissolved after some time, there is a much livelier demand for preservatives against impregnation than for means for its encouragement. Pills or pessaries of oblong shape, the composition of which Hurgronje does not report, are sold by doctors to be introduced by the men into the meatus.[65] More frequently, however, midwives introduce them into the vaginas of their clients. "The midwives are so sure of the success of their treatment that they habitually make contracts binding themselves to return the money if the drugs fail of their desired effect. Each of these midwives has her own special ingredients, the compounding of which is her secret, a secret imparted only to her slave girls." The midwives claim to have a method of contraception effective for one, two or three years, and another permanently sterilizing. The temporary preservatives are called *tasbîrah*. When permanent sterility is desired the woman requests that she be made into a *baghlah*, or female mule. Hurgronje adds[66] that the concubines are more inclined to use the temporary than the permanent techniques.

In the absence of more detailed information, little can be said of the effectiveness of these techniques; but it is interesting to note that some are employed. Might it not be possible that the female suppository was physically occlusive at least to some extent?

[64] C. Snouck Hurgronje, *Mekka in the latter part of the 19th century.* Trans. by J. H. Monahan, Leyden: E. J. Brill; London: Luzac & Co., 1931, pp. vi, 3–309.
[65] *Ibid.*, Eng. trans., p. 105.
[66] *Ibid.*, Eng. trans., p. 109.

§5   EUROPE DURING THE MIDDLE AGES

It is not easy to account for the great infusion of magic and superstition in the discussion of contraceptive techniques as reported in writers on the Continent belonging to the late Middle Ages. Doubtless the heritage was through Rome (e.g., Pliny) rather than through Islamic medicine. For, when the best of the Greek and Roman knowledge began to flow back into Europe through the Arabs, we have, as a consequence of forces operating also on the Continent, the Renaissance in literature, science and medicine.

Surely, it is an established fact that we have found nothing comparable to the accounts of Soranos and Aëtios; nothing that equals that of such writers as 'Ali ibn 'Abbās, Ibn Sīnā, Ismā'īl al-Jurjānī, and Ibn al-Jamī', Rāzī, or even Ibn al-Baiṭār. It may even be doubted whether Europeans in the late Middle Ages knew as much about contraceptive medicine as the ancient Hebrews and Egyptians. Certainly, the point is debatable. And though it would be fallacious to attribute the circumstance to a single factor, it is difficult to avoid the conclusion that the rise of Christianity, especially in the form of the dominance of the Catholic Church, was essentially responsible. Service to the City of God was the central object of life, salvation in the hereafter rather than on earth. This is not to suggest that the Church neglected to cultivate medicine. It did; but the objects were quite different from those of modern scientific medicine. According to the dominant ideal of the Middle Ages all discovery had to square with the ethical outlook, the religious dogma, of the Church. Science was subservient; small wonder it was decadent. And what was true of science in general was true of contraceptive medicine. There was much of value in the mediaeval synthesis; but if ethics and science are to join hands in the future, as many thoughtful people hope, it will have to be a new synthesis on a new level. One of the greatest questions concerning the future is whether this is possible.

The low level of knowledge of anti-conceptional technique during the Middle Ages outside of Islam is well shown in the remaining sections of this chapter.

(5a)   Albert the Great, Arnold of Villanova, Constantine the African

Albert the Great[67] (1193–1280), the Dominican philosopher, teacher and theologian, was one of the most learned men, and perhaps one of the greatest alchemists, of the Middle Ages. He cultivated medicine as a necessary adjunct of a monastic education, and in the course of doing so made references to contraceptive recipes, though these seem to be quite devoid of rational foundation. This is not surprising when one contemplates the

---

[67] For an excellent discussion of the life, thought, scientific activity and literature by, upon, and critical of, Albert the Great, see Sarton, *op. cit.*, ii, 934–944.

enormous reach of Albert's intellectual endeavor. Though he wrote a series of encyclopedic treatises dealing with various branches of natural science, philosophy, and theology, many works attributed to him, including those containing contraceptive recipes, are apocryphal. Even allowing for the apocryphal literature, his productive efforts were miraculous. Sarton's opinion seems shrewd when he says that in spite of Albert's original judgment, and in spite of his prodigious energy, his work is no real encyclopedia, no organic synthesis, but rather a compilation. If it does credit to his enormous energy and intelligence, it may hardly be described as the product of creative genius, for Albert contributed little to genuine intellectual progress.[68] Albert's main work is best viewed as an attempt to assist the integration of Aristotelian knowledge with Latin culture. A weaker theologian than St. Thomas, but a better scientist, Albert's contribution to the history of contraception is worthy only of passing mention. The recipes which have so far come to light, which appear in his apocryphal works, are essentially magical. Of these, one instance may be cited. Albert believed that if a woman would spit thrice in the mouth of a frog, or eat bees, she would not become pregnant.[69] Qusṭā ibn Lūqā,[70] a Christian of Greek origin (tenth century), though having an Arabian name, also avowed that spitting thrice in the mouth of a frog would prevent conception. During the Middle Ages the belief was prevalent that holding a pebble of jasper in the hand during coitus would prevent conception.[71] This would be as ineffective as the method not infrequently used in China and India for centuries: Many Chinese and Indian women believe that if they remain passive during coitus,[72] so that they do not enjoy normal connection, they will not become pregnant. The Chinese refer to this as *cong-fou*.[73] The rate of births in these countries is eloquent testimony to the ineffectiveness of such a recipe.

[68] Sarton, *op. cit.*, ii, 935.

[69] See the apocryphal works, *De secretis mulierum item de virtutibus herbarum lapidum et animalium* (Amsterdam, 1565, pp. 329) and *De mirabile mundi* as well as the account which follows below in the text from a French source. Albert's *Historia animalium* was written in imitation of Aristotle. Thomas Aquinas was one of Albert's disciples. A contemporary writer says that he was doubtless with justice charged with necromancy. See George F. Fort, *Medical Economy During the Middle Ages* (New York: Bouton, London: Quaritch, 1883), p. 312.

[70] Qusṭā ibn Lūqā was a physician, philosopher, astronomer and mathematician who flourished in Bagdad and died in Armenia c. 912. The name Qusṭā is exceedingly rare in Arabic; it is probably a Syriac corruption of the Byzantine name Constans or Constantine. See Sarton, i, 602; Leclerc, *Histoire*, i, 157–159.

[71] Dawson, "Early Ideas Concerning Conception and Contraception," in [Stopes?] *Medical Help on Birth Control*, p. 200.

[72] *Cf.*, the text of Ibn Sīnā on avoiding simultaneous orgasms.

[73] Iwan Bloch (pseud. for Eugen Dühren), *The Sexual Life of Our Times*. (*Engl.* ed. from 6th Ger. ed.) Ch. xvii.

Related to passivity as a measure one may recall the statement by Ibn Sīnā (Avicenna) that avoidance of a simultaneous orgasm will prevent conception.[74]

Arnold of Villanova,[75] a writer of the second half of the thirteenth century, "abundantly recognizes," says Fort, "the power of lettered characters when sprinkled with blood in the hands of an unforgiving rival, totally to transform the enticements of the nuptial chamber."[76]   This sounds like a magical anaphrodisiac.   Arnold also revived the prescription of Soranos in declaring that

If a woman drinks in the morning for three days two minas of water in which smiths quench their forceps, she will be sterile permanently.[77]

And Fort avows that nuns not only made attempts by the use of amulets and talismen, to prevent conception, but produced abortion:

Nuns and consecrated women residing in convents, whose time was employed in embroidering fine textures and attiring themselves in bridal vestments to attract the attention of strange men, after having glided down the fascinating slope of human impulses, instead of relying on the presumed puissance of religion, had recourse to the more practical method of restoring their virginity by medicinal potions—a practice placed under the ban as early as the year 798, by a Carlovingian rescript [*Lex Salica*, Tit. XXI, lex 4].   In some instances erring sisters bore amulets or applied the preventative talismanic influence of a sacred shirt or girdle, to suppress the manifestation of conventual irregularities.   The bold [contraceptive] recommendation of mediaeval medical professors against the legitimate

---

[74] See *infra* p. 142.

[75] Arnold of Villanova (Arnaldus de Villa Nova, or Villanovanus, also Bacuone or Barchione, i.e., of Barcelona) was born near Valencia c. 1234–1250.   After studying medicine at Naples, he travelled extensively, practising in Paris, Montpellier, Barcelona and Rome.   He died in 1311.

This Catalan physician was an alchemist, astrologer, diplomat, social reformer and visionary.   Approximately 123 treatises, most of them short, have been attributed to him, but many are apocryphal.   Sarton (*op. cit.*, ii, 893) refers to him as "one of the most extraordinary personalities of mediaeval times."   Though he realized the value of natural science and had some slight conception of the experimental point of view; and though he occasionally seemed opposed to magic and sorcery, "his own works are full of superstitious ideas." (Sarton, ii, 893).   None the less, he enjoyed fame as a medical practitioner and was consulted by Aragon kings and the popes.

In view of the above facts, it is not strange that Arnold's views on contraceptive technique were, so far as they are now known, worthless.

For a list of the most important works attributed to Arnold, see George Sarton, *Introduction to the History of Science*, ii, 894–900.

[76] Fort, *Medical Economy*, note, p. 294, citing Villanova, *De Maleficiis*, col. 1529.

[77] "Si mulier bibat quod libet mane per tres dies duas minas aquae, in qua fararii extingunt forcipes suas steriles sit in perpetuum."   Arnold Villannov., *Breviarii Additiones*, Lib. III, c. 5, col. 1338.

results of these frailties, attests the extent of an evil justly regarded by the Church as a most heinous crime.[78]

Fort, moreover, suggests that the nuns sometimes followed the prescriptions of Arnold and Constantine the African.

A number of recipes, mainly magical, for the prevention of conception, are to be found in a treatise ascribed to Albert bearing the title *The Admirable Secrets of Albert the Great*.[79]   Many of these recipes which follow have become more or less traditional in the folk medicine of Europe:

(1) If one soaks up in a piece of cloth the oil of the barberry tree, and if one applies it to the left temple of a woman, she will not conceive while it is there.[80]

(2) The ancients say that if a woman hangs about her neck the finger and the anus of a dead foetus, she will not conceive while they are there.   The same result will be achieved if she drinks sheep's urine or the blood of a hare; or if she hangs around her neck the anus of the hare.[81]

(3) If one wishes that a woman be not sexually desirous of men, it is necessary to take the penis of a wolf, to take the hairs of his eyelids, and those under his beard, to have them burned, and then to make the woman drink the results without her knowing anything about it.[82]

(4) It is also said that if one cuts off the foot of the female weasel, leaving her still alive, and if one puts this foot about the neck of a woman, she will not conceive while she wears it; and that if she takes it off she will become pregnant.[83]

(5) If one takes the two testicles of a weasel and wraps them up, binding them to the thigh of a woman who wears also a weasel bone on her person, she will no longer conceive.[84]

Little Albert advises as follows in order to turn women away from the sexual act:

(6) Reduce to a powder the sexual organ of a red bull, and give a crown's weight of this powder in a bouillon composed of veal, of purslane and lettuce.[85]

[78] Fort, *op. cit.*, p. 280.

[79] *Les secrets admirables du Grand Albert . . . suivis du Trésor des merveilleux secrets du Petit Albert*. Réédition par Marius Decrespe. Paris: Guyot. n. d., pp. 190. This work cannot be located in any library of the United States. I am indebted to Dr. Paul Delaunay of Le Mans, Sarthe, France, for work on this source.

[80] *Ibid.*, p. 67.

[81] *Ibid.*, p. 68.

[82] *Ibid.*, p. 69.

[83] *Ibid.*

[84] *Ibid.*, p. 70.

[85] *Ibid.*, p. 113.

In order to make men incapable of conceiving, Little Albert advises as follows:

Take the penis of a newly killed wolf, and, coming near the [house] door of the one whom you wish to render sterile, you will then call him by his own name; and as soon as he has replied, you will tie up the said penis of the wolf with a string of white thread; and he will be rendered impotent in regard to the act of Venus just as much as if he were indeed a eunuch.[86]

(5b) *Frater Rudolphus' Fourteenth Century Manuscript, De officio cherubyn.*

An interesting report on the magical contraceptive practices prevalent in the late Middle Ages among the early Germans, is contained in a fourteenth century manuscript of eighteen parchment sheets on deposit in the University of Leipzig library, the contents of which have been described in considerable detail by Franz.[87]   It bears the title, *Liber de officio cherubyn.* The second part alone remains to us.   The manuscript deals primarily with the proper guidance of the flock by the priest, and with the practice of confession; and, while essentially theological in content, is noteworthy also for its practical observations on the cultural history of the times.   A keen observer of the life of the people, the author, who was probably the Minorit, Rudolphus de Bibraco (Biberach near Ulm), believed the religious interests of the people were jeopardized by their superstitious customs. Hence he admonishes the clerics to root them out regardless of the forms they take.   Among the superstitions reported are the following:

Those who desire to prevent birth and conception do a great many fantastic things. When they sit or lie down they sometimes put a number of fingers under them, thinking they will be free from conception as many years as they put fingers under them.   A substance which they call their "flower" they place in an elder tree, saying: "You will bear for me and I will bloom for you."[88]

Evidently Frater Rudolphus understood that this act of sympathetic magic did not help the women to prevent conception, for he immediately adds:

And yet the tree blooms, and the woman bears children with pain.   [Some] of this "flower" they throw away, in order not to conceive.   Some of it likewise they give in water to a dog, a pig, or a fish in order that they [the women] may not conceive.[88]

---

[86] *Ibid.*, pp. 112–113.

[87] Adolph Franz, "Des Frater Rudolphus Buch *De officio cherubyn,*" *Theologische Quartalschr.*, lxxxviii (1906), 411–436.

[88] *Ibid.*, p. 427.   The original of the passage reads as follows: "Conceptum et partum impedire uolentes plurimas faciunt fantasias.   Cum sedent vel iacunt, quandoque ponunt sub se aliquos digitos credentes se tot annos liberas a conceptu, quot [for quod] digitos sub se ponunt.   Quidam florem suum vocant, in arborem sambuci mittunt, dicentes: Porta tu

(5c) Book of the Cyranides

In an equally superstitious way the *Book of the Cyranides*,[89] a compendium of ancient lore on the virtues of animals, stones and plants, says that the left testicle of the weasel

placed in mule skin, and worn, prevents conception. It is necessary to write on the mule skin these words IΩΑ′, ΩΙΑ′, ΡΑΥΙΩ, ΟΥ,″ ΟΙ″ ΚΟΟΧΡ. Remove the testicles as the moon goes down, and leave the weasel living; and give its testicles to be worn in the muleskin; it will serve as a sort of philtre, invincible and agreeable, against conception.[90]

Further

If a woman . . . wears [the heart of a salamander] attached to her knees, she will not conceive.[91]

(5d) Drugs, Gems and Stones

The drinking of drugs to prevent conception was somewhat prevalent during the Middle Ages, as it is in many parts of the world today to provoke abortion. It was believed, for instance, that the prolonged and methodical use of sabine (*Juniperus sabina*) would prevent conception.[92]

Many writers have referred to the supposed special powers of gems and stones. There are gems to induce continence. For example, a lapidary of the second quarter of the thirteenth century says that "the emerald is very potent against [not only] storms," but "also against male sexual desire."[93]

Little need be said about the irrationality of these recipes. They are of interest chiefly in showing that the *desire* to prevent conception was characteristic of the Middle Ages in Europe, when the Church was more dominant than at present. Were the desire for prevention not present, it is difficult to see how these superstitions could have persisted so long.

---

pro me, ego floream pro te. Et tamen arbor floret et ipsa parit pueros cum dolore. De eodem flore suo proiciunt, ne concipiant; de eodem dant cani aut porcello aut pisciculo in aqua, ne concipiant." The heading of the chapter (9th) is "De sortilegiis puellarum et malarum mulierum." Love charms are also discussed in the chapter. Chapter 8 deals with the birth and care of children and the superstitions associated therewith.

[89] Probably translated from Greek into Latin by Paschal the Roman (Pascalis Romanus) in 1169. The Greek text with a French translation will be found in F. de Mély, *Les Lapidaires de l'Antiquité et du Moyen Age* (vols. 2 and 3, Paris, 1898–1902). *Cf.*, Lynn Thorndike, *History of Magic*, ii, 229–235; George Sarton, *op. cit.*, ii, 347.

[90] *Livre des Cyranides*, p. 77.

[91] *Ibid.*, p. 91.

[92] Letter of Dr. Paul Delauney of Le Mans, France, to the author. *Cf.*, also von Oefele, *Die Heilkunde*, ii (1898), 277.

[93] L. Pannier, *Les Lapidaires français du Moyen Age des XII, XIII et XIV Siècles*, p. 245.

(5e)   The Catholic Church as Represented by St. Thomas Aquinas

It is hardly possible to trace the development of any subject through the Middle Ages without devoting some attention to the Catholic Church which was chiefly responsible for the cultural unity of that interesting period.   Inasmuch as it will not be possible to consider here in detail the relation of the mediaeval Christian church to contraception, this procedure has been followed: St. Thomas Aquinas (1225–1274) has been taken as typical.   For his views on contraception became those of the Catholic Church; and the doctrines of the Catholic Church on contraception have been modified little, if at all, from that day to this.   Despite the fact that Aquinas has no place in the history of medicine, we cannot understand the development of contraceptive thought during the Middle Ages unless we recognize the influence of his doctrines on the Catholic Church, and, through the church, upon the masses.

The spirit of scientific inquiry was foreign to Aquinas's whole temper of thought.   His contribution to the history of science is negligible—virtually nil.[94]   He holds some place in the history of philosophy, government and economic theory; but he has no place in medical history.   Since he was primarily concerned with re-interpreting Aristotle, and in reconciling Aristotelian and Muslim knowledge with Christian dogmatics, we would not expect him to have faced the problem of the control of human fertility with the open mind of a scientist.   In respect to his attitude toward contraception St. Thomas was not the good Aristotelian he proved to be in nearly every other field of knowledge, for Aristotle, it will be recalled, reported on contraceptive technique in his *Historia Animalium*, even if there is no evidence that he approved the practice.   St. Thomas, who wrote a volume in imitation of Aristotle's *Historia*, avoided a discussion of technique, and, we may deduce, condemned such practices.   They were not permissible according to his theological presuppositions.

Aquinas's chief work is the *Summa Theologica* (c. 1267 to Aquinas's death).   Of interest to us is also his *Summa Contra Gentiles* (1258– to 60 or 1264).   The bulk of his writings is enormous.   There are many old

---

[94] Sarton says (*op. cit.*, ii, 914–915) of him "though interested in science, he [St. Thomas] utterly failed to understand its true spirit and methods, and no scientific contribution can be credited to him.   Indeed his mind was far too dogmatic to be capable of disinterested scientific curiosity.   His master, Albert, was a more genuine man of science than he was . . ."

"St. Thomas was a clear and forceful expositor, eclectic with regard to his sources, but as firm as a rock with regard to his own dogmatic purposes. . . . Within the unbending frame of Christian dogmatics he offers us a complete and well-ordered explanation of the world."

editions of the *Summa Theologica*, but an edition of twenty volumes has been published in London recently translated by the English Dominican Fathers. Likewise, there is a new edition of the *Summa Contra Gentiles*.[95]

Aquinas condemned birth control, says Father John A. Ryan, on the ground that it was "against nature and therefore morally wrong."[96] The condemnation is, however, perhaps more implicit than explicit.[97] I am indebted to Father John A. Ryan for the following "free and condensed" translation of relevant passages. In the *Summa Theologica* we read:

In so far as the generation of offspring is impeded, it is a vice against nature which happens in every carnal act from which generation cannot follow.[98]

Likewise in the *Summa Contra Gentiles*:

The inordinate omission of semen is against the good of nature, which is the conservation of the species; hence, after the sin of homicide, by which human nature actually existing is destroyed, this kind of sin, by which the generation of human nature is impeded, seems to hold second place.[99]

The doctrines of Aquinas became the doctrines of the Catholic Church. They were incorporated in the general body of theology. Despite early attempts to censor the general body of Thomistic theology, Thomism became the official doctrine of the Dominican Order four years after Aquinas's death (1278). During the Council of Trent (1545–1563) the *Summa Theologica* was placed on the altar with the Holy Scriptures and the Decretals.[100]

The movement toward the recognition of Thomism as an integral part of Catholic doctrine culminated when Leo XIII (1878–1903) issued the encyclical *Aeterni Patris* (1879). Later (1880), St. Thomas was proclaimed the patron of all Catholic schools. Leo XIII also ordered the publication of a

---

[95] The *Opera Omnia* have been edited by S. E. Fretté and Pauli Maré (Paris, 1871–80, 34 volumes). The most authoritative edition, still incomplete, is the Leonine (Rome, 1888–1926, vols. i–xiv have appeared). Both the *Summa Theologica* (London, 1911–1925, 20 vols.) and the *Summa Contra Gentiles* (London, 1923–28, 20 vols.) have been translated by the English Dominican Fathers. See Ryan, *op. cit.*, for further references.

[96] John A. Ryan, Art. on Aquinas in *Encyclopedia of the Social Sciences*, ii, 148.

[97] This is also the view of Father John A. Ryan (U. S. A.) who, at my request, had a search made of St. Thomas's works. Father Ryan reports that no explicit statement "has been brought to light;" he thinks this not "surprising inasmuch as such practices were apparently not prominent in his time." (Letter dated November 17, 1930.) Just how "prominent" these were is not known.

[98] *Summa Theologica*, Secundae 2 ae, Question 154, Article I.

[99] *Summa Contra Gentiles*, Bk. iii, ch. 122. *Cf.*, also Question 154, Art. XI and Art. XII.

[100] Sarton, *op. cit.*, ii, 916.

new edition of St. Thomas's works.   Thus has St. Thomas gradually come
to be recognized "officially as the intellectual guide of the Roman Catholic
Church."   Leo XIII's efforts were furthered by his successors: Pius X
(1903–1914), Benedict XV (1914–1922).   The recent encyclical of the
present Pope (Pius XI, 1922–   ) on *Casti connubii* (Jan. 1931), dealing
with marriage problems, clearly lays down a Thomistic doctrine on birth
control.   "It is thus sufficiently clear," says Sarton, "that Thomism is the
official philosophy of the Roman Catholic Church; that it is as authoritative,
for the members of that Church, as anything can be, short of the dogmas
themselves."[101]

§6 THE EFFECTIVE RÔLE OF CONTRACEPTION IN THE MIDDLE AGES PROBABLY SMALL

Since Aquinas's doctrines became incorporated with the doctrine of the
Catholic Church, it is not difficult to infer what the attitude toward contraceptive medicine would be on the part of Catholic mediaeval and modern
writers on that subject.   *It is abundantly clear, however, that even in the
Middle Ages, the era of greatest dominance of the Church, when Europe was
culturally unified and dominated by custom almost to the point of stagnation,
the Church never succeeded in preventing the application of contraceptive knowledge.*   It should not be inferred from such a statement that contraception
was generally practised during the Middle Ages.   It is highly probable
that it was not.   On the other hand, it is equally probable that, even though
the economic, social and religious mores of the populace favored large families, some use was made of the popular remedies handed on by oral tradition and in medical literature.   Physicians also must have made, perhaps
only in rigorously selected cases, some use of contraceptive technique.   It
is difficult to believe that all the contraceptive knowledge that came down
from the Greeks, Romans and Arabs failed to find application.

Was contraception applied sufficiently in the Middle Ages to affect seriously the natality figures?   Here we are necessarily in the dark, since there
were, of course, no censuses, much less birth-rate calculations in the period
under examination.   Even if we had such data, we could only make inferences from them.   *The soundest conclusion seems to be that, prior to late
modern times, say 1800 in western civilizations, much later in eastern civilizations, the numbers of a people on a given territory have been determined by
various factors affecting natality and mortality, independently of attempts
artificially to control conception.*   Much, if not most, of the information
popularly current on contraception throughout the whole historical period

[101] *Ibid.*, ii, 917.

has been ineffective.   What the physicians knew is another n.
of this ineffectiveness was necessarily due to the infusion of magic
ogy into all branches of knowledge in the Middle Ages.   In the folk
of Europe, the subject of the next chapter, we see this tendency pers
It may be that the development of the condom or sheath, so readily acc
ible even in cultures that ostensibly mention contraception only in furtive
whispers, has done more than almost any other force to displace many of
the nonsensical—though, upon occasion, brilliant and effective—contraceptive folk practices.

AGES

atter. Much
and astrol-
medicine
sting.

169

CHAPTER VII

BELIEFS AND LAY LITERATURE
FROM 1400 ON

§1 MAGICAL FOLK MEDICINE

SIDE by side with rational methods of controlling conception, such as the condom (Chapter VIII), there have persisted in the folk beliefs and folk medicine of Europe down to our day the superstitions of antiquity and of the Middle Ages. Many will be reported in this section. Often fantastic, they may try the endurance of the reader; but a smooth, readable account of the scrappy materials available is difficult to produce without sacrificing our first object—accurate recording and restrained interpretation. Completeness and classification of these materials are difficult. Much of this folklore passed orally and was never recorded. The very furtiveness with which it was undoubtedly passed from woman to woman renders most such ideas inaccessible to the compiler.

In German folk medicine one finds majoram (*Origanum maiorana*), thyme (*Thymus vulgaris*), parsley[1] (*Petroselinum sativum*), and lavender (*Lavendula officinalis*) recommended in tea form not simply as an abortifacient but also as a contraceptive.[2] Rosemary and myrtle have still a symbolic application; for the former is worn on the breast by the bride, and myrtle in the form of a wreath with the idea that these will protect against pregnancy.[3] Folk poetry has accordingly grown up around these simples.

The root of the worm fern (?) (*Wurmfarn*, or *Aspidium filix mas*), has also been used to produce abortion and to render women sterile. At least the German people have thought it had this latter effect.[4] Tartar women have used the seeds of these fern plants for the same purposes.[5] In German folk medicine one also finds brake (*Adlerfarn* or *Pteris aquilina*) mentioned to prevent pregnancy and cause miscarriage. Francus de Franchenau

---

[1] We have seen that an American Indian group used parsley. See ch. i, n. 47.

[2] Hovorka and Kronfeld, *Vergleichende Volksmedizin*, i, 33–35. *Cf.*, Aigremont (pseudonym?) *Volkserotik und Pflanzenwelt* (Halle, 1908–1909. 2 vols.), i, 134 and i, 149.

[3] Hovorka, *loc. cit.*

[4] Aigremont, ii, 20.

[5] Ploss-Bartels, *Das Weib*, i, 543. Cited by Aigremont, ii, 20.

accordingly dubbed it "prostitute root" (*Hurenwurz*).⁶ This use dates back at least to Dioscorides.

According to symbolic or sympathetic magic the seeds of many *fruitless* trees, drunk as a tea, would render a woman sterile. Fruitlessness would provoke fruitlessness. The notion that like produces like is a very old primitive belief—one prevalent in many savage, and in some highly civilized societies; and, as Winternitz says, the principle of *similia similibus curantur* prevails throughout the entire range of folk medicine.⁷

Seitz and Mathiolus, for example, have shown that even until relatively late times the German people believed that drinking willow tea made one sterile. This notion doubtless came down from the Romans. The German women thought, in addition, that if the tea were drunk boiling hot, it would drive away all desire for, and inclination to, unchastity. Willow is mentioned as productive of sterility in an early eighteenth century treatise on *Women's Diseases* (1709) by R. D. Carolus Musitanus, from Chapter IV of which (On Sterility) the following is extracted:

Many are the drugs which dispose of or impede semen, or cause the abortion of the foetus. Amongst those which destroy semen and prevent conception is willow, which does not weaken the appetite of small women (muliercularum) so much as poisons do, for which reason it mitigates excessive salacity, if first, truly tender willow shoots are cut off, for thus there flows a liquor; when it is shaped into a little lump and drunk by a woman it is efficacious, so that never is love deemed stronger, but if a potion of willow be drunk by a woman on an empty stomach several times, it induces sterility. It is said that either crocus or mint prevents conception, if introduced into the vagina immediately after intercourse. Borax combined with the willow drink, taken internally before or shortly after intercourse, is said to be an impediment to conception; there is a common saying that camphor prevents love, and consequently emasculates, whence the little verse:

"Camphor through the nostrils by its odour castrates men."

But we know the opposite of camphor, for it renders "sumetes" more lustful. Also, when a suppository of black helkbore [hellebore] with castoreum is inserted following intercourse, conception is prevented. And if a woman did conceive, the fruit would be destroyed.⁸

Note that in the above passage ineffective means to be taken by the mouth are emphasized, but that a suppository of black hellebore with castoreum is to be inserted *after* intercourse. If such a suppository has any effectiveness when inserted prior to coitus, it seems reasonable to infer that this

---

⁶ Aigremont, *ibid.*

⁷ Moritz Winternitz, "Witchcraft in Ancient India," in *Indian Antiquary* (Bombay), March, 1899. Also separate.

⁸ R. D. Carolus Musitanus, *De Morbis Mulierum*, 1709, ch. iv, De sterilitate, pp. 100–101.

would be greatly reduced if the medication did not take place until after. And herein, we may point out, lies one of the essential differences between contraception prior to 1900 and contraception after that period: We now have more experience enabling us to sift the effective from the ineffective, the harmless from the harmful. This is not to suggest that the sifting process is now complete, especially as regards reliability; far from it. But in recent years even popular writers have automatically—not through any special pains of their own—been saved from such confusions as were common, indeed well nigh universal, in the Middle Ages.

To his prescriptions on willow Musitanus adds:

> Passionate coitus is to be avoided, for it is unfruitful. Sometimes the woman does not draw back her buttocks [as Soranos directs], and conquers, as is the custom of Spanish women, who move their whole body while they have intercourse, from an excess of voluptuousness (they are extraordinarily passionate), and perform the Phrygian dance, and some of them passionately sing a song, which in Spanish is called "Chaccara," and on account of this [sic] Spanish women are sterile.[9]

This passage is of interest chiefly in showing the persistence into the eighteenth century of the influence of Soranos; it shows the persistence of the medieval and Christian notion that if one really enjoys coitus there must be dire results—in this case sterility. The general acceptance, we may remark, of this false Christian dogma is perhaps as much responsible for the prevalence in our own time of marital disharmony and hence of divorce as any single factor. Thus has Christianity helped to create what it at bottom deplores—the separation of married partners.

Hovorka and Kronfeld,[10] following perhaps the suggestion of von Oefele,[11] think that some of the substances reported above and used in folk medicine to prevent conception may be partially effective by causing a catarrh of the uterine canal. Many are supposed to contain an ether oil which might hinder conception through the nexus mentioned. Very little is known about this subject, and it merits investigation. It is not inconceivable that a thorough inquiry by medical science into the effectiveness of many recipes commonly thought by anthropologists and others to be magical may teach us much about modern contraception. Such a study might also throw light upon variations in fertility in various cultures at different epochs in the past.

Lammert reports that in many localities the superstition prevailed, even

---

[9] *Ibid.*, p. 111.

[10] Hovorka and Kronfeld, *op. cit.*, i, 34.

[11] See article II in *Die Heilkunde* (1898), pp. 273–284, on "The Pharmacological Possibility of Influencing Fertility."

as late as the end of the eighteenth century, that, if an unmarried maiden ate pears or medlars (*Mespilus germanica*—the fruit of a small Asiatic tree related to the apple family) grafted on to hawthorn branches, she would not become pregnant.[12]

An early eighteenth century writer, John Gustave Rudolph,[13] reports superstitious practices designed to induce sterility: The suspension of hare dung and mule's hide over women's beds; the suspension over women of children's teeth caught in silver plates before they fall to the ground;[14] the throwing away by a woman into a river of as many seeds as she desires years to avoid pregnancy.

In the account of contraception during the Middle Ages we noticed the mention, in the *Additional Letters* of Arnold Villanova, of a prescription of Soranos calling for the internal use "of water in which smiths quench their forceps." Fossel reports that in Steiermark (East Austria) the same prescription has been followed by simple folk in late modern times. These people believe that, if the solution mentioned is drunk after every menstrual period, it will induce sterility; as will also the partaking of tincture of lead, English balsam, bee honey, and purgatives of all kinds, and especially aloes and myrrh.

In the hope that it might throw some light on the effectiveness of the prescription calling for the internal use of the water from smithy's fire buckets, an investigation is being made to determine whether or not it contains lead or some other sterilizing agent. It is known that lead does have such an effect; and Dr. R. L. Dickinson informs me that during the war, some women actually preferred work in factories where lead was used in the expectation, often warranted, that it would render or keep them sterile.

The continuity of another idea is noteworthy. It will be recalled that Hippocrates noted that corpulence interfered with fertility.[15] Likewise in Steiermark corpulence has been considered, since the very oldest times, a hindrance to conception.[16]

The observation of Hippocrates was certainly a shrewd one in the absence of even our limited modern knowledge of endocrinology. For there is

[12] G. Lammert, *Volksmedizin und medizinische Aberglaube in Bayern*, p. 157.

[13] Joannes Gustav Rudolphus, *Dissertatio medico-iuridica ae venenis sterilitatem inducentibus* (Wittenberg, 1731? based on ed. of 1709), ch. xxxviii.

[14] *Cf.*, Ibn al-Baiṭār, *op. cit.*, ii, 455 (No. 1560). If one takes, before it falls, the tooth of a child who is losing his teeth, and puts it in a silver leaf, and [if] a woman carries it, it will prevent her from conceiving.
Quoted from *Proprietés* of Ibn Zuhr.

[15] Haeser, *Lehrbuch* (1875), p. 202. On account of the corpulence of Scythian women the Greeks considered them unfruitful.

[16] V. Fossel, *Volksmedicin*, p. 48.

frequently an increase in obesity after the menopause, when the ovaries cease functioning. The endocrine cause for sterility sometimes involves obesity. This association between obesity and low fertility or even sterility shows the insight of some writers of the antique world. It shows also how such observations may enter into folk tradition without any seeming reason therefore, and yet have a certain foundation in fact.

According to Jaworskij, the South Russian women of the Skaler mountain range in Galicia use the following magical contraceptive receipts:

(1) A young girl, in order to prevent children, takes a few drops of her first menstrual blood, and lets it flow into a hole in the first egg of a young hen. She then buries the egg near the table in the room. There the egg remains for nine days and nine nights. When the egg is taken up, it will be found to contain worms with black heads. She will have as many children as the egg contains worms. If she throws the egg with the worms in it into the water, she will have the children; if she throws it into the fire, they will burn up once and for all.[17]

(2) The menstrual blood of wives is taken and put on flax lint. This is then tied into ten knots in ten "corners," rolled together, and worn for nine days and nine nights. During the night it is carried under the right arm, and during the day under the left knee. Thereafter it is buried in the earth in the main corner of the room while these words are recited three times: "I do not bury you for one year, but for eternity!" Then this woman will not have any children.[18]

Kaćser reports that Slovak women drink, with contraceptive intent, softened walnut leaves and saffron in water. With the same purpose in mind they carry club-moss (*Lycopodium clavatum*) in their clothes.[19] Other Slovak women are less naïve: They use linen rags to occlude the os. (See below.)

Gurewitsch and Woroschbit[20] have recently shown in their account of

[17] Juljan Jaworskij, "Malthusianische Zaubermittel," *Zeitschr. f. Österr. Volkskunde*, iv, 47.

[18] *Ibid.*, On the tying of "newly-wed knots" (novorum nuptorum ligaturae) *cf.*, Joannes Gustav Rudolphus, *Dissertatio*, ch. xiii, pp. 13–14. The Latins called the magicians who tied knots in thread or shoestrings during a marriage ceremony *Fescennini*. The symbolism of closing the bar on the door was also carried out for the same purpose.

For many centuries knot-tying was employed, especially by males, to render coitus unfruitful. The medieval Hebrew verb was *asar*, the French "nouer l'aiguillette"; in German these knots were called "Nestelknüpfen." *Cf.*, Solomon Gandz, "The Knot in Hebrew Literature," *Isis*, xiv, 194.

[19] Mory Kácser (of Luki, Hungary), *Originalbeiträge über Volksmedizin in Ungarn.* Cited by Hovorka and Kronfeld, *Vergleichende Volksmedizin*, ii, 523. *Cf.*, Aigremont, *op. cit.*, ii, 92.

[20] Z. Gurewitsch and F. Grosser, *Probleme des Geschlechtslebens* [in Russian, Staatsverlag der Ukraine, 1930, pp. 259] and *Materialen zur ukrainisch-russischen Ethnologie* [Lemberg, 1906, Bd. viii]. Cited by Z. Gurewitsch and A. J. Woroschbit, "Das Sexualleben der Bäuerin in Russland," *Zeitschr. f. Sexualwissenschaft*, xviii (May, 1931), 51–74, espec. pp. 69–70.

the sexual life of farming women in the Ukraine that *coitus interruptus* (Onanismus) is widespread among them.   These reporters also state that many other means are employed for the prevention of conception.[21]   The view is also current among the girls and women of the Ukraine that if they have coitus with many men at short intervals they will be thereby protected from impregnation.

According to Krebel, Russian women, to prevent conception, drink an infusion of saxifrage (*Locopodium clavatum*); or they drink a glass of warm water.[22]   The leaves of arum and the roots of saxifrage were, according to an Upper Palatinate legend, drunk by the daughters of the hero Attila in order to remain sterile.[23]

Some women of Siberia believe that, if they take a certain amount of white lead as soon as their menses appear, it will prevent conception until the next menses.[24]   This would be ineffective unless lead were taken in regular doses, in which case, if the doses were beyond tolerance, poisoning might result.   Trjić reports[25] that among peasant Rumanian women living in Serbia (called by the Serbs "valsi;" the Walachen?) the belief is prevalent that:

If a woman wants to remain childless, she ought on no account to sleep with her husband during the time of menstruation; but outside of the period she may always have coitus with him provided that she boils down an herb called *jarba starba* (chick weed, or *Stellaria media*), and drinks the decoction on an empty stomach. She will then not become pregnant.

The magical use of one's fingers plays an interesting rôle in the history of ritualistic, ineffective contraception.   It may be recalled that the fourteenth century observer, Frater Rudolphus, noted that women thought they would not conceive if they sat or lay down on a certain number of fingers, according to the number of years they wished to be free from pregnancy.   Superstitions of this nature have persisted for centuries, and still operate in some quarters of Europe.   Hovorka reports[26] one form of this ritual as practised by Serbian women: they place as many fingers in a child's first bath water as they desire years of freedom from pregnancy.   Krauss gives us a different variant: the bride, while riding in the wedding coach, sits on her fingers.[27]

[21] *Zeitschr. f. Sexualwissenschaft*, xviii, 70.

[22] R. Krebel, *Volksmedizin und Volksmittel verschiedener Völkerstämme Russlands.* Leipzig und Heidelberg, 1858.

[23] G. Lammert, *Volksmedizin*, p. 158.

[24] Hovorka and Kronfeld, *op. cit.*, ii, 524.

[25] Trjić on "Das Geschlechtsleben der Rumänen in Serbien" in *Anthropophyteia.* vi, 150–161.   See p. 157.

[26] *Op. cit.*, ii, 524.   Serbian women also close the house door with the legs of a newly-born infant.   This "closes" the mothers to impregnation.

[27] Cited by Ploss-Bartels, *Das Weib*, ii, 301.

Lammert reports the folk belief that:

> If a woman carries on herself the finger of a premature child, or if she drinks the urine of a ram or of a hare, or wears hare dung, she will not conceive. The same is the case if a thorn is extracted from the foot of a living weasel and a woman wears it.[28]

This prescription is reminiscent of recipes numbered two and four extracted from "The Admirable Secrets of Albert the Great" to be found on page 163.

Linné reports that in Gottland and Öland the young wife, after divorce, is able to limit the number of expected children by touching her womb with her fingers! Though the theory behind this practice is not exactly clear, one gathers that the woman thinks she will have only as many children as she uses fingers. There seems to be no question here of lathering the cervix.[29] The practice is somewhat similar to that indicated by Truhelka as operating among Bosnian peasants. When a Bosnian woman mounts into a saddle, she shoves the fingers under her belly girdle—one for each year. If she puts both hands under, she will remain sterile forever.[30] Of a similar type is the superstition of the Serbian women that they will remain childless if they raise, with the *whole hand*, the vessel containing their wedding bath water, and place it before the fire. If a few fingers are used, they will have a corresponding number of children.[31]

Still other magical rituals are reported as accepted by Serbian women. They throw a certain number of glowing coals into the bath water saying: "When these pieces of coal begin to burn again, I shall bear a child." Later, when they want a child, they throw the coals into the fire. As they begin to burn again, they feel themselves becoming pregnant on the spot. Then there is the symbolic magic of closing locks, doors, etc. Some Serbian women lay on the church floor in front of the aisle a wide-open padlock and key. Then they walk between them, and turn around saying, "When I open the lock again, I shall conceive a child."

The folk medicine of Europe reveals many other symbolico-magical methods for preventing conception. Some of these have been collected by Ploss-Bartels in their monumental and informing work, *Das Weib*.

Various peasant groups have at different times believed that, if a woman would throw various objects such as kernels of grain, apples, stones, wooden pegs or nails into a neighboring well, spring or river, she would remain free from pregnancy. One or two instances have already been reported in this

---

[28] G. Lammert, *op. cit.*, p. 158.

[29] For a discussion of this method of prevention, see Dickinson and Bryant, *op. cit.*, p. 74.

[30] Ploss-Bartels, *op. cit.*, ii, 300–301.

[31] Krauss, cited by Ploss, *ibid.*

account. Magyar women, in order to remain childless, fill, before coitus, an open padlock with poppy; then they put it in the nearest well.[32] In lower Bavaria the spotted orchid (*Orchis maculata*) is used to prevent conception. This plant has two subterranean bulbs shaped like a hand. They are dug up and thrown into water. The older clod floats; the one more recently developed sinks. The former is used by the Letts to induce sterility.[33] My understanding is that this ineffective magical means is resorted to mainly by unmarried girls in order that they might not become pregnant by their lovers.

Turning the wheel of the grain mill backward four times at midnight, being a reverse process, is supposed to prevent conception. Another symbolico-ritualistic procedure is to lay under the mill as many wheat kernels as one expects children. Another is for a woman to go to the graves of her sisters and call out three times over the graves, "I don't want any more children."[34]

According to Demeter Dan the Rumanian bride who wishes to remain childless during her married life, places, during the wedding ceremony, as many roasted walnuts in her bosom as she wishes to remain years without children. After the wedding, the nuts are buried in the earth.[35]

These practices, almost without exception ineffective, are simply symbolic magic and popular superstition. But the frequency and persistence with which they appear, now in this period, now in that; now in this geographical location, now in that, show that women of all times have longed to control their maternal, biological function; that they have wanted both fertility and sterility, each in its appointed time and place. This fear of slavery to pregnancy has been to many women like a ghost stalking the corridor of time, always present, yet always elusive; sometimes placated, more often threatening. Often, pathetically enough, women have hit upon the ineffectual and the injurious; and only lately has science consciously begun to help them.

Certain customs in existence among the simpler peoples of Europe in late modern times may have been influenced by the availability in cities of certain articles and drugs. For this reason it may be questioned whether the practices reported in the next two paragraphs really come under the classification of folk medicine. In the case of the use of the sponge reported below we suspect some urban influence. However, the practices are placed here for want of a better classification.

[32] Hovorka, *op. cit.*, ii, 524.
[33] *Ibid.*, i, 35.
[34] Ploss-Bartels, *Das Weib*, p. 300.
[35] Hovorka, *op. cit.*, ii, 524.

Mr. Horst von Einsiedel, a former German exchange student to the United States, has informed me that rural women in Southeastern Poland and in the Ukraine have the habit, when they come to the market once a year, of providing themselves with a small sponge which they use to prevent conception.   They are purchased of apothecaries, one of whom so informed Mr. Einsiedel.   This rural population is largely Russian Catholic.   But the ban of the Church seems to have little effect upon the sexual customs of these farming women, who are of the European peasant type that live in the same room with their cattle.   No information is available on how long this has been the usage.   My *guess* is that it is rather recent, and that it has been influenced by the practices of city folk.

Though it seems almost unbelievable, Byloff, in a very recent report,[36] avows that in eastern Austria, especially in the rural Alpine districts of Styria, arsenic is used not only to produce abortion but with contraceptive intent.   There is a high rate of arsenic poisoning in the region.

§2   CONTRACEPTION IN EROTIC LITERATURE

Does the whole range of erotic literature throw any light upon the history of folk contraceptive practices?   The few data available will be introduced here before discussing the more rational methods known to European folk medicine.   The medical techniques of the erotic treatises are perhaps best classed as folk literature in the sense that they were usually written by laymen.   Further, from the standpoint of classification, not enough is known about contraception in these sources to justify separate treatment in an independent chapter.   In effectiveness these prescriptions occupy a position intermediate between those discussed in §1 and those treated in §3.

It is probable that the erotic literature of the ages contains nothing new on contraceptive technique, nothing, that is, not to be found in the great medical tradition traced in this book.   Some experts on erotic literature whom I have questioned believe that erotic treatises contain virtually nothing on prevention.   This is not quite accurate, for some discussion appears.   In general, however, this literature has not been searched for this inquiry.   It would seem highly probable that the great medieval Arabic writers on sex devoted attention to it.   This literature has never been searched from this point of view, and ought to be a fruitful source for investigation.

Little light is also thrown on the history of contraceptive practices by the literature on phallicism.   A preliminary survey of Goodland's *Bibliography*

[36] Fritz Byloff, "Die Arsenmorde in Steiermark," *Monatschr. f. Kriminalpsychol. u. Strafrechtsreform*, xxi (1930), 1–14.

of Sexual Rites and Customs[37] which details the contents of some nine thousand books and articles, seems to offer few promising leads for this research.

(2a) Nefzaoui, *The Perfumed Garden*

This sixteenth century Arabian manuscript,[38] which has been translated into French, is not a scientific but an erotic treatise. Though the author discusses the most lascivious and obscene questions,[39] the translator avows that Shiek Nefzaoui is prompted by a desire to serve mankind. Al-Ṭabarī, a great Persian historian and physician of the first half of the tenth century, is quoted; and there is other evidence that the work is largely based on much older Arabic, Persian, and Indian sources.

Only two contraceptives are mentioned by Nefzaoui, and these are very old. It is stated[40] that alum introduced into the vagina, or placed on the penis before coitus, dries and narrows the vagina, and prevents the seed from reaching the uterus. Used too frequently, it makes a woman sterile. Anointing the male member with tar (goudron vegitale) will remove from the male seed the faculty of engendering.[41]

It may be provisionally stated that there is no mention of contraception in Aretino's works.

(2b) Brantôme, *The Life of Gallant Ladies*

The Abbé de Brantôme's detailed picture of the unblushing and undisguised profligacy of the court life of his time (d. 1614) touches upon the subject.[42] He says:

There are some who have no desire to receive the seed, like the noble lady who said to her lover, "Do what you will, and give me delight, but on your life have a care

[37] R. Goodland, *A Bibliography of Sex Rites and Customs.* London: Routledge, 1931. New York: Horace Liveright, 1931, pp. 752, quarto.

[38] Cheikh Nefzaoui, *Le Jardin Parfumé.* Paris: Bibliothèque des Curieux, 1922, pp. 278 (translated in 1850 by Baron R———). Copies seem to be scarce in the U. S. A. The library of the New York Academy of Medicine, however, possesses a copy. Harvard has only one edition, and that is very different from the one used here.

[39] The author says: "I swear by God, verily the knowledge herein is necessary; only the shamefaced ignoramus, enemy of all science, would refuse to read it, or would ridicule it."

[40] P. 232.

[41] It is stated that tar placed in the vagina will produce an abortion. Cinnamon on a tampon of linen in the vagina will bring about the fall of the foetus—"with the permission of God most high."

[42] Pierre de Bourdeille [Abbé de Brantôme, d. 1614], *Das Leben der Galanten Damen* (*La Vie des Dames Galantes*). Leipzig: Deutscher Verlagsactiengesellschaft, 1904. (Translated by Willy Alexander Kastner.)

to let no drop reach me." Then the other [partner] must watch out for the right moment.[43]

Brantôme also relates how Count de Sauzay, a slave, was captured by the Algerians; how the wife of the slave's master, chief priest of the mosque, seduced the slave, but insisted that "no drop enter her." In both instances the reference is probably to *coitus interruptus*.

More interesting from the standpoint of the social diffusion of such knowledge and of such practices is the statement by Brantôme that a proper (i.e., effective) means against pregnancy was known to the apothecaries of his time; and that they helped to shield unmarried girls.[44]

(2c)   Casanova, Mémoires

The use of a gold ball intravaginally, during the middle of the eighteenth century, is of some interest since one meets with it only in Casanova's (1725–1798) *Mémoires*. In the same source there is rather frequent mention of the sheath (see next chapter). Casanova avowed (August 1760) that such 60 gr. balls[45] served him successfully for fifteen years; further that they never became displaced during coitus:

It is sufficient for the ball to be at the base of the temple of love when the loving couple carry out the sacrifice. The antipathetic power given to this metal by an alkaline solution in which it has been placed for a certain time, prevents all fertilization. But, says the friend, movement may displace the ball before the end of the libation. . . . This is an accident which need not be feared, provided one exercises foresight.[46]

Casanova reports having purchased three such balls for six quadruples (about $100) of a Genevese goldsmith. Helbig,[47] a recent observer, agrees with Casanova as to the antipathetic power of gold in an alkaline solution; but Helbig is mistaken. There is hardly a more inert metal than gold; and there is no reason to suppose that the gold ball had any chemical effect, though, if it could stay in position, it might conceivably have a slight

---

[43] *Ibid.*, p. 40.

[44] P. 374. Abortion by the use of drugs is also mentioned. *Cf.*, also pp. 136, 374. Brantôme observes that "What often holds back maidens [from coitus] is the fear of pregnancy." This suggests, as one may infer on other grounds, that few, if any, really reliable methods of prevention were *generally diffused* in the sixteenth century.

[45] They had a specific gravity of 19 and a diameter of 18 mm.

[46] *Mémoires de Jacques Casanova de Seingalt, écrites par lui-même* (Bruxelles, 1863), iv, ch. 9, pp. 198 ff. It is purely a matter of convenience to classify this use of the gold ball under folk medicine. There is no record of the gold ball elsewhere.

[47] C. E. Helbig, "Zur Geschichte der mechanischen Vorbeugemittel gegen Schwangerung und geschlechtliche Ansteckung," in Krauss's *Anthropophyteia*, x, 11.

mechanical effect.[48]   But even this remains to be demonstrated.   Would it tend to fall out by virtue of its weight?   I know of no evidence that the gold ball was used during the Middle Ages.   References to it have not been met with in literature.   Helbig thinks it unreliable, and thus accounts for a lack of dissemination of the idea.   It has never been tried in clinical series; theoretically, it hardly merits such trial.

It may be noted in passing that Dr. Konikow reports[49] a block pessary (see sketch) which operates on a somewhat similar principle.   The principle seems to be one of physical occlusion of the os.   Will it do so regardless of its position in the vagina?   If it is displaced by the phallus, does another concave surface tend to occlude the cervix, being shoved into position by pressure of the vaginal walls?   Dr. Konikow thinks not.   She says, "In actual practice this apparatus is by no means certain to cover the cervix; its bulk and shape can cause irritation to the female and male organs.   It is rather an instrument of torture than a preventive.   An article has appeared in the *Journal of the American Medical Association* reporting a case in which this cubical pessary caused a fistula between the bladder, rectum, and vagina."[50]

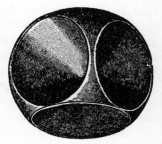

Dr. Konikow rightly labels the block pessary "a curiosity."   Certainly it plays no part in the recommendations of the world's clinics; nor have I known it to be reported in any series of cases recording the use of various contraceptive methods prior to a clinical visit (see Chapter XIII).   However, it is advertised in some cheap, American women's magazines as for sale through the mail.   Regarding the age of the block pessary nothing is known.

Casanova reports a curious use of the lemon supposed to detect a venereal infection on the part of women.[51]   He suggests that the mucous membrane of the labia and of the introitus be daubed with half a lemon.   While this is hardly a certain test of infection, any raw surface, a sore or chancre would smart.   And it may be remarked that half a small lemon from which the juice has been extracted might, as Casanova describes it, make a reasonably efficacious cervical cap.

[48] This is the judgment also of Dr. Stuart Mudd, Head of the Department of Bacteriology, University of Pennsylvania Medical School, who kindly rendered an opinion at the author's request.

[49] A. F. Konikow, *Physicians' Manual of Birth Control* (New York: Buchholz, 1931), p. 97.

[50] *Ibid.*, pp. 95–96.

[51] *Mémoires*, iv, ch. 13, p. 307.

§3 MORE EFFECTIVE FOLK PRACTICES

Let us now consider some of the more rationally founded, more effective methods found in the literature of European folk medicine and folk beliefs. German-Hungarian women in Banat, in order to prevent conception, were accustomed to apply disks made of melted beeswax one centimeter in thickness and approximately five to ten centimeters in diameter.[52] One of these they would introduce into the vagina, pressing it up against the os. Is this practice to be likened not so much to the suppository as to the more recent German practice of first taking a mould of the cervix and then fashioning an individual cervical cap? Beeswax will not melt and flow at body temperature. Banat women have also practised *coitus interruptus* and *coitus inter femora*.[53] Unmarried men in the valley of the Styrian Oberland sometimes induced women with whom they had extra-marital relations to use linen rags to occlude the os. This substitute for the sponge has been in use for many years.[54] Likewise Slovak women, just before coitus, stuff the vagina with cloth, and go out with the idea that they are all the more certainly protected from pregnancy the larger the number of men with whom they have sexual traffic.[55] Since we have found a similar practice in vogue among the natives of the Kasai Baisin, Central Africa (see Chapter I), and since there is no reason to believe that the vaginal use of rags by the natives was a result of white contact, we may conclude provisionally that this contraceptive method is very old.

A practice similar to that of the German Hungarian women just mentioned is that used by Constantinople women, who, according to Rigler, insert a sponge moistened with diluted lemon juice.[56] This would seem to be one of the most effective contraceptives to be found in the whole range of literature on folk medicine. Recent research by Voge has shown that citric acid is much more efficient as a spermicidal agent than lactic acid, now so widely employed. In fact the use of a sponge moistened with lemon juice is, like the use of beeswax, so clever, that one may legitimately

[52] Of the date I cannot be certain. Beeswax was in use certainly during the nineteenth century, but concerning its antiquity I have no knowledge. The Greeks were such beekeepers, and had such extensive knowledge of the use of vaginal suppositories that it seems quite strange that nothing has to date been found in their literature relating to the application of beeswax for this purpose.

[53] Hovorka and Kronfeld, *op. cit.*, ii, 523.

[54] V. Fossel, *op. cit.*, p. 48. Cited by Hovorka, ii, 523.

[55] Mory Kaćser, *Originalbeiträge über Volksmedizin in Ungarn.* Cited by Hovorka, ii, 523.

[56] Lorenz Rigler, *Die Türkei*, Wien, 1852. Cited by Hovorka, ii, 525. J. G. Rudolph [in his *Dissertatio medica-iuridica* (1709). I used the Wittenberg, 1731 ed. See viii, p. 7.] declared that the juice of the lemon would prevent pregnancy. *Cf.*, also material *infra* on Casanova's *Mémoires* [vol. iv, ch. 13, p. 307].

doubt whether it belongs in the folk-belief class at all. But perhaps it is a triumph of the trial and error process. The Constantinople women, after coitus, replace the sponge thus impregnated with citric acid, with a paste made from aloes, rue, and rubber; or else they rub the os with tobacco juice.

A folk contraceptive of unusual interest in the contemporary United States is the use of lard by women in the Central States (the so-called Corn Belt where hogs are raised). My informant is a well-known sociologist who prefers to remain anonymous.

Coitus interruptus is doubtless the most popular, widely diffused method of contraception. It is generally prevalent among European working class people, and has been for centuries. In view of its general diffusion it seems odd that one writer should refer to it as the *usus italicus*. It is no more an Italian than a French or American practice. My study in 1927 of the records of the first 234 patients to pass through the Liverpool Women's Welfare Centre showed that, whenever any method was employed prior to the clinic visit of the wife, withdrawal was most frequent.[57] The safe period, significantly enough, was not mentioned once. In 44 per cent of the instances (102 cases out of 234) an attempt to prevent births was admitted. Of these 59, or 58 per cent, used *coitus interruptus*. That this sample is representative is shown by similar evidence being collected at other clinics. At the clinics where trouble is taken to inquire into the sexual habits of the patients and their husbands, I have found this, upon inquiry, to be confirmed. One gathers the same impression by a perusal of the periodical literature. And why should this not be the case? The method is accessible, cheap, easy, and its injuriousness probably exaggerated, even by those more or less well-informed on contraception.[58]

§4 SUMMARY

The notions of the populace on contraceptive technique have been, until late modern times, essentially magical. Though more rational methods are recorded in the literature of folk medicine; and though *coitus interruptus*

---

[57] *Eugenics Review*, xx (1928), 159. *Cf.*, recent data by R. Pearl, E. Charles, H. Stone. *Cf.*, ch. xiii, *infra*.

[58] Though scientific questions are not to be decided by vote taking, it is interesting to note that Dr. Gertrude E. Sturges, an investigator for the National Committee on Maternal Health, found that among fifty-nine French medical men best qualified to judge its merits, "more than two-thirds considered *coitus interruptus* harmless, or probably harmless. Two-thirds of the gynecologists so voted, and four-fifths of the sixteen neurologists." [Dickinson and Bryant, *op. cit.*, p. 58.] Much nonsense has indeed been written on this subject even by those who should have known better. *Coitus interruptus* is ordinarily to be condemned on utilitarian and hedonistic grounds, rarely on the ground that it does nervous injury. The main reason why it should not be used lies in the fact that better methods are now available.

is probably nearly as old as the group life of man, methods essentially effective are rare.

Regarding the means of communication of what little was known this may be said. Popular views were passed on orally rather than in writing. This may partially account for some bizarre notions. Generally speaking, the simple peasant folk of Europe were little accustomed to consult physicians about any matters until just before their death. A European peasant woman would no more contemplate the desirability of consulting a physician to limit her family than the majority of the populace even in our day will consult a physician for a common cold. If this is true, folk contraceptive practices were self-perpetuating by oral tradition, little influenced by the best knowledge of medicine.

Again we must remember that until quite late in history only the best contraceptive prescriptions in medical tradition had any *raison d'être*. They, almost alone, were effective. And the *best* medical practices are almost never—especially before the rise of improved methods of communication[59]—those in general use. This fact is not peculiar to the history of contraception. It is true of virtually all branches of medicine. This separation in development of folk medicine and classical medicine accounts, along with the self-amplifying nature of any oral tradition, for the more magical nature of folk contraceptive ideas and practices.

Most common perhaps are the prescriptions to be taken by the mouth as well as various magical rituals. Often these are on no higher level than those of savages. Various forms of symbolic magic (e.g., use of fingers) are involved. The use of seeds or leaves of fruitless trees seems to involve symbolic implications. In this manner willow plays a prominent rôle, and is rather frequently mentioned. Musitanus (in 1709) mentioned the use of a suppository of black hellebore and castoreum after coitus; also the avoidance of passionate coitus. The last view is very old. But it was reinforced by Christian dogma to the effect that the genuine enjoyment of coitus was satanical. Christianity is now reaping the results of its suppression of the art of love in an increased divorce rate.

For centuries one can trace prescriptions using dung, smith's fire-bucket water (Soranos); and the association between corpulence and sterility is very old (Hippocrates).

No attempt has been made to survey erotic literature for this history. The Arabic sources, as yet mostly untranslated and unpublished, ought to be especially rich; but such a search must be a separate task. The alum and tar of Nefzaoui's sixteenth century manuscript go back to classical and

---

[59] E. g., "inexpensive" medical journals and books, the growth of many medical libraries, etc.

Oriental sources; likewise with Brantôme's report of *coitus interruptus*. The report of the gold ball by Casanova seems, so far as present knowledge goes, to be quite unique in literature; but Casanova's report of the sheath goes back, of course, to Fallopius's *De Morbo Gallico* (1564) and possibly, but not certainly, to Imperial Rome. Thus, one is forced to the provisional conclusion (pending an elaborate survey of the literature) that the erotic literature of the ages contains nothing new when compared with the great body of medical literature having its culmination in all that is best in the modern healing art.

One should not conclude that all the contraceptive practices of the simple folk of Europe in bygone centuries were magical, ineffective. Excluding the use of a sponge by the rural women of Southeastern Poland and in the Ukraine—a usage perhaps influenced by the urban mores of recent development—we may recall the use of beeswax intravaginally by German-Hungarian women in Banat. Whether the beeswax is used as a suppository or as a specially moulded cervical cap is uncertain.

Coitus interruptus is widely diffused, and must be classified as rational in conception, and, in some measure, reliable. Stuffing the vagina with cloth or linen rags is reported among Slovak women and some female inhabitants of the Styrian Oberland. The practice of some Constantinople women of soaking a sponge in diluted lemon juice and using it as a vaginal tampon is theoretically not surpassed in reliability by any modern clinical contraceptive. Probably it was never widely diffused, or the results of use would have shown up in a low birth rate (assuming that the motives for its use were widely diffused). Citric acid ranks high as a spermicide.

The persistence of the folk practices detailed above suggests additional proof of the main thesis of this book: that the human race has in all ages and in all geographical locations *desired* to control its own fertility; that while women have always wanted babies, they have wanted them when they wanted them. And they have wanted neither too few nor too many. This is the great "paradox" of the biological history of man. In reality, however, it is no paradox at all. It is merely one phase of the dialectic of history.

What is new is not the desire for prevention, but effective, harmless means of achieving it on a grand scale. The older effective techniques were never until recently democratically diffused; and even that process is still going on.

CHAPTER VIII

HISTORY OF THE CONDOM OR SHEATH

§1 INTRODUCTION

WHETHER from the standpoint of numbers used or availability for use by the modern public, the condom, or male covering, is undoubtedly the most important contraceptive instrument of our day. When we realize that (1) approximately 1,500,000 individual condoms are manufactured daily in the United States, an annual production of about 317,000,000;[1] that (2) approximately three million decisions[2] are made daily by the married couples of the United States as to whether or not they shall use contraceptives, we get some conception of the importance of this whole matter. Further, my analysis of more than 27,000 instances of the use of contraceptives prior to first visits to birth-control clinics—and that means in virtually all instances prior to any special medical advice on contraception—shows that the condom was used in roughly one-quarter of the instances. Douching had the same popularity—witness the advertisements in women's magazines on "feminine hygiene" and the full-page advertisements in mail-order-house catalogues—even though the ever-popular withdrawal led. So far as extra-marital relations are concerned it seems a safe guess that the condom is the chief instrument used. The vulcanization of rubber revolutionized transportation. Will it revolutionize morals and sexual relations? Time will give the safest verdict; but the answer seems clearly in the affirmative.

It is worth while, therefore, to inquire a little into the history of the condom.

Passing mention may be made of the fact that many primitive peoples, as well as the early Egyptians, used various forms of penis protectors, not for contraceptive purposes but for protection against tropical diseases (like condirus and bilharzia) against insect bites, as badges of rank or status, as amulets to promote fertility, for decoration, or for modesty.

[1] Report of Mr. Randolph Cautley to the National Committee on Maternal Health. See Norman E. Himes and Randolph Cautley, article on "Condom" in the forthcoming *Encyclopedia Sexualis*. New York: Dingwall-Rock, 1936.

[2] Robert Latou Dickinson and Louise Stevens Bryant, *Control of Conception*, p. 1. This figure is based on an estimate of the number of fertile married couples living in the U. S. A. in 1925.

From these it was but a step to cover the penis as a prophylaxis against venereal infection; and the earliest sheaths of contraceptive form were undoubtedly used for that purpose, at least as early as the sixteenth century. Only later, say about the eighteenth century (so far as we now know), were they used for the prevention of conception. The prophylactic linen glans condom of Fallopius (1564) gradually became a full covering using the caeces of various animals.

The real revolution did not come, however, until the vulcanization of rubber by Goodyear in the U. S. A. or by Hancock in England (1844). Then the rubber product, owing largely to its cheapness, virtually displaced the membranous condom. Latterly, that is, within the last decade, the industry has experienced a second revolution, the introduction of the latex condom. We shall return to this subject later.

How far back can the condom be traced? The early non-contraceptive coverings were all made of some non-skin-like material. Not until the second century do we have any record of a sheath of skin-like materials.

§2 EARLY HISTORY OF THE CONDOM

(2a) *The Legend of Minos and Pasiphae. Was the Sheath Used in Imperial Rome to Prevent Conception?*

A difficult problem of historical interpretation arises in connection with the Minos-Pasiphae legend as it relates to the early use of a goat membrane. According to the account that has come down to us in Antoninus Liberalis's *Metamorphoses* (forty-first, "The Fox"), Prokris, daughter of Erechtheus, abandoning her husband, Cephalus, as a result of a quarrel, took refuge with Minos, the King of Crete. Now, inasmuch as the semen of Minos contained serpents and scorpions, all the women who had cohabited with him had been injured. For this reason he married Pasiphae, who was immune against infection because she was the daughter of the King of the Sun. Inasmuch as this union remained sterile, Prokris sought a remedy in the following:

She slipped the bladder of a goat into the vagina of a woman. Into this bladder Minos cast off his serpent-bearing semen. Then he went to find Pasiphae, and cohabited with her.[3]

In this manner Pasiphae conceived not only Ariadne and Phaedra, but also two other daughters and four sons.

Helbig,[4] who first called attention to this myth in relation to the history

---

[3] Antoninus Liberalis, *Sammlung von Verwandlungen* (übersetzt von Friedrich Jacobs, Stuttgart, 1837), pp. 141–142.

[4] C. E. Helbig, "Ein Condom im Altertume," *Reichs-Medizinal-Anzeiger*, xxv (1900), 3. See *La Chronique Médicale*, xii (1905), 141, for a translation into French by Klotz-Forest.

of the condom (in this instance it was a female sheath), contends that "if religious legends reflect in any degree the practices and customs of an epoch," one must conclude that "in imperial Rome the bladders of animals were used to receive the sperms of men during coitus with the purpose of protecting women against the consequences [pregnancy or infection?]." Seven years later (1907) Helbig complained that his interpretation had been misunderstood; that the myth concerned itself not with the prevention of conception, but with the induction of pregnancy and with protection against infection.[5] If the latter is the proper interpretation, as seems probable,[6] the responsibility would seem to be largely Helbig's for using a vague term ("consequences"). But nothing is gained by an attempt to allocate responsibility. Whatever the motive for the use of the goat bladder, it seems quite possible that it was employed.

Both Streich and Helbig believe that Liberalis did not correctly report the facts, holding that King Minos himself wore the sheath; that, in short, a male and not a female sheath was employed. They think that Liberalis was misled in his description, owing to the unfamiliarity of ancient writers with such procedures.[7] This imputation of naïveté to the ancients appears somewhat far-fetched. But it seems impossible now to go behind the original versions of Liberalis and others. No doubt some sheath, male or female, was used in imperial Rome, though we know nothing of the extent of such use. In the absence of more positive knowledge we must assume that it was not in common use.

(2b)   *The Linen Sheath of Fallopius* (1564)

The first known published description of the condom is to be found in the work of the great Italian anatomist, Fallopius, who in his *De morbo gallico*,[8] first published in 1564, two years after the author's death, described a linen sheath. (See Figure XI for a photostatic reproduction of the appropriate page in Fallopius's work.) This sheath, cut to shape for the glans, Fallopius, one of the early authorities on syphilis, claims to have invented.[9]

---

[5] C. E. Helbig, "Zu dem Schrifttume über den Condom," *Reichs-Medizinal Anzeiger*, xxxii (1907), 405–407; 424–426. See especially pp. 405–406.

[6] Nevertheless, Rondibilis (pseudonym?) accepted the view in 1919 (*Progrès Médicale*, February 8, 1919) that the goat bladder was used to prevent conception.

[7] *Reichs-Medizinal Anzeiger*, xxx (1900), 3. Arthur Streich, "Zur Geschichte des Condoms," in *Sudhoff's Archiv. f. Gesch. d. Med.*, xxxii, 209–213.

[8] Gabrielle Fallopio, *De Morbo Gallico liber absolutismus* (Patavii, i.e., Batavia), ch. 89 on "De praeservatione a carie Gallica," p. 52.

[9] Helbig (in Krauss' *Anthropophyteia*, x, 8) contends that Fallopius' invention was not a forerunner of the condom; but as Streich points out, Helbig elsewhere contradicts himself. Helbig's accounts seem to me inaccurate on several points.

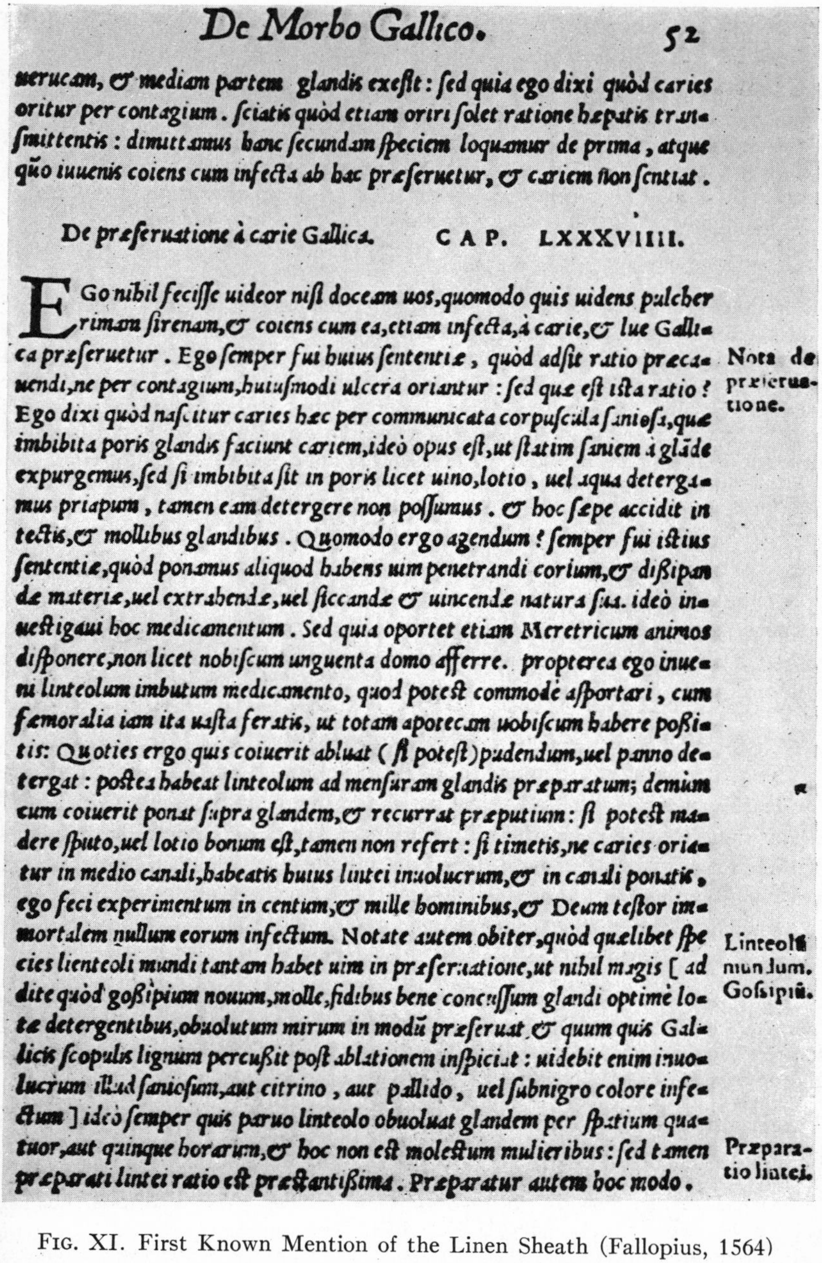

De Morbo Gallico.   52

werucam, & mediam partem glandis exest: sed quia ego dixi quòd caries
oritur per contagium. sciatis quòd etiam oriri solet ratione hæpatis trut-
smittentis: dimittamus hanc secundam speciem loquamur de prima, atque
quo iuuenis coiens cum infecta ab hac præseruetur, & cariem non sentiat.

De præseruatione à carie Gallica.   CAP. LXXXVIIII.

Ego nihil fecisse uideor nisi doceam uos, quomodo quis uidens pulcher
rimam sirenam, & coiens cum ea, etiam infecta, à carie, & lue Galli-   Nota de
ca præseruetur. Ego semper fui huius sententiæ, quòd adsit ratio præca-   præseruu-
uendi, ne per contagium, huiusmodi ulcera oriantur: sed quæ est ista ratio?   tione.
Ego dixi quòd nascitur caries hæc per communicata corpuscula saniosi, quæ
imbibita poris glandis faciunt cariem, ideò opus est, ut statim saniem à glade
expurgemus, sed si imbibita sit in poris licet uino, lotio, uel aqua deterga-
mus priapum, tamen eam detergere non possumus. & hoc sæpe accidit in
tectis, & mollibus glandibus. Quomodo ergo agendum? semper fui istius
sententiæ, quòd ponamus aliquod habens uim penetrandi corium, & dissipan
de materiæ, uel extrahendæ, uel siccandæ & uincendæ natura sua. ideò in-
uestigaui hoc medicamentum. Sed quia oportet etiam Meretricum animos
disponere, non licet nobiscum unguenta domo afferre. propterea ego inue-
ni linteolum imbutum medicamento, quod potest commodè asportari, cum
femoralia iam ita usta feratis, ut totam apotecam uobiscum habere possi-
tis: Quoties ergo quis coiuerit ablaut (si potest) pudendum, uel panno detergat: postea habeat linteolum ad mensuram glandis præparatum; demum
cum coiuerit ponat supra glandem, & recurrat præputium: si potest madere sputo, uel lotio bonum est, tamen non refert: si timetis, ne caries oriatur in medio canali, habeatis huius lintei inuolucrum, & in canali ponatis,
ego feci experimentum in centum, & mille hominibus, & Deum testor immortalem nullum eorum infectum. Notate autem obiter, quòd quælibet spe   Linteolī
cies lienteoli mundi tantam habet uim in præseruatione, ut nihil magis [ad   mundum.
dite quòd gossipium nouum, molle, sidibus bene concussum glandi optimè lo-   Gossipiū.
tæ detergentibus, obuolutum mirum in modū præseruat & quum quis Gal-
licis scopulis lignum percussit post ablationem inspiciat: uidebit enim inuolucrum illud saniosum, aut citrino, aut pallido, uel subnigro colore infe-
ctum] ideò semper quis paruo linteolo obuoluat glandem per spatium qua-
tuor, aut quinque horarum, & hoc non est molestum mulieribus: sed tamen   Præpara-
præparati lintei ratio est præstantissima. Præparatur autem hoc modo.   tio lintei.

Fig. XI. First Known Mention of the Linen Sheath (Fallopius, 1564)

In Chapter 89 "On Preservation from French Caries [Syphilis]" we find the following:

Quoties ergo quis coiuerit abluat (si potest) pudendum, uel panno detergat: postea habeat linteolum ad mensuram glandis praeparatum; demum cum coiuerit ponat supra glandem, et recurrat praeputium: si potest madere sputo, uel lotio bonum est, tamen non refert: si timetis, ne caries oriatur in medio canali, habeatis huius lintei inuolucrum, et in canali ponatis, ego feci experimentum in centum, et mille hominibus, et Deum testor immortalem nullum eorum infectum.

This, in translation, reads as follows:

As often as a man has intercourse, he should (if possible) wash the genitals, or wipe them with a cloth; afterward he should use a small linen cloth made to fit the glans, and draw forward the prepuce over the glans; if he can do so, it is well to moisten it with saliva or with a lotion; however, it does not matter: If you fear lest caries [syphilis] be produced [in the midst of] the canal, take the sheath of this linen cloth and place it in the canal; I tried the experiment on eleven hundred men, and I call immortal God to witness that not one of them was infected.

Fallopius avowed that one advantage of this instrument was that it could be carried in the trouser pocket. It was fitted over the glans, and the prepuce then drawn over it. This was, of course, recommended for protection against infection. After Fallopius' mention of the condom for this purpose it passed down in the enormous European literature on syphilis. (Some of this literature is referred to in §3 in which the origin of the word condom is discussed.)

(2c)   Seventeenth and Eighteenth Century Sources

The next important mention in literature of the condom is, so far as one can learn, that made in 1671 in the letters of Mme. de Sévigné (1626–1696) to her daughter, the Countess of Grignan. Mme. de Sévigné here speaks of the sheath made of gold-beaters skin as "armor against enjoyment, and a spider web against danger."

An early eighteenth century English physician, Daniel Turner, in his work on *Syphilis* speaks of

. . . the *Condum* being the best, if not the only Preservative our Libertines have found out at present; and yet by reason of its blunting the Sensation, I have heard some of them acknowledge, that they had often chose to risk a *Clap*, rather than engage *cum Hastis sic clypeatis*. [With spears thus sheathed.][10]

Turner gives us no description of the instrument, condemns by implication its use, and furnishes no hints on the etymology of the word.[11]

---

[10] Daniel Turner, *Syphilis. A Practical Treatise on the Venereal Disease* (London, 1717), p. 74. Fourth ed. (London, 1732), p. 107; 1724 ed., p. 84.

[11] Turner does, however, say that "Dr. *Sharp*, as well as the *Wolverhampton* Surgeon,

Astruc, writing in 1736, nineteen years after Turner, speaks of great debauchees who, in England,

have been employing for some time sacs made of fine, seamless membrane in the form of a sheath [scabbard] and called in English condum.[12]

(2d) A Theory of Origin

A plausible theory of the origin of the condom is that a medieval slaughter-house worker first conceived the idea that covering the penis with the thin membranes of some animal would protect one against venereal infection. Perhaps someone tried it, found himself protected, communicated the idea to others.

It seems unlikely that the sheath was used as early for contraception as for prophylaxis. Use for the prevention of conception seems definitely later. The slaughter-house theory of the origin of the sheath seems as reasonable as any since it fits into the trial and error method of learning—a method used since time immemorable and one which always will be used, the "rationalists" and planners to the contrary notwithstanding. Are we to credit the statement of Fallopius that he invented the glans condom? Regarding other contraceptive techniques one finds so many claims to "invention" that one becomes aware of the necessity of discounting such claims.[13] I am disinclined to credit Fallopius's statement. Probably the real inventor hit upon the idea by accident, is unknown, and never will be known.

§3 ORIGIN OF THE WORD CONDOM

Many are the theories that have been evolved to account for the origin of this word. In the literature of venereology it is most commonly stated that the condom was invented by, and named after, one Dr. Condom or Conton, a physician at the court of Charles II (1660–1685). A variant story has it that he was a physician living at the time, but not attached to the Court. Still another version declares that Charles II was beginning to be annoyed at the number of his illegitimate children; and that Dr. Condom invented the instrument for Charles, in return for which Charles, with great gratitude, knighted him. Others have said that the "inventor" was not a

---

with two or three others behind the Curtain, stand Candidates with Dr. C——n, for the Glory of the invention." 1724 ed., p. 84. Turner adds " . . . the Bait being like to catch Fools, the *Secret* has since multiply'd."

[12] *De Morbis Venereis*, 1736. French translation by Le Pileur.

[13] Examples are Knowlton's statement that he first used alum; Edward Bond Foote's statement that his father, Edward Bliss Foote invented the cervical cap. Several other cases could be cited.

physician at all but a mere courtier of Charles II.[14]   Painstaking efforts to trace the existence of such a physician have failed.[15]   Ferdy gave attention to the matter; and Havelock Ellis[16] made an investigation on his own account.

Let us trace to their sources the origins of these mistaken views, show the wide-spread adoption of them, and finally, examine the validity of other attempts to account for the etymology and philology involved.

The word Condum first appears in Turner's treatise on *Syphilis* (1717).[17] One finds in Bachaumont's diary entry for December 15, 1773 these words supposed to be addressed to a former ballet dancer who had become a prostitute:

> You know the use of the *condon* . . .
> The *condon* my daughter, is the law and the prophets.[18]

A London dictionary of street language mentions the word *Condum*[19] in 1785. Girtanner refers to it in 1788,[20] followed by F. Swediaur in 1801.   Swediaur seems to have been the first to have introduced the statement, later generally copied by German textbook writers and authors of encyclopedia articles, that the invention of the caecal-condom so honored the inventor that he found it necessary to change his name.[21]   There is no original source which enables us to check the statement; and the view deserves rejection in the absence of more positive evidence.   It was probably Girtanner (1788) who started the erroneous statement in the German literature to the effect that the sheath was invented by Dr. Condom during the reign of Charles II.

[14] Prof. Joseph Hyrtl of Vienna (in *Handbuch der Topographischen Anatomie*, Wien ii, 212, 7th ed.) thinks the instrument should be called *Gondom*, that being, in his opinion, the name of the chevalier at Charles II's court.

[15] Dr. Rollins of the Harvard English Department, an authority on this period in English literature, informed me in oral conversation that he is not aware that Pepys in his diary ever mentioned a Dr. Condom or the instrument itself.   He added that much of the shorthand diary has never been translated.

Iwan Bloch assures Ferdy likewise on the same point (*Chronique Médicale* xii (1905), 535).   Bloch says that neither John Evelyn nor Samuel Pepys, the two chief memoir writers of the reign of Charles II, made any mention of a Dr. Condom, Condon, or Conton. Bloch wrote Ferdy that "the origin of *Condom* has remained up to this time [1903] an unsolved riddle." (*Ibid.*)

[16] Havelock Ellis, *Studies in the Psychology of Sex* (Philadelphia: Davis, 1924), vol. vi on *Sex in Relation to Society*, p. 600.

[17] Daniel Turner, *loc. cit.*

[18] Cabanès, *Les Indiscrétions de l'Histoire* (Paris, 1903), p. 121 f.

[19] [Francis Grose], *A Classical Dictionary of the Vulgar Tongue*. London: Hooper, 1785.   A new edition edited with a biographical and critical sketch has been issued by Eric Partridge, London: Scholartis Press, 1931.

[20] *Abhandlung*, p. 280, f.

[21] *Traité*, p. 102 f.

How Girtanner, the great authority on syphilis, introduced the error—Astruc, on whom Girtanner built, does not affirm it—will be told in §4, since treatment of this point is more convenient there.

The view that the device was named after its inventor, one Dr. Condom, then crept into literature, and was repeated by many nineteenth century physicians and lay authors, among whom were Cullerier,[22] Merat,[23] Langelbert,[24] Proksch,[25] Wilde,[26] Nysten, Littré,[27] Power, W. Sidgwick,[28] Dühren,[29] Robley, Dunglison,[30] Thompson, Moll[31] and many others. They all speak of a Dr. Condom. Possibly they borrowed from Swediaur, and have simply perpetuated an error. A pseudonymous English Neo-Malthusian writer of the mid-nineteenth century, Anti-Marcus,[32] repeats the same statement. Even C. J. S. Thompson repeats it in our time.[33] I am inclined to think it a myth; but confess that disproof is impossible. But neither is proof possible.

Ferdy at first believed[34] that the word condom was derived from the name of a French village in the Department of Gers. Later he rejected this,[35] deriving *condum* from *condus*, the former being the accusative of the substantive *condus* (*condere*, to conceal, protect, preserve). Ferdy conjectures[36] that *condus* was probably used in the accusative form in an early Latin

[22] *Dictionnaire des Sciences Médicales*, 1820–21. Article on "Syphilis."

[23] *Ibid.*, Article on "Redingotes."

[24] *Dictionnaire de Médicin*. Article on "Condom."

[25] Proksch said in 1872 that Dr. Conton was the first to recommend the use of lamb intestines as a preservative against syphilis. For this purpose a piece of intestine of the desired length was cut from a killed animal, cleaned, dried, and then rendered soft and pliable by rubbing with fine oil and bran (J. K. Proksch, *Die Vorbauung der Venerischen Krankheiten*. Wien, 1872, p. 48).

[26] Friedrich Adolph Wilde, *Das weibliche Gebär-unvermögen* (Berlin, 1838), p. 316.

[27] *New Sydenham's Society's Lexicon*, ii, (1882). Cited by G. Pernet in "Notes sur les préservatifs de la syphilis á travers les âges," in *Ann. des Mal. Vénériennes*, (Paris) 1907, pp. 740–741.

[28] *Le Marquis de Sade et son Temps* (Berlin, Paris, 1901), p. 211.

[29] "Le Médecin Condom a-t-il existé?" *La Médicine Internationale Illustrée*. Paris, April and May, 1901.

[30] Dunglison says [in his *Dictionary of Medical Science*, 1904 (23rd ed.) p. 274] that the condom was named "from its proposer, Dr. Condom." He lists armour, French letter and Cytherean shield as synonymous.

[31] *Handbuch* (Leipzig), p. 451.

[32] Anti-Marcus, *Notes on the Population Question*. London: J. Watson, 1841. This historically important little tract is virtually unknown in the United States. At least I have never seen it cited in the population literature produced here.

[33] C. J. S. Thompson, *Quacks of Old London* (London: Brentano's, 1928), p. 273.

[34] Hans Ferdy, *Limitation voluntaire morale*, p. 176, note 1. Bloch (Dühren, *Sexual Life of our Time*) repeats this statement. It is probably erroneous.

[35] Hans Ferdy, "Contribution à l'étude historique du 'Coecal-Condom,'" *Chronique Médicale*, xii (1905), 535–537. See p. 537.

[36] *Ibid.*, p. 537.

treatise on syphilis; and since *condus* meant one who collects or preserves something, the term may have been used in the sense of a receiver of semen to prevent venereal infection. Ferdy thinks the word *condum* then became corrupted in common speech to condom, *condon* or *conton*. He is convinced, and this seems quite possible, that the term condom is not of English origin (unless, we should add, it is a proper name). Ferdy's theory seems hardly acceptable.

Richter has still another theory.[37] Not only was *condum* latinized from a Greek neuter form, but the word has a Persian origin, Zὼ, *kendü* or *kondü*, referring to a long vessel made of the intestines of animals, and used for storing corn or grain. Richter thinks a learned Latin scholar of the Middle Ages jokingly gave the name *condum* to the animal-vessels used to prevent conception. Accordingly, he does not think any English "inventor" had to change his name because of opprobrium. Here again we have a problem for philologists to settle. The theory seems hardly more credible than Ferdy's.

A Harvard friend of mine, a young philologist of unusual competence, made, at my request, an independent and *de novo* investigation of the philology of *condom*, and reported that he could "find nothing reliable." He concluded that "It must have been originally a proper name." The story of Charles II is repeated, but with the additional remark that he (the philologist) does not "know how reliable this story is."

It is interesting to note how each of two nations refuse to accept the "honor" of association with it. The French call the condom "la capote anglaise" or English cape; the English have returned the compliment; to them it is the "French letter."

§4 THE CONDOM IN THE EIGHTEENTH CENTURY

It would seem reasonable to suppose that the houses of prostitution made, during the eighteenth century, and perhaps in an earlier period, considerable use of male sheaths. It is said that these houses were veritable arsenals of them.[38] It is also probable that prostitutes personally sold them. Madame Gourdan had special purveyors.[39]

De Sade, an eighteenth century writer, says Madame de Saint Ange recommended condoms and sponges.[40] The sponge, it may be remarked, was rarely mentioned in the literature from the time of the Talmud to Francis Place, whose favorite method it was. However Jeremy Bentham recommended its use for reduction of the poor rates as early as 1797.

[37] Paul Richter, "Beiträge zur Geschichte des 'Kondoms,'" *Zeitschr. f. Bekampfg. d. Geschlechtskrankheiten*, xii, (1911) 35–38.

[38] Rondibilis, *op. cit.*

[39] *Correspondance de Madame Gourdan dite la Petite Comtesse.* Bruxelles: Uzanne, 1883.

[40] Eugene Dühren, *Marquis de Sade et son Temps*, pp. 384–387.

(4a) Casanova

Casanova (1725–1798) knew and used the condom.[41] He had several appellations for the sheath: "The English riding coat" (redingote anglaise); "the English vestment which puts one's mind at rest" (un vêtement anglais qui met l'âme en repos);[42] "the preservative sheaths" (les étuis préservatifs);[43] and in still another connection he speaks of them as "assurance caps" (callotes d'assurances).   Elsewhere he refers to "preservatives that the English have invented [sic] to put the fair sex under shelter from all fear."[44]

Casanova relates that on All Saints Day in 1753 he purloined from the secretary of a Viennese nun her provision of preservatives, and substituted for them a bit of poetry; but he let himself be moved by her entreaties, and returned to her "that which is so precious to a nun who wishes to make sacrifices to love."[45] Upon another occasion at Marseilles, Casanova, about to enter into relations with a public woman, did not fail to make known his fear of a possible infection.   Thereupon, she offered him "un vêtement anglais" which "met l'âme en repos."   Casanova refused it because "the quality was too ordinary;" whereupon she offered him a finer one at three francs, a kind which "the tradeswoman sold only by the dozen."   Casanova decided to take the entire dozen, and proceeded to try them out on a young domestic of fifteen years.[46] With their use Casanova seems to have been satisfied.   They have not disappointed him; nor have they suddenly broken.   The worst that he can say against them is: I do not care "to shut myself up in a piece of dead skin in order to prove that I am perfectly alive."[47] Casanova used sheaths not only to prevent infection, but to avoid impregnating his women.   He seems, moreover, to have tested them for imperfections by inflating them with air.

(4b) Writers on Syphilology

Girtanner,[48] investigator of syphilis and contemporary of Casanova, writing in 1788, said, in the course of describing five means of preventing venereal infection:

It is necessary in the meanwhile that I cite once more one of these means, because today it is considered a current custom and considered infallible by the debauchees

---

[41] For Casanova's use of the gold ball as a contraceptive see elsewhere within.

[42] *Mémoires* (Bruxelles, 1863), iv, 313 f.

[43] *Ibid.*   Cited by Helbig, *Reichs-Medizinal-Anzeiger*, xxxii, 424.

[44] As quoted by Rondibilis in *Progrès Médical*, xxxiv (1919), 56–58.

[45] *Mémoires* (Paris, Flammarion), iv, 352–353.

[46] *Ibid.*, iv, 222 and 281; v, 357.

[47] As quoted by H. Ellis.   *Studies*, vi, 600.   Ellis is in error in thinking that Casanova made no use of these instruments—a slip which could easily be made even by an investigator of Ellis's erudition.

[48] Christoph Girtanner, *Abhandlung über die Venerische Krankheit* (Göttingen, 1788), i,

who go to excess.   On this occasion I proved, as I have proved in other passages in this work, how difficult it is to speak on the subject which I treated, to fulfill the duties of a doctor who should let nothing pass in silence which can be of interest to the human race and at the same time guard against offending modesty.   The German language appears too chaste to furnish decent words on subjects so shameful.   Meanwhile the matter is too important to allow it to pass in silence. I wish to speak of the fish membranes which serve to protect the man's member during copulation.   This shameful invention which suppresses and annihilates completely the only natural end of cohabitation, namely procreation, *comes from England, where these instruments were used for the first time under the debauched reign of Charles II.   Even today they bear the name of their inventor;* [italics mine] they diminish pleasure and annihilate the natural end of cohabitation; finally they are insufficient to assure immunity, for the least hole will permit contagion.   And again it may happen that during coitus the membrane may tear by a strong strain.

Girtanner also avowed that fish-skin condoms were openly sold in Paris, London, Berlin, and St. Petersburg.   "The negligence of the police," he complained, "who do not seek to prevent the sale of an invention so shameful and so detrimental to repopulation, is, in truth, inconceivable."[49]   Monseignor Brown, testifying before the first English Birth-Rate Commission, declared that condoms were in use in London at the time of the great fire (1666).[50]   Brown's source is unknown.

Girtanner's source was apparently Johannes Astruc, one of the physicians of Louis XV, whose classic treatise on venereal disease first appeared in 1738.   For Girtanner speaks of Astruc's treatise as his "model."   Girtanner quotes part of the following from Astruc:

I hear from the lowest debauchees who chase without restraint after the love of prostitutes, that there are recently employed in England skins made from soft and seamless hides in the shape of a sheath, and called condoms in English, with which those about to have intercourse wrap their penis as in a coat of mail in order to render themselves safe in the dangers of an ever doubtful battle.   They claim, I suppose, that thus mailed and with spears sheathed in this way, they can undergo with impunity the chances of promiscuous intercourse.   But (in truth) they are greatly mistaken.[51]

280–282.   Up to 1788 Girtanner was a physician in Pyrmont.   In 1789 he emigrated to Göttingen where he compiled medical works, and wrote on the French Revolution.

[49] *Ibid.*, i, 280–282.

[50] *Report of the National Birth Rate Commission* (Second ed. London, 1917), p. 184.

[51] Johannes Astruc, *De Morbis Venereis* (Paris, 1738), bk. iii, ch. ii, §2, p. 209.   The passage reads: Audio a perditissimis ganeonibus, qui meretricios amores effrenate sectantur, adhiberi nuper in Anglia folliculos a tenui et inconsutili pellicula in vagine formam confjctos et Anglice Condum dictos, quibus congressuri obvolutum penen loricant, ut a periculis pugnae, semper dubiae tutos se praestent.   Autumant scilicet ita cataphractos histisque eo modo clypeatis se vulgivagae veneris discrimina subire impune posse.   Sed errant quidem maxime.   [All in italics.]

It should be noted that while Astruc avows the instruments are "called condums in English," he says nothing about their being named for an English physician. It would seem, therefore, that Girtanner introduced the error—for such it probably is—that the device was given the name of a physician living in the time of Charles II.

(4c) English Handbills of the Eighteenth Century

In the latter part of the eighteenth century handbills were distributed in London advertising the sale of "cundums," stating where they could be purchased. Grose, a satirist of the period, liked to expose the quacks of his time; and he speaks of a Mrs. Philips "modestly" offering "her wares, prepared with the result of thirty-five years of experience. This public-spirited matron [sic] informs us, that after ten years retirement from business, she has resumed it again, from representations, that since her recess, goods comparable to what she used to vend cannot be procured."[52] It seems that a handbill or advertisement issued as early as 1776 by Mrs. Philips offered sheaths for sale at the Green Canister in Half Moon Street in the Strand; and that after having acquired a competence she retired from business.[53] She evidently sold out to a Mrs. Perkins. It is difficult to piece together, from the conflicting evidence preserved by Grose, the facts regarding subse-

---

[52] [Francis Grose], *A Guide to Health, Beauty, Riches and Honour* (second ed. London, 1796), p. iii. (First ed. 1783 according to B. M. Catalogue.) That Grose had a satirical purpose in making this collection of advertisements is evinced by the following statement in his introduction (p. viii):

> In fine, kind reader, from these premises my assertion seems incontrovertibly demonstrated, namely, That if we are not healthy, beautiful, rich, and wise, we have only our own incredulity or negligence to blame for it, since the means of these blessings are daily offered to us, with many other advantages, set forth at length in the following collection [of handbills, advertisements, etc.], which, it is hoped, will make us set a proper value on our native country, and inspire foreigners with a due reverence for Old England.

[53] [Francis Grose], *Classical Dictionary of the Vulgar Tongue* (London: Hooper, 1785), has the following to say under

> CUNDUM, the dried gut of sheep, worn by men in the act of coition, to prevent venereal infection, said to have been invented by one Colonel Cundum. These machines were long prepared, and sold by a matron of the name of Philips, at the Green canister in Half-moon-street, in the Strand. That good lady having acquired a fortune, retired from business; but learning that the town was not well served by her successors, [she,] out of a patriotick zeal for the public welfare, returned to her occupation, of which she gave notice, by diverse hand bills, in circulation in the year 1776.

Note that these "machines" are mentioned only as preventives of infection. It is highly probable, however, that they were used also in the eighteenth century for the prevention of conception. The 1823 edition of Grose's *Dictionary* omits this word.

Mrs. PHILIPS, who about ten years left off busineſs, having been prevailed on by her friends to reaſſume the ſame again
upon repreſentations that, ſince her declining, they cannot
procure any goods comparable to thoſe ſhe uſed to vend ;——
begs leave to acquaint her friends and cuſtomers, that ſhe has
taken a houſe, No. 5, Orange-court, near Leiceſter-fields, one
end going into Orange-ſtreet, the other into Caſtle-ſtreet, near
the Upper Mews-gate.——To prevent miſtakes, over the door is
the ſign of the Golden Fan and Riſing Sun, a lamp adjoining
to the ſign, and fan mounts in the window, where ſhe continues to carry on her buſineſs as uſual.——She defies any one
in England to equal her goods, and hath lately had ſeveral
large orders from France, Spain, Portugal, Italy, and other
foreign places. Captains of ſhips, and gentlemen going
abroad, may be ſupplied with any quantity of the beſt
goods on the ſhorteſt notice.

☞ It is well known to the public ſhe has had thirty-five
years experience, in the buſineſs of making and ſelling machines,
commonly called implements of ſafety, which ſecures the
health of her cuſtomers : ſhe has likewiſe great choice of ſkins
and bladders, where apothecaries, chymiſts, druggiſts, &c.
may be ſupplied with any quantity of the beſt ſort.——And
whereas ſome perſon or perſons pretending to know and carry
on the ſaid buſineſs, diſcovering the preference given to her
goods ſince coming into buſineſs again, have induſtriouſly
and maliciouſly reported that the Original Mrs. PHILIPS is
dead, and that ſuch perſon or perſons is or are her ſucceſſors
(which is entirely falſe and without the leaſt foundation), and
hath and doth, or have and do, utter or deliver out in the
name of Philips, and as from her warehouſe, a moſt infamous
and obſcene hand-bill or advertiſement ; the public are hereby
aſſured, that ſuch perſon or perſons is or are a mere impoſtor or
impoſtors, and that the real original Mrs. PHILIPS lives and
carries on her buſineſs in Orange-court aforeſaid, and not elſe-
where (as can be teſtified by many who daily ſee her behind
her counter), and that ſhe hath no concern whatſoever in the
buſineſs publiſhed by ſuch hand-bills of theirs, notwithſtand-
ing the impudent uſe of her name thereto affixed ; and neither
prepares or vends, or ever did or ever will prepare or vend,
any other goods than thoſe above ſpecified. She alſo ſells all
ſorts of perfumes. The following lines are very applicable
to her goods :

> To guard yourſelf from ſhame or fear,
> Votaries to Venus, haſten here ;
> None in my wares e'er found a flaw,
> Self preſervation's nature's law.

FIG. XII. Mrs. Philips's Eighteenth Century Handbill or Advertisement.
Source: F. Grose, Guide (1796) pp. 10–11.

quent events. Mrs. Philips probably re-entered business after selling out to Mrs. Perkins, and this caused resentment on the part of the latter. This would explain the war of handbills (Figures XII, XIII and XIV). Mrs. Philips opened her new shop at 5 Orange Court near Leicester Fields. Interesting from the standpoint of diffusion is the statement that she has "lately had several large orders from France, Spain, Portugal, Italy and other foreign places." She boasts in her advertisement of thirty-five years of experience. A wholesale trade seems to have been operated by her, for we learn that she is prepared to supply "apothecaries, chymists, druggists,

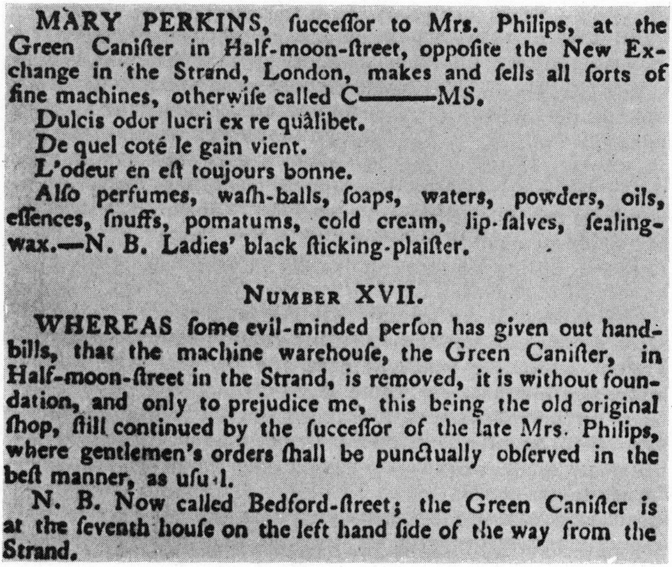

MARY PERKINS, succeffor to Mrs. Philips, at the Green Canifter in Half-moon-ftreet, oppofite the New Exchange in the Strand, London, makes and fells all forts of fine machines, otherwife called C————MS.

Dulcis odor lucri ex re quàlibet.

De quel coté le gain vient.

L'odeur en eft toujours bonne.

Alfo perfumes, wafh-balls, foaps, waters, powders, oils, effences, fnuffs, pomatums, cold cream, lip-falves, fealing-wax.—N. B. Ladies' black fticking-plaifter.

NUMBER XVII.

WHEREAS fome evil-minded perfon has given out handbills, that the machine warehoufe, the Green Canifter, in Half-moon-ftreet in the Strand, is removed, it is without foundation, and only to prejudice me, this being the old original fhop, ftill continued by the fucceffor of the late Mrs. Philips, where gentlemen's orders fhall be punctually obferved in the beft manner, as ufual.

N. B. Now called Bedford-ftreet; the Green Canifter is at the feventh houfe on the left hand fide of the way from the Strand.

FIG. XIII. Mrs. Perkins's Handbill. Source: F. Grose, *Guide* (1796) p. 13

etc." Another handbill states that "Ambassadors, foreigners, gentlemen, and captains of ships, &c. going abroad, may be supplied [from "Mrs. Philips's Warehouse"] with any quantity of the best goods [condoms] in England, on the shortest notice and [at] the lowest price."

Thompson, who is aware of Mrs. Philips's trade, says that condoms "were originally made from the dried gut of a sheep and were first [sic] sold at two [London] taverns near Covent Garden, viz., the *Rummer* and the *Rose*, the latter hostelry in Russell-street being a famous meeting place in Stuart times."[54] Since the statement is undocumented, the source is unknown.

[54] C. J. S. Thompson, *Quacks of Old London* (London: Brentano's, 1928), p. 273.

No one knows of what material they were "first" made, much less at what particular place they were "first" sold.

The eighteenth century sheath was a descendant of the linen sheath of Fallopius, if not of the Roman, goat-bladder sheath reported by Antoninus Liberalis. After Fallopius the caeces of lambs, sheep, calves, goats, and

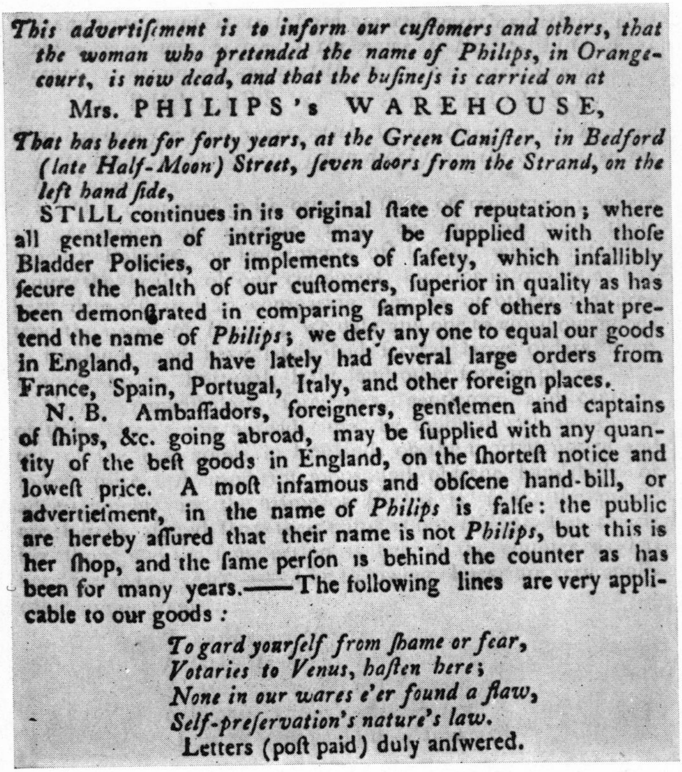

This advertifement is to inform our cuftomers and others, that the woman who pretended the name of Philips, in Orange-court, is now dead, and that the bufinefs is carried on at

Mrs. PHILIPS'S WAREHOUSE,

That has been for forty years, at the Green Canifter, in Bedford (late Half-Moon) Street, feven doors from the Strand, on the left hand fide,

STILL continues in its original ftate of reputation; where all gentlemen of intrigue may be fupplied with thofe Bladder Policies, or implements of fafety, which infallibly fecure the health of our cuftomers, fuperior in quality as has been demonftrated in comparing famples of others that pretend the name of *Philips*; we defy any one to equal our goods in England, and have lately had feveral large orders from France, Spain, Portugal, Italy, and other foreign places.

N. B. Ambaffadors, foreigners, gentlemen and captains of fhips, &c. going abroad, may be fupplied with any quantity of the beft goods in England, on the fhorteft notice and loweft price. A moft infamous and obfcene hand-bill, or advertiefment, in the name of *Philips* is falfe: the public are hereby affured that their name is not *Philips*, but this is her fhop, and the fame perfon is behind the counter as has been for many years.——The following lines are very applicable to our goods:

> *To gard yourfelf from fhame or fear,*
> *Votaries to Venus, haften here;*
> *None in our wares e'er found a flaw,*
> *Self-prefervation's nature's law.*
> Letters (poft paid) duly anfwered.

FIG. XIV. Advertisement of Mrs. Philips's Warehouse. Source: F. Grose, *Guide* (1796) p. 12.

perhaps other animals were employed. Probably the fish bladder condom is a figment of the imagination.[55] And the female condom is virtually a museum specimen. I have never known a patient to use one. They are thick and dull sensation.

[55]Girtanner and a writer in the *Real Enzyclopädie der ges. Heilkunst* (Wien, 1885), iv, 431, considers it a reality. If the air bladder of some fishes was used, no authority for such usage has been found.

§5   THE CONDOM SINCE THE VULCANIZATION OF RUBBER

Widespread, common use of the condom, however, had to await the vulcanization of rubber, first successfully carried out by Goodyear and Hancock in 1843–44.[56] This lowered costs so materially that the condom immediately won a place for itself.[57] Thereafter virtually every late nineteenth century treatise, and certainly every twentieth century treatise, dealing with technique gave it a prominent place. There are at least a hundred such pamphlets and volumes; and no useful purpose would be served by citing the literature, for many of them are mentioned in Part Five, which discusses briefly the developments since 1800.

The use of liquid latex and the introduction of automatic machinery has cheapened the condom still further in the last decade. Sales are enormous. There are no statistics available of the number manufactured in England and Germany, but in the United States sales approach 317 million annually. In fact it has recently come to light in an American Circuit Court of Appeals that one American manufacturer sold 20,000,000 in *one year* to druggists and doctors.[58] J. Schmid of New York says that the fifteen chief manufacturers in the United States produce a million and a half a day. Harmsen reports[59] that one German firm put twenty-four million rubber condoms on the market every year. He declares that since the war there has been an extraordinary increase in their use in Germany. Though the birth-control clinics seldom recommend the condom,[60] it is increasingly used by the general populace, doubtless because

---

[56] As early as 1872, Proksch (*op. cit.*, pp. 50–51) proposed the feasibility of rubber condoms. It is difficult to credit the statement of Streich [*Sudhoff's Archiv. f. Gesch. d. Med.*, xxii (1929), 210] that the rubber glans condom was first introduced into Europe from America through the World Exposition held in Philadelphia in 1876. Must Yankee inventive genius be credited with this also? I doubt it; yet the fact that rubber was first vulcanized here may lend credence to the view. The English claim Hancock invented the process, but the honor is generally (and I believe correctly) attached to Goodyear's name.

[57] Though those made in our time of animal membranes are undoubtedly superior in strength, they have never, for economic and sanitary reasons, proved as popular. Butherand and Duchesne give a description of the manufacture of condoms in *Lyon Médicale*, Oct. 21 and 28; Nov. 4, 1877.

[58] The official citation is Youngs Rubber Corporation, Inc., v. C. I. Lee & Co., et al, 45 Federal Reporter, 2nd Series, 103. *Cf.*, Morris L. Ernst, "How We Nullify." [New York] *Nation*, cxxxiv, 113–114 (January 27, 1932). See p. 114.

[59] In Sanger and Stone [Eds.], *Practice of Contraception*, p. 153.

[60] The Cambridge, England, clinic and the Russian clinics are exceptions. Since this was written the English clinics are using sheaths increasingly. A recent statistical study by Enid Charles supports well, though I do not think it conclusively proves, the thesis that the condom is the most reliable contraceptive we have. Havelock Ellis took this view many years ago.

it is cheap, easily available, generally known, and also the best protection against infection. The height of mechanized diffusion of contraceptives seems to have been reached in one respect in Germany and Holland, where for many years condoms have been sold by coin slot-machines! In the United States vending machines have likewise been introduced; and more are sold in gasoline stations and tobacco shops than in drug stores. Thus enters a new problem in social control.

§6 MODERN ECONOMIC ASPECTS OF THE INDUSTRY[61]

We have spoken of the revolution following the vulcanization of rubber, which caused, in turn, all but the disappearance of the skin condom. Sales and use expanded enormously, facilitated by substantially lowered costs. In the last half decade (1930–1935) the industry has experienced another technological revolution: the manufacture of condoms from liquid latex instead of from crepe rubber. We have noted the sales results. It remains now to sketch certain other aspects of this change: the processes involved, the problems of distribution, cost, competition, price and quality; the methods of testing.

The processes of modern manufacture are of interest. The substitution of liquid latex for crepe rubber is one of the most important recent technical changes, the introduction of automatic machinery being another. The latex is the whole sap of the rubber tree, suspended in water, concentrated by evaporation, stabilized by ammonia. Until recently rubber condoms were made of crepe rubber masticated and dissolved. There were difficulties incident to mastication, solution and fire hazard. Now all American manufacturers save one has ceased to make the "cement" rubber condom of crepe rubber. The latex product resists aging from three to five years, is odorless and often thinner. The new process requires constant attention of highly skilled chemists and technicians since the use of colloidal suspensions in this industry is new. Even the old processes have been so modified through changes in compounding, and in the use of the "hot" cure instead of the "cold" cure utilizing sulphur chloride gas, that the newer product does not deteriorate so rapidly. Accompanying these changes has been the introduction of continuous, automatic machinery which has also contributed to lower costs and hence to a doubled market. (See below for an estimate of prices and the total value of the output of the industry.)

In the Killian process, glass tubes (also called "forms" and "bottles") about 14 inches long and $1\frac{1}{4}$ inches in diameter dip into tanks filled with

---

[61] Parts of this section are extracted from a report of Mr. Randolph Cautley to the National Committee on Maternal Health, and almost the entire section is based on his report.

ivory-colored latex at the rate of 1 per second on each side of a dual machine which operates 24 hours per day. Rotating smoothly through the compound, they gather a dripping film of latex and rise out of the tank elevating their angle with the continuous chain to which they are attached, distributing the running liquid evenly about the blunt end of the form and preventing the formation of a drop at the tip. They are dried by hot air, dipped a second time, and dried again. The protective bead or ring at the open end is then rolled by rotating cylindrical brushes, after which vulcanization takes place in a long overhead hot air duct followed by a hot water bath. The films of latex are partially dried and dusted with talc, and are then stripped from the forms by brushes quite like the bead-rollers but so placed as to roll the condoms completely off the forms whence they fall to continuous belt-conveyors. The belts take them into an adjacent room and deposit them on a table where women unroll and snap them to remove the wrinkles (induced by the rolling) before they have time to result in permanent sticking. Meanwhile the glass forms have been cleaned by having passed through brushes and hot water, and are beginning to dip again. The entire conveyor, about 500 feet long, and containing about 4,000 glass forms in two series, one on either side of the machine, is driven at a constant rate of speed by two large cogs set about 250 feet apart in a completely air-conditioned room.

The Shunk process differs principally in the method of dipping and in the method of cure. Where the Killian machine rotates the forms through the compound at an angle of 45° with the level of the fluid, the Shunk unit dips the forms vertically into the compound through the elevation and lowering of the compound tanks, and the forms remain perfectly stationary except for rotation. The compound runs down the form and forms a hard, thick tip at the very end of the condom. The process is not completely automatic, in that labor is required to transfer the forms back and forth between the dipping machine and the conveyor, which unifies the whole process. The forms, instead of being fastened to one conveyor, are divided into units of 24, each unit being a separate board or rack. Four of these racks are placed on the dipping arm and taken off after the dipping. Finally, after vulcanization in hot water, the forms and condoms are cooled by a spray of cold water before dipping. The Killian machine is the larger of the two, being adapted to produce 1200 gross per day, while the Shunk unit will produce in the neighborhood of 700 gross per day.

Each step in the compounding, dipping and curing presents opportunities for wide variations in the properties of the resulting condoms. The pH, viscosity and ingredients of the compound are especially important in their influence upon the final product. Continuous agitation of the compound is sometimes necessary to prevent "creaming," a condition in which the rubber particles rise to the top as do the fat particles in milk.   Humidity and temperature must be controlled in the dipping, and the temperature of the cure or vulcanization is also quite important.   Particles of dust, oil or other foreign matter in the compound at the time of dipping conduce to defective condoms.   The cure affects the aging characteristics and other physical properties.   With a viscosity too high, the compound is likely to permit the formation of fine bubbles, which in the finished condom are seen as holes, thin spots and blisters.   Weight, size, thickness, elasticity, tensile strength, aging quality, resistance to abrasion, reaction with physiological fluids, reaction with lubricants, porosity, presence of foreign matter, etc., are all determined by the technological processing, equipment and supervision.

American condoms are generally much thinner than the European product, for the latter are predominantly of the "cement" type.   Those produced in air-conditioned rooms are remarkably free from dirt and foreign matter.

The patents of the industry are chiefly in the hands of three competing producers; and while there has been talk of a patent pool this has not materialized.

Production costs and prices are of importance.   Figures on manufacturing costs are extremely difficult to obtain, and they vary, of course, not only with efficiency in production, with control of patents, but with size of overhead (generally speaking, the smaller the output the larger the overhead), with care taken in testing, means of marketing, etc.   It is a common economic phenomenon that marketing costs are high in relation to manufacturing costs.   This is illustrated very well in the industry under consideration.   In a preliminary cost estimate[62] of $2.17 per gross, distribution is roughly as follows: $1.30 is for salesmen, a conservative estimate; 41¢ for overhead (perhaps higher than average); and 20¢ for raw materials.   The small balance is for stamping, rolling, packaging, etc.   Testing costs vary between nothing and 23¢–25¢, with an average probably around 5¢.

Distributors all over the country can now buy bulk condoms from the leading manufacturers for less than 50¢ a gross, and most of them are sold in bulk by manufacturers to distributors who then resell them, using their own brands and packages.   There are countless numbers of brands on the market varying greatly in quality and selling to the retailer mainly from 50¢ to $1.50 a gross, though some run as high as $5.50 or $10.80 a gross.

Retail prices vary greatly in this anarchical industry.   One brand sells at retail 3 for 75¢.   The retail price of a gross is $36.   These can be pur-

---

[62] Of tentative value only.   It is very difficult to get at cost figures in the industry.

chased from the manufacturer for $6. Is it any wonder that the druggists are being undersold, and that today retail druggists sell only about one-third of the condoms annually produced in the United States? In the face of these economic facts it hardly seems possible that the trade can be restricted to regular retail drug outlets.

It is estimated that the druggists sell in the vicinity of 700,000 gross annually at an average price of around $16 per gross, or approximately $11,000,000. Other retail outlets and peddlers sell about 1,400,000 gross annually at an average price of about $10 per gross, or about $14,000,000 per year. Thus we have an annual retail value of $25,000,000. At the price of 3 for 50¢, or $24 a gross retail, the annual sales to consumers would be valued at roughly $50,000,000. But since the present average price, under the conditions of cut-throat competition prevailing in the industry, is probably nearer $12 a gross or $1 per dozen, the annual value of sales to consumers is probably nearer $25,000,000 annually. An annual export quota of about 200,000 gross must be allowed for in estimating domestic consumption.

As is often the case in a modern industry a few producers have cornered the major portion of the market. The three leading manufacturers are responsible for 70 per cent of the daily production; the leading four for 80 per cent; the leading six for 88 per cent of the output; and all others for 12 per cent.

In this anarchically competitive industry emphasis is upon production at a low price rather than upon quality of output. Price factors have likewise led to a more than proportional increase in sales through non-drug-store channels (pool rooms, food stores, gasoline stations, etc.). Drug stores are being undersold. They have considered condoms "whisper items," and have consequently insisted on margins of profit approaching those on drugs. It is a common saying in the drug trade that the sale of condoms pays the store rent.

There are four chief methods of testing; a fifth is used in England. (1) During the "Flip Test" an operator sits at a table with bulk condoms at her left elbow using her right hand to pick up individual condoms. As they fill with air this is imprisoned in the tip end by a scissor-like action of two fingers of the left hand. The entire condom is thus elongated and the tip distended. This is supposed to show up holes and facilitate rejection of those containing wrinkles or creases. Sometimes the condom is turned over. However, holes, weak spots and dirt specks are not well perceived by this method of testing, which is the least satisfactory of the methods now in use. None the less, this is all the testing most "tested" condoms ever get. (2) An operator fills a dozen condoms with air from a compressed air jet, squeezing them against the body, bursting some and leaving others intact. Visual examination may or may not follow. (3) An operator blows down a condom held vertically with open end up, imprisons some air, and turns the inflated tip to the cheek to detect air streams. (4) A cheek test follows full inflation. At the same time there is a visual examination for dirt, wrinkles, creases, etc. There is a careful, deliberate visual examination of the condom inflated and uninflated, about 15 seconds being spent upon each one. This is the best test in general commercial use in the U. S. A. today. (5) The following test is used by an English manufacturer. Condoms are inflated to about 6 x 8 inches and placed on moving belts about 5 or 6 inches apart. As they are carried slowly across the room—transit occupies 20 to 30 minutes—those which become deflated because of holes or defects drop to the floor between the belts. Several distributors in this country employ visual examination before a frosted glass pane. The laboratory of a certain manufacturer occasionally tests for tensile strength by stretching a portion of his product on a vertical rod; another claims to inflate every third condom with smoke, the outpourings of which are more readily visible.

Testing by the consumer is usually difficult because of his inexperience. Inflation with water and breath are commonly used. The disadvantage of the latter is that exhalation into the condom sometimes causes the powder thereon to form a sticky paste and thus to cover up defects. The percentage of condoms which meet high standards of manufacture vary greatly with different brands. And even some of the good ones are not uniformly good. The habits of consumers militate against effective purchasing of quality products only. These devices are usually purchased rolled, and never examined until the crucial moment. Until the habits of consumers change, it is probably not likely that manufacturers and distributors will consider it commercially advisable to maintain more rigid testing standards.

It seems clear from the data presented above that the economic, social and medical problems of the production, sale and distribution of condoms are considerable. Certainly we have in the greatly increased use of this instrument nothing short of a revolution in the sexual relations of mankind. How astounded Fallopius would be, could he return to earth and observe what a change has taken place since he invented his linen glans covering! Little did he realize how social forces would catch up his invention and improve and diffuse it until its use became common knowledge. This process of democratization is the subject of the next Part.

PART FIVE

DEMOCRATIZATION OF TECHNIQUE SINCE 1800 IN ENGLAND AND THE UNITED STATES

CHAPTER IX

THE EARLY BIRTH-CONTROL MOVEMENT IN ENGLAND AND THE UNITED STATES

§1 RECAPITULATION AND INTRODUCTION

UP TO this point attention has been focussed on contraceptive practices and methods in various cultures prior to the nineteenth century. We have shown that the *desire* to control conception is a universal social phenomenon, a constant element, as Pareto would say, in group cultural life. We have shown, further, that this is true even at those times and in those cultures where such a desire is overlaid with disdain of sterility, and where we find present powerful mores making for rapid reproduction as, for example, among the ancient Hebrews and in the Orient. More than this, not only the *desire*, but some *knowledge* of control is a more or less constant element in the sense that some methods, though not always effective ones, are usually present. It is not affirmed that in early cultures this knowledge was generally diffused. That cannot be proved. In fact, all the evidence we have points to the contrary. The truth is rather that until recently the general diffusion of genuinely effective methods in no way met human expectations. There was a great gap between desire for control and effective prevention. The proof of this lies partly in the somewhat greater predominance of such positive checks as infanticide and abortion in early as compared with modern cultures.

It was in the nineteenth century in Western societies, especially in England, Germany and France that contraceptive practices spread most rapidly.[1] The reasons need not be analyzed in detail; but factors associated with growing industrialization, urbanization, lessened ecclesiastical authority, and greater freedom for women have played a major rôle.[2] My present

---

[1] My prediction is that there will be a rapid diffusion in the Orient during the twentieth century. But whether it will be as rapid as in western Europe during the nineteenth century remains to be seen.

[2] See *infra* ch. xiii, §6. For one thoughtful analysis of motives see James A. Field, *Essays on Population and Other Papers* (Edited by Helen Fisher Hohman, Chicago: University of Chicago Press, 1931), chs. xi and xii. Field was a first-class investigator of the phases of the population problem he chose to develop. He was, at the time of his death, the world's greatest authority on the history of Neo-Malthusianism. My estimates of the book are to be found in *Eugenics Review*, October, 1931, and in the *Jour. Pol. Econ.*, February, 1932.

object is rather to sketch briefly the literature dealing with the development during the nineteenth century of contraceptive technique, and to trace the socialization of this knowledge.

Contraceptive knowledge always has been, and still is to some extent, the possession essentially of the upper, more privileged classes. Since Place's propaganda this information has, at an accelerating rate, spread to the working and less privileged classes. *This is the most important new aspect of birth control*; and it is this process that I call socialization, or democratization. What once existed almost exclusively for the classes will soon be a reality for the masses.

It is impossible to write exhaustively on technical developments during the nineteenth century. First, such an account would require several hundred pages. Second, we are more interested in the social diffusion of knowledge as the chief characteristic of the period. Third, in earlier chapters of this work techniques have been examined in detail in order to show that the desire for prevention and also some knowledge of actual techniques were present in many different cultures at various epochs; present, in fact, throughout the entire range of social evolution. Such detailed treatment is not necessary for the nineteenth century since all informed students of recent social changes are agreed that contraceptive practices have been present in Western societies since 1800. In fact, such practices have been more widespread in Western cultures since 1800 than in any major cultures at any period in the world's history. It is likewise hardly necessary to labor the point that there has been great improvement in the effectiveness of these devices since 1800, especially since about 1870. Nevertheless, some attention will be devoted to the methods mentioned by the more important of the earlier nineteenth century figures; and in some cases, the development of a writer's ideas (especially if he or she is important, e.g., Owen, Knowlton, Besant etc.) on technique will be traced. Information, whenever available, on the circulation of tracts and books will also be introduced, as this is the chief means we have of studying the cultural diffusion of this knowledge prior to the founding of the birth-control clinics.

Approximately two hundred mechanical devices, all based upon a few basic principles and varying only in details, are now being used in Western cultures. This is exclusive of chemical agents in douches or soluble pessaries, and exclusive of ineffectual magical procedures which still survive from the earliest times. Virtually all of these techniques either originated in, or were considerably developed during the nineteenth century except possibly the condom, suppositories, *coitus interruptus* and *obstructus* and the tampon with or without medication. There is little mention of douching before Knowlton. Certainly the device that has found most universal acceptance clinically, the vaginal diaphragm (or Mensinga or Dutch pessary[3]), in combination with a spermicidal paste or jelly was an invention of the nineteenth century (1880). As early as 1838 a German gynecologist, F. A. Wilde, had recommended a cervical rubber cap specially moulded by taking a wax impression of the parts (see discussion of Wilde on pp. 318–20). It is evidently the prototype of the rather widely-used modern cervical cap now made in many different materials, soft rubber being the most common.

The chemistry of contraception has been considerably developed in this period, especially in the past few years by Voge and Baker whose works (see Bibliography) the reader should consult for the best researches on this subject. Chemical investigation is destined to see still greater developments since it is one of the most promising fields. Immunization through spermatoxins or hormones lies in the future, perhaps the distant future; yet it may revolutionize contraception. So much for recent and possible future developments.

Turning now to the nineteenth century writers on technique, we shall mention the names of certain English, American, and German writers who have made contributions to this field. It happens that the four chief authors writing in English in the period 1823–1850—Francis Place, Richard Carlile, Robert Dale Owen, and Dr. Charles Knowlton—were also the world's chief early theorizers in this field. Regardless of whoever may have preceded them in literature by way of mention of contraceptive practices, these writers initiated the social theory which surrounds this subject; and though some of their views have required modification or even rejection, they have for the most part steadily gained ground until today they are accepted by the majority of economists and sociologists. They are now supported by the weight of authority on the subject.

Stress upon the social and economic desirability of birth control is a characteristic of the nineteenth century, and hardly ante-dates it. This generalization is exceedingly important. Medical discussion is old; the economic and social justification, the body of doctrine known as Neo-Malthusianism, is new. There was some, though little, Neo-Malthusian theory before Malthus.[4] This is possible since Malthusian theory did not begin with Malthus. But

---

[3] There are many trade names such as Ramses, Rantos, Durex, etc. It is also sometimes called the Haire pessary since Dr. Norman Haire, Harley Street physician, popularized it in England about 1922. Haire has done much to push this improved technique in England, and was among the first to use it there.

[4] Jeremy Bentham advocated use of the sponge method of birth control to reduce the English poor rates as early as 1797, a year before Malthus published his *Essay*. See the passage in Arthur Young's *Annals of Agriculture*, xxix, 422–423. Pamphlet ed. p. 31. See my article on "Jeremy Bentham and the Genesis of English Neo-Malthusianism" in the Historical Supplement to the *Economic Journal* January, 1936.

the point which cannot be too strongly emphasized is the late development of the economic and social case for birth control as compared with the medical case. I am speaking now of the literature. I have shown in Chapter I that some preliterate or "savage" people sometimes saw a connection between too many children and individual, family or tribal poverty. But these people, of course, left no literature. It is in this sense, and with these qualifications (which rather prove the rule), that one may legitimately claim that the medical case for birth control is old, the economic and social case new. The latter characterized especially the theory of the nineteenth century.

Until a few years ago many informed people believed that the modern birth-control movement, as a social movement, began with the prosecution in London in 1877–79 of Bradlaugh and Besant for publishing Dr. Charles Knowlton's *Fruits of Philosophy*. As early as 1910,[5] however, Professor James A. Field published an interesting and able paper demonstrating that England had a fairly extensive birth-control propaganda in the eighteen twenties led by Francis Place (1771–1854). In this model of historical-economic research Field showed that Place was probably the anonymous author (since corroborated) of the "Diabolical Hand Bills"—as they were later dubbed—distributed among the working populace by various surreptitious methods. Field thought that Robert Owen, the New Lanark philanthropist and founder of the coöperative movement, was involved in the authorship.[6] But later research has definitely eliminated him from complicity in the affair.[7]

§2   FRANCIS PLACE (1771–1854) FOUNDER OF THE BIRTH-CONTROL MOVEMENT

Though many preceded Francis Place[8] in discussing the technique of contraception, he seems to have been the first to venture, at first alone and unaided, upon an organized attempt to educate the masses. *Place holds, therefore, the same position in social education on contraception that Malthus holds in the history of general population theory*. Malthus had approximately twenty predecessors, yet economists and sociologists concede that he was

[5] James A. Field, "The Early Propagandist Movement in English Population Theory," *Bull. Amer. Econ. Asso.* 4th Series, 1911, i, 207–236. Reprinted in *Essays on Population*, pp. 91–129.

[6] *Essays*, p. 49, and elsewhere. (See "Owen" in index.)

[7] Norman E. Himes, "The Place of John Stuart Mill and of Robert Owen in the History of English Neo-Malthusianism," *Quart. Jour. Econ.*, xlii (1928), 627–640.

[8] The best general biography of Place is Graham Wallas' *Life of Francis Place*, London: Longman, 1898; Allen & Unwin, 1918. There is a readable, short biography of Place by Wallas in the *Dictionary of National Biography*. There is also a Fabian Society tract.

the first to treat the subject of general population theory systematically. So it was Place who first gave birth control a body of social theory.

A self-taught workingman who rose to prominence in English political life through sheer dint of heroic effort, Place was a friend of Thomas Wakley, the medical reformer who founded, and who for many years edited, the *Lancet*. It was a daring innovation in the history of economic thought—less significant in the history of medical thought—when, in 1822, Place published his *Illustrations and Proofs of the Principle of Population* (Himes ed. 1930), the first treatise on population in English to propose contraceptive measures as a substitute for Malthus' "moral restraint."

There is still a widespread misconception, especially outside the circle of economists and sociologists, as to the exact meaning of the term "moral restraint." It never implied restriction on intercourse within the married relationship, but rather postponement of marriage until the contracting parties were able to support possible offspring. (For the reasons why Malthus condemned birth control, see my edition of Place's *Population*, pp. 283–298.)

(2a) Place's Handbills and Propaganda

Still more courageous was Place's dissemination among the working classes of contraceptive handbills. Place called the attention of statesmen, working-class leaders, the editors of newspapers and of other influential citizens to the need for contraceptive instruction. By clever and sometimes by subterranean methods, Place and his assistants succeeded in widely distributing these medical handbills. In 1823 they received considerable circulation not only in London, but in the industrial districts of the North; while the discussions which ensued caused them to be reprinted in several radical journals of the period.[9]

Copies of the handbills are still preserved in the so-called Place Collection in the Hendon repository of the British Museum. They exist in two forms, printed and manuscript. The three printed forms are addressed respectively "To the Married of Both Sexes,"[10] "To the Married of Both Sexes in Genteel Life,"[11] and "To the Married of Both Sexes of the Working People."[12] The first two were neatly printed on a single sheet about 5 by 9 inches, while the third was a four-page pamphlet approximately 3 by $5\frac{3}{4}$ inches. Still another draft addressed "to the mature reader of both sexes"[13]

---

[9] Notably in Carlile's *Republican*, in T. J. Wooler's *The Black Dwarf*, in Carlile's *Every Woman's Book*, etc. They even had a limited circulation in America; but that is a separate story.

[10] Place Collection, lxi, part ii, p. 43.

[11] *Ibid.*

[12] *Ibid.*, p. 42.

[13] *Ibid.*, lxviii, p. 103.

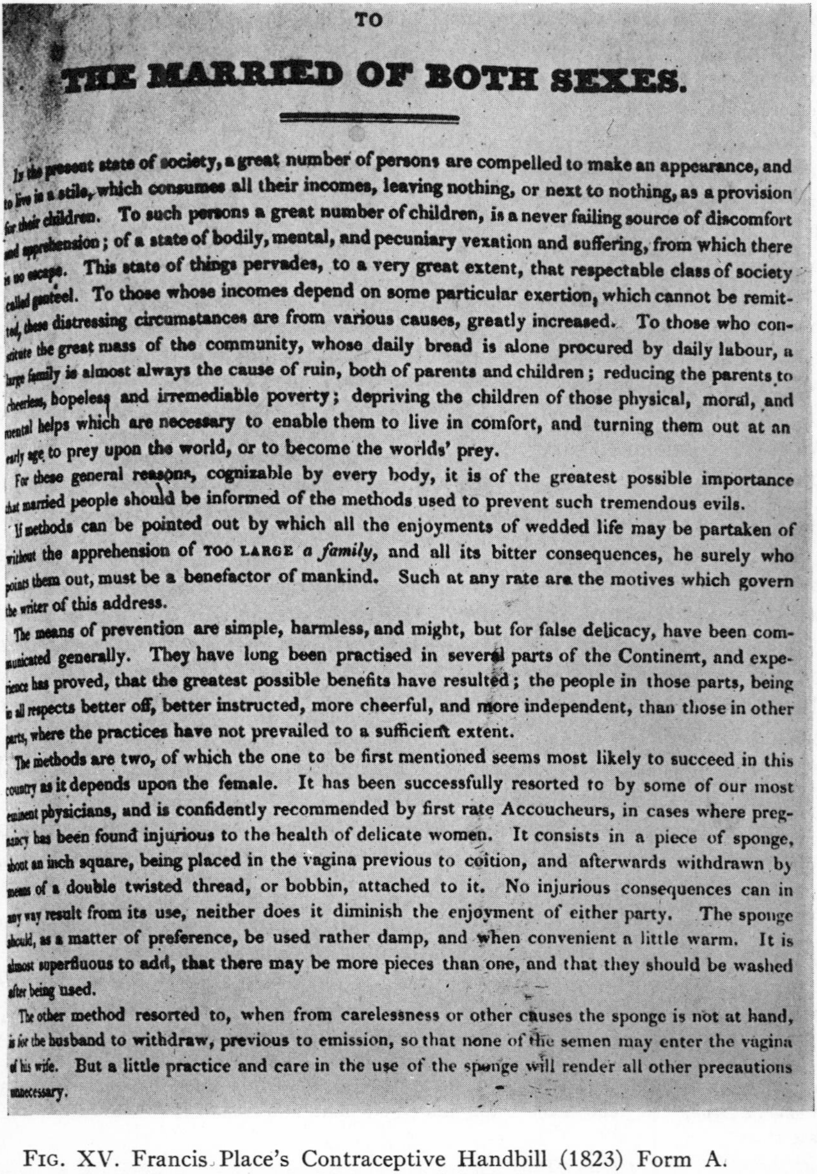

TO

THE MARRIED OF BOTH SEXES.

In the present state of society, a great number of persons are compelled to make an appearance, and to live in a stile, which consumes all their incomes, leaving nothing, or next to nothing, as a provision for their children. To such persons a great number of children, is a never failing source of discomfort and apprehension; of a state of bodily, mental, and pecuniary vexation and suffering, from which there is no escape. This state of things pervades, to a very great extent, that respectable class of society called genteel. To those whose incomes depend on some particular exertion, which cannot be remitted, these distressing circumstances are from various causes, greatly increased. To those who constitute the great mass of the community, whose daily bread is alone procured by daily labour, a large family is almost always the cause of ruin, both of parents and children; reducing the parents to cheerless, hopeless and irremediable poverty; depriving the children of those physical, moral, and mental helps which are necessary to enable them to live in comfort, and turning them out at an early age to prey upon the world, or to become the worlds' prey.

For these general reasons, cognizable by every body, it is of the greatest possible importance that married people should be informed of the methods used to prevent such tremendous evils.

If methods can be pointed out by which all the enjoyments of wedded life may be partaken of without the apprehension of TOO LARGE a family, and all its bitter consequences, he surely who points them out, must be a benefactor of mankind. Such at any rate are the motives which govern the writer of this address.

The means of prevention are simple, harmless, and might, but for false delicacy, have been communicated generally. They have long been practised in several parts of the Continent, and experience has proved, that the greatest possible benefits have resulted; the people in those parts, being in all respects better off, better instructed, more cheerful, and more independent, than those in other parts, where the practices have not prevailed to a sufficient extent.

The methods are two, of which the one to be first mentioned seems most likely to succeed in this country as it depends upon the female. It has been successfully resorted to by some of our most eminent physicians, and is confidently recommended by first rate Accoucheurs, in cases where pregnancy has been found injurious to the health of delicate women. It consists in a piece of sponge, about an inch square, being placed in the vagina previous to coition, and afterwards withdrawn by means of a double twisted thread, or bobbin, attached to it. No injurious consequences can in any way result from its use, neither does it diminish the enjoyment of either party. The sponge should, as a matter of preference, be used rather damp, and when convenient a little warm. It is almost superfluous to add, that there may be more pieces than one, and that they should be washed after being used.

The other method resorted to, when from carelessness or other causes the sponge is not at hand, is for the husband to withdraw, previous to emission, so that none of the semen may enter the vagina of his wife. But a little practice and care in the use of the sponge will render all other precautions unnecessary.

FIG. XV. Francis Place's Contraceptive Handbill (1823) Form A.
Source: Place Collection, Brit. Mus. Vol. lxi, Pt. II, p. 43.

TO

THE MARRIED OF BOTH SEXES

IN

Genteel Life.

—◆●●◆—

AMONG the many sufferings of married women, as mothers, there are two cases which command the utmost sympathy and commiseration.

The first arises from constitutional peculiarities, or weaknesses.

The second from mal-conformation of the bones of the Pelvis.

Besides these two cases, there is a third case applicable to both sexes: namely, the consequences of having more children than the income of the parents enables them to maintain and educate in a desirable manner.

The first named case produces miscarriages, and brings on a state of existence scarcely endurable. It has caused thousands of respectable women to linger on in pain and apprehension, till at length, death has put an end to their almost inconceivable sufferings.

The second case is always attended with immediate risk of life. Pregnancy never terminates without intense suffering, seldom without the death of the child, frequently with the death of the mother, and sometimes with the death of both mother and child.

The third case is by far the most common, and the most open to general observation. In the middle ranks, the most virtuous and praiseworthy efforts are perpetually made to keep up the respectability of the family; but a continual increase of children gradually yet certainly renders every effort to prevent degradation unavailing, it paralizes by rendering hopeless all exertion, and the family sinks into poverty and despair. Thus is engendered and perpetuated a hideous mass of misery.

The knowledge of what awaits them deters vast numbers of young men from marrying and causes them to spend the best portion of their lives in a state of debauchery, utterly incompatible with the honourable and honest feelings which should be the characteristic of young men. The treachery, duplicity, and hypocrisy, they use towards their friends and the unfortunate victims of their seductions, while they devote a large number of females to the most dreadful of all states which human beings can endure extinguishes in them to a very great extent, all manly, upright notions; and qualifies them to as great an extent, for the commission of acts which but for these vile practices they would abhor, and thus to an enormous extent is the whole community injured.

Marriage in early life, is the only truly happy state, and if the evil consequences of too large a family did not deter them, all men would marry while young, and thus would many lamentable evils be removed from society.

A simple, effectual, and safe means of accomplishing these desirable results has long been known, and to a considerable extent practised in some places. But until lately has been but little known in this country. Accoucheurs of the first respectability and surgeons of great eminence have in some peculiar cases recommended it. Within the last two years, a more extensive knowledge of the process has prevailed and its practice has been more extensively adopted. It is now made public for the benefit of every body. A piece of soft sponge about the size of a small ball attached to a very narrow ribbon, and slightly moistened (when convenient) is introduced previous to sexual intercourse, and is afterwards withdrawn, and thus by an easy, simple, cleanly and not indelicate method, no ways injurious to health, not only may much unhappiness and many miseries be prevented, but benefits to an incalculable amount be conferred on society.

FIG. XVI. Francis Place's Contraceptive Handbill (1823) Form B. Source: Place Collection, Brit. Mus. Vol. lxi, Pt. II, p. 43.

is preserved in manuscript on both sides of a single sheet of paper $6\frac{1}{2}$ by $7\frac{1}{2}$ inches. The handwriting of the manuscript draft is not that of Francis Place. There is reason to believe that it was written by one Benjamin Aimé, a London instrument maker. These handbills (see Figures XV, XVI,

2

TO THE

MARRIED OF BOTH SEXES

OF THE

WORKING PEOPLE.

———◆———

THIS paper is addressed to the reasonable and considerate among you, the most numerous and most useful class of society.

It is not intended to produce vice and debauchery, but to destroy vice, and put an end to debauchery.

It is a great truth, often told and never denied, that when there are too many working people in any trade or manufacture, they are worse paid than they ought to be paid, and are compelled to work more hours than they ought to work.

When the number of working people in any trade or manufacture, has for some years been too great, wages are reduced very low, and the working people become little better than slaves.

When wages have thus been reduced to a very small sum, working people can no longer maintain their children as all good and reepectable people wish to maintain their children, but are compelled to neglect them;—to send them to different employments;—to Mills and Manufactories, at a very early age.

The misery of these poor children cannot be described, and need not be described to you, who witness them and deplore them every day of your lives.

Many indeed among you are compelled for a bare subsistence to labour incessantly from the moment you rise in the morning to the moment you lie down again at night, without even the hope of ever being better off.

The sickness of yourselves and your children, the privation and pain and premature death of those you love but cannot cherish as you wish, need only be alluded to. You know all these evils too well.

And, what, you will ask is the remedy ?

How are we avoid these miseries ?

The answer is short and plain : the means are easy. Do as other people do, to avoid having more children than they wish to have, and can easily maintain.

What is done by other people is this. A pice of soft sponge is tied by a bobbin or penny ribbon, and inserted just before the sexual intercourse takes place, and is withdrawn again as soon as it has taken place. Many tie a piece of sponge to each end of

XVII) seemed of such unusual interest that I caused them to be reprinted in the *Lancet* in 1927.[14]

Though the appeal of the handbills was essentially economic, they are not without medical and sociological interest. Not only are techniques detailed, but we probably have here the first good discussion of indications in the literature.[15] While the Talmud had not only mentioned the use of

[14] Norman E. Himes, "The Birth Control Handbills of 1823," *Lancet*, August 6th, 1927, p. 313 ff. Reprinted in part, but with a somewhat incorrect text by the *Birth Control Review*, xi (Nov. 1927), 294–295.

[15] For indications in preliterate societies see the summary of ch. i *infra*.

spongy substances many centuries before Place but had also favored medical if not economic indications, the Talmudic indications were partly magical. They were much mixed with Hebraic rites and law. Place's indications were free from such entanglements.

3

the ribbon, and they take care not to use the same sponge again until it has been washed.

If the sponge be large enough, that is; as large as a green walnut, or a small apple, it will prevent conception, and thus, without diminishing the pleasures of married life, or doing the least injury to the health of the most delicate woman, both the woman and her husband will be saved from all the miseries which having too many children produces.

By limiting the number of children, the wages both of children and of grown up persons will rise; the hours of working will be no more than they ought to be; you will have some time for recreation, some means of enjoying yourselves rationally, some means as well as some time for your own and your childrens' moral and religious instruction.

At present every respectable mother trembles for the fate of her daughters as they grow up. Debauchery is always feared. This fear makes many good mothers unhappy The evil when it comes makes them miserable.

And why is there so much debauchery? Why such sad consequences?

Why? But, because many young men, who fear the consequences which a large family produces, turn to debauchery, and destroy their own happiness as well as the happiness of the unfortunate girls with whom they connect themselves.

Other young men, whose moral and religi-

4

ous feelings deter them from this vicious course, marry early and produce large families, which they are utterly unable to maintain. These are the causes of the wretchedness which afflicts you.

But when it has become the custom here as elsewhere, to limit the number of children, so that none need have more that they wish to have, no man will fear to take a wife, all will be married while young—debauchery will diminish—while good morals, and religious duties will be promoted.

You cannot fail to see that this address is intended solely for your good. It is quite impossible that those who address you can receive any benefit from it, beyond the satisfaction which every benevolent person, every true christian, must feel, at seeing you comfortable, healthy, and happy.

FIG. XVII. Francis Place's Contraceptive Handbill (1923) Form C.
Source: Place Collection, Brit. Mus. Vol. lxi, Pt. II, p. 42.

(2b) Methods Recommended in the Handbills

The form first issued, that addressed "To the Married of Both Sexes," mentioned *coitus interruptus* as well as the sponge. The second and third drafts refer only to the sponge; while the uncirculated manuscript draft mentions as an alternative to the sponge, a tampon of "lint, fine wool, cotton, flax, or what may be at hand." We are informed in the first handbill that "the use of the sponge will render all other precautions unnecessary." The third goes so far as to suggest that "the means for preventing conception are easy." The condom is conspicuously absent.

(2c) *Place's Social and Medical Justification of Contraception*

Economic indications are given greater stress than medical indications, though the latter are by no means minimized. The whole appeal centers around the prevention of poverty, and raising the standard of living of the masses. Contracted pelves and constitutional weakness are mentioned.

Whether written by Place alone or by Place with the assistance of others, the handbills were in advance of modern medical opinion in maintaining that economic indications held a coördinate place with medical indications for contraception. Place argued that birth limitation among laborers would make them scarcer in the labor market, and raise the rate of wages.[16] But he insisted that even should wages rise from other causes, the good effects in raising the standard of living would be nullified, if the working class reproduced too rapidly. And though he based much of his argument upon the long-since-refuted wages-fund theory,[17] the gist of his argument remains sound, supported by the weight of authority in modern economic theory. Place argued that if trade unionists could raise their wage rates by restricting the number of apprentices, the working-class, as a whole, could, if a program of responsible parenthood were only adopted, increase the total share of the national income destined to be paid it.

Place found Malthusian moral restraint no solution at all to the over-population possibility then thought to be immediately at hand. In his opinion it would never be widely adopted; it involved too great a strain upon human nature. Moreover, it was unnecessary, in order to keep population within reasonable control, for man to deny himself the pleasures of the most cherished intimacies of married life.

The vital statistics of the Western World corroborate Place's prediction that moral restraint would never be widely adopted; for, taking large populations as units, it is true to say that, except for the past few years, when the dissemination of birth-control knowledge has become quite general, there has been no tendency for marriages to be postponed.[18] Many who

[16] We would now say "rates of wages" since there is no general wage rate for all classes of laborers.

[17] Lest it be thought by those unacquainted with the history of economic thought that Place was alone in erroneously accepting the validity of the wages-fund theory, it may be remarked that the best minds in orthodox economic theory of the period accepted the wages-fund theory as valid. One needs only mention James and John Stuart Mill, Ricardo and McCulloch. See F. W. Taussig, *Wages and Capital* for the best exposition of it, and for the best account of its final demise.

[18] For data on the U. S. A. see Ernest R. Groves and William F. Ogburn, *American Marriage and Family Relationships.* New York: Holt, 1928, pp. xiii, 3–497.

think otherwise have been misled. They have focussed upon the postponement resulting from lengthened education in a limited group. They forget that on the lower end of the social scale modern machine technology has made it possible for members of the working class to earn almost their maximum income at an early age, thus inducing early marriages. One tendency seems to have counteracted the other; so that the average age of marriage of the total population has remained for a century virtually unchanged. Malthus's recommendations have, therefore, not yet been widely adopted. And in so far as Francis Place may have foreseen this fact, *his prediction is one of the most remarkable that the history of social science records.* It may be noted, however, that in recent years there has been a tendency toward early marriage. I agree with Ogburn that this is largely a consequence of the diffusion of birth-control knowledge.

Place knew all about birth control inducing earlier marriage. Postponement led, in his opinion, to vice and prostitution. There was nothing new in this view; it had been presented by the church for centuries as one of the secondary reasons for marriage as an institution. Place argued that, if contraception were universally adopted, early marriages would become more general; and that the incidence of the sex diseases would be reduced. Better sexual adjustments in marriage would also result, since one who married early would more easily adapt his or her personality to that of the partner. Place probably got this idea by reading the works of Benjamin Franklin.[19]

Place, being in intimate contact with the forces influencing working-class welfare, argued also that large families were a cause of child labor. Many who have written on the subject since Place have come to similar conclusions. In fact, many economists are of the opinion that it was the passage of legislation restricting child labor that has had much to do with the growth of family limitation. It has been one of a number of changes which have made large families less advantageous to parents. The raising of educational standards, and hence costs, has operated in the same direction. By the operation of many social forces children have become less an economic asset and more an economic responsibility than formerly.

There is no reason to believe that Place was supported by the medical profession in his attempts to teach the working class both the theoretical

[19] For a full account of Franklin's influence on Place, see my article on "Benjamin Franklin on Population. A Re-examination with Special Reference to the Influence of Franklin on Francis Place," to appear in the *Econ. J.*, Historical Supplement, January, 1937. Franklin and Charles Knowlton are both exceptions to the proposition that usually the nexus of influence in social theory in this period was from Europe to the United States rather than the reverse.

need for, and the actual means of carrying out contraception. But there is abundant evidence (in Place's manuscripts still preserved in the British Museum) that, upon detailed points, he repeatedly sought the advice of physicians. Place writes a newspaper editor: "I have taken pains in my enquiries on this subject ... amongst surgical and medical [as well as] amongst intelligent elderly women, and especially with two respectable, clever women who are or were matrons at public lying-in hospitals."[20] Richard Carlile informs us that Place "studied anatomy in the regular way."[21] In one of the handbills, for instance, he advised us that "some respectable persons in the metropolis of this country, of both sexes, among whom are included many medical men of the first rank, have inquired after a means [of controlling conception] which is here unfolded." The second handbill avows that "accoucheurs of the first respectability and surgeons of great eminence have in some particular cases recommended" the methods suggested for preventing conception. It would be interesting to know just whom Place had in mind.

(2d)   Place's Immediate Disciples: Richard Carlile, Richard Hassell and William Campion

Curiously enough there was no legal interference with the early propaganda. Despite the wide distribution of the handbills; and despite a protest to the Attorney General by a woman who received a bundle of handbills with an anonymous request that she distribute them, no prosecution followed. Nor were Carlile's works prosecuted. Carlile, Place's most intrepid follower, had published in 1825 his *What is Love?*.[22] Reprinted in 1826 as *Every Woman's Book; or, What is Love?*,[23] the pamphlet enjoyed a large circulation. There was a shorter edition abridged by Godfrey Higgins.[24] Though this was more frank than refined, and though Carlile spent, at one time or another, several years in jail for free speech offenses on charges of

---

[20] Ms. Letter, Place to MacLaren. Place Collection, lxii, p. 165. The whole letter is published in my edition of Place on *Population*, pp. 309–312. Punctuation mine.

[21] *Old Monthly Magazine*, May, 1835. See Place's "Notes on Surgery and Medicine" in Brit. Mus. ADD. Mss. 27, 828 (vol. iv, sec. 5).

[22] *Republican*, xi, No. 18.

[23] *Every Woman's Book; or, What is Love?* was first published under this title in February, 1826. Of authentic, complete editions I know of the whereabouts of only two copies, both of which are cf the fourth edition (1826). One is in the Chicago collection of the late Professor James A. Field who, fortunately for scholarship, cherished such rare items; the other is in the Goldsmiths' Library of the University of London. I have caused a photostatic copy to be placed in the Harvard Library.

[24] Unique copy in the Seligman Collection now on deposit at the Columbia University Library.

blasphemy,[25] he never ran afoul the law as a consequence of his birth-control activity. The same immunity was shared by T. J. Wooler, radical editor of the *Black Dwarf*. He was never hailed into court for publishing the handbills in his periodical.

The worst that leaders of the educational campaign suffered was public abuse. They were castigated at the hands of certain fly-by-night periodicals, at least one of which, the *Bull Dog*, was founded for the express purpose of vilifying Place, Carlile, and Bentham. The scandals and exposures which ensued upon the handbill diffusion, and the discussions which followed were numerous. Place was publicly dubbed "the master spring that moves the whole infernal machine."

EVERY WOMAN'S BOOK:

OR,

WHAT IS LOVE?

Fourth Edition.

LONDON:

PRINTED AND PUBLISHED BY R. CARLILE,
62, FLEET-STREET.

1826.

Two disciples of Place, Richard Hassell and William Campion, whom I have labelled the Newgate Neo-Malthusians, owing to their incarceration in Newgate prison as a consequence of assisting Carlile in his free-press struggle, discussed extensively the social and economic aspects of birth control. This they did in their periodical, *The Newgate Monthly Magazine*, edited while they were still in prison. Unlike Place and Carlile, Hassell and Campion avoided the medical aspects of the subject, and confined their

---

[25] See the *Republican, Lion*, and other periodicals edited by Carlile. Also William H. Wickwar, *The Struggle for the Freedom of the Press. 1819–1832*. London: Allen & Unwin, 1928.

efforts to public instruction on the general need of population control. Both were self-taught workingmen whose educational opportunities had been exceedingly limited; yet their treatment of birth control is often illuminating and well-reasoned.   They added little, however, to the doctrines of their teacher, Place.

In educating Carlile to the need for birth control, Place had great difficulty, for the former was preoccupied with other reforms, and believed the causes of working-class misery lay in other directions than unrestrained reproduction.   Once Carlile accepted Place's point of view, there was no restraining him.   In Place's copy of the *Bull Dog* definite marginalia are to be found in Place's handwriting stating that he made an effort to dissuade Carlile from publishing *What is Love?* at least in the *particular form* in which it was submitted to Place.

Carlile's *Every Woman's Book* may have been coarse and somewhat naïve; but it is significant in that it is the first little book in the English language frankly discussing the economic, social and medical aspects of birth control. The coarseness, if not excusable, is at least comprehensible when one reflects that Carlile had been, as a youth, underprivileged; that he just "grew."[26] Like Place, his teacher, Carlile had risen by heroic efforts from the squalor and murk of his youthful surroundings.

Between 1820–30 the subject had been discussed in many periodicals. Place's handbills and Carlile's practical pamphlets had been distributed by thousands.   Other working-class reformers were induced to take up the subject.   Carlile made a speaking tour which, though concerned primarily with freethought subjects, occasionally brought to other communities the knowledge that birth control was an actuality.   Carlile was not infrequently heckled on his birth-control views, even though he may have come to discuss the immoralities in the Old Testament.   Upon one occasion at Bath a few listeners were so violently opposed to his taking the platform that *Every Woman's Book* was publicly burned, and the author pelted out of town.

(2e)   The Effect of Place's Propaganda upon the English Birth Rate

One is naturally led to inquire: How effective was the English campaign of the eighteen twenties?   There is no reason to suppose that it had any immediate and substantial effect upon the English birth rate.   The increase of population is not a fair test of the extent of the propaganda in this period because the phenomenal increase of population during the nineteenth century was, as is now known to all vital statisticians and demographers, more

---

[26] See George Jacob Holyoake, *The Life of Richard Carlile*.   Several editions.

a result of a declining death rate than of an increasing birth rate.[27] The sum and substance of the matter seems to be this: Though the educational campaign that Place led had no immediate and measurable effect upon British society as shown by the birth rate, none the less, by re-sowing the seeds of a new branch of thought, by re-vitalizing it through cross-fertilization with sociology, economics and philosophical radicalism, the propaganda released forces which, buttressed by a rising standard of living, by the emancipation of women and by growing rationalism, set in motion one of the most remarkable, revolutionary, *organized* social movements of which history makes record. Doubtless the tendency towards controlled parenthood which has taken place since 1822 has been essentially the result of social forces beyond the control, or even the guidance, of any individual or group of individuals.[28]

§3 THE OLD VS. THE NEW IN THE HISTORY OF CONTRACEPTION

The organizational element which Place introduced was absolutely new so far as present knowledge of the history of this subject goes. The validity of this conclusion cannot be doubted. Whether it will need eventually to be overthrown as a consequence of new contributions to knowledge remains to be seen. In the meantime the fact that the organizational element is new should be noted by those who always talk about the antiquity of this and that in tones calculated to suggest that nothing new ever happens in social experience. *The desire to control conception is very old. Contraception as a genuinely effective instrument is new; as a diffused social habit or as a democratized social institution it is new.* Further evidence on the validity of this last point will be presented later.

With the passage of the Reform Bill in 1832, and of the new Poor Law in 1834, and with the death in the same year of Malthus, the social ferment, set in motion by the French Revolution and by the economic disabilities facing England in the post-Napoleonic period of readjustment, died down. As the clamor for social reform waned, interest in birth control declined.

This is not to gainsay that there was a quiet penetration of the new knowledge throughout all classes of society. Doubtless this took place. But after the handbill propaganda of 1823–27, there was little activity by way of formal dissemination until the re-issue in England of two American pamphlets, one by Robert Dale Owen, another by Dr. Charles Knowlton. At this point it is necessary to interrupt the chronicle of the English history in order to make clear certain American developments.

[27] For one demonstration, see G. Talbot Griffith, *Population Problems of the Age of Malthus.* Cambridge: Cambridge Univ. Press, 1926, pp. 276.
[28] *Cf., infra*, ch. xiii, §6.

§4   AMERICAN BEGINNINGS: ROBERT DALE OWEN AND CHARLES KNOWLTON

The American birth-control movement, which was initiated in America in the period 1828–1832 by Robert Dale Owen and Dr. Charles Knowlton, was an indirect result of the work of Place and Carlile.   English writers influenced American authors, and these in turn had a very considerable influence upon the social diffusion of contraceptive knowledge in England. Elsewhere[29] the circumstances have been traced which led Robert Dale Owen (1801–1877), eldest son of Robert Owen, to publish in New York in 1830 his *Moral Physiology*,[30] the first[31] little book published in America on birth control.   This eloquent and refined tract filled an immediate need.   It went through several editions within a year; and 75,000 copies were sold in America and England by the time of Owen's death (1877).

(4a)   Owen's Discussion of Technique

The chief method recommended by R. D. Owen was *coitus interruptus.* Though this would involve sacrifices, they would be insignificant compared with the benefits resulting.   Case studies were presented to show the good effects of its adoption.[32]   Owen denied that men would not adopt *coitus interruptus;* he believed that public opinion could enforce it.   It resulted in less violence to the social feelings than celibacy: and was that not widely prevalent?   To the charge that birth control was unnatural, Owen replied that the same was true of the thwarting of many human wishes.   Its wide adoption in France was a guarantee of its practicability.   Its practice might be impossible for some temperamental, strongly-sexed men; but such cases were rarer than commonly supposed.

Carlile had recommended partial withdrawal; but Owen considered this "not an infallible preventive."[33]   The sponge method, said Owen, was not only of "doubtful efficacy;" it was "physically disagreeable."[34] Carlile was in error in thinking that the sponge was widely used in France as a contra-

---

[29] Norman E. Himes, "Robert Dale Owen, the Pioneer of American Neo-Malthusianism," *Amer. J. Soc.*, xxxv (1930), 529–547.

[30] Robert Dale Owen, *Moral Physiology; or, a brief and plain treatise on the population question.*   Fourth edition.   New York: Wright & Owen, 1831, pp. iv, 5–72.   See Bibliography for a list of editions.

[31] However, our Puritan forefathers were evidently acquainted with *coitus interruptus* as may be inferred from the fact that Governor Bradford, in his [*History*] *Of Plimmoth Plantation* [*Colony*] (1630–1650), made reference to the attempt by a local minister, one Lyford, to prevent conception.   See Figure XVIII and my "Note on the Early History of Contraception in America," *New Eng. J. Med.*, ccv (August 27, 1931), 438–440.

[32] So far as is known, Robert Dale Owen published in *Moral Physiology* (New York, 1830), the first birth-control case histories.

[33] *Ibid.*, p. 66.

[34] *Ibid.*

ceptive. Had Carlile had an opportunity to discuss the subject with French physicians, declared Owen, he could have established this fact. It may be inferred from that observation that Robert Dale Owen, who as a young man had been educated in Switzerland, and who had travelled with his father in France, had discussed conception control with physicians in France.

The baudruche, or condom, Owen thought "inconvenient." All he had heard from physicians and private individuals led him to believe that, as

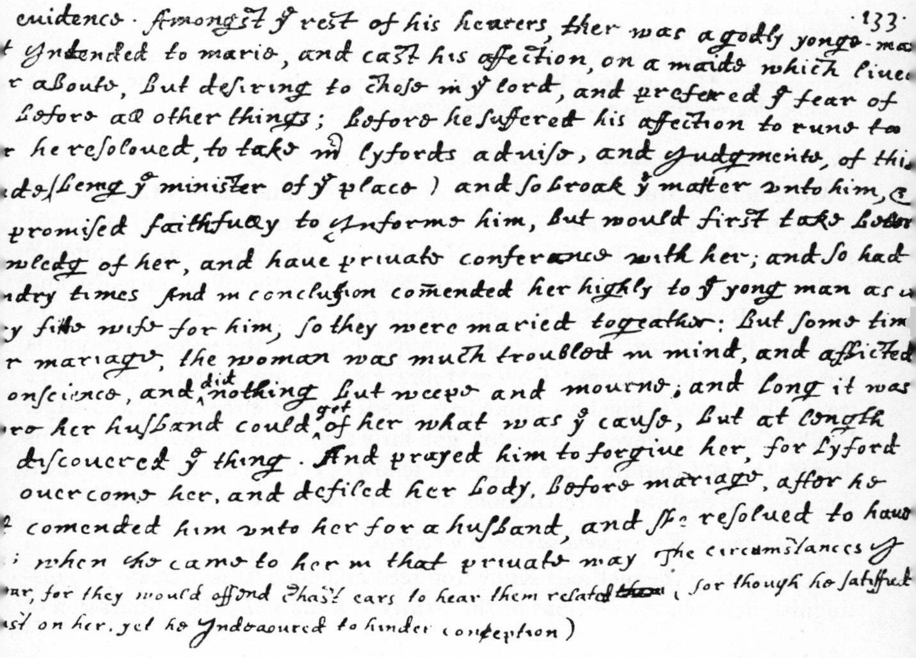

evidence. Amongst ye rest of his hearers, ther was a godly yonge man .133. yntended to marie, and cast his affection, on a maide which lived ther aboute, but desiring to these in ye lord, and preferred ye fear of before all other things; before he suffered his affection to rune too farr he resolued, to take mr lyfords aduise, and yudgments, of this (he being ye minister of ye place) and so broak ye matter vnto him, he promised faithfully to enforme him, but would first take better knowledg of her, and haue priuate conference with her; and so had sundry times, and in conclusion comended her highly to ye yong man as a very fitte wife for him, so they were maried togeather: But some time after mariage, the woman was much troubled in mind, and afflicted in conscience, and did nothing but weepe and mourne; and long it was before her husband could get of her what was ye cause, but at length she discouered ye thing. And prayed him to forgiue her, for Lyford had ouercome her, and defiled her body, before mariage, after he had comended him vnto her for a husband, and she resolued to haue him when he came to her in that priuate way The circumstances of *... for they would offend chast ears to hear them related ... for though he satisfied lust on her, yet he yndeauoured to hinder conception)*

Fig. XVIII. Reference to the Prevention of Conception in Governor Bradford's manuscript: [*History*] *Of Plimmoth Plantation* [*Colony*] Date: 1630–1650. Source: Original MS. on Deposit in State House Library, Boston, Massachusetts.

regards health, the method was "perfectly innocent." To the objection that it placed control in the hands of the man, Owen naïvely remarked that the "only effectual defence for women is to refuse connexion with any man *void of* honour."[35] If this were done, a public opinion regardful of the rights of women during the sexual intimacies would gradually be developed.

[35] *Ibid.*, p. 67.

(4b) Inevitability of Birth Control

Such a change in manners was as inevitable as the gradual adoption of birth control itself.

In the silent, but resistless progress of human improvement, such a change is fortunately inevitable. We are gradually emerging from the night of blind prejudice and of brutal force; and, day by day, rational liberty and cultivated refinement, win an accession of power. Violence yields to benevolence, compulsion to kindness, the letter of the law to the spirit of justice: and, day by day, men and women become more willing, and better prepared, to entrust the most sacred duties (social as well as political) more to good feeling and less to idle form—more to moral and less to legal keeping.

It is no question whether such reform will come: no human power can arrest its progress. How slowly or how rapidly it may come, *is* a question; and depends, in some degree, on adventitious circumstances.[36]

(4c) Charles Knowlton (1800–1850)

More notable from the standpoint of ultimate influence was the publication of the *Fruits of Philosophy*[37] by Dr. Charles Knowlton. This appeared anonymously, "By a Physician" in New York in 1832; and was reprinted,[38] undoubtedly by Abner Kneeland, the Boston free-thought journalist and editor, at Boston in 1833. No copy of the first edition is extant (known to me only by a court record), but a unique copy of the second edition is preserved in the Harvard College Library's treasure room. Knowlton's tract, like Owen's, filled an immediate need; and its circulation was large. Unlike Owen, however, Knowlton got into trouble with the courts—this despite the fact that he was a respected fellow of the Massachusetts Medical Society, and despite the restrictions he placed on the sale of his book.[39]

(4d) Methods Recommended by Knowlton

In discussing the methods Knowlton recommended, it is necessary to distinguish between the editions of the *Fruits of Philosophy* the publication of

[36] *Ibid.* Note the error of unilinear and inevitable (as opposed to cyclical) progress in the passage. Owen was certainly an optimist.

[37] By a Physician, *The Fruits of Philosophy; or, the private companion of young married people.* New York, (Jan.) 1832. Probably 32 mo.

[38] Charles Knowlton, *The Fruits of Philosophy: or the private companion of young married people. Second edition with additions.* Boston, 1833. There are approximately thirty-five issues and nearly as many editions of this work. Most of the large libraries have only one edition (see Bibliography).

[39] The writer hopes to publish shortly a monograph on Knowlton. Little research has been done on his life and influence. See Norman E. Himes, "Charles Knowlton's Revolutionary Influence on the English Birth-Rate," *New Engl. J. Med.*, cxcix (Sept. 6, 1928), 461–465. There are brief biographical accounts by the writer in *Dict. Amer. Biog.*, x, 471–472; *Ency. of the Social Sciences*, viii, 585.

which he supervised, and for which he was therefore personally responsible, and those editions to which additions have been made by others. The edition used in the discussion which follows is that published in Boston in 1877 (tenth edition with additions), being a reprint (sold by subscription) of the 1839 edition,[40] the last edition for which Knowlton himself is known to be responsible.

Perhaps it is no exaggeration to say that Knowlton's treatment of contraceptive technique is the first really important account after those of Soranos and Aëtios. At least there is no denying that it was the first reasonably full account published in the United States. Knowlton's book was more detailed than Owen's; more complete than any modern treatise until the appearance of certain recent medical manuals. As we shall see presently, however, the distinction, historically, achieved by the *Fruits* rests more upon its social influence than upon any notable advance in treatment of medical technique.

Knowlton's chief method was douching,[41] the rubber pessary being unknown at the time (1832), since its development had to await the vulcanization of rubber in the 'forties. Solutions of alum and of "astringent vegetables, [such] as white oak bark, hemlock bark, red rose leaves, green tea, raspberry leaves or roots" were recommended.[42] When leucorrhoea was present a solution of sulphate of zinc[43] was advised. When relaxation was present a combination of zinc and alum he thought most suitable. When there was tenderness of the parts, a solution of sugar of lead was advised.[44] "Perhaps as a general thing, a solution of saleratus [sodium bicarbonate or baking soda] is the best and most convenient thing to use."[45] Knowlton was "quite confident that a liberal use of pretty cold water would be a never-failing preventative."[46]

---

[40] The title differed from that on earlier editions. It now reads: *Fruits of Philosophy, or the private companion of adult people. Tenth edition with additions.* Boston: Published by subscription, 1877. Mr. N. R. Campbell, the Cambridge antiquarian book dealer, now deceased, whose father was a medical publisher in Boston, informed me just before his death that the 1877 edition of the *Fruits* was issued, possibly through his father, but at all events by someone on the initiative of a group of professors at the Harvard Medical School. It is perhaps significant that the Library of the Harvard Medical School is the only public repository known to possess a copy of this edition. There is another in my collection. Campbell sold one to William James, an admirer of Robert Dale Owen; but I have not been able to trace James's copy since the dispersal of his library.

[41] Owen's method, *coitus interruptus*, he believed "not sure." *Fruits*, 1877, p. 78.

[42] *Ibid.*, p. 80.

[43] We now know that zinc sulphate acts too slowly to be an efficient spermicide. It is a more effective treatment of some forms of leucorrhea.

[44] *Ibid.*

[45] *Ibid.*

[46] *Ibid.*, p. 81.

Knowlton's advice regarding the concentration of these solutions was not as cautious as it might have been. He knew that individual tolerance varied; but he complained that people did not have small scales and weights handy; and apothecary shops were, in those days, inaccessible to many families. Necessarily, therefore, he had to resort to rule of thumb prescriptions. He therefore suggested that each woman use the solution as strong as she could bear it without producing disagreeable sensations.[47] He did, however, mention the following doses:

1. Of Alum, to a pint of water, a lump as large as a large chestnut.
2. Of Sulphate of Zinc,[48] to a pint of water, a large thimble full.
3. Of Sal Eratus, to a pint of water, two common sized *even* teaspoons full.
4. Of good Vinegar, to a pint of water, four or five greatspoons full.[49]
5. Liquid Chloride of Soda, to a pint of water, four or five greatspoons full.[50]

A little "spirits" may be added to the solutions to prevent freezing.[51] The woman should douche two or three times freely within five minutes of coitus.[52] There are specific directions for proper syringing. He observes: "No doubt a very small quantity of semen lodged anywhere within the vagina or within the vulva, may cause conception, if it should escape the influence of cold, or some chemical agent."[53] Knowlton did not believe that vinegar had been recommended before, but thought it useful owing to its handiness and harmlessness. He also thought it "quite effectual"[54] as indeed it is. Pearlash and sal-soda would work, if used in weaker solutions than saleratus. When the woman is syringing, she should take care that the room is not too cold.

(4e) *His Notions Regarding Originality*

Under the conviction, firmly but possibly erroneously held, that he originated douching as a contraceptive, Knowlton writes:

Any publication, great or small, mentioning the syringe (or anything else that operates upon the same principle) as a means of preventing conception—whatever liquid may be recommended—is a violation of my copyright. . . . I never should have written any such book as this but for my discovery of this plan. I have devoted much time and thought to the leading subject of this work. I have done

---

[47] *Ibid.*, p. 82.

[48] Sulphate of zinc acts too slowly to be an effective spermicide. See Dickinson and Bryant, *Control of Conception*, p. 45.

[49] So far as I can recall, this is the first mention of vinegar since Aëtios. See p. 92.

[50] *Fruits* (1877), p. 82.

[51] We may recall that not so many homes were well heated in Knowlton's day.

[52] *Ibid.*, p. 83.

[53] *Ibid.*, p. 84.

[54] *Ibid.*

so under a strong conviction that I was rendering a signal service to frail and suffering humanity; and if the result of my labors be worth anything, it is my property; but if worthless, no one ought to sell it for a price, even if it were not secured to me.[55]

One may suspect that others before Knowlton (1831 or 1832) mentioned douching; but if such is the case, search of the literature has not revealed it.

In Knowlton's opinion the above methods had the following advantages: they were sure, cheap, harmless, would not cause sterility, and involved no sacrifices during coitus.[56] Moreover, control was thus placed in the hands of the woman where, for good reasons, it ought to be. Place and Knowlton seem to have been among the first to stress the desirability of placing control in the hands of the wife.

(4f) The Scientific Viewpoint in the Works of Owen and Knowlton

One ought not to leave the subject of techniques discussed by Owen and Knowlton without pointing out the fact that, whatever limitations their treatment of the subject may have from a modern point of view, it was at least an American beginning. Moreover, both made conscientious, consistent efforts to follow the scientific point of view. This cannot be said for most of their successors. Knowlton speaks of "the caution that ought to be exercised against drawing conclusions from a too limited number of facts or cases."[57] He may have been right when he said: "Hasty conclusions from a limited number of facts have done more to retard the progress of science than incredulity."[58] The whole of Knowlton's case for contraception from the medical, social and economic viewpoints is exceptionally well-reasoned and balanced.[59] So far as the general sociological theory is concerned one finds, after a hundred years of progress, few statements to which one can take serious exception. The same is also true of Owen's Moral Physiology.

In the early part of his book Knowlton asks his readers, though they may be under the impression that the discussion of the subject of contraception may be neither useful or good, to divest their minds of preconceived opinions and to follow him into a discussion of its merits. He avows that it is a "subject of too great and abiding influence to be passed over without a serious and impartial examination. I am perfectly willing that the anti-con-

---

[55] Ibid., p. 89.

[56] Ibid., p. 85.

[57] Ibid., p. 81.

[58] Ibid., p. 73.

[59] The same is true of his pre-Galtonian views on positive and negative eugenics. See Norman E. Himes, "Eugenic Thought in the American Birth Control Movement a Century Ago," Eugenics, ii (May, 1929), 3–8 and plate.

ception art stand or fall according to its merits, but I do desire that these merits be inquired into before judgment is passed—I do desire that the reader will try to divest himself of all prejudice—if sensible he has any—and go along with me into an examination of its merits and demerits."[60] Likewise Robert Dale Owen, tiring of metaphysical speculation on the theory of conception[61] without constant reference to the facts of experience, says in 1831:

> I leave these and fifty other hypotheses as ingenious and as useless, to be discussed by those who seem to make it a point of honour to leave no fact unexplained by some imagined theory; and I descend at once to the *terra firma* of positive experience and actual observation.
>
> It is exceedingly to be regretted that mankind did not spend some small portion, at least, of the time and industry which has been wasted on theoretical [i.e., purely speculative] researches, in collecting and collating the *actual experience* of human beings.[62]

For idle speculation, especially when it had lost contact with experience and observation, Owen had little respect.   To it, and to the reluctance of individuals to communicate their sex experiences to physicians Owen attributed much of the ignorance of his time.   "Many physicians," continues Owen, "will positively deny that man possesses any such power [over the reproductive instinct as I have affirmed to be possible].   And yet, if the thousandth part of the talent and research had been employed to investigate this momentous fact, which has been turned to the building up of idle theories, no commonly intelligent individual could well be ignorant of the truth."[63]

§5   THE PERIOD OF QUIET PERCOLATION IN ENGLAND: FROM THE DEATH OF MALTHUS (1834) TO THE BRADLAUGH-BESANT TRIAL (1877–1879)

(5a)   *Early Influence in England of the Fruits of Philosophy*

Though there was an immediate demand for the *Fruits of Philosophy*, it is estimated that not more than ten thousand copies were sold in the U. S.

---

[60] *Fruits of Philosophy* (1877), p. 4.

[61] Before the discovery of the microscope through which Hamm, student of Leeuwenhoek (1632–1723), first saw spermatozoa in 1677, theories of generation numbered not scores but hundreds.   This discovery very much narrowed the field of tenable hypotheses. In fact it was not until the middle of the nineteenth century that the general connection between spermatozoa and impregnation was fully realized.   These considerations, incidentally, have a bearing on the validity of the contentions of those anthropologists who strongly insist that preliterate peoples generally understand the physiology of conception. See ch. i.

[62] *Moral Physiology* (Fourth ed., 1831), pp. 59–60.

[63] *Ibid.*, p. 60.

up to 1839. By 1834, however, it had been reprinted in London by James Watson, intrepid publisher of freethought literature; in subsequent decades by John Brooks, Austin Holyoake, Holyoake & Company, F. Farrah, and Charles Watts. For forty years this six-penny, paper-covered pamphlet circulated quietly and unobtrusively, selling probably not more than a thousand copies a year. Between 1834 and 1876 the circulation of the English editions was approximately 42,000 copies. It was not until a prosecution in 1877–79, that Knowlton's pamphlet was to achieve the notoriety that now surrounds it. Before turning to that important episode, however, it is necessary to consider events which transpired in the interval.

(5b) Anti-Marcus and "M. G. H."

It has been stated earlier in this account that with the passage of the Reform Bill in 1832 and the Poor Law in 1834, the public agitation for birth control died down. This was followed by a period of quiet infiltration. Nothing of account seems to have been published until the appearance of Anti-Marcus's *Notes on the Population Question* (1841).[64] The identity of the author remains to this day a mystery. There is nothing original in the pamphlet from the medical, economic or sociological standpoints. The author followed Richard Carlile in recommending the sheath and *coitus interruptus*. Likewise he followed Knowlton by mentioning vaginal douches with solutions of sulphate of zinc, of alum, or pearlash, or of any salt acting as a spermicide.[65] Place's method, the sponge,[66] was mentioned, as was also the sheath.[67] Owen was extensively quoted. It is quite possible that the *Notes* contains the first mention of the condom in strictly contraceptive pamphlet literature.

The circulation of the *Notes* is unknown. Only one edition has ever been traced; and from its great rarity[68] nowadays one might safely conclude that it never had great influence in England in spreading contraceptive knowledge. In America and on the Continent it is virtually unknown.

Since its influence, like the *Notes*, was modest or negligible, one may mention here—though it really belongs to the period of a few decades later—the publication of an interesting mid-century English contraceptive pamphlet by one "M. G. H.," entitled "Poverty: Its Cause and Cure."[69] This

[64] Anti-Marcus, *Notes on the Population Question*. London: J. Watson, 1841, pp. 44.

[65] *Ibid.*, p. 27.

[66] *Ibid.*, p. 21.

[67] *Ibid.*, pp. 21–22. Carlile had mentioned the "condam" in *Every Woman's Book* (London, 1826), p. 37.

[68] A photostat has been made for the Harvard Library. Copy in the author's collection.

[69] M. G. H., *Poverty: its cause and cure. Pointing out a means by which the working classes may raise themselves from their present state of low wages and ceaseless toil to one of*

penny pamphlet probably went through several issues and was widely distributed.   While it is of interest chiefly for its theoretical support of the prevention of conception, it does not overlook instruction in technique. It especially recommends the introduction "of a piece of fine sponge, slightly soaked in tepid water, and of sufficient size, in such a way as to guard the womb from the entrance of the male semen during sexual connection.   This might be followed by an injection of tepid water."[70]   The other methods mentioned are withdrawal, the sheath, injections immediately after inter-course, and a sterile period.[71]   The sponge and the sheath are considered "most certain."   But injections and use of the sterile period, as well as the sponge, "are the least open to objections in other respects."[72]   The pamphlet shows unmistakable internal evidence of having been designed for distribu-tion among working men and the general populace.

With Anti-Marcus's *Notes* and M. G. H.'s *Poverty*, there stands in about the same class, from the standpoint of influence, an anonymous pamphlet, published in 1868 under the title "The Power and Duty of Parents to Limit the Number of their Children."   (London, 1868, pp. 11)   It has not been possible to find a copy of this on public deposit, but Stopes says[73] that it mentions as contraceptive methods the safe period, coughing, sneezing,

---

comfort, dignity and independence; and which is capable of entirely removing, in course of time, the other principal social evils. London: E. Truelove, n.d., pp. 16, 1d.   This was probably first published between 1854–61.   It is reviewed by Barker in the *National Reformer*, ii (No. 63), 9 (July 27, 1861).   The author's personal copy is probably a late edition, since it contains an advertisement of the twenty-second edition of the *Elements of Social Science*.

Efforts to determine the author have been, up to date, without avail.   Here are the various theories: Miss Vance, a rather intimate co-worker with Charles Bradlaugh, told me before she died that she thought the pamphlet was written by "Mentor" Holyoake, a son of George Jacob Holyoake.   However, the elder Holyoake had no son by this name but did have a son, Malthus Questell Holyoake.   It could also have been by John Maughan or George Drysdale.   The author, whoever he was, appeals to traditional Malthusianism and to orthodox classical economic theory, and was acquainted with the Neo-Malthusian writ-ings of Place, Carlile, Owen, Knowlton, George Drysdale, and Austin Holyoake.   He refers to A. Holyoake's "Large and Small Families."

[70] *Ibid.*, p. 13.

[71] *Ibid.*   "The avoidance of connection, from two days before, till eight days after, the monthly courses—at which time impregnation is far most likely to occur."   Probably through an error, "M. G. H." is here garbling George Drysdale's recommendation of the sterile period.   See p. 234.   M. G. H. is recommending that individuals abstain from coitus at the very time Drysdale said was the sterile period.   But Drysdale guessed wrong. When it exists, the sterile period just precedes the onset of menstruation.   The modern physician will not counsel use of a sterile period, first because it is unreliable and not to be used particularly in cases where pregnancy is contra-indicated, second because, if such a period really exists, it is not simple to determine it for each patient.   *Cf.*, p. 416 n. 33.

[72] *Ibid.*

[73] Marie C. Stopes, *Contraception* (1925), p. 291.

jumping, violent exercise, injections immediately after coitus, withdrawal, and the "interposition of some material [in front of the os]; but such artifices are not recommended."

(5c)   George Drysdale

Owing to the great influence of his writings, Dr. George Drysdale occupies a most significant place in the medical history of contraception.   In 1854 he published his *Elements of Social Science*,[74] a radical treatise on sex education, critical of the institution of marriage, warmly advocating the principles of Malthusianism and of classical political economy.   Though the volume ran to six hundred finely printed pages, only five and one-half pages were devoted to the technique of "preventive sexual intercourse."[75]   There is reason to believe that Drysdale's knowledge of contraceptive technique was mainly theoretical.   When he wrote the *Elements* he was a student of medicine.   The comparative amount of space devoted to the different topics discussed demonstrates what can be established on other grounds, namely, that he was less interested in contraceptive methods than in building up the case, medical and economic, for birth limitation.   In his view it was the main, long-run "cure" for poverty and low wages.   Drysdale and Place differ from most post World War writers on conception control in stressing the urgency of population limitation.

The warm reception given the *Elements* resulted in an enormous circulation.   Up to 1904, after which the book went out of print, thirty-five English editions had appeared; and it was translated into at least ten European languages.

(5d)   Methods Recommended by Drysdale

Drysdale mentioned five techniques.   Following Place, he preferred the sponge; but he seems to have been the first[76] to recommend this method in combination with a douche of tepid water.   Partly on the authority of Raciborski[77] and M. Bischoff, Drysdale gave considerable approval to a

---

[74] *The Elements of Social Science; or physical, sexual and natural religion.   An exposition of the true cause and only cure of the three primary social evils: poverty, prostitution, and celibacy.*   By a Doctor of Medicine.   London: Edward Truelove, 1887 (26th ed. enlarged, 65th thousand), pp. 604.   The first edition, of which no copy is known to be extant, was "By a Student of Medicine."   Rather frequently Drysdale contributed general articles on economics and Malthusianism to the *National Reformer*, Bradlaugh's paper.   These articles were signed "G. R.," an abbreviation for *George Rex*, which he had been dubbed as a student.

[75] *Elements* (1887), pp. 347–350; 513–514.

[76] He is the first so far as my present knowledge goes.   Did others before George Drysdale recommend this well-known combination?

[77] Adam Raciborski, *Traité de la Menstruation*.   Paris, 1868, and other books on physiology.

sterile period (from two or three days before menstruation to eight days after).[78] While Drysdale did not consider resort to a sterile period infallible, it would, in his view, materially reduce the likelihood of conception. Actually about the seventh or eighth day after is the period of high fertility; the few days preceding, a period of low fertility, other factors remaining equal. Withdrawal, continued Drysdale, was "physically injurious,"[79] interfered with pleasure and caused nervous disorders. The sheath was unaesthetic, dulled enjoyment, and even produced impotence![80] The use of the sponge, followed by a douche with tepid water, was the best means known to him.[81] This was non-injurious, would not interfere with the pleasure of coitus, and placed control in the hands of the woman. The efficacy of this method was not fully known, but doubtless better methods could be devised in the future. This was all the more reason why obstacles to research should speedily be overcome.[82]

Drysdale gave only cautious approval to the safe period (or mid-period, as it is often, but less accurately termed). He says "It results from my investigations, that, though there may not be periods . . . when conception is physically impossible, there are nevertheless periods, when it is infinitely less likely to happen than at others."[83]

Regarding the douche, Drysdale observed that it was Wagner's opinion that the movements of spermatozoa cease in pure water.[84] Wagner and Drysdale thus anticipated the recent research of Voge. Dickinson and Bryant summarize Voge's work on this point in this statement:

Water is a strong inhibitor of motility, but it must be in three times the volume of the sperm and mixed with it to kill instantly, and no such quantity will stay within the vagina. After washing out the vagina immediately following coitus, however, the wetness remaining should have some effect on any minute quantity of sperms not washed away. Water in a douche used before coitus is not effective.[85]

Dr. George Drysdale long preceded Stopes and other writers of our day in discussing the advantages and disadvantages of particular contraceptive

---

[78] *Elements*, p. 348. For an authoritative modern statement on the *tempus ageneseos* see Robert L. Dickinson, "The 'Safe Period' as a Birth Control Measure. A Study and Evaluation of Available Data," *Amer. Jour. Obst. & Gyn.*, Dec., 1927. Since the reprint of the National Committee on Maternal Health is no longer available readers may refer to the summary in R. L. Dickinson and L. S. Bryant, *The Control of Conception*, pp. 54–57.

[79] *Elements* (1887), p. 349.

[80] *Ibid.*

[81] *Ibid.*, p. 350

[82] *Ibid.*

[83] *Ibid.*, p. 348.

[84] *Ibid.*, p. 350.

[85] R. L. Dickinson & L. S. Bryant, *Control of Conception*, p. 45. *Cf.*, Cecil I. B. Voge, *Chemistry of Contraception*.

methods. Knowlton, and to a lesser extent Place and Carlile, were also early in giving attention to this subject. Such critical discussions, did not, it may be mentioned, ante-date 1820.

(5e) *Some Writers Influencing Him*

Dr. George Drysdale had no little knowledge of the Malthusian and Neo-Malthusian literature of the first three-quarters of the nineteenth century—probably a better knowledge than any English writer of the period (1850) not excepting J. S. Mill. It is clear from many passages in his *Elements* that he was influenced by many writers of economic and medical literature, prominent among whom were the classical economists and the early nineteenth century Neo-Malthusians. To mention but a few, there were Malthus,[86] James Mill,[87] J. S. Mill,[88] Garnier,[89] Dunoyer,[90] Senior,[91] J. B. Say,[92] Cairnes[93] and McCulloch[94] among economists; Place,[95] Carlile,[96] "R. H." [i.e., Richard Hassell],[97] Knowlton,[98] R. D. Owen,[99] Anti-Marcus,[100] and Truelove,[101] among the avowed Neo-Malthusians; and among physicians, Pouchet,[102] Raciborski,[103] Naegele,[104] Bischoff,[105] and especially (as regards the methods Drysdale recommended) Ashwell.[106] Among two score others

[86] *Elements* (1887), passim.

[87] *Ibid.*, pp. 508, 513.

[88] See the chapter (pp. 315–330) on "Mr. Mill and Others on the Law of Population." *Cf.*, pp. 506–534; 535–587.

[89] *Ibid.*, p. 513.

[90] *Ibid.*, p. 527. Dunoyer was Professor of Political Economy at Paris, and for many years chief editor of the *Journal des Économists*.

[91] *Ibid.*, p. 511.

[92] *Ibid.*, p. 521.

[93] *Ibid.*, p. 510.

[94] *Ibid.*, p. 510.

[95] *Ibid.*, p. 512, 513.

[96] *Ibid.*, p. 513, 518.

[97] *Ibid.*, p. 518.

[98] *Ibid.*, p. 513.

[99] *Ibid.*

[100] *Ibid.*

[101] *Ibid.*

[102] *Ibid.*, p. 348.

[103] *Ibid.*, pp. 347, 513.

[104] *Ibid.*, p. 348.

[105] *Ibid.*

[106] *Ibid.*, p. 349. The Ashwell referred to is probably Dr. Samuel Ashwell, author of *A Practical Treatise on Diseases Peculiar to Women* (London, 1884, 8°, first ed. 1828?). I have not yet been able to find any passages on contraception in the 1844 edition of Ashwell (the only one available to me). Perhaps such passages appeared in earlier editions. If so, the matter deserves research to determine the place of Ashwell in the medical history of contraception in England during the nineteenth century. His name is never mentioned in our day.

were Legoyt,[107] H. Martineau,[108] a writer in the *Penny Encyclopedia*,[109] and one in *Ree's Cyclopedia*.[110]

(5f)   Early Influence of Charles Bradlaugh and Dr. George Drysdale

One who coöperated closely with George Drysdale was Charles Bradlaugh,[111] later an M.P. His public advocacy of contraception began as early as 1860, when he was just starting the *National Reformer*. An acrimonious dispute over birth control between Bradlaugh and Joseph Barker, his co-editor, led to a severance of relations.[112] Barker claimed that Bradlaugh gave unqualified approval to all the teachings in Drysdale's *Elements*. Such was not the case; but Bradlaugh, in the columns of the *National Reformer*, had recommended the work to readers as worthy of their thoughtful perusal. He, of course, agreed with Drysdale's Neo-Malthusian views, and himself published articles and tracts on Malthusianism and Neo-Malthusianism.[113] But Bradlaugh never wrote on the medical aspects himself.

---

[107] *Elements*, p. 524.

[108] *Ibid.*, p. 515.

[109] *Ibid.*, p. 511. The writer avowed that "to recommend early marriage without recommending preventive measures, is just to recommend that poverty should be increased."

[110] *Ibid.*, p. 511.

[111] The best biography is that by Bradlaugh's daughter, Hypatia Bradlaugh Bonner, *Charles Bradlaugh. A Record of His Life and Work*. London: T. Fisher Unwin, 1895, vol. i, pp. xiv, 1–400; vol. ii, pp. ix, 1–440. Other editions are available. See especially vol. ii, chs. ii, iii, iv. See also J. M. Robertson, *Charles Bradlaugh*. London: Watts, 1920, pp. vi, 1–122. George Jacob Holyoake wrote an account in 1891; and there is the "libellous" life by Charles R. Mackay (*Life of Charles Bradlaugh, M.P.* London: Gunn, 1888, pp. 468). See also Reynaert in *Revue Générale*, 1882. Adolphe S. Headingly, *The Biography of Charles Bradlaugh*. Sec. ed. revised. London: Remington, 1880. London: Freethought Publishing Co., 1883, pp. 195. George Standring wrote a penny pamphlet on Bradlaugh's life published by the Freethought Publishing Co. in 1881. There are still other accounts, but the biography by Mrs. Bonner, Bradlaugh's daughter, though perhaps somewhat marred by an attempt to clear his name from the abuse heaped upon it, is the most complete and informing account.

[112] See the *National Reformer* for the period and Joseph Barker's periodical, *The People*. Barker was in no position to cast stones. He published some really coarse material on sex.

[113] "Jesus, Shelley, and Malthus: An Essay on the Population Question," *National Reformer* [abbreviated herein as N. R.], June 8 and 15, 1861. First appeared as a pamphlet in June, 1861 [so "Iconoclast," (i.e., Bradlaugh) says in a note to correspondents in N. R., June 22, 1861]. There must have been numerous editions. In 1883 there was an edition bearing the title "Jesus, Shelley and Malthus; or, Pious Poverty and Heterodox Happiness." London: Freethought Publishing Co., 63 Fleet St., 2d. I have never found a copy of a pamphlet entitled either (a) "What has the Population Question to do with Parliamentary Reformers?" or (b) "Poverty and Parliamentary Reform" (1863). In the N. R. for April 25, 1863 (p. 5, col. 3) this is announced for publication on May 8, 1863. Another notice below refers to the second title, and gives the date as May 15, 1863. If it

In the 'sixties, Drysdale, over the initials "G. R.," contributed to the *National Reformer* some well-reasoned articles on Neo-Malthusianism, then

---

ever saw the light, "Iconoclast" tried to demonstrate therein "that the political rights of the masses can never be thoroughly attained until the people themselves investigate the conditions of their existence as affected by the operation of the law of population"—by which Bradlaugh meant "as affected by excessively large families." See "Moses and Malthus" in N. R. March 7, 1863. "Labour's Prayer" first appeared in the N. R., vi, 338 (May 8, 1865); vi, 356–7 (June 4, 1865); vi, 377–8 (June 11, 1865). It was probably reprinted the same year; and was issued as late as 1882. It is not in the British Museum, and is exceedingly rare. The author has only this edition: London: Annie Besant and Charles Bradlaugh, n.d. [1882?] pp. 8. Bradlaugh says (N. R., xx, 169, Sept. 15, 1872 in a correspondence column in reply to "J. H.") that both the pamphlets, "Labour's Prayer" and "Why do Men Starve?" "urge the same propositions" as those to be found in Austin Holyoake's "Large and Small Families." Austin Holyoake, like his brother George, who was one of the greatest reform figures in English nineteenth-century history, advocated, in the pamphlet mentioned, Neo-Malthusian principles. Bradlaugh's "Why do Men Starve?" is exceedingly rare. So far as I know no copy exists at the present time in any public repository not excepting the British Museum, Bodleian, Library of Congress, etc. My copy bears the date 1882 (London: Annie Besant and Charles Bradlaugh, pp. 8), which suggests that it was at least occasionally reprinted many years after its first appearance. Another early, rare Malthusian article by Bradlaugh, and which in tract form is not known to be on public deposit, is "Poverty and its Effects on the Political Condition of the People." It is announced in the N. R. April 25, 1863 (p. 5, col. 3). Shortly afterward, Bradlaugh relinquished the editorship, on account of ill health, to Watts. The article appears in the issue of May 30, 1863 on the first page unsigned, which would erroneously suggest that Watts was the author. It is first advertised as a pamphlet in the N. R. Jan. 16, 1864, but it *may* have been reprinted in 1863.

In the N. R. for June 14, 1862 appeared a report of an interesting lecture delivered by Bradlaugh at the Hall of Science before Freethinkers on "Malthusianism and its Connection with Civil and Religious Liberty." In this address Bradlaugh mentioned the abuse he received for his "Malthusianism." He avowed that so long as men were poor, they could not know what civil and religious liberty is; hence they would not fight for it. He pleaded for a thorough examination and discussion of Malthusianism. Speaking of his Malthusian views, he added prophetically, so far as his future activity was concerned: "I affirm to you that I shall persist in their advocacy until I have compelled fair and complete discussion of them." This promise he kept fifteen years later when he fought a valiant struggle in the courts for the right to publish without interference contraceptive literature. The circumstances of his re-issue of Knowlton's *Fruits of Philosophy* is related in the text on following pages. Here our main purpose has been to show, by citing the detailed evidence, that Bradlaugh was an avowed Neo-Malthusian for a quarter of a century before his famous legal defence.

Bradlaugh's early medium of expression, the *National Reformer*, did more to spread Malthusian and Neo-Malthusian teachings than any other periodical published prior to 1900 save the *Malthusian*. The *National Reformer* was read mainly by Secularists and Freethinkers. In the form of non-periodical literature the writings of J. S. Mill and Miss H. Martineau were perhaps most influential in spreading Malthusian teachings (in the rather strict sense).

euphemistically called Malthusianism.[114]   He founded in the same decade a
Malthusian League for non-medical propaganda purposes; but the time was
not yet ripe for it, and the flower of his youthful enthusiasm withered from
the cold.   It was not until after the prosecution of Bradlaugh and Besant
that the Malthusian League was able to find genuine public support, found
a journal (the *Malthusian*), and finance the publication of propaganda
tracts.   That was in 1879.   From 1860 on, Dr. George Drysdale and
Charles Bradlaugh seem to have coöperated considerably in forwarding
the public discussion of Neo-Malthusianism.

Bradlaugh's real service, however, to the popular dissemination of contraceptive information was in 1877, when he decided to re-issue the Knowlton pamphlet.   The period 1834–1876 was, in fact, one of quiet, limited
circulation.   But the publicity attending the Bradlaugh and Truelove
prosecutions changed this limited percolation downward of contraceptive
knowledge into something hardly less than an inundation.

[114] This was the euphemistic word for birth control, contraception, etc., with this difference: There was a doctrinal difference in emphasis.   The post-Malthusian writers, styled
Neo-Malthusians, usually stressed the need of population restriction.   Though they
considered, and gave some attention to, the health side, it was, with the exception of some
writers, always secondary.   The presence in their social reasoning of the wages-fund
fallacy, now long since thrust into the discard, was also a differentiating ear-mark, at least
before the 'seventies.

CHAPTER X

DEMOCRATIZATION BY PUBLICITY

§1 THE BRADLAUGH-BESANT TRIAL (1877–1879)

The circumstances of this prosecution may be briefly summarized as follows: One Henry Cook of Bristol, who, it has been alleged,[1] interleaved obscene pictures with a Charles Watts edition of Knowlton's pamphlet, was, as a consequence, sentenced to two years imprisonment at hard labor. Charles Watts, the London publisher, was in turn prosecuted, but upon pleading guilty, got off comparatively easily. However, Charles Bradlaugh, and Annie Besant,[2] his co-worker in the Freethought movement, believed the pamphlet to be not only decent but highly useful. They felt that if their Freethought predecessors, whom they were accustomed to laud and esteem, had been distributing obscenity for the past forty years, and if their generation had just awakened to the fact, the less that was said about those predecessors the better. A test case seemed desirable in order to settle the legality of sale of the pamphlet. Having resolved to defend the right of publishing Knowlton's work, Bradlaugh and Besant organized the Freethought Publishing Company for the express purposes of reprinting it and pushing the sale. The London police were notified of the time and place of intended distribution. Upon arrest, the defendants were first tried at the Guildhall. After the case was taken to the Central Criminal Court, it went to the Court of Queen's Bench (High Court of Justice) on a

[1] See *Annie Besant: An Autobiography* (London: T. Fisher Unwin, Sec. ed., n.d.), p. 206.

[2] The best biographies are the following: Gertrude Marvin Williams, *The Passionate Pilgrim. A Life of Annie Besant*. New York: Coward-McCann, 1931, pp. 382. [Accurate in recording and finished in style. For present writer's review see *Birth Control Review*, October, 1931, pp. 280–282 under the title "Earlier Days of Birth Control."] Geoffrey West, *Mrs. Annie Besant*. London: Gerald Howe, 1927, pp. 89. New York: Viking Press, 1928, pp. 174. [The English edition is in the "Representative Women" series edited by Francis Birrell. Brilliantly written. The writer's estimate of the book will be found in the *Birth Control Review*, March, 1930. Both the above contain brief accounts of the Knowlton trial.] Mrs. Besant has herself written: *Autobiographical Sketches*. London: Freethought Publishing Co., 1885. [These first appeared in Mrs. Besant's periodical, *Our Corner* (1883–1888), a periodical which accepted G. B. Shaw's early novels when no one else would publish them.] *Annie Besant. An Autobiography*. London, [1893]. There are other, less useful biographies. The above are the chief and best summary sources.

writ of certiorari, and was there tried before Lord Chief Justice Cockburn.[3]
A lucid and cogent argument on the desirability of getting contraceptive
information to the poor was presented by Mrs. Besant, while Bradlaugh,
who was an able lawyer, was successful in quashing a somewhat adverse
decision.   In this manner the case of *Regina v. Charles Bradlaugh and Annie
Besant* ended victoriously, and the right of publication was vindicated.

The social effects of the publicity attending this prosecution were nothing
less than revolutionary.   But before considering these it would seem desirable to consider another trial of similar nature.

§2   THE TRIAL OF EDWARD TRUELOVE (1878–1879)

Another prosecution of the same period that forwarded the spread among
the masses of contraceptive knowledge was the trial[4] of Edward Truelove,
aged and esteemed Freethought publisher, for issuing Owen's chaste and
refined, but somewhat hortatory *Moral Physiology* and J. H. Palmer's tract
of a similar nature.[5]   Truelove had published both, and had exhibited them
in his shop window at 256 High Holborn, London.   This incurred the dis-
pleasure of the Society for the Suppression of Vice; and, upon its complaint,
the police, in May, 1877, seized two hundred and twenty copies of *Moral
Physiology* and twelve hundred copies (most of the supply?) of *Individual,
Family and National Poverty*.[6]

On Tuesday, May 22, 1877, the case came before Mr. Vaughan of the
Bow Street Police Court on two summonses: one charging Truelove with a

[3] For a report of the trial, see, *The Queen v. Charles Bradlaugh and Annie Besant*.
London: Freethought Publishing Co., n.d. (1878), pp. ii, 3–324.   The official citation is
2 Q.B.D., 569.   Reversed by 3 Q. B. D., 607.

[4] See the stenographic report separately published under the title *The Queen v. Edward
Truelove for publishing the Hon. Robert Dale Owen's "Moral Physiology" and a pamphlet,
entitled "Individual, Family and National Poverty."* London: Edward Truelove, 1878,
pp. viii, 1–125.   There is an account in the *National Reformer* (Feb. 3 and 10, 1878).
Cf., the paper of James A. Field on "Publicity by Prosecution," *Survey*, xxxv, 599–601
(Feb. 19, 1916).   Reprinted in Field's *Essays* as ch. vii.   The fact that we have no
scholarly accounts of the Bradlaugh-Besant and Truelove trials is a serious hiatus in our
knowledge of this social movement.   This subject will be treated in a future volume.

[5] J. H. Palmer, *Individual, Family and National Poverty.   Reasons why in every family
the number should be regulated; the methods that have been proposed, extensively adopted, and
found to answer for doing it, together with a few valuable hints for the young.*   Second ed.
London: Truelove, 1875, pp. 17.   This pamphlet is exceedingly rare.   Palmer mentions
no new methods.   He referred to the French letter or condom (unsafe and inconvenient);
to the sponge as suggested by Drysdale, and to injections (i.e., douches) of a solution of
sulphate of zinc or of alum as advocated by Knowlton.   He considered withdrawal,
coupled with the use of a sponge and douche, the only certain method.   The public
influence of the pamphlet was small.

[6] *National Reformer*, xxix (1877), 308.

misdemeanour at common law, the other demanding destruction of the seized pamphlets. Bradlaugh, representing the Bradlaugh-Besant Defence Committee, which was backing Truelove, put up £50 bail for Truelove's appearance at the Central Criminal Court. There was a second hearing before Vaughan, but as the case of *Regina v. Bradlaugh and Besant* was still *sub judice*, it was agreed to postpone the Truelove case until a decision was reached in the Bradlaugh case. Truelove entered into an agreement not to sell any of the prosecuted works in the interim.

On February 1 and 2, 1878 the case came before the Queen's Bench Division of the High Court of Justice. With the details of the counts and of the arguments pro and con we are not concerned. Our present purpose is rather to show the manner in which ill-advised prosecution "socialized" or democratized birth control knowledge. The prosecution attempted to prove that the pamphlets would have an injurious effect on the minds of the young, and that such an influence was intended by the authors and publishers. Purity of motive and a desire to discuss important questions of public policy—in this instance the need for population control—were not mitigating circumstances. For the defence Professor W. A. Hunter argued ably.

The jury was out two hours, failed to agree, and was discharged. The London *Times* indicated that the disagreement was due to the stubbornness of one juror;[7] but the *National Reformer*, the more reliable source in this instance at least, claimed that five had voted "not guilty."[8]

The second trial came before Barron Pollock in the Central Criminal Court. In the interval between the first and second trials a defence fund had been raised, largely through the publicity given the case in the *National Reformer*. The case was argued; the jury was out for forty minutes, and returned with a verdict of guilty. Sentence was then imposed: Four months in prison without hard labor; and, inasmuch as Truelove had made a profit on the sales, a fine of £50 was added.

The storm then broke. A hue and cry was raised in liberal and radical circles. Radical journals bristled with denunciation of the Society for the Suppression of Vice. Annie Besant scored the society and the prosecution in the *National Reformer*.[9] She was convinced, as were many others, that a great injustice had been done an innocent, pure-minded publisher of Freethought literature, aged nearly seventy. Charles Watts joined in the public defence of Truelove and the book.[10]

[7] London *Times*, February 4, 1878, p. 11.

[8] *National Reformer*, xxxi (1878), 1051. See N. R., xxxii (1878), 235 for a legal summary of the various steps in the trial.

[9] *National Reformer*, xxxi (1878), 1237.

[10] *Secular Review and Secularist*, i, 305.

Several efforts were unsuccessfully made to obtain an appeal on a writ of error. At South Place Chapel the Reverend Moncure Conway spoke in terms of severe condemnation of the proceedings against Truelove; and the congregation signed a memorial requesting his release.[11] Again, through the diligence of the *National Reformer*, a number of other memorials, praying for the release of Mr. Truelove, were sent to the Home Secretary, but without avail. The National Secular Society now took up the case, and produced memorials for Truelove's speedy release. Previous to the sentence, the Society had taken little interest in Truelove's predicament. Its periodical, the *Secular Review*, had always been a little shy of mixing Secularism and Neo-Malthusianism.[12] But now it declared:

We have forwarded our own Petition, [and] also the signature of some hundreds of our friends, to the Home Secretary, praying for the release of Mr. Truelove. The members of the British Secular Union throughout the country have been, we are pleased to see, exceedingly active in endeavouring to obtain a remission of the sentence. We are willing to receive any subscriptions on behalf of Mr. Truelove, and will undertake that all money so received shall reach the proper quarter direct[ly].[13]

The Home Secretary, however, was not to be moved. He evidently thought it inadvisable to interfere with the courts by lightening Truelove's sentence.

Thwarted in their attempts to appeal the case and then to shorten the sentence by use of special powers of the Home Secretary, Truelove's supporters now did all they could, without much success, to make him as comfortable during incarceration as circumstances would permit.[14] The *National Reformer* sarcastically remarked that "Such privileges are reserved for real criminals like Colonel Baker, who have the honour to be friendly with royalty."[15]

When Truelove was released on September 12, 1878 there was occasion for much rejoicing. He was met by a large crowd, and celebrations followed.

[11] *National Reformer*, xxxi (1878), 1276.

[12] This was the point of view also of George Jacob Holyoake, a thorough-going Neo-Malthusian. His relation to the development of Neo-Malthusian doctrine needs only to be mentioned here. In a number of publications from 1860 on Holyoake not only showed his interest in the general subject, but publicly favored it in debates and in print. But he never was the fighter Bradlaugh was. In another volume Holyoake's work will be traced in detail.

[13] *Secular Review and Secularist*, i, 245.

[14] Truelove complained bitterly of the severity of the prison discipline. He was fed water and gruel. He was not permitted to see anyone save his counsel; and request for outside medical aid was also refused.

[15] *National Reformer*, xxxi (1878), 1336.

The matter of destruction of the pamphlets dragged on in the courts for several months.   On October 3, 1878, the seized pamphlets were ordered destroyed by the Bow Street Police Court;[16] but on April 26, 1879, the case came up before the Sessions House on appeal.   After still more delays on points of law, destruction was finally ordered.

§3   EFFECT OF THE BRADLAUGH-BESANT AND TRUELOVE PROSECUTIONS IN DEMOCRATIZING CONTRACEPTIVE KNOWLEDGE

The social effect of these two trials upon the public mind was electric. The Bradlaugh-Besant trial went far to make legal the *general*, free distribution of contraceptive knowledge, and thus established a situation quite different from that prevailing in the United States.

There can be no doubt that the publicity gave wide advertising to the idea that contraception was possible.   Millions of people learned of more effective methods.   We can judge this only by two circumstances: (1) the enhanced circulation of works containing instruction on contraception; (2) the halving of the English birth rate since 1876.

The validity of the second point is so well established as hardly to require a demonstration.   If needed, this may most summarily be shown by Dr. C. V. Drysdale's chart[17] (Figure XIX) brought up to date.   Democratization of contraceptive knowledge is further shown by the increased diffusion of contraceptive literature following the prosecutions.   To this we now turn.

It has been stated previously that prior to 1876 the circulation of the *Fruits of Philosophy* approximated only a thousand copies annually, despite the regular advertisement of it in Freethought journals.   In the three and a half years after that trial (up to August 28, 1881) 185,000 copies of the Freethought Publishing Company edition were sold at sixpence each.   More than this, the notoriety of the trial caused several editions to be issued in provincial towns: in Sheffield, Wakefield and Newcastle among others. Other publishers beside Bradlaugh and Besant reprinted the pamphlet in London; and possibly additional English editions were issued at this time which I have not been able to trace.   None of these editions are in the British Museum or other important public repositories; and the proof of their existence has been possible only by resort to private collection (see

[16] *Ibid.*, xxxii (1878), 235, 250–252.

[17] It first appeared to my knowledge in Dr. C. V. Drysdale's "The Empire and the Birth Rate," *Jour. Royal Colonial Institute* (1914); and was reprinted as a Malthusian League tract, (reprint pp. 4).   It was also printed on the program of the Malthusian League annual dinner in 1927 when Mr. J. M. Keynes was chairman and Annie Besant the chief speaker.   Prof. Ross, republished it in his able *Standing Room Only?*

Bibliography). At about the same time French and Dutch translations appeared.

Probably the sale of the miscellaneous English editions other than the Bradlaugh-Besant edition, reached 50,000 to 100,000. Adding the smaller

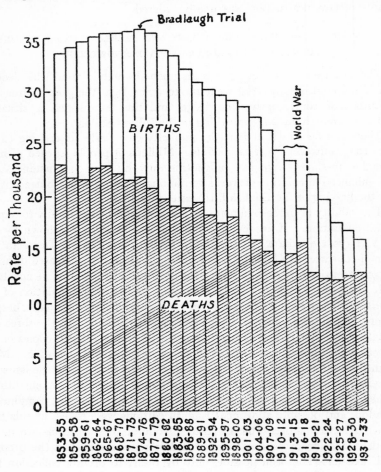

Fig. XIX. Birth, Deaths and Natural Increase in England and Wales Since the Bradlaugh-Besant and Truelove Prosecutions. By Three-Year Periods—1853–1933.

figure to the circulation already reached by the Bradlaugh-Besant edition, we have a total of 235,000 attained in a relatively short period. If one were to include the English circulation, reached before 1876 (42,000), the total would be 277,000.

How much the notoriety of this legal tussle increased the sales of a score of similar tracts we have no means of ascertaining, but there is every reason to believe that there was a substantial upward movement in the numbers distributed, and that this was out of all proportion to the increase in the number and literacy of the population. The *National Reformer*, in reprinting full accounts of the trial in the Guildhall, mentioned the titles of many other books giving similar information, some issuing from esteemed publishers. The circulation of these may have been increased.

Shortly after the right of publication of medical information on contraception was clarified in England by legal decision, the Knowlton pamphlet was replaced by Annie Besant's *Law of Population*.[18] This elucidated in even greater detail than the *Fruits of Philosophy* methods of controlling conception. Mrs. Besant's tract was first issued in January, 1879 (though possibly late in 1878), to replace the out-of-date Knowlton treatise. Chapter I dealt with "The Law of Population," Chapter II with "Its Consequences," Chapter III with "Its Bearing upon Human Conduct and Morals," while the fourth chapter was entitled "Objections Considered."[19] With the non-medical portion of Mrs. Besant's treatise we need not concern ourselves here inasmuch as this will find exposition and critical analysis in a subsequent volume. Though Mrs. Besant's treatment of contraception was thoroughly Malthusian, it was essentially sound both as regards her elucidation of Malthusian principles and her discussion of the tendency of population pressure to cause poverty, misery, low wages, child labor, etc. In later editions of the pamphlet Mrs. Besant devoted more attention than in early editions to refuting the contentions of her socialist friends who were, on the whole, antagonistic to Neo-Malthusianism.

After considering at some length her reasons for believing that family limitation is a duty, Mrs. Besant observes:

It remains, then, to ask how is this duty to be performed? It is clearly useless to preach the limitation of the family, and to conceal the means whereby such limitation may be effected. If the limitation be a duty, it cannot be wrong to afford such information as shall enable people to discharge it.

There are various prudential checks which have been suggested, but further investigation of this intricate subject is sorely needed, and it is much to be wished that more medical men would devote themselves to the study of this important branch of physiology.[20]

[18] Annie Besant, *The Law of Population: Its Consequences, and Its Bearing upon Human Conduct and Morals.* London: Freethought Pub. Co., n.d. [1879], pp. 3–48.

[19] The dedication is interesting: "To the poor in great cities and agricultural districts, dwellers in stifling court or crowded hovel, in the hope that it may point out a path from poverty, and may make easier the life of British mothers, to them I dedicate this essay."

[20] *Ibid.*, p. 31.

(3a)   Techniques in Annie Besant's "Law of Population"

It is interesting to follow, through the many editions of the *Law of Population*, the development in Mrs. Besant's treatment of contraceptive technique. The discussion immediately following is based upon what I believe to be the first issue of that pamphlet.

Nearly two pages are devoted to a discussion of the safe period which, we are informed, "is not certain."[21] Withdrawal is considered "absolutely certain as a preventive,"[22] but Mrs. Besant rather shrewdly adds:

A few among the French doctors contend that the practice is injurious, more especially to the wife; but they have failed, so far as we can judge, in making out their case, for they advance no proofs in support of their theory, while the universal practice of the French speaks strongly on the other side.[23]

We are informed that "there is but little doubt" that Knowlton's check' syringing with a solution of sulphate of zinc or alum, was an "effective one."[24] She observed that "there are many obvious disadvantages connected with it as a matter of taste and feeling."[25] "The same remark applies to the employment of the *baudruche*, a covering used by men . . . "[26] She adds:

The check which appears to us to be preferable, as at once certain, and in no sense grating on any feeling of affection or of delicacy, is that recommended by Carlile many years ago in his "Every Woman's Book."[27]

The sponge, therefore, was Mrs. Besant's favorite check; and this preference appears in the first issues of the pamphlet. This method, it will be recalled, had been preferred by Place, Carlile's instructor. It was only in later editions of the *Law of Population* that vaginal suppositories were recommended—perhaps as a result of the influence of Dr. Allbutt. Dr. Marion Sims is referred to in the first issue as recommending the use of a "'small wad of cotton, not more than an inch in diameter' . . . secured with a string for its removal."[28] This, too, had been mentioned by Place. Mrs. Besant's advice that the cotton wadding should be worn during the day and removed at night seems odd. Prolonged nursing is condemned as detrimental to health. A popular medical writer, Dr. Chavasse, is quoted

[21] *Ibid.*, p. 33.
[22] *Ibid.*
[23] *Ibid.*, pp. 33–34.
[24] *Ibid.*, p. 34.
[25] *Ibid.*   Presumably Mrs. Besant has in mind aesthetic objections.
[26] *Ibid.*
[27] *Ibid.*
[28] *Ibid.*, p. 35.   This quotation was eventually dropped in later issues.

on the extent of injuries supposed to be caused by prolonged nursing. According to Chavasse it seemed to cause nearly every disease to which human flesh is heir. Chavasse's extreme views are reminiscent of Bergeret's and Tissot's discussions of the horrible results of masturbation (which they referred to as Onanism). Abortion is, of course, condemned by Mrs. Besant,[29] though medical testimony is adduced to show that this is sometimes medically indicated, and therefore necessary.

Chapter III closes with a peroration on the Utopian effects of the general adoption of the preventive checks just outlined. There can be no doubt that Mrs. Besant over-stated and therefore weakened her case; but it is only scant justice to her courageous pioneering efforts to recall that those were fiery days of hot and irresponsible calumniation of anyone who undertook even the most indirect and tactful public support of preventive measures. It was natural enthusiasm and self-defence that prompted Mrs. Besant to claim more than she needed; and, considering the violence of some of the opposition,[30] Mrs. Besant's moderation and good temper are rather striking.

As later editions of the *Law of Population* were called for, improvements were made in the account on technique. For example, the edition known as the "Seventieth Thousand" [1882] contained a special appendix amplifying the earlier treatment. Mrs. Besant there informs the readers that "Experience has proved that the checks mentioned in the preceding pages are none of them absolutely certain in their action."[31] Conversation with "one of the most eminent of London physicians,[32] who has paid great attention to this matter, with a view to discover[ing] some definite protection for those women who are the subjects of distortion of the pelvis, and to whom labor often means death," led Mrs. Besant to the belief that douching failures were usually caused by the lack of use of a reverse current syringe. Mention is then made of the name of a syringe believed to meet these re-

[29] *Ibid.*, pp. 35–36.

[30] Typical of the abusive and satirical literature are the following: Peter Agate, M.D. [pseud.], *Sexual Economy as Taught by Charles Bradlaugh, M.P., With Addendum by Saladin.* London: W. Stewart, n.d., pp. 54. Rare. See also the Mackay and Headingly biographies of Bradlaugh referred to in ch. ix, n. 111. Bradlaugh was subjected to more abuse than Mrs. Besant, though she received more than her share. It was sufficiently unbecoming in Victorian times for a woman to appear on the public platform, much less to advocate "Malthusianism" in a public print sold at a low price. There were also a few impersonal but childish attacks on the Knowlton pamphlet itself.

[31] *Law* (Seventieth Thous., n.d. [1882]), p. 49.

[32] Dr. Palfrey, as appears from the appendix to the ninetieth thousand of the *Law*. After quoting Dr. Palfrey's letter, Mrs. Besant adds: "Dr. Palfrey informed me that in his practice he continually recommended the use of this check to married women, and that it has been very largely and very successfully adopted."

quirements. Information on where it might be purchased was also included. A recommendation not in earlier editions was that regarding douching solutions.[33]

In the one hundred tenth thousand of the *Law of Population*, which appeared in 1887, Mrs. Besant still further modified the account of technique.[34] She declared at the outset that the most reliable checks are the soluble pessary [suppository], the India-rubber pessary [cervical cap], and the sponge.[35] Note that the rubber cervical cap and the suppository had by now [1887] taken coördinate rank with the sponge in Mrs. Besant's mind. After stating where these might be obtained (reference is made to an advertisement on p. 48), Mrs. Besant declares:

There is no difficulty in the use of any one of these three checks; they are, I believe, thoroughly reliable if ordinary care is used to place them in position; and they have enormous advantage of being entirely in the hands of the woman and of being absolutely unobtrusive.[36]

The sponge may be soaked in a solution of twenty grains of quinine to a pint of water. The woman is also recommended to douche with a solution

[33] Instead of a solution of alum or of sulphate of zinc being used, in the manner mentioned in the text, a dessert spoonful of a powder—composed of sulpho-carbolate of zinc and dried sulphate of zinc, of each 1 ounce, alum 4 ounces—is recommended. Care must be taken that these drugs be reduced to a *perfectly fine powder*. The better plan is to dissolve the quantity of the powder just named in a few ounces of boiling water to ensure its perfect solution, to pour this solution when cool into a bottle and keep it ready for use, adding the solution to a pint of tepid, or in hot weather cold, water at the time of using the syringe, and this is the quantity to be used on each occasion.

As a matter of caution the solution must be kept from the reach of children or curious persons, and it is wise to label the bottle in which the solution is kept, "Poison." (p. 49).

[34] The following new material is, in part, used to introduce the subject:

There are various prudential checks which have been suggested, but further investigation of this intricate subject is sorely needed, and it is much to be wished that more medical men would devote themselves to the study of this important branch of physiology. The main difficulty in the way is the absurd notion that prudential checks are obscene, and very few doctors have the courage to face the odium that would arise from a frank treatment of the subject. Some medical men do, at the present time, recommend the use of checks to their female patients, but even these would hesitate ere they openly dealt with the subject. The consequence of this unfortunate state of things is that much doubt hangs over the efficacy of the checks proposed, and all that can be done is to state what these checks are, adding a word of recommendation on those which have proved most successful in practice. (Besant, *Law* (110th thous.), pp. 31–32.)

[35] *Law* (1887), p. 32.

[36] *Ibid.*, p. 32.

of quinine (ten grains to a pint of water) in the morning before removing the cap.[37]   Quinine was the supposed active agent in Rendell's suppositories in a cocoabutter vehicle.   Nowadays quinine is not preferred as being irritating to some women.   Furthermore, recent research by Voge and Baker has shown that its spermicidal power is low.

For the first time in the *Law* reference is also made to Allbutt's the *Wife's Handbook* and to the use of an artificial sponge.[38]   In discussing the douche, Mrs. Besant here incorporated material which she had, in preceding issues, inserted in the appendix.   Hence this issue (110th thousand, 1887) is without an appendix.

Mrs. Besant warns her readers that "there is much uncertainty attending the use of all these injections.   If the spermatozoa have entered the womb before the injection is used, conception may occur, and though many women have found this check satisfactory, there are also many failures marked against it.   There are also many obvious disadvantages attending its use."[39] She states that the use of withdrawal and the mid-period, though "very widely used . . . cannot be regarded as so satisfactory as those [checks like the suppository, rubber cap, and sponge] which depend on closing the entrance to the womb."[40]   The same condemnation of abortion and prolonged suckling appears.

The discussion of technique which followed in succeeding issues of the *Law of Population* remained, so far as one can at present determine, substantially the same as in the issue of the one hundred tenth thousand. Noteworthy is the absence of mention of the vaginal diaphragm or pessary of the Mensinga type.   Undoubtedly when Besant spoke of the rubber pessary,[41] she meant the cervical cap.   One finds illustrated English advertisements of the cervical rubber cap but not of the Mensinga pessary in the 'eighties.   The Mensinga had reached Holland from Germany by the early eighteen eighties, but apparently not England.

The influence of the *Law of Population* was remarkable.[42]   Up to 1891,

[37] *Ibid.*, p. 33.

[38] *Ibid.*

[39] *Ibid.*, p. 34.

[40] *Ibid.*

[41] This vague term should never be used in our time save in a generic sense; and even then it is well to avoid its use.

[42] As early as 1884 Mrs. Besant wrote (p. iii) in the introduction to the ninetieth thousand:

> FOUR-AND-A-HALF years have passed away since this little book was first issued; it was written for the poor, in the hope that by the information therein given—information long familiar to and long acted upon by the wealthier classes of society— poor men and women might make the home happy, and rear in respectability and comfort a limited number of children, children who should hereafter bless the parents

that is within twelve years after its first issue, 175,000 copies were sold in England at sixpence each. It was reprinted in America[43] as well as in Australia, where an unsuccessful attempt was made to prosecute it.[44] It was translated into German, Dutch, Italian, French and doubtless other languages. When Mrs. Besant became a theosophist, and temporarily renounced her Neo-Malthusian views, the pamphlet was withdrawn. At that time, other publishers, wishing to continue the sale, offered a liberal sum for the copyright, but Mrs. Besant refused to sell it.

The *Law of Population* and similar pamphlets were sometimes bound together with advertisements on separate sheets stating where the reader could procure modern contraceptive supplies.

Returning to the extent of the circulation of contraceptive literature given currency by virtue of the notoriety of the Bradlaugh and Truelove prosecutions, one finds that in the period 1876–1891 a minimum of 410,000 copies of only two pamphlets (the *Fruits of Philosophy* and the *Law of Population*) were distributed. There is no means of estimating the increased circulation of Owen's *Moral Physiology*, but there can be little doubt that the notoriety of the trial increased its circulation.

We have stated above that in this period Dr. George Drysdale's *Elements of Social Science*, first published in 1854, was making notable strides toward reaching its ultimate goal of thirty-five English editions, and translation into at least ten European languages. We shall make mention below of

---

whose wisdom and forethought had given them a fair chance in the life-race. That hope has been largely realised. During these years fifty thousand copies of the book have found their way into English homes; across the Atlantic it has found warm welcome, and very large American editions have been sold. It has been translated into German, Italian, French, Swedish, and Dutch, and has thus spread over the Continent of Europe, while the English edition has been largely sold in Hindustan, Australia, and New Zealand. A circulation so wide is the sign of the need which this pamphlet has striven to supply.

[43] New York: Butts [188-], and San Francisco, 1893. If there were any prosecutions of the American issues I have never heard of them.

[44] In Australia, the pamphlet was prosecuted as obscene, and Mr. W. W. Collins, who assumed responsibility for publishing it, was condemned by a magistrate. The case was then carried to the superior court, and the conviction quashed by Justice Windeyer. In England, it was never prosecuted; nor was its circulation in any manner interfered with. See, *Mr. Justice Windeyer on the Population Question. An abridgment of the judgment delivered in the Supreme Court of New South Wales by Mr. Justice Windeyer, Senior Puisne Judge, 12th December, 1888*. London: [Malthusian League], pp. 7. See also, *Is Limitation of the Family Immoral? A judgment on Annie Besant's "Law of Population," delivered in the Supreme Court of New South Wales, by Mr. Justice Windeyer, Senior Puisne Judge*. London: Freethought Pub. Co., 1889, pp. 26. *Cf*., Ex parte Collins. N. S. W. St. R. 497 (1888).

Dr. H. A. Allbutt's the *Wife's Handbook*, which appeared shortly after the Bradlaugh prosecution. In this instance also there is no accurate means of estimating circulation, but we know that it went through many editions rapidly. The work was constantly revised, probably by anonymous individuals employed by the later publishers. By 1927 it had passed the half million mark. This figure represents sales. Never was it distributed gratuitously.

One might go on to trace the circulation of numerous other tracts and books, some of which had been quietly circulated to a modest extent before the trials, but which suddenly found a more interested reading public after the notoriety of the prosecutions. Probably not less than a million tracts furnishing elaborate contraceptive information were sold in England between 1876 and 1891, when Mrs. Besant ceased the publication of her *Law of Population*. It is not inconceivable that the figure might be two millions.

It is not at all unlikely that the prosecutions of this period were at least partially responsible for the introduction into England of more reliable contraceptive methods. The advertisements mentioned above frequently offered for sale such appliances, and, barring the eighteenth century advertisements of the sheath made in the form of handbills by Mrs. Philips, they are the first English commercial advertisements dealing with contraceptives that have come to my attention.

Dr. Henry A. Allbutt, who suffered some rough handling by the Medical Council, may have been responsible for the introduction of the rubber cervical cap. The date is probably the early 1880's. While this point cannot be considered as yet established, it would seem quite probable that the Knowlton prosecution occasioned so much publicity as to increase the effective demand for an improved contraceptive device. If the publicity did not actually cause the introduction of the article, it probably enhanced the market for it.

It is no part of my argument that the democratization of contraceptive knowledge in the 'eighties was solely a consequence of the prosecutions of Bradlaugh, Besant and Truelove. Many circumstances made the time ripe for the socialization of this information. Chief among them was no doubt the notoriety of the trials.

Just as the trials called birth control to the attention of the lay public, so Dr. Allbutt's publication of a medical pamphlet drew the medical profession into the very vortex of the movement.

(3b) The Allbutt Incident (1887)

About 1884 or 1885 Dr. H. A. Allbutt, a Leeds physician and a Fellow of the Royal College of Physicians of Edinburgh, published a six-penny pamphlet entitled the *Wife's Handbook*.[45]   It was a decent, popular medical treatise designed to diffuse among the general populace hygienic knowledge, but especially information on pre-natal care and the management of the baby.   Inasmuch as the author believed that there were many cases in which contraceptive information was medically indicated, he added to the inexpensive pamphlet a chapter (vii) on "How to Prevent Conception when Advised by the Doctor."   According to the author's own story we are assured that his motives in publishing the work were of the very highest: to prevent poverty, destitution, prostitution, misery and marital discord— inevitable concomitants of reckless reproduction.   A thorough-going Malthusian and Neo-Malthusian of the Drysdale school—Allbutt was evidently much influenced by Drysdale's *Elements of Social Science*—this Leeds physician believed that the diffusion of contraceptive knowledge among poor women would not only promote health and happiness but actually save many lives.   He would dispel the fog of ignorance by a popular educational campaign.

Considering the period in which it was written, the pamphlet contains a rather good survey on technique.   We find mentioned here, in addition to the safe period[46] (failed in five[47] per cent of the cases), withdrawal ("hurtful to the nervous system in many persons"), injections (alum, quinine, "Palfrey's Powder," quinine[48] or vinegar[49] solutions), sponges or tampons, the Mensinga vaginal diaphragm and the cervical cap.   Allbutt observed that he knew "a great many cases . . . where injections . . . have failed in preventing conception."[50]   This was particularly true of plain water douches. Noteworthy in the light of recent research is the special recommendation of a vinegar solution.   When properly used it is quite effective.   Use of the sponge alone without medicaments sometimes resulted in failures; but we are told nothing of failures with medicated sponges.   The sheath was a "very certain check."[51]

Though most of the techniques mentioned by Allbutt had been discussed

---

[45] H. Arthur Allbutt, *The Wife's Handbook: how a woman should order herself during pregnancy, in the lying-in room and after delivery. With hints on the management of the baby, and on other matters of importance, necessary to be known by married women.*   Fourth ed.   London: Forder, 1887, pp. 58.   The third edition was published in London by W. J. Ramsey in 1886, pp. 45.   Probably the first edition appeared about 1884 or 1885.   To date, copies of the first and second editions have not been traced.

[46] Five days before and eight days after menstruation.

[47] Actually the percentage is very much higher.

[48] Twenty grains to a pint of water.

[49] One part to six of water.

[50] *The Wife's Handbook* (1887). p 48

[51] *Ibid.*, p. 49.

by predecessors, his reference to the Mensinga diaphragm seems to be the first in a birth-control tract published in English. If there were earlier notices in any of the medical journals published in English, such notices have not come to my attention. Allbutt, and not N. Haire, is thus to be credited with making it known in England. Haire however, did much to popularize its use among physicians after 1922.

Allbutt furnishes tolerably adequate instructions for its use, and gives the address of a retailer. In England at that time it seems to have been made in only three sizes. Now there are twenty or thirty. Instructions are likewise given for the use of the "check pessary," or cervical cap. Rather modern is the suggestion that in its hollow there should be placed a compound of vaseline,[52] cocoa butter, and quinine. Also very modern is the mention by name of Rendell's soluble pessaries (suppositories).[53] This is the trade name of one of the oldest manufacturers in England. The word of caution regarding their use which Allbutt includes is worthy of attention: "It is but right to say that these pessaries are at present only on trial. Time will show whether they can be relied upon to prevent conception. My opinion is that they will do all their inventor claims for them."[54] An artificial sponge or tampon is mentioned "containing in its center a friable capsule filled with slightly acidulated quinine solution." The medicament is freed by squeezing the sponge and breaking the capsule. Allbutt condemned the internal use of arsenic and other drugs to produce impotence, and declared unreliable the method used by some Italian women of coughing to expel the semen.[55] One is impressed in Allbutt's favor upon reading the footnote attached to Chapter VII: "When a woman is advised by her doctor not to conceive on account of the state of her health, she had better consult him as to which of these methods of prevention would be best in her particular case."[56]

In 1887, a few years after the publication of the *Wife's Handbook*, Mr. Joseph Latchmore, secretary of the Leeds Vigilance Association, protested

[52] Since it causes rubber to deteriorate, vaseline is no longer recommended.

[53] *Ibid.*, p. 50.

[54] *Ibid.*

[55] Allbutt reports that Dr. Giovanni Tari, a physician of Naples, was informed by an Italian priest that poor women in Italy thought they could prevent conception by sitting up in bed directly after intercourse and coughing. Tari was of the opinion that this method was suitable in most cases. Allbutt, however, thought it ineffective for several reasons, among others that the ridges in the vagina would prevent the semen from being wholly expelled. It is interesting to note that this method was noted by Soranos in the first century and Aëtios in the sixth. The persistence of the idea is an interesting example of the continuity of a contraceptive practice for centuries.

[56] P. 47, note.

to medical societies; whereupon the Royal College of Physicians of Edinburgh, of which Allbutt was a member, served, through the Fellows, an indictment upon Allbutt accusing him of having "published and exposed for sale an indecent publication, titled *The Wife's Handbook*, and having published, and attached thereto, advertisements of an unprofessional character, titled 'Malthusian Appliances'." Albutt was summoned to appear, presumably to show cause why his name should not be stricken from the register. However, the Malthusian League, which was founded shortly after the Bradlaugh-Besant prosecution, took up Allbutt's case, and protests were addressed to the College from all parts of Great Britain, and from France, Germany, Holland, Italy, India, and Jamaica. It seems that the Edinburgh Fellows either transferred the case to the General Medical Council in London or dropped the charge. According to Allbutt's own account, it was the latter.[57] In 1887, Dr. Allbutt's case was heard before a committee of the General Medical Council, Dr. Allbutt being represented by Mr. Wallace (barrister), and the prosecution being conducted by Mr. Muir Mackenzie, legal adviser of the Council. Wallace justified Allbutt, and called attention to a list of over seventy petitions, many of them from medical and scientific societies, presented to the Council from all parts of Europe. There was a difference of opinion among members, he noted, whether Dr. Allbutt should be condemned; his motives were unimpeachable. The verdict was, however, as follows:

In the opinion of the Council, Mr. Allbutt has committed the offence charged against him; that is to say, of having published, and publicly caused to be sold, a work entitled *The Wife's Handbook*, in London and elsewhere, at so low a price as to bring the work within the reach of the youth of both sexes, to the detriment of public morals. Secondly, the offence is, in the opinion of the Council, "infamous conduct in a professional respect." Thirdly, the Registrar is hereby ordered to erase the name of Mr. H. A. Allbutt from the Medical Register.[58]

Inasmuch as one of Allbutt's chief motives in writing the *Wife's Handbook* had been to diffuse contraceptive information among the masses, he now avowed that he would not give up. Instead, he appealed to the country as one unjustly treated by the General Medical Council, as indeed a martyr to Neo-Malthusianism, and published a pamphlet (*Artificial Checks*) in defense of his position. Allbutt liked to make it appear that his sole offence had been to publish a hygienic pamphlet, allegedly indecent, *at a low price*. But the case was not so simple as this. Without attempting any final adjudication of the matter, the following circumstances seem relevant. Allbutt was diffusing medical knowledge in a form generally not approved

[57] H. A. Allbutt, "Artificial Checks to Population" (London, 1889), p. 28.
[58] *Ibid.*, p. 7.

by physicians—the issuance of popular medical treatises. Trade-marked articles of various kinds were recommended to the general public. Though the edition of the *Wife's Handbook* of 1886 (third) contained advertisements of contraceptive supplies, and though Allbutt rigorously condemned abortion in his pamphlet, the brochure in which he defended himself against treatment by the General Medical Council contained two advertisements of retail distributors of abortifacient pills. There is, however, no evidence known to the writer that advertisements of abortifacients appeared in the early issues of the *Wife's Handbook*. Since the Council was much concerned about the effect of the distribution of the pamphlet upon public morals, it is not irrelevant to observe that Allbutt specifically declared in this work that "this chapter . . . is intended to be read in the privacy of the chamber by married women or by those contemplating marriage, and is not intended for the publicity of the streets or to satisfy the curiosity of the vicious."[59]

Allbutt appealed to the public through addresses, his defence pamphlet, and by means of the assistance of the Malthusian League. But the case of the General Medical Council seems never to have been presented to the general public. In sum, it is difficult to say how much weight the committee of the Council placed upon unprofessional conduct, such as advertising, and how much upon the diffusion, outside of the medical office, of information allegedly injurious to public morality. It is a matter of public record, though, that other physicians have been rather severely dealt with by Medical Ethics Committees of Medical Councils and Academies for diffusing contraceptive information even when advertising was not an issue. This is a highly controversial subject, and doubtless each case must necessarily be determined on its merits. It is of the utmost importance to the public that the standards of the medical profession should be protected, that commercialization should be avoided, that the publicity seekers should be duly guided and restrained. Many zealous medical advocates of contraception have sometimes made matters unnecessarily difficult for themselves by running counter to the accepted methods of control. On the other hand, it is probably safe to say that Councils and Academies have been somewhat reluctant, at least in some cases, to view the problems of ethics and of control before them in broad social terms.

Striking Dr. Allbutt's name from the Medical Register was quite without the disciplinary effect intended. On the contrary, it merely spurred Allbutt to renewed efforts, and fanned the flames of the propaganda. At least one newspaper publicly defended him: The *Pall Mall Gazette* declared on November 28, 1887 that the decision was "one of the most glaring illustrations

---

[59] *The Wife's Handbook* (1887), p. 51.

of professional prejudice and human folly." Whether this position was extreme is not for the writer to adjudicate. He only knows that Allbutt now became a martyr; that the *Wife's Handbook* increased tremendously in circulation; that it was subsequently translated into many European languages. In England it has sold by hundreds of thousands down to this very day, having been constantly revised and brought up to date. When the writer was in England in 1927 investigating the birth-control clinics, he purchased a copy of the pamphlet which was then in its fiftieth edition or five hundred thousandth copy. Since the pamphlet was then much out of date, it probably did some harm as well as good. It was still permeated with advertisements. In various editions it bore somewhat changed titles.[60]

§4 NOTORIETY AND A CRISIS PROMOTE ORGANIZATION: THE MALTHUSIAN LEAGUE (1878–1927)

The Bradlaugh prosecution led to the founding of the Malthusian League in 1878[61] and of its journal the *Malthusian* (1879–1922). Dr. Charles Drysdale, brother of George Drysdale, became the League's first president,[62] and Mrs. Annie Besant the first secretary.[63] It might more accurately have

[60] The title of the French edition was *Le Livre de l'Épouse.*

[61] 1878, not 1877, is the correct date of the founding. It should, however, be recalled that in the early sixties a group had been organized, but the attempt was abortive. The time was not yet ripe for it. See p. 238.

[62] Dr. Charles was the president from 1878 to his death in 1907. Chief among his Malthusian and Neo-Malthusian writings were, besides his contributions to the *Malthusian*, the following: Malthusian League Tracts Nos. 1, 2, 5, 6 and 9, mentioned in a note following. "Debate on Infanticide, in the Harveian Medical Society of London, May 17th 1866," reprinted from the *Med. Press and Circular,* June 13, 1866, London, 1866, pp. 12. [Touches upon evils of large families.] "The Population Question at the Medical Society of London; or, the mortality of the rich and poor. A paper read at the society with the debate." London: Standring, 1879, pp. 12. *The Life and Writings of T. R. Malthus.* London, 1887 (1st ed.), 1892, (2nd ed.). *The Population Question According to Thomas R. Malthus and J. S. Mill.* London: William Bell, 1878. London: Standring, 1892. [See especially Chapter VII (pp. 74–87) on the "Prosecution of Malthusian Works."] "The Cause of Poverty. A Paper read at the National Liberal Club on 21st October, 1890." London: Standring, 1891. "Medical Opinions on the Population Question." London: Standring, 1901, pp. 32. "Clerical Opinions on the Population Question." London: Standring, 1904, pp. 19. For a biographical sketch of Dr. Charles Drysdale see the 1905 edition of George Drysdale's *Elements of Social Science,* and George Standring's *Republican,* xii, 25–26.

[63] Also active was Dr. Alice Drysdale-Vickery, the English feminist leader and wife of Dr. Charles Drysdale. In the critical days from 1877 onward, when it required great courage for any physician, much less for a woman physician, she took an active part in the public support of contraception. She gave medical testimony at the Bradlaugh-Besant trial, later contributed to the *Malthusian,* wrote a pamphlet on "Early Marriages and Limited Families," and subsequently became president of the Malthusian League. She

been called the Neo-Malthusian League, but that English word had not yet been coined.[64]   Its objects at this time were primarily to gain a public hearing for Malthusianism (and Neo-Malthusianism).   Even a sober discussion of Malthus's doctrines was more or less tabu in the English public prints of the mid-nineteenth century.   At this time the League made no attempt at medical instruction.   But lectures were held and pamphlets distributed.[65]   We have seen that the League assisted in the Allbutt case. Largely through the iniative of Dr. Charles R. Drysdale, a Medical Branch of the Malthusian League was formed about this time; and in August, 1881 an International Medical Congress was held in London.   Upon that occasion the Medical Branch of the Malthusian League called a meeting of

---

shared for many years the fine sacrifices of the Drysdale family in working steadfastly for the general welfare of the working classes of Great Britain. It was my pleasure to meet her in 1927, and though she was then in advanced years, her mind was still keen. (In addition to "Early Marriages" see Dr. Vickery's address before the Ligue Malthusienne de Femmes.   Branche de la Fédération Humaine.   Paris: Ligue de la Régénération Humaine, n.d., pp. 12. A Woman's Malthusian League.   London: Standring, n.d., pp. 8.)

[64] The word Neo-Malthusianism was apparently first used in English by J. M. Robertson in the early eighteen eighties.   At least it is the first use of which I have record.   See my paper "Note on the Origin of the Terms Contraception, Birth Control, Neo-Malthusianism, etc." in *Med. Jour. & Rec.*, cxxxv (1932): 495–496.

[65] The series of Malthusian League tracts first printed were the following.   No attempt has been made to list the later and better known pamphlets.

No. 1. C. R. Drysdale, M.D., "The Principle of Population," pp. 4.

No. 2. C. R. Drysdale [Ed.] "The Struggle for Enjoyable Existence."

No. 3. James Laurie, "The Limitation of Families: A Discussion on the 'Happiness of the Community as Affected by Large Families,'" pp. 8.

No. 4. Henry Arthur Allbutt, M.D., "Evils Produced by Over-Childbearing and Excessive Lactation," pp. 4.

No. 5. C. R. Drysdale [Ed.] "Great is Truth, and it will Prevail."

No. 6. C. R. Drysdale, "Presidential Address Delivered . . . July 18, 1878," pp. 8.

No. 7. Anon. "The Bondsmen of these Our Days," [1879] pp. 8.

No. 8. ——? —— "The Cause of Poverty."

No. 9. Charles R. Drysdale, "Large Families and Over-Population."   [1879 Presidential Address.]   pp. 12.

No. 10. Annie Besant, "The Social Aspects of Malthusianism."   [1881], pp. 8. [This originally appeared in the Malthusian, vol. i, No. 1.]

These pamphlets are now rare—exceedingly rare.   My collection seems to be the most complete in any known public or private repository.   Evidently these little pamphlets were hardly ever saved.   Yet some contain important historical data.

The writer's collection also contains what is probably the most complete collection of annual reports of the League.   These were likewise not saved even by the League itself. In my library there is also a complete set of different issues of the medical leaflet and pamphlet (1913 and later).   The Library of Congress has another set, complete or nearly complete.   I am inclined to think that there are not more than two or three such sets extant.

British and foreign physicians for the purpose of discussing Malthusianism and parental prudence. Thirty or forty medical practitioners attended, the chair being occupied by Dr. C. R. Drysdale.[66] A number of letters were read from several absent physicians, expressing their hope that the conference would be successful in bringing Neo-Malthusian doctrines to the attention of the medical profession. Dr. Guye of Amsterdam, secretary of the International Medical Congress of 1879, declared himself fully in favor of Neo-Malthusian doctrines. He held that all classes should endeavor to limit their families.

It might well be claimed that the Conference of 1879 was a genuine forerunner of the Zürich Conference of 1931. This, too, was a conference essentially of physicians, but there was this difference between the two conferences: clinics had developed after the war in the United States, England and Germany; and many of these sent representatives with papers in 1931.

It was not until 1913 that the League prepared for public distribution with due precautions, a leaflet (subsequently a pamphlet)[67] on technique. Beginning in 1879, a journal, the *Malthusian*, discussed family limitation mainly from the economic standpoint. This periodical continued until 1922 when the name, and to a considerable extent, the editorial policies were changed. The *Malthusian* became the *New Generation*. It is still published. In 1927 the League disbanded with a celebration dinner. It considered its work finished. Membership had never been large, and there had generally been annual deficits covered by the Drysdales and a few large donors. With the general acceptance of birth control after the World War, with the newspapers devoting scores of columns monthly and billboard headlines to birth control, there seemed little advantage in making further financial sacrifices. Then, too, Marie Stopes's new organization, the Society for Constructive Birth Control,[68] founded in 1921, seemed more in keeping with prevailing socialistic sentiment; it was less economic and more sentimental in its appeal. It soft-pedalled the appeal to classical

[66] Little has been said in the present volume about the fine pioneering work of Charles R. Drysdale. His career will receive more adequate attention in a subsequent volume treating the economic and social history of contraception. Though he was a physician, and though he seems to have been mainly responsible for the founding of the Medical Branch of the League, Dr. Charles R. Drysdale's career seems to me essentially economic in significance. He was a dyed-in-the-wool Malthusian, and wrote not so much from the medical, as from the Malthusian viewpoint (see preceding note or Bibliography for a list of his writings).

[67] *Hygienic Methods of Family Limitation.* For details on issues, see Bibliography under MALTHUSIAN LEAGUE, COMMITTEE OF. Also B. Dunlop and N. Haire.

[68] It publishes the *Birth Control News*, largely the personal organ of its editor, Dr. Marie C. Stopes.

economics, and stressed birth control as a health and eugenic measure. George Standring preceded Stopes in this emphasis in his short-lived periodical, *Birth Control*, published in 1919.

Between 1880 and the present, especially since the war, the number of writers on birth control in England has been so considerable that one cannot hope to mention them all. Chief among those who have influenced opinion recently are Stopes, Harold Cox, Julian Huxley, Harold Wright, Norman Haire, Helena Wright, C. P. Blacker, Lord Buckmaster, Lord Dawson of Penn, C. J. Bond, Dean Inge and many others. The works of some of these are mentioned in the bibliography. Other titles associated more properly with the social history will appear later. Here attention is merely directed to the fact that the efforts of these writers have furthered the socialization of birth control.

Elsewhere will be found a brief account of the international Neo-Malthusian conferences held in the past few decades.[69] These interest-groups did much to further birth control on an international scale.

It is necessary now to return to developments in the United States in the period following Owen and Knowlton.

---

[69] Norman E. Himes, "Birth Control in Historical and Clinical Perspective," *Annals of the Amer. Acad.*, March, 1932. *Cf.*, F. H. Hankins article on "Birth Control" in *Encyclopedia of the Social Sciences*, ii, 559–565. Hankins' article is one of the best brief accounts on birth control in print. Most of the articles on contraception in other encyclopedias are third-rate performances.

CHAPTER XI

MID-NINETEENTH CENTURY AMERICAN WRITERS

§1 INTRODUCTION

IN AN earlier chapter it has been shown that Place and his disciples gave an impetus to the birth-control movement in the United States. We observed further that there was a boomerang action, and that Robert Dale Owen and Charles Knowlton eventually had considerable influence upon thought and conduct in England. Attention will now be directed to certain American authors of the second half of the nineteenth century whose influence was almost exclusively American.

With one exception there are no scholarly monographs[1] to which one may turn for treatment of the writers about to be considered; even the medical histories and the recently-published and detailed *Dictionary of American Biography* omit virtually all of the men of interest for contraceptive development and socialization. These circumstances, the inaccessibility of the source materials, and the fact that my efforts in the past have been directed mainly at studying the development of English Neo-Malthusianism in the nineteenth century, have combined to render the following account much less adequate than it ought to be. Doubtless there are many gaps that need filling; but in a work covering the development of birth control throughout the entire range of social evolution, it has not been possible, in the present state of our ignorance, to cover the American medical history thoroughly. It can only be hoped that the subject has been advanced somewhat. Years of research will be required to fill in the details. Until this is done, premature generalization is a little hazardous. Perhaps the main outlines, conclusions and evaluations herein will find support in later detailed research; perhaps some will need modification.

The individuals considered in this chapter, all physicians save Noyes, are A. M. Mauriceau, J. Soule, John Cowan, R. T. Trall, John Humphrey

---

[1] One may except Dr. F. M. Vreeland's unpublished doctoral thesis in sociology on *The Process of Reform with Especial Reference to Reform Groups in the Field of Population* (University of Michigan, 1929) even though it is mainly devoted to a study of the history of the American Birth Control League as it throws light on the reform process. The reason I except this is that it contains some information on early figures in the American birth-control movement.

Noyes, Alice B. Stockham, Edward Bliss Foote, Edward Bond Foote, and "W. S. W." Incidental mention is made of Daniel Winder and Harry Knox Root. A following chapter (XII) will continue the medical history of contraception in the United States during the second half of the nineteenth century, but in that chapter there is special emphasis not on the writers of books and pamphlets but on contributors to medical journals, especially on contributors to the earliest medical-journal symposia.

In addition to the writers just mentioned, birth control was advocated, in the second half of the century, by certain erratic and odd people connected with various other reforms. Some were of doubtful character. The policies advocated ranged from anarchism and free love to conservative evangelical religion. Among these defenders of birth control were Mrs. E. B. Duffey,[2] Lois Waisbrooker, Ida Craddock, Emma Goldman, Ben Reitman, Abner Pope, Jay Fox, Abe Isaak, Mattie Sawyer, Moses Jull and perhaps Isabel Beecher Hooker, and Hannah Macy Hinshaw. Space considerations as well as a sense of perspective do not permit more than a passing reference to them in the present account.[3] Some information about them is given in Dr. F. M. Vreeland's thesis[4] and in Dr. Victor Robinson's *Pioneers of Birth Control*.[5] The American writers in the period under consideration, especially those not considered in the following account, never reached the level of theoretical discussion attained by the English writers.

Likewise, there is no detailed analysis here of the work for birth control of De Robigne M. Bennett, Ezra Heywood, Robert Ingersoll and Moses Harman. It will be convenient to devote brief attention to them in connection with the early legal struggles and the social history. None of them was a physician, and they are of small significance for the medical aspects of contraception.

[2] Mrs. E. B. Duffey, *What women should know. A woman's book about women containing practical information for wives and mothers.* Philadelphia, 1873. This recommends the sterile period, the only one known to the author. *The Relations of the Sexes* has a section on the limitation of offspring. The author also wrote books on etiquette and dress.

[3] The same is true of Thomas Ewell, M.D., U. S., Navy surgeon who, writing in 1807, recommended as a preventive measure "embracing only in vessels filled with carbonic acid or azotic gas." (Art. on "Generation" in *Medical Repository*, iv (1807), 131–133). Ewell thought the fertility of Negroes high (which it is not) because they frequently had coitus in the open air. Oxygen or pure air (not to be found in beds) promoted fertility—hence the bizarre contraceptive.

[4] *The Process of Reform with Especial Reference to Reform Groups in the Field of Population* (unpublished thesis, University of Michigan, 1929), pp. 31–56.

[5] Victor Robinson, *Pioneers of Birth Control*. New York: Voluntary Parenthood League, 1919, pp. 107.

§2 A. M. MAURICEAU

Even a summary of the diffusion of contraceptive information in America during the nineteenth century should make at least some mention of Mauriceau's *Married Woman's Private Medical Companion* (1847).[5a] Mauriceau who described himself as a "Professor of Diseases of Women," and who maintained an office at 129 Liberty Street, New York City, was probably a quack. At best he was a popularizer of medical knowledge.[6] There is internal evidence that Mauriceau lived in France, and moved to this country. In the edition used in the present investigation (1851), pages 104–156 are devoted to the prevention of conception. Page after page is quoted from Robert Dale Owen with scarcely a mention of his name.[7] Mauriceau complains that Owen is unaware of Desomaux's method of contraception. Desomaux, it would seem, was a French physician, who used a "French secret" for the prevention of conception. For this method Mauriceau had an exclusive distribution agency (sic) for the United States. The fee was ten dollars. We are piously informed by the author that it was with some reluctance that he was induced to accept the exclusive agency. He was so overwhelmed, however, with testimonials to the efficacy of the method, and so impressed with warm expressions of gratitude and thankfulness for its helpfulness, that he decided to be of assistance to the American people in this matter.

Its efficacy [avows Mauriceau] is beyond question, as in Europe, among the higher classes especially, it is universally used . . . of late among all classes. Thousands of married persons have for years used it with invariable success. . . . The principle

---

[5a] A. M. Mauriceau, *The Married Woman's Private Medical Companion, embracing the treatment of menstruation, or monthly turns, during their stoppage, irregularity, or entire suppression. Pregnancy, and how it may be determined; with the treatment of its various diseases. Discovery to prevent pregnancy; the great and important necessity where malformation or inability exists to give birth. To prevent miscarriage or abortion when proper and necessary to effect miscarriage, when attended with entire safety. Causes and mode of cure of barrenness, or sterility.* The first edition evidently appeared in New York in 1847. A copy is on deposit in the Surgeon General's Library. I have used the 1851 edition. The Boston Medical Library owns a copy dated 1855, and the Surgeon General's Library has, in addition to the first edition, other editions dated 1849, 1854, and 1855. These reprintings suggest that the work was in popular demand.

[6] The author states in his Preface that the object of his work is "to extend to every female, whether wife, mother or daughter, such information as will best qualify her to judge of her own maladies [sic] and, having ascertained their existence, [to teach her how to] apply the proper remedies." (p. iii) This is a sort of home medical book.

[7] Owen never took out a copyright on his *Moral Physiology*, and permitted anyone to reprint the work, but requested that copy be submitted in order that he might not be misquoted.

upon which it prevents conception is to neutralize[8] the fecundating properties in semen, and it preserves and conduces to the health of the female by eradicating all predisposition to sexual weakness, fluor-albus, or whites, the falling of the womb, &c., and restores and maintains ... elasticity and firmness of the generative function. ... [9]

Mauriceau also claimed that his method was indispensable in cases of malformation, deformed pelvis, and a low state of health.

We are not told exactly what the method is, but it would seem to be not a French pessary or cervical cap, but rather douching with some secret solution. It is possible that it was a suppository.

Mauriceau's method of treatment of the subject brands him as a quack[10] rather than as a *bona fide* member of the medical profession. But his work is of interest to us in the undoubted influence which his book must have had in the late forties and in the decade of the fifties. It is extremely doubtful if Robert Dale Owen would have approved the use by Mauriceau of long extracts from his *Moral Physiology*. The whole tone and temper of the *Medical Companion* is not in accord with the good taste Owen always showed in his writings on this subject.

Mauriceau is also of importance as a forerunner of the popular medical books by Dr. E. B. Foote, and Dr. E. B. Foote, Jr., and other early American medical writers partial to contraception to whom attention will be given after Trall.

A popular home medical encyclopedia somewhat similar to the volumes later issued by E. B. Foote was Harry Knox Root's, *The People's Lighthouse of Medicine*, the fourteenth edition of which was published in 1856. Did this first appear in the 'forties? It recommended (p. 155) the condom and "prevention powders" presumably to be used in douching. The circulation of this book is not known to me.

A pamphlet of unknown influence dating from the late 'fifties and presumably discussing technique was the *Marriage Chart* "By an Ohio Physician," most likely Dr. Daniel Winder.[11] What seems to be a unique copy in the possession of the Library of Congress is temporarily, perhaps perma-

---

[8] The phaseology here (to neutralize the fecundating properties in semen) is Knowlton's. It suggests that Knowlton also influenced Mauriceau, who never mentioned his name.

[9] Punctuation slightly altered.

[10] Abortifacients are referred to on pp. 16–17 where Mauriceau speaks of M. Desomaux's "Portuguese female pills." In the Chapter on "Sterility" the author states that "Morand's 'Elixir'" will prove "infallible," "if the case is curable." (p. 234) This "elixir" he advertised for sale in his office.

[11] By an Ohio physician, A rational or private marriage chart. For the use of all who wish to prevent an increase of family. Mansfield, O., 1858.

nently, "lost." The same is true of G. W. Warren's *A Confidential Letter to the Married*, which the Library of Congress still has indexed under prevention of conception. It was published at Cleveland, Ohio in 1854 (pp. 28). I know nothing of its content, for no other copy is available. But it is worth recording here as a pamphlet of the 'fifties.

§3 J. SOULE

In about the same category with Mauriceau, though probably less influential, is to be placed J. Soule, M.D. The full title[12] of his seventy-two page pamphlet, *Science of Reproduction and Reproductive Control*, which seems to have appeared in Cincinnati, Ohio, about 1856,[13] rather well typifies its contents. Only the last of the four parts will be of concern here, since this section alone treats of contraceptive technique and indications. But a general description is in order: Part I deals with "The Imperative Duty of Some to Have No Children," and with the "Duty of All to Limit Their Families According to Their Circumstances." Part II is of interest chiefly in showing how liberal views on the prevention of conception could be mixed in a single volume with antiquated unscientific opinions, based largely on Tissot, regarding the frightful evils of masturbation and the "inhuman practice" of having sexual intercourse at certain times. Part III deals with the "Philosophy of Conception." The last few pages are devoted to answering objections to birth control, and contain nothing new. So much for a general description.

Regarding his purpose in publishing the pamphlet, Soule says,

I write this book, first, because society wants it and needs it, and therefore ought to have it. Second, because there is no work [sic] in which this subject is fully and philosophically presented. These are sufficient reasons to fully justify the writing of any work.[14]

Later in the pamphlet Soule says "I make no apology for introducing my book into society, for I believe it will be a blessing to the race."[15]

---

[12] J. Soule, *Science of Reproduction and Reproductive Control. The Necessity of some Abstaining from having Children—The Duty of all to Limit their Families according to their Circumstances Demonstrated. Effects of Continence—Effects of Self-Pollution—Abusive Practices. Seminal Secretion—Its Connection with Life. How to Preserve Youthful Vigor, and How to Attain to the Acme of Physical, Moral, and Intellectual Perfection. Laws and Philosophy of Impregnation. With an Explanation of the Seminal Animalculae, and Female System. With all the Different Modes of* PREVENTING CONCEPTION, *and the Philosophy of Each.* Closing Remarks by the Author. Illustrated with Engravings. By Dr. J. Soule. Stereotyped edition. [Cincinnati, Ohio, c. 1856], pp. 72.

[13] This is the estimated date on the Library of Congress card. The copy of the work in that library is the only one which has been located to date.

[14] *Ibid.*, p. 7.

[15] *Ibid.*, p. 69.

This is followed by a discussion of contraceptive technique and indications which discussion is a part of the justification, of course, of publication. There is treatment of the safe period (unsafe), the prevention of ovulation, withdrawal, the condom, expulsion of the semen by exercise or injections, the sponge, douches with tannin water or plain cold water. Internal remedies may cause sterility, but none of these should be taken without medical advice. Soule mentions the following drugs as destroying spermatozoa: opium, prussic acid, iodine, strychnine, and alcohol. How these drugs, some of which are certainly dangerous, were to be used, Soule does not say. In that respect his work may have had unfortunate results. He thinks that cold water is preferable to warm in douches—a view certainly not held in our time—and, interestingly enough, mentions contraceptive powders as being sold in the U. S. A. in the 'fifties, presumably to be added to douches.

We are modestly told that Soule's book furnishes the reader "all the information on this subject that is worth knowing, and much that is not published in any other work."[16] We are informed further that "no other work in the English language" discusses the subject so fully! The work "embraces all that is published, in all other works on this subject, and more."[17]

Soule's treatise contained only fragmentary mention of what would now be considered indications. The Malthusian or economic indication is mentioned, as are also malformations and diseases of the ovaries, and likelihood of hereditary transmission of disease, mental or physical. Those married persons also need contraception who are unable to transmit to their offspring healthy and vigorous constitutions; likewise the unhappily married. Hence there is stress on positive as well as negative eugenics. The scope of the present work does not permit discussion of the legitimacy of indications for contraception, but they ought to be stated as a matter of historical record. The inclusion, however, of the unhappily married is so unusual among writers on contraception in this period that it is worthy of special emphasis. Just what was in Soule's mind is not clear; perhaps he felt that those who were not well adapted to one another would not be likely to provide a suitable psychic environment for the training and upbringing of children. Also such marriages are more likely to be broken and to leave children without the usual guidance of two parents. But only the germs of these ideas are in Soule's work. None the less, the fact that he considered marital disharmony an indication for contraception shows how far in advance of even contemporary medical opinion Soule was. Is this the first mention in medical literature of this indication? The writer can think of no prede-

[16] *Ibid.*, p. 69.
[17] *Ibid.*

cessor at the moment.   Naturally there will be differences of opinion as to the wisdom of the indication.

That Soule had been influenced by Malthusian thought, and that there is implicit in his doctrine the idea of spacing, is clear from the statement that "Those who ought to have children, have no right to have more children than they can properly care for. . . ."[18]   "The happiness of a woman is seriously undermined if she has to bear one child rapidly after another.   It also creates economic difficulty for the husband."[19]

Soule was quite possibly a writer of less than ordinary attainments.   His arguments are often weak, illogical, and half-informed; but his conclusions were sometimes sound.   The value of the sound points is at times reduced by overstatement, as when he expects too much of birth control by way of eliminating crime and abortion.[20]   Despite these defects, there seem to be certain new emphases in his little book.   Soule's treatise is rare, and there is no evidence that his influence was other than very nominal.

§4   JOHN COWAN

Another writer of limited importance, heretofore overlooked, is John Cowan, M.D., who published in 1869, that is, four years before the first Comstock Law was passed, a treatise[21] containing a chapter on the "prevention of conception."[22]   Cowan is best described as a popularizer and "pot-boiler.[23]   His account of contraceptive technique, though unsatisfactory, must have played some rôle—no one can estimate just how much—in popularizing contraceptive knowledge.   He reports that "To compass the end of prevention all manner of means are and have been used, but, as a rule, all tending more or less to the physical and spiritual harm of the individual."[24]   The Oneida perfectionist's method (*congressus reservatus*) is described as expressing a low and animal nature, and as injurious to health. The Biblical method (*coitus interruptus*) is "beastly" and does not differ from self-abuse.   We are then told that continence is the only sure method. "The employment of coverings for the male organ, made of rubber or gold-

---

[18] *Ibid.*, p. 10.

[19] *Ibid.*, p. 14.

[20] See statements on p. 14.

[21] John Cowan, *The Science of a New Life*.   New York: Cowan & Co., 1869, pp. 9–405.

[22] Ch. x, pp. 108–113.

[23] Other titles from his pen were: *The Use of Tobacco vs. Purity, Chastity and Sound Health*.   New York: Cowan & Co., 1870, pp. 76.   *Self-Help in the Attainment of Perfection of Character and Success in Life*.   New York: Cowan & Co., 1870.   Cowan also wrote a book on *Disease of the Heart*, no doubt of a popular nature.

[24] *Science of a New Life*, p. 109.

beater's skin, is certainly effectual;"[25] but they dull sensation, are animal, and irritate the vagina. "The use by the woman, of sponge or rubber pads, placed against the mouth of the womb, to prevent the entrance of the sperm, are somewhat used, and widely advertised and sold under many different names by quacks."[26] They prevent pleasure (sic), and are not reliable owing to the possibility of misplacement.[27] Cold-water douching "may or may not be successful," and is inadvisable on other grounds. Prolonged lactation should be avoided as unreliable and undesirable. Drugs were not only ineffectual but injurious. Then "there are other methods of prevention, and some of them [are] more disastrous in their effects than any enumerated, the rationale of which it is useless to mention."[28]

Cowan was not well-informed, in that he stressed the "physical and spiritual harm" of the use of contraceptives, but his book must have spread some enlightenment and some erroneous notions regarding prevention.[29] Though the book seems never to have been quoted, and though Cowan's influence must have been modest, he deserves a small place among the mid-nineteenth century American writers on birth control. The first edition of *The Science of a New Life* seems to have appeared in 1869; other issues in 1870 and 1871. In the 'seventies Cowan's work seems to have died a natural death, but it appeared in a revised edition, without the chapter on prevention, in New York in 1915 (see Bibliography). It is possible that the Comstock Law of 1873 caused a temporary suspension, if such was the fact.

§5   R. T. TRALL (1812–1877)

An American writer of some English influence in the mid-nineteenth century was R. T. Trall. His *Sexual Physiology*[30] was first published in America in 1866, and went through three editions in the year issued. Twenty years later (1886) it was in its fortieth thousand. The Appendix to Trall's *Hydropathic Encyclopedia* (1852 or 1853) mentions the safe period, and justifies the voluntary control of parenthood. Despite Trall's influence, his thinking was often illogical and his views contradictory. One

---

[25] *Ibid.*, p. 110.

[26] *Ibid.*

[27] The same objection is heard in our time. If the sponge is large enough, the likelihood of failure from this cause is much reduced.

[28] *Ibid.*, p. 112.

[29] There is another book by Cowan presumably discussing prevention that I have not seen. It is: *What All Married People Should Know.* Chicago: Ogilvie, 1903.

[30] R[ussell] T[hacher] Trall, *Sexual Physiology; A Scientific and Popular Exposition of the Fundamental Problems in Sociology.* Glasgow, 1866. There are about twenty cards in the Library of Congress on Trall. He wrote on popular physiology, hygiene, hydrotherapy, vegetarianism, temperance reform, and even elocution.

cannot even be certain that he is genuinely to be ranked among the birth-control pioneers of the nineteenth century. Undoubtedly Stopes makes too much of his importance.[31] Yet, on the other hand, some of his more pious statements may have been included to disarm criticism.

Trall seems to have held that a woman had an absolute right to determine when she should, and when she should not conceive. However, in discussing the danger of too frequent pregnancies, he declares that abstinence is the only remedy[32]—hardly a very progressive viewpoint even for 1866. Later he states that abstinence is "not always possible, nor is it always proper."[33] If sexual intercourse is restricted to the mid-period, he avows, pregnancy will seldom occur. But this method is not infallible.[34] Any obstruction placed against the os, preventing the seminal fluid from coming into contact with the ovum, will be an infallible [sic] preventive. A piece of soft sponge introduced as high in the vaginal canal as possible will, when it is kept in position, prove a sure preventive. "These suggestions," Trall declares, "may enable the ingenious woman to adopt some device on emergencies that will accomplish the object."[35] In connection with a discussion of the manner in which impregnation takes place Trall mentions, as contraceptive methods, coughing, sneezing, jumping [!], cold water douches, and massages [!] which may be used to cause the uterus to contract quickly. He does not, however, hold that these methods will prevent conception in all cases.[36] Referring to the "movement cure" practiced, according to his statement, in the Friendly Islands and in Iceland, Trall writes:

Some women have that flexibility and vigor of the whole muscular system that they can, by [an] effort of will, prevent conception. They can, by a voluntary bearing-down effort so compress the abdominal muscles upon the pelvic viscera as to cause the uterus to contract with a degree of force that expels the impregnated egg, or at least causes it to be moved from the point where impregnation occurred.[37]

[31] Stopes speaks of Trall's discussion of technique as "not bettered until two or three years ago"; (truly an amazing statement); and of the book as dealing "profoundly with matters of sex and marriage," and as "being packed with extraordinarily valuable deductions." (*Contraception*, 1923, p. 289; 1925 ed., pp. 327–329; 1931 ed., p. 301.) Far from being an excellent treatment of the subject, as Stopes implies, it was a mere muddleheaded vulgarization of it. Stopes also speaks ("Early Days of Birth Control," p. 17) of Trall as the author of an article entitled "New Theory of Population" in the *Westminster Review*, 1852. This was, of course, by Herbert Spencer. Trall only reprinted it!

[32] *Ibid.*, pp. 203–204. This fact, coupled with the pious tone of the book, may account for the fact that Trall's work escaped the vigilance of Comstock's crusade.

[33] *Ibid.*, p. 205.

[34] *Ibid.*, p. 206.

[35] *Ibid.*, pp. 212–213.

[36] *Ibid.*, p. 209.

[37] *Ibid.*, p. 211.

If this is not a figment of Trall's imagination, the method mentioned is an abortifacient, and may not properly be classified among contraceptives. For the practice, as described above, is carried out only after the ovum is fertilized.   One wonders if this is related to the practice reported in Chapter I as employed in Southeastern Asia.   Perhaps the purpose is there somewhat different; to cause retroversion or anteflexion of the uterus.   If it is similar, this is an interesting instance of the persistence throughout the range of social development of a practice intended to prevent reproduction or even fertilization.

§6   MALE CONTINENCE AND KAREZZA

(6a)   John Humphrey Noyes (1811–1886) and Male Continence

Though Noyes's significance is perhaps more economic and eugenical than medical, this account would be incomplete without reference to his experiment in "scientific propagation" and to his special method of conception control.   Noyes was the founder of a communistic colony of the voluntary type (a type not to be confused with what is now commonly known as communism) bound together by religious doctrines known as Perfectionism.[38]   His followers eventually settled near Oneida, New York, adopted a community of goods and a system of "complex marriage," including "stirpiculture" (from stock, root), according to which members of the colony voluntarily gave Noyes, or a committee, authority to arrange matings for the purpose of biologically improving the stock.   Noyes seems to have had the power of choice most of the time; but in selecting mates he was exercising no rights not signed over to him.   In the early days of the stirpicultural period (1869–1879 inclusive) piety seems to have been the chief basis of selection; only later were health and intelligence emphasized; and I am not sure that they were ever the main or exclusive basis of selection.

The community's method of conception control is also of interest.   Male Continence (other names, Karezza, Magnetation Method, more properly, *coitus reservatus*) consists in normal, unclothed entry followed by movements but not ejaculation.   Too close an approach to the climax is intentionally avoided, and, as is not so commonly understood about this method, detumescence takes place intravaginally until normal circulation is restored. It is claimed by the adherents of male continence that, when detumescence takes place inside rather than outside, there are no harmful effects,

---

[38] Hence the group was often known as the "Perfectionists" or "Oneida Perfectionists." They were called Perfectionists because they believed that as they came into perfect communion with Jesus Christ most of the world's troubles would disappear—not only sin but death itself.

nervous or otherwise. The method differs from withdrawal, or *coitus interruptus*, in that this last is usually followed by ejaculation.

The idea first occurred to Noyes in 1844. An inquiry from a medical student led him to put his views in writing in 1866; and so frequent were the requests for a reply that Noyes printed it in leaflet form.[38a] Not until 1872, however, was his chief tract on birth control, *Male Continence*, published.[38b] Noyes stood not only for controlled paternity but for scientific human reproduction, for what would now be called eugenics, for the sexual rights of women,—for these at a time when such views scandalized. In viewing conception control and eugenics as necessary concomitants to fundamental social reform, he anticipated much of the best thought of ensuing decades. As early as 1848 Noyes had said:

We are not opposed to procreation. But we are opposed to involuntary procreation. We are opposed to excessive and, of course, oppressive procreation, which is almost universal. We are opposed to random procreation, which is unavoidable in the marriage system. But we are in favor of intelligent, well-ordered procreation. . . . We believe the time will come when involuntary and random procreation will cease, and when scientific combination will be applied to human generation as freely and successfully as it is to that of other animals.[38c]

As an expression of insight and conviction this is a remarkable statement for its period. Owen and Knowlton had expressed similar views in different language; and it is probable that Noyes obtained from Robert Dale Owen the idea that sexual union had a love as well as a reproductive function. Undoubtedly the idea is very old; but he had read Owen's *Moral Physiology*.

Noyes doubtless believed, as many still do, that he originated the idea of *coitus reservatus*. But that is extremely doubtful. In fact it is probably not true. References to the index of this work will show earlier mention of the practice of *coitus reservatus*. However, Noyes probably wrote more about it than anyone up to his time; and he was quite probably the first to give male continence a theoretical and doctrinal setting. We have seen (p. 127) that a Japanese teacher, Kaibara, urged suppression of the male orgasm in the mistaken belief that it would increase longevity. But I know of no evidence that Noyes held any such belief.

In a medical evaluation of male continence it is important to distinguish between two problems: (1) its usefulness to the community; (2) its useful-

[38a] John Humphrey Noyes, *Male Continence; or Self-Control in Sexual Intercourse. A A Letter of Inquiry Answered.* Oneida, New York, 1866.

[38b] John Humphrey Noyes, *Male Continence.* Oneida, New York: Office of the Oneida Circular [a colony journal], 1872, pp. 24; 1877, pp. 32.

[38c] Declared in 1848, but published in February, 1849 in the "First Annual Report of the Oneida Community."

ness for us.   Perhaps Noyes knew only of withdrawal and obstructus in the early days; if so, by 1870 he had come to reject condoms, sponges and "lotions" as "unnatural, unhealthy and indecent, and of course destructive to love."   [*Oneida Circular*, viii (1870), 212.]

In an age of modern techniques male continence would seem to have little merit as a contraceptive technique, whatever may be said for it as a variant in the art of love.   My judgment is that the majority of informed medical opinion would disapprove it as a contraceptive technique.   Certainly it leaves something very important out of the sexual relation.   Writers on contraceptive technique and its history generally condemn *coitus reservatus*.   Some of these writers may go too far in mentioning nervous disease as a probable result; but one might theoretically expect it to predispose to nervous tension at least.   At all events, it is unphysiological, contrary to the sexual pattern of the male developed over a long historical period, a pattern now well-ingrained, as indeed it is in all copulating animals. I do not believe this pattern can be lightly opposed.   Anyhow, what is its advantage in this day of reliable contraceptives?   Normal coitus with climax is probably the most intense joy in human experience.   Why crucify mankind on a cross of religious mysticism?   Only the leadership of Noyes's magnetic personality and great religious devotion could induce normally-sexed people to adopt such a régime.   It is safe to say that the hedonistic impulses of mankind will make the general spread of male continence impossible.   It involves a strain on human nature which can easily be avoided in our time, whatever the limited knowledge of the Community members.

It is as a contraceptive technique that I have criticized male continence. It may well have merit as a variation in the art of love; but that is not under adjudication here.   I am inclined to think, however, that the Oneida Community stands out historically as perhaps the only group experiment, at least in the Western World, placing great emphasis upon full satisfaction of the woman, and this in a culture dominated by male attitudes.

Reports are available on the health and longevity of colony members. A Syracuse gynecologist, Dr. Van der Warker, found no injurious effects of male continence after physical examinations made in 1877;[38d] and Theodore R. Noyes, M.D., John Humphrey's son, reporting after twenty-two years, contended that nervous diseases were far below the average for the country."[38e]

It is certain that infant and general mortality were low.   Of the sixty-two

---

[38d] Ely Van der Warker, "A Gynecological Study of the Oneida Community," *Amer. J. Obst.*, August, 1884.   Dr. Van der Warker was a professor of high standing.

[38e] Theodore R. Noyes, *Med. Gazette*, October 22, 1870.   See also, "Report on the Health of Children in the Oneida Community."   Oneida, New York, 1878, pp. 8.

births in the stirpicultural period (1869–1879 inclusive), four were still-births, and some were unauthorized by the committee.   There was only one death under one year, a phenomenally low incidence of infant mortality for that, or even the present, period.   There was one death at seven years; another at nineteen.   Of the fifty-eight live births, fifty-five thus reached twenty or more years.   As late as 1921, when Dr. Hilda Noyes reported on mortality at the Second International Congress of Eugenics,[39] fifty-two survived.   At the present time (November, 1935) forty-six remain, and the oldest is sixty-six.   In fact, in the sixty years since the middle of the stirpi-cultural period, there have been but twelve deaths among the original fifty-eight live births.

This represents an extraordinarily low mortality experience.   Back in 1921 Edwin W. Kopf, then assistant statistician of the Metropolitan Life Insurance Company, studied the mortality experience of the stirpicultural children using a Scandinavian method applicable to small groups, the ratio of actual to expected mortality.   He found that the Oneida Community experience was "only 25 per cent of that which would have occurred if the total Registration Area death rates had prevailed, only 32 per cent of a typical rural mortality experience, and 24 per cent of the total New York state experience."   "In general," he added, "I believe it is safe to say that two-thirds fewer deaths occurred among this Oneida Community group than if a typical rural experience of recent times had prevailed."   He explained the experience as follows: "One may conclude that the hardy New England stock represented in these Oneida Community matings, and the exceptional intelligence applied to Community domestic and personal hygiene, have shown results in a low mortality experience without precedent in the history of modern sanitary science."[40]

This extraordinarily interesting social experiment foundered on the rocks of internal dissension and external religious bigotry and persecution.   As Noyes aged, his powers of leadership declined.   The younger generation and new recruits came to have, in an expanding age of science, less fervor for Noyes's religious doctrines.   Hence the main bond of union was weakened.   When Noyes and the older men began selecting the younger women that was the beginning of the end.   Not only several young men, but some of the young women, then began to oppose non-monogamy; and the system

[39] Hilda H. Noyes & George W. Noyes, "The Oneida Community Experiment in Stirpiculture," in *Eugenics, Genetics and the Family*, being vol. i of the Proceedings of the Second International Congress of Eugenics, New York City, September, 1921.   Baltimore: Williams & Wilkins, 1923.

[40] Ms. letter to Dr. Hilda H. Noyes, March 26, 1921.

of complex marriage, devised to reform marriage "in the world," resulted only in wrecking the community.[40a]

External pressure, however, played a substantial, if inferior, rôle. Opposition to complex marriage was aroused in upper New York state clerical circles mainly through the activity of a misguided and ultra-pious Hamilton College professor. Prosecution and even special legislation was threatened. Prosecution on the ground of bigamy would have been impossible; for no marriages had taken place. A small portion of the public and even some of the newspapers openly sympathized with Noyes as a victim of bigotry. But the demagogues, as so often happens, carried the day and Noyes was spirited into a forced "exile." Noyes was now a feeble old man, broken in spirit and will, by a combination of circumstances quite beyond his control. The story of his retreat, as told by Parker,[40b] is one of the most touching and dramatic episodes in the history of social experiment in this country. The flag of biogtry and public misunderstanding had now been nailed to the mast. Noyes had paid the penalty for courageously acting on advanced views in a world that appreciates all too lightly the social value of toleration.

Society will pay for this blunder for a long time to come. By this statement I do not mean to imply that I approve all the measures of the experiment. But difference from me, as Terence once remarked, is not the measure of absurdity. It may well be that complex marriage is impossible for any group. On that the verdict of history is not, in my view, yet in. At all events, there is no gainsaying the fact that the Oneida Community was the most interesting eugenical experiment ever tried.[40c] On the birth

[40a] It seems quite conceivable that in another age of greater social and ethical maturity the mores may view with a broader tolerance such a system of complex marriage as Noyes suggested. Though pair marriage, or monogamy, has existed in virtually every society, even in those in which polygamy has been sanctioned, a perfectly rational society would carry Noyes's ideas further and not only take great pains about matings but would adopt eutelegenesis.

Eutelegenesis may be defined as the use, through artificial insemination, of especially well selected male seed for the fertilization of equally wisely-chosen potential mothers for the purpose of improving the human stock. A beginning in artificial insemination is already being made in the instance of biological failure of the male. Eutelegenesis has one advantage over complex marriage: it does not interfere with the well-established institution of monogamy. Will society ever be rational enough to adopt the essentials of eutelegenesis? Or will this idea be demagogically branded as "the ethics of the barnyard applied to human relations." For an interesting article on the subject, see Herbert Brewer, "Eutelegenesis," *Eugenics Review*, xxvii, 121–126 (July, 1935).

[40b] Robert Allerton Parker, *A Yankee Saint. John Humphrey Noyes and the Oneida Community*. New York: Putnam, 1935.

[40c] For further information, see Havelock Ellis, *Studies*, vi, 553–554; 617–622; John Humphrey Noyes, "Essay on Scientific Propagation," *Modern Thinker*, 1870 (also reprinted by the Oneida Community); Anita Newcomb McGee, "An Experiment in Human Stirpiculture," *Amer. Anthrop.*, October, 1891; Parker, *op. cit.*

control side, the verdict of Dr. Robert L. Dickinson is worthy of much weight.   In an unpublished letter to Dr. Hilda H. Noyes, he wrote: "The Oneida Community experience is, as far as I can judge, the only long-continued, deliberate, organized, and consistent experiment in birth control by a group of intelligent people using a single method, combined with physical examinations to check up the effects of health."   Further, I am informed by a reliable source that four-fifths of the children were planned.

Some may hold the view that Noyes's views on sex were merely unconsious rationalizations induced to quiet a New England conscience in the presence of a strong sex urge, revolting against the restraints of monogamy, and impelled to express itself under conditions of variety.   But even if this contention is granted—and I am not at all sure that it should be—nothing can alter the record of his courage and insight along many lines.

From exile Noyes advised the community to renounce complex marriage in deference to public opinion, and tense was the atmosphere when that letter was read in public meeting in the community hall.   Noyes's advice was accepted, and community of goods was likewise given up.   Members married, but a few mothers could not immediately find mates because they were committed to others.   Women who had never felt personal insecurity before, under hated communism, now faced it "in the world."   This was just one more phase of the tragedy.

The colony had been economically successful for thirty-two years.   The members—upright, law-abiding, God-fearing citizens, whom everyone respected who ever had personal contact with them, who made honest goods and kept their contracts as solemn obligations—were now called upon to readjust their entire lives.   As voluntary communism was renounced, a joint stock company was set up (now the well-known Oneida Ltd., manufacturers of Community silver plate), and the assets of the stock company distributed equitably among the former members, apportioned partly on the basis of the number of years of membership, partly on the basis of the property brought to the original community.   Children were given a guarantee up to sixteen years of age in proportion to the earnings of the company; and at the age of sixteen each child was endowed with a bonus of $200.

Thus ended one of the most interesting experiments of its kind.   Originality and courage, if not genius, had been forced into exile.   A great spirit had been broken.   But what did it matter so long as "civilization" and "public morality" had been saved for the future?

(6b)   Alice B. Stockham and Karezza

Noyes's method was popularized in the 'eighties and 'nineties under different names (Karezza and sedular absorption) by Dr. Alice Stockham, who was considerably influenced by Noyes. She was a popular medical writer whose chief works were *Karezza, Parenthood*, and *Tokology*. Her treatises have little scientific value, but find a place here inasmuch as they had a modest influence in diffusing, together with much mysticism on religion and marriage, an undesirable form of birth control.[41] Whether the medical historian or sociologist approves of such literature or not, if it has even a modest influence, it is worthy of passing mention in a detailed history. Moreover, my estimate of Stockham's significance is much more modest than that accorded her by some other writers. It is therefore desirable that Stockham's place in the history of birth control be put on record even if her niche in history is hardly very secure.

Stockham believed that Karezza (prolonged coitus without emission) was the scientific method of controlling conception. The book by that title is permeated with mysticism, a queer kind of religionism and with much sentimental idealism. Quite possibly the cheap sentimentality of Stockham's literary output—Stockham would call it spirituality—was a factor in preventing prosecution. Though *Karezza* and the other books were never very frank in discussing contraceptive technique, some of the editions mentioned methods, but only to condemn them.

Although *Tokology* is mainly devoted to such subjects as impregnation, the hygiene and diseases of pregnancy, abortion, menstruation, the change of life, etc., passing reference is given to the prevention of conception. A comparison of various editions shows that the texts varied. For example, in the 1885 American edition there was no discussion of preventive means, but the 1887 edition mentioned withdrawal, the syringe, drugs (i.e., medicated douches), and "sedular absorption." We are told that withdrawal causes nervousness, dyspepsia, insomnia, and uterine disorders.[42] But prolonged coitus without emission never has bad effects! "Drugs that are used to destroy the germ are usually injurious, and cannot accomplish the purpose beyond the vagina."[43] Stockham adds that "Some of the appliances sold for this purpose [prevention] are a sure prevention by mechanical interference. If the material is pliable, the only possible injury is from preventing complete interchange of magnetism, and the harm is considered a more negative than a positive one."[44] The author usefully indicates the

[41] Even as late as 1915 Margaret Sanger published a pamphlet on "Magnetation Methods of Birth Control," New York, n.d., pp. 20, c. 1915. This was the Noyes-Stockham method. Mrs. Sanger was not long, however, in learning better methods. Since the technique is just as "natural" as use of the unestablished sterile period, it is a wonder Catholic writers have not made more use of it. I understand, however, that it is officially sanctioned.

[42] *Tokology* (1887), p. 325.

[43] *Ibid.*, p. 326.

[44] *Ibid.*

erroneousness of the idea that, if a woman avoids orgasm, she will not become pregnant. The 1897 edition discusses withdrawal, the syringe, "withholding," sedular absorption but not appliances.

In the Toronto edition of *Tokology* the last chapter called a "Familiar Letter" discusses the limitation of offspring. We are told that birth control is a "subject of frequent inquiry."[45] Few women, we are assured, would abuse such knowledge if they possessed it. Though women shrink from forced maternity, and from the bearing of children under unusual burdens, in general, they desire adequate reproduction. She declares that it is her professional experience that "more women seek to overcome causes of sterility than to obtain knowledge of limiting the size of the family."[46] Withdrawal is again condemned.[47] Stockham objects to the use of the syringe and describes drugs (medicated douches) as "usually injurious."[48] If the woman avoids orgasm that will not protect her. Regarding the safe period we are informed that women can "usually depend upon this law."[49] The core of Stockham's point of view is perhaps best expressed in the following sentence: "Believing in the rights of unborn children, and in the maternal instinct, I am consequently convinced that no knowledge should be withheld that will secure proper conditions for the best parenthood."[50]

It is difficult to estimate the true influence of *Tokology*, but the elder Foote seemed to think that it did much to extend a knowledge of the particular birth-control practice recommended. This seems quite possible because the earliest edition which I have happened to trace is one published in 1885. This was marked as the twenty-ninth edition. Even if it were only the twenty-ninth issue, this suggests a certain popularity.

Even more influential than Trall and certainly more so than Noyes and Stockham were Dr. Edward Bliss Foote and his son, Dr. Edward Bond Foote, whose works, especially those of the elder Foote, enjoyed an enormous circulation, thus doing much to prepare the public mind for changes in opinion which many have erroneously assumed to be a phenomenon of our generation solely.

§7 EDWARD BLISS FOOTE (1829–1906)

The elder Foote was born in Ohio in 1829, became a printer's devil at 16, later a journalist, and at twenty a journal editor. By his twenty-fifth year he had become an assistant and secretary to a botanical specialist,

---

[45] *Tokology* (Toronto), p. 323.
[46] *Ibid.*, p. 324.
[47] *Ibid.*, p. 325.
[48] *Ibid.*, p. 326.
[49] *Ibid.*, p. 324.
[50] *Ibid.*

and alternated between medical work and editorial endeavors on a daily paper in Brooklyn. He graduated from the Pennsylvania Medical University in 1858, and shortly afterward published his first book, *Medical Common Sense.*[51] In the preparation of this work he was assisted by two other physicians.

Edward Bliss Foote is of interest to us chiefly for his advocacy of the prevention of conception in *Medical Common Sense*, in *Plain Home Talk*,[52] in his *Home Encyclopedia*,[53] in his periodical the *Health Monthly*, (1876–1883) and especially in a little pamphlet on technique entitled *Words in Pearl*. This was printed in pearl type, hence the name. The pamphlet is rare, and a wide search has not revealed a copy.[54] But we know from discussions appearing elsewhere in Foote's works that *Words in Pearl* discussed not only techniques but indications. He argued that contraception was desirable in certain cases of constitutional ill health, of predisposition to insanity, physical deformity and pauperism. Note that he included economic as well as medical and eugenic indications. It is probable that this pamphlet had the same hereditarian, eugenic approach to be found in Foote's other writings.

The so-called Comstock law of 1873, the federal statute prohibiting the distribution through the mails of contraceptive information, was hardly enacted when Foote, in response to a decoy letter sent from Chicago under a false name, mailed a copy of *Words in Pearl*. As a result he was, in January, 1876, indicted in the U. S. District Court of New York. He was held in $5000 bail to appear on trial at the May term of the court. The case was heard in June, and on July 11, 1876, he was found guilty. He was fined $3000, but the costs amounted to approximately $5000.

Judging by the number of letters which Dr. Foote is reported to have received, sympathy with his predicament was quite general, at least in liberal-minded circles. Foote appealed, through his periodical, the *Health Monthly*, for assistance in paying his fine; and by October, 1876 some three hundred donors had responded. Foote avowed that had a general business

[51] Edward Bliss Foote, *Medical Common Sense*. New York: Murray Hill Pub. Co., 1858, 1863, 1870, etc.

[52] *Plain Home Talk* . . . New York: Wells & Coffin. San Francisco: Bancroft, etc., 1870 and many later editions. The titles of various editions varied.

[53] *Dr. Foote's Home Cyclopedia of Popular Medical, Social and Sexual Science, Embracing His New Book on Health and Disease . . . Also Embracing Plain Home Talk on Love, Marriage and Parentage.* New York: Murray Hill Publishing Co., London: Fowler, 1901. *Home Encyclopedia* . . . was the title of the 1902 edition.

[54] There is no copy filed with the Foote record in the U. S. District Court, Southern District, in New York City. And no library seems to have it. Can readers assist me by locating a copy?

depression not existed, the full amount of the fine would have been covered by donations. Commenting upon the trial in the same journal, Foote declared that, while he had been fairly treated by the judge, jury, and even by Comstock, he felt "equally convinced that the law under which he was convicted goes too far, [that it] is too vague, and . . . [that it] interferes with the practice of medicine, as well as [with] the laws of health, vitality, and physiology."[55]

After the prosecution, Foote continued to practise medicine. It is probable that he was never in first-rate standing with the profession. This may have been a consequence partly of his radical views, partly of medical popularization, and partly because he held some unorthodox views. He fought as valiantly for the freedom of discussion as for the freedom of the physician to give contraceptive advice when in his judgment it was desirable.

In his more popular works, such as *Plain Home Talk* and the *Encyclopedia* as well as in a pamphlet entitled "The Physical Improvement of Humanity"[56] Dr. Foote confined his efforts to advocacy of control and to the desirability of legislative reform. He devoted a pamphlet to an attack on the Federal statute.[57]

After the prosecution, Foote became more cautious. The table of contents in the 1881 edition of *Plain Home Talk* mentions pages 876–880 as dealing with the "prevention of conception." But Foote explains later that this section had to be expurgated on account of a "piece of meddlesome impertinence on the part of hasty lawmakers."[58] In lieu of his medical discussion of contraception he explains at some length the Oneida community's system of "male continence" as advocated by John Humphrey Noyes.

Many of Foote's works were exceedingly popular both in this country and in England. Several of his books were translated into German and even into the Scandinavian languages. So popular had his treatises become that by 1886 the stereotyped plates for *Medical Common Sense*, first published in 1858, were worn out; new ones were required. The book was accordingly revised, and went through many editions.

Many of the arguments commonly heard in our times for contraception were well known to, and advocated by Edward Bliss Foote. We have already touched upon those mentioned in *Words in Pearl*. In another

[55] *Health Monthly*, i (1876), 18.

[56] "The Physical Improvement of Humanity: A Plea for the Welfare of the Unborn." New York: Murray Hill Publishing Co., 1876, pp. 16.

[57] " . . . A Step Backward. Written by E. B. Foote . . . in Reviewing Inconsiderate Legislation, concerning Articles and Things for the Prevention of Conception." New York: Issued by the Author [Murray Hill Pub. Co.], 1875, pp. 16.

[58] *Plain Home Talk* (1881 ed.), p. 876.

pamphlet, the "Physical Improvement of Humanity," Foote denied the immorality of the use of contraceptives, and declared that their employment was preferable to excessively large families among the poor. Planned motherhood was preferable to accidental reproduction. If families are so large that parents cannot provide sufficiently for their children, the latter are likely to suffer from lack of nourishment and care. It was particularly important that parents with hereditary mental or physical disorders should use conception control.[59] Contraception would also diminish the incidence of disease.[60] Continence is impractical.[61] Perhaps his point of view on contraception is best expressed in this sentence: "In brief, I would, if possible, so fix things that none but the healthy people should procreate at all, and that wives should procreate only at will."[62] Foote seems to have been early in expressing the opinion that a decrease of numbers resulting from contraception would be compensated by an improvement in quality. This view has been much stressed in recent decades by those associated with the English Malthusian League and the American Birth Control League. The proposition needs to be carefully stated to avoid fallacy. It is true only up to a certain point.

Foote predicted that popular sentiment would eventually change so that the prevention of conception would be encouraged rather than prohibited by law. He believed that in this instance legislation was interfering on the wrong side.

It is possible that Foote invented the cervical rubber cap. So his son claimed;[63] and though one may be hesitant about accepting the claim, I know of no evidence to doubt it. I do not remember that Foote ever mentioned the cap in his popular literature, but it may have been described in *Words of Pearl*, which is unobtainable now. I cannot recall that the rubber cervical cap is mentioned in the literature prior to Foote Sr. Wilde, however, had described in 1828 in Germany either a vaginal diaphragm of rubber or a cervical cap (see 318–320).

[59] Edward Bliss Foote, "The Physical Improvement of Humanity" (New York: Murray Hill Pub. Co., 1876), p. 7.

[60] *Ibid.*, p. 9.

[61] See also a "Reply to the Alphites, Giving Some Cogent Reasons for Believing that Sexual Continence is not Conducive to Health." New York: Murray Hill Pub. Co., 1882, pp. 39.

[62] *Ibid.*, p. 12.

[63] E. B. Foote, Jr., says that "the best mechanical means yet devised, though commonly described as a 'French' article, was really invented and elaborated in the office of . . . Dr. E. B. Foote Sr." (*Radical Remedy*, 1889, pp. 59–60). My guess is that the "French pessary" rather than the "French letter" is here referred to. It seems a little improbable that Foote, Jr. would claim that his father "invented" the condom.

§8   EDWARD BOND FOOTE (1854–1912)

Somewhat less influential than the elder Foote was his son, Dr. Edward Bond Foote. He was born in East Cleveland, Ohio, August 15, 1854. His mother, Catherine G. Foote, had been a New England school teacher. Following preparatory work at Charlier Institute in New York, he entered Columbia University where his major work was done in science. About the time of the prosecution of his father, young Foote graduated from the College of Physicians and Surgeons winning the Sequin Prize for the best report on certain lectures on the diseases of the nervous system. He then founded, and edited with his father, the *Health Monthly*.

Like his father, young Foote was a strong believer in freedom of discussion—he founded the Free Speech League—and openly advocated contraception and the desirability of repealing the Comstock legislation. As early as 1886, he published in pamphlet[64] form a general discussion on contraception. It gave no details on technique. In the *Radical Remedy* Foote opposed reckless propagation on medical, hygienic, hereditarian, and economic grounds.

There was also a Malthusian element in Dr. Foote's reasoning. He held that the Malthusian principle of increase must be recognized as theoretically sound. Though population pressure was not a characteristic of the United States in his time, there was no guarantee that such a situation might not occur in the future. At all events, it is desirable on other grounds to reduce the sum total of reckless, haphazard propagation—productive of vice, misery, and crime. There is too much waste in human reproduction. Too many children are born in circumstances where mortality rates are high, and under conditions which are in themselves conducive to high mortality. It would be better to reduce the number of births and to save more of them. This would be an economy of effort. In other words, as far back as the eighteen eighties, Dr. Foote was protesting against the phenomenon now known as pregnancy waste. There is a strong hereditarian and eugenic point of view in Dr. Foote's discussion. He points out, for instance, the eugenic function of jails, asylums, and institutions which check the reproductive power of criminals, of the insane, and of other defectives. He protested on eugenic grounds against the too free use of parole inasmuch as this nullified the eugenic effects of isolation.

Undoubtedly the best statement of young Dr. Foote's views on contraception are those published in the *Critic and Guide* in 1910, two years before his death:

[64] Edward Bond Foote, *The Radical Remedy in Social Science; or Borning Better Babies through Regulating Reproduction*. New York: Murray Hill Pub. Co., 1886, pp. 122. (Bibliog.)

First—Under all circumstances contraception is preferable to abortion, and should as far as possible be substituted for it.

Second—The waste of seed which is not permitted to fructify, is, in the human species, better than a waste of the products of conception.

Third—When it is discovered that a married woman can not bear a child with safety, it is better to contracept than to abort.

Fourth—When a woman has borne several children, has all she can properly attend to, or is physically broken down by excessive child-bearing, contraception is wise.

Fifth—When, because of ill-health of husband or wife, or other cause making it, in their opinion, unwise to propagate, it is justifiable to contracept.

Sixth—Deciding when to have children, and when not to have them, is a purely family affair, to be decided by the only two persons directly interested.

Seventh—The improvement of human stock, like that of live stock, requires that births should be [the] result of design rather than accident.

Eighth—There is enough parental instinct, fatherly and motherly feeling, to insure the perpetuation of the race and of the best specimens of it.

Ninth—The virtue worth preserving is not that which merely depends upon fear of consequences; and where it [virtue] is lacking, fear does not save.

Tenth—Reckless reproduction and over-population are concomitants, if not direct causes of poverty, pauperism, prostitution, drunkenness, crime, imbecility, insanity, infanticide, etc., etc.; regulation of reproduction would be one effective remedy, and, for the present, contraception is essential to that regulation.[65]

These doctrines, sound on essential points, were remarkably in advance of those held during the period by the overwhelming number of Foote's American medical colleagues.

§9 W. S. W.'s ANONYMOUS PAMPHLET

A bona fide American medical pamphlet[66] of uncertain date (perhaps c. 1870–90), by one "W. S. W.", undoubtedly a physician, treats of contraception in discussing the conditions of women endangering life during parturition. The author contends that wherever abortions are repeatedly required, where miscarriages occur in succession, or when a woman cannot give birth to a living child, the prevention of conception is indicated. It is not only moral for the physician to inform women of the means; it is his duty:

Under such circumstances it is the physician's *duty*, and eminently in accordance with the dictates of humanity and justice, *to warn such parties of their condition and the attendant dangers, and to place at their disposal a safe and efficient means of*

[65] E. B. Foote [Jr.], "A Summary of My Views on the Prevention of Conception," *Medico-Pharmaceutical Critic and Guide*, xiii (1910), 408. Punctuation slightly altered.

[66] W. S. W., "Conditions of the Female Organs of Generation in which Pregnancy Endangers Life," n.d., n.p., pp. 3–41. While it is possible that this item may be a reprint from a medical journal, it is doubtful.

Preventing future Pregnancies altogether—rather than allow them to repeatedly subject themselves to the necessity of submitting to Operations which have been shown to *endanger their own lives,* and to be inevitably fatal to their *Offspring,* . . .

As an *alternative* we much prefer *preventing* as many recurrences of this necessity for Feticide, as a previous knowledge of the patient's incapacity enables us to do; and we believe the Physician would perform a higher moral duty by giving such [a] woman the proper means and instructions to avoid in the future the pregnant state altogether—thus enabling her to preserve her health and strength—than he does by allowing her to test the capacity of her endurance under the ordeals of repeated Operations for the procurement of Abortion, Premature Labor, or Embryotomy.[67]

So far as methods are concerned, W. S. W. recommends a medicated "cone" to be inserted before coitus, or, as we would now say, a medicated suppository. We are not told what the medication should preferably be.

§10   LACK OF LEADERSHIP OF THE MEDICAL SCHOOLS AND EARLY CONDEMNATION OF BIRTH CONTROL

Doubtless there were many men on faculties of medicine teaching in the last century who personally approved prevention. Few, however, seem to have spoken out frankly in its support,[68] *and not one of them did anything to advance the subject.* This seems an astonishing fact; yet, from another point of view, it is not remarkable. For it has always been true that for one man who advances knowledge or diffuses advanced knowledge, there are a hundred job holders. This is true even of our leading universities today in every branch of science. The proportion alone may not be so great as formerly, but even that is open to doubt.

One way to gain a reputation for supermorality a few decades ago was to condemn birth control in portentous tones with much moral exhortation to purity, and in violent language. Though the day for this has unfortunately

---

[67] *Ibid.*, pp. 36–37.

[68] An exception was Professor Edward H. Clarke, Professor of Materia Medica in the Harvard Medical School (*Bost. Med. & Surg. Jour.*, Dec. 1, 1870, p. 350). When Clarke's approval appeared in print, Professor H. R. Storer of the same institution promptly disagreed (*Gyn. Soc. Jour.* (Boston), June, 1871, p. 351).

A still more notable exception than Professor Clarke, was a case of interference by the governing body of Cornell University in the publication by a medical professor there of a chapter on birth-control technique in a little volume entitled "What Young People Should Know." The author was Dr. Burt G. Wilder, Professor of Neurology and Vertebrae Zoölogy. When the volume was published in 1874, the chapter was omitted on request of the governing body of the institution. This statement was publicly made by Professor Wilder in 1918 (*Med. Rev. of Rev.*, 1918, p. 139). He tells us that "Later, however, the subject was freely presented in special lectures to the members of several graduating classes." This would place the Cornell Medical School as one of the first institutions in the country, and perhaps the first, to impart instruction in contraceptive technique.

not passed, people seem a little less gullible now. Even the man on the street seems to possess something akin to Freudian insight. This super-morality—it is really a pseudo-morality—is not quite so dead as the old emotionally-charged religious revivals, but nearly so.

No attempt has been made in this brief account of the development and diffusion of contraceptive technique in the U. S. A. during the nineteenth century to include such condemnations. The reason is that such writers made no contribution either to the advance or diffusion of knowledge; and that is what this treatise deals with. A few instances should be cited, however, lest it be supposed that even in the nineteenth century we were without such an intellectual plague, such a travesty upon logic and common sense.

After directing attention to two moderate condemnations, one in 1860, the other in 1890, mention will briefly be made of some of the less sober litera-ture. The first is from the pen of August K. Gardner, M.D., writing in 1860:

Local congestions, nervous affections and debilities are the direct and indisputable results of the *coitus imperfecti, tegumenta extaria, ablutiones gelidae, infusiones astringentes, et cetera,* as commonly employed by the community, who are so ignorant on all these matters, and who are in fact substituting for one imaginary difficulty in prospect, a host of ills that will leave no rest or comfort to be found. . . .[69]

This has at least the merit of aiming to state the facts.

This could not be said, however, for the unscientific, reactionary position taken in 1890 by Dr. John B. Reynolds, then president of the American Gynecological Society, in his address on "The Limiting of Childbearing among the Married."[70] Approaching the subject with a strong theological bias, he advocated large families at least for normal people in good health free from inherited disease. He opened this discussion with the following statement:

We will shut wholly out of view the misleading issues [sic] drawn from the family of the drunkard, the improvident, the phthisical, or the insane, and will equally

[69] *The Knickerbocker*, iv, 49. This was in 1860. In 1866 Professor H. R. Storer of Boston published an essay entitled "Why not? A Book for Every Woman." The pur-pose was to prevent abortion, and the essay won an A.M.A. gold-medal! In the preface to the second edition Storer says that "methods of prevention are uniformly injurious, and that, of all of them, incomplete intercourse, by whatever way effected, is probably the worst." Two decades later, E. B. Foote, Jr., took him to task for making no exception even for severe medical or eugenic indications. (*Radical Remedy in Social Science*, 1889, p. 66.)

[70] Pamphlet reprinted from the *Trans. Amer. Gyn. Soc.*, Sept., 1890. *Cf.,* also *Bost. Med. & Surg. Jour.*, Dec. 1, 1870, p. 350. Also January, 1871, p. 58.

forget every case in which, for medical reason, sound and well-considered, pregnancy ought to be interdicted or seldom allowed.[71]

If the physician is "to shut wholly out of [his] view" such cases, one wonders what types of cases he is to assist in this connection. Presumably the answer is that he is not to assist them at all. It may be argued, I suppose, that Reynolds was not so much condemning contraception when use is guided by physicians, as use for non-medical reasons. Yet the whole tone and implication of his presidential address is that physicians should have nothing to do with the nasty business. It seems doubtful, therefore, if the passage in smaller type above can be liberally interpreted. That Reynolds' view was definitely a function of his conservative viewpoint in general is suggested by his opposition to what we would now call the sex education of children. "Curious interest in that subject," he wrote, "will only be set at rest by the sexual relation itself. . . ."[72] He avowed that sex education necessarily promoted low moral standards.

Less restrained than Gardner and Reynolds were a group of writers of whom one Dolan and one McArdle are typical. Reference to the last two names in the Bibliography will show that each of these men published an anti-birth-control article in a medical journal which was widely reprinted in other medical journals. Evidently the authors, in a propaganda spirit, had sent the manuscript to several journals without advising the editors thereof that it had been published previously. These articles so "distinguished" as to "merit" several reprintings, no one has ever heard of since.

In the seventies the diatribes of one of the worst writers the subject has ever had, Bergeret, were being circulated in this country. Bergeret had a complex against "Onanism" and "conjugal frauds." His books, originally published in French[73] had an enormous circulation for many years in many languages.[74]

Men like Tissot and Bergeret are of importance in the medical history of contraception not because they ever wrote much sense on the subject, but because their sensational, unscientifically-deduced conclusions on the injuriousness, medically and socially, of the use of contraceptives profoundly supported the prejudices of many men who have sat on Royal Commissions to investigate declining birth rates. Similarly they have influenced Catholic

---

[71] *Ibid.*

[72] *Ibid.*, p. 15.

[73] *Les Fraudes dans l'Accomplissement des Fonctions Génératrices.* Fourteenth edition, Paris, 1893. There are many earlier editions.

[74] An American edition of this period was *The Preventive Obstacle or Conjugal Onanism.* Trans. from the third French ed., New York: Turner and Mignard, 1870, pp. 182.

writers and many others who started with preconceived notions. Following in the footsteps of Tissot, Bergeret and their school are many contemporary writers who condemn contraception in violent language and in the most irresponsible manner. A considerable number of these writers are Catholics, whether medical men or not. They are first and foremost religious protagonists; only later, if at all, scientists. Violent and vulgar condemnation of contraception of the character I have in mind is not infrequently heard when Catholics assemble before legislative committees to condemn a bill calculated to liberalize the statutes. And many are the Catholic books of the same calibre printed in our day. Not infrequently the quotations used are simply dishonest, sentences being lifted from their context to give the reader an erroneous idea of the original writer's opinions and scientific conclusions. It is only fair to add that not all Catholic treatises are written in this manner. Since most of these books belong to a period later than that under examination, they will not be specified here.

What is important to realize is that the writers of this school are not entitled to a hearing in scientific circles any more than are witch doctors or primitive medicine men. The reasons are first, that they are usually uninformed, second, that their assumptions and methods are unscientific. Note that I did not say that these writers are not entitled to a hearing. I said they are not entitled to a hearing in scientific circles. Yet they have had their way for nearly a century—perhaps longer—and it is time that medicine regained its classical birthright. It is time that we refused to be stampeded and cajoled by Roman metaphysics. It is time that physicians in this country began to take the traditional viewpoint of classical medicine, the viewpoint of Soranos and Aëtios. Many are the signs that there has been a steady drift in this direction in recent years. And there are many signs (see later pages) that the tendency will strengthen for some time yet. The first stages of that drift in the form of contributions to medical-journal symposia are sketched in the next chapter.

CHAPTER XII
LATER MEDICAL WRITERS

§1   MEDICAL JOURNAL AUTHORS

HAVING reviewed some of the independent treatises on birth control published by American physicians in the second half of the nineteenth century, we shall now consider the place of medical journals in facilitating the instruction of physicians and the helpful exchange of views among them.

It may be considered an established generalization that the medical journals gave space to conception control much later than separately published books and pamphlets. This might be expected on theoretical grounds, since the journals have to represent a more conservative consensus of attitude. They cannot give space to subjects taken up by every fly-by-night brochure until the subject is seen to merit a genuine place in their pages. Even then journals have to proceed cautiously for a thousand medical claims are made for one that will stand rigid scientific examination. This is not the only circumstance that has made the medical journals cautious, but it is probably the major one. Some have even suggested that physicians have opposed birth control because of the feeling that a declining birth rate would reduce their incomes. The analysis is probably erroneous, but that it has troubled some physicians not only unconsciously but consciously is shown by a recent letter published in the *Journal of the American Medical Association* inquiring what the effect of diffused birth control would be on medical incomes. So much remains to be done to get adequate medical service to the masses that it would seem that there need be no worry about incomes being reduced by a declining birth rate. In the first place those who reproduce responsibly not only demand more medical service than those who reproduce irresponsibly, but they are better able to pay for such service. It is the spawning poor who secure most of the free assistance. So much for a brief analysis of factors delaying the appearance of articles on birth control in medical journals.

(1a)   O. E. Herrick

One of the earliest articles published in this country on contraception, and one which led to subsequent discussion by others, was that of O. E. Herrick in the *Michigan Medical News*[1] of 1882. It is of interest for the medical

---

[1] O. E. Herrick, "Abortion and Its Lesson," *Mich. Med. News*, v (1882), 7–10. Herrick lived in Grand Rapids.

history of contraception because of its strikingly liberal and well-informed point of view for that period in the development of American medicine. The main emphasis of Herrick's article is that legislation and moral suasion have failed to prevent widespread abortion, and that the best preventive of this is diffused contraceptive knowledge.[2] Herrick was, however, like many who have followed him, overly optimistic about diffused contraception entirely eliminating self-induced abortion.

Herrick held that no woman should be forced to become an unwilling mother. He upbraids those "medical teachers and writers [who] have pandered to the notion spread among the people by the priesthood, that it is their [women's] duty to raise many children,"[3] and who have stressed the danger to health of the use of preventives. Much of the talk about "congestive pathology is a myth." As a matter of fact, since many of the diseases of women are associated with childbearing, the incidence of these diseases would be reduced if offspring were limited.[4] There are large numbers of couples, married for many years, who have practiced prevention during the whole course of their married life without injury.[5] Herrick informs us that in an article published some months before in the same journal he touched upon the subject of prevention and adds

Since that time, I have received numerous letters from physicians endorsing the position taken, and asking me to give them what I considered some of the best methods of preventing conception. These letters show that a portion of the profession see the necessity of dealing with this matter by some other method than by telling their patients to 'let nature take its course' . . . [6]

He then cites a typical letter.

Herrick's discussion of contraceptive technique is solely of historical value; he admits that he knows little about the subject, but presents for the benefit of other medical-journal readers what information he has. He prefers douching as "the only sure preventive,"[7] but contradicts himself on the value of the unmedicated douche.[8] The medicament preferred is carbolic

[2] *Ibid.*, p. 9.

[3] *Ibid.*, p. 9.   Punctuation mine.

[4] *Ibid.*

[5] *Ibid.*, p. 9.

[6] *Ibid.*, p. 9.   Punctuation mine.

[7] *Ibid.*, p. 9.

[8] "Injections as ordinarily used are very unreliable, if only water is used, but if carbolic acid is added to the water, and it is used immediately after connection, it will often prevent conception. Injections properly used, if of nothing but pure water, are an absolute protection." (p. 9) Herrick here furnishes us with a bit of humor. For assistance in douching he recommends a "Comstock Syringe," which he tells us, was respectfully dedicated to the manufacturers to Anthony Comstock after he prosecuted them for sending the device through the mails with directions for use. Comstock was defeated in the legal battle. *Cf.*, E. B. Foote, *Radical Remedy* for the same story.

acid (with no warning against too strong a solution), but other medicaments are mentioned.[9]

In failing to warn against acid solutions that were too strong Herrick may have been under the erroneous impression that the medical profession could control such a private practice. It is to Herrick's credit, however, that he observed the importance of adequately distending the vagina during the flushing process, a point not touched on by the earlier writers, such as Knowlton. In the second century Soranos had warned against the use of irritating medicaments. Many modern writers object to douching, partly because daily use might affect the normal flora of the vagina, partly because over-crowded housing conditions usually make it difficult where there is limited privacy. What is more important, sperms can get out of reach of a douche in half a minute, if they land on the os.

No sooner had Herrick declared that the injections provided "an absolute protection," than an anonymous physician "E. H.", writing in the same journal, the *Michigan Medical News*, corrected Herrick by pointing out that "all means will fail in some cases."[10] E. H. felt that "skin coverings" worn by the male were "almost an absolute protection."[11] This writer not only contradicts himself, but makes the same error that Herrick did. E. H. holds the sucking-in theory by the cervix, and thinks that for this reason any syringe is liable to fail. We now know it can fail for other reasons. He states that the safe period cannot be relied upon, and that while prevention is simple for some women, it is difficult for others.

Besides the medicated and unmedicated douche, Herrick mentions withdrawal (the oldest means and without bad effect, except for the diminution of pleasure), the sponge, and "womb veil."[12]

In the issue of the *Michigan Medical News* for February 10, 1882, there appeared a letter from Dr. Charles Ambrook, of Boulder, Colorado, who thanked the editor for publishing Herrick's article, agreed with Herrick's opinions in essentials, and affirmed that it was "possible to discuss this question from a natural stand-point, to reason from facts,"[13] and to maintain the scientific attitude. Ambrook speaks unequivocally in favor of voluntary motherhood, and thinks it about time that the medical profession took a new departure on this question. While no family is complete with-

[9] Such as "plumbi acetas, zinci sulphas, [and] acid salicylicum." (p. 9)

[10] *Ibid.*, p. 37.

[11] *Ibid.*

[12] *Ibid.*, p. 10. "The introduction of pieces of sponge into the vagina before connection, has proved to be ineffectual sometimes; and I have also known women to be disappointed who placed confidence in a 'womb veil' [cervical cap or diaphragm]." The term womb veil is ambiguous. Sometimes it may have meant a female condom.

[13] *Ibid.*, p. 37.

out children, they should not swarm like rats. The medical profession has "been too much in the habit of putting the question aside as one for religion to deal with."[14] Indications are merely touched upon: a woman with tuberculosis should not bear children, not only because she is likely to die, but because this would leave other children motherless. Ambrook did not hesitate to state that he believed that involuntary maternity was positively correlated (as we would now say) with crime, intemperance, pauperism, and domestic discord.

(1b) Symposium in Medical and Surgical Reporter (1888).

So far as our present knowledge goes, the first symposium[15] held in an American medical journal on the subject of the prevention of conception took place in the *Medical and Surgical Reporter* (Philadelphia) in 1888 as a consequence of an editorial[16] which appeared in that journal during the same year. The editorial declared that while the subject demanded "discretion" for its discussion, "even so delicate a subject may be regarded with too much timidity. . . ."[17] It added that "No medical man of any experience can fail to know that the propriety and feasibility of preventing conception engages, at some time or other, the attention of a large proportion of married people in civilized lands, . . . [that] there is danger that an undue dread of discussing it frankly in medical circles may deprive medical men of the means of properly directing a disposition which cannot be ignored, and which, in the present state of human nature and civilization, it seems impossible to eradicate."[18] After references to the principles of Malthus, which are based essentially upon economic considerations, the editorial observes that many women complain of the hardships entailed by too frequent childbearing. "The question of preventing conception is one which demands chaste . . . but also fearless consideration" on the part of those who bear the chief burden of reproduction—women.[19] Moreover, the subject is intimately connected with "marital and family felicity. The woman who lives in dread of her husband's sexual appetite cannot satisfy him as a wife, and, with this poison in her life, must find it hard to be a kind and wholesome mother to her children."[20]

---

[14] *Ibid.*, p. 36.

[15] This is on the assumption that the discussion in the *Michigan Medical News* six years before is not to be considered a symposium.

[16] *Med. & Surg. Rep.*, (Phila.), lix, (1888), 342–343.

[17] *Ibid.*, p. 342.

[18] *Ibid.*

[19] *Ibid.*

[20] *Ibid.*

It will not do to cover up such a state of affairs with euphemisms. Those who know what goes on in the privacy of many a home, as physicians only know it, know that the dread of pregnancy and child-bearing has wrecked the peace of thousands of households, and led to . . . [desperate resort to abortion].

Impressed with this fact, we invite our readers to discuss in these pages, as wise and thoughtful physicians, the importance of the prevention of too frequent conception. Opinions may differ as to what constitutes too frequent conception, or as to the desirability of interfering at all with the course of nature in sexual matters, but we believe that a candid study of the subject is an urgent need of the present day, and hope that the REPORTER may do something toward meeting this need, difficult and delicate as the task may be.[21]

The first to respond by venturing his opinions was Dr. W. R. D. Blackwood of Philadelphia. He agreed that the subject was "of vast importance to the profession and general public alike." It was unfortunate that its discussion was taboo among physicians "partly from indifference, but largely from absolute cowardice in those capable of writing intelligently about it." In previous discussions there had been altogether too much of an injection of the religious and moral aspects of the subject. After making clear the distinction between abortion and the prevention of conception, Blackwood affirms:

I state my belief honestly and fearlessly, that under proper conditions the PREVENTION of conception is not only proper *per se*, but that *it is imperatively demanded under certain circumstances*.[22]

Blackwood mentioned as indications "inherited" syphilis, scrofula, and tuberculosis, mental weakness and insanity. Blackwood refuses to consider valid the argument that interference with nature's processes is morally and physically wrong; that continence should be employed in such instances. He affirms that "It will not do to say that a man *can* control his sexual appetite, and that he *must* do it. Some men cannot, and many who are supposed to do so are simply apt in concealing their indulgence from public gaze."[23] If prostitution is to be eradicated, it can only be done by encouraging judicious marriages. The lot of women should not be a continual round of impregnation, delivery, and lactation. "The land is full of wretched, broken-down women today whose lives have been wrecked because they have become mere machines for the reproduction of the race, and if the race is degenerating, as many think it is, it is worth careful consideration whether or not something in the way of controlling the quantity would not enhance the quality of the product. . . . To me the matter reduces itself to a choice between foeticide and prevention. The one is an indefensible crime—the other a necessity."[24]

Dr. Thomas A. Pope of Cameron, Texas, the second contributor to the symposium, also favored prevention.[25] Though population in the United States was increasing rapidly both by natural increase and by immigration, we need not fear Malthusian over-population for a long time. Prevention was, however, a question which the medical profession would have to face eventually. From the medical standpoint too frequent childbearing caused the weaning of the preceding child, thus increasing death hazards. He observed that "very frequent conception is now mostly confined to the poorer class. The rich, in town and country, already limit the number of their offspring. . . ."[26] Then "there are very many women who ought not to bear children because their children are likely to be diseased in body or mind, and, if they survive childhood, will be a burden to themselves and society."[27] Knowledge of the prevention of conception would undoubtedly reduce the maternal death-rate. The mental anxiety and worry of too frequent childbearing makes many women prematurely old. Pope doubted whether woman should "become a mere machine for the propagation of the species." Such she would be without birth limitation. Absence of control often means a neglect of the children because the mother is unable to give them proper care. Then, too, the net average income of most families in the United States is such that they are unable to rear large families properly. It is only cruelty for a man or woman with little visible means of support to give a large family a heritage of poverty, ignorance, and excessive toil. "If the number of children were limited, better opportunities and better care would be [possible] for all, and all [sic] could have a start in life so fair that success would come to all who deserved it."[28] Crime would be decreased because there would be fewer offspring of vicious parentage. Moreover, training would be better. Taken as a whole, the point of view of Pope and Blackwood is extraordinarily progressive and well-informed for the U. S. A. in the eighteen-eighties.

Pope then referred to a contribution in the *American Journal of Obstetrics* in which the author complained of the frequency of resort to Onanism and of its dangers. Pope countered these observations by introducing statements by Dr. J. Ford Thompson in the same journal[29] in which he pointed

[24] *Ibid.*, p. 396.   Punctuation mine.
[25] Thomas A. Pope, "Prevention of Conception," *Ibid.*, lix (1888), 522–525.
[26] *Ibid.*, p. 523.
[27] *Ibid.*
[28] *Ibid.*, p. 524.
[29] *Amer. Jour. Obst.*, Sept. 1888.

out that much pseudo-science had been talked by those who stressed "the danger and injuriousness of preventive methods." In Thompson's judgment, the condom, douche, withdrawal, as well as "the use of the hood by the woman" were all non-injurious.

In the issue of November 10, 1888, Dr. L. Huber of Rocky Ford, Colorado, supports the liberal views of those who preceded him in the symposium, and affirms that "There is a continuous demand made upon the physician to prevent conception. . . ."[30] He reports also that there is "a prevailing practice among the laity to prevent conception. . . ."[31] Unfortunately much pseudo-scientific literature is being distributed. "Now, why should there not be," he asks, "a preponderance of good and reliable books . . . on so general and so important a subject [instead of so much trash]?" Huber anticipates R. L. Dickinson and the late Whitridge Williams in declaring that "The demand upon the practitioner to prevent conception is an unquestionable fact. Under these circumstances, it is the duty of the profession to define more clearly what conditions justify and what do not justify interference, and then to settle upon some safe, efficient measures to meet the demand. As this work is pushed forward, criminal interference [in the form of abortion], so general and flagrant nowadays, should decline or cease altogether."[32] This subject should be taken up bravely and prudently by medical men and not shunned as it has been in the past. "If medical men leave it entirely to those who discuss it from unworthy motives, they cannot be held wholly guiltless of the consequences."

The next letter, signed X. Y. Z.,[33] is of interest chiefly as demonstrating the unwise counsel of an eminent Philadelphia physician who, when he was asked to advise a woman in frail health on account of nervousness, recommended that the husband use withdrawal. It is reported that the husband also, as a consequence, became a nervous wreck. It was effective, however, for three years so far as pregnancy was concerned. X. Y. Z. believed that the physician made a grave mistake in recommending *coitus interruptus*, and wants to know if no better advice is available.

There was more piety than science in the viewpoint of Dr. Isaac Peirce of Tazewell, Va.[34] Yet he believed that the subject should be approached with candor and frankness, and a decision made on the basis of the individual conscience. He disagreed with Blackwood's contention that the diffusion of preventive knowledge would reduce the incidence of prostitution. On

[30] *Med. & Surg. Rep.*, lix (1888), 580.
[31] *Ibid.*
[32] *Ibid.*, p. 581.
[33] *Ibid.*, p. 600.
[34] *Ibid.*, pp. 614–616.

the contrary, it would "bring about a worse state of affairs."[35] It might, however, reduce suffering, pauperism, and the neglect of illegitimate children. If men possessed knowledge of prevention, seduction would be facilitated. "I shudder," says Peirce, "at what would be the result of the promiscuous prevention of conception, even with the idea of stopping criminal abortion, pauperism, and suffering of illegitimate children. I believe that if we put into the hands of men a ready and sure means of preventing conception, there will be more prostitutes, fewer marriages, and more disease among women."[36] Peirce thinks that it has been the fear of increasing syphilis and gonorrhea which has prevented the medical profession from diffusing contraceptive knowledge in the past. "It has been the fear of instituting a process which we could never hope to control, and which would in a short time become so universal and popular as to admit of no check, that has made cowards of the medical profession . . . [He adds]: Should we ever prevent conception? and, if so, when should we interfere? What is a ready and sure means of effecting the object? and how shall we keep the matter in our own hands?"[37]

Note the implications of the last question. Peirce believed that a large number of physicians and laymen would take the view that it was morally wrong to interfere with the natural process of conception; that a woman who marries should accept the risks of pregnancy and childbearing and bear the consequences as best she can, making no protest against allowing her husband his "rights," and being prepared even to fill a premature grave should fate so determine! Such a callous point of view is nothing short of treason to the best traditions of medicine. Whenever religious preconceptions interfere with the scientific practice of the healing art, they should be discarded. Unless this is done, the physician is incompetent to just that degree and unworthy to be permitted by the state to practise his art.

For one so ignorant of the subject, Peirce's discussion of indications is curiously advanced. He calls for a definition of indications and goes so far as to agree with Blackwood that prevention should be used in order to avoid the birth of children who might "inherit" syphilis, scrofula, tuberculosis, epilepsy, or imbecility; and agrees that in such cases prevention "is imperatively demanded."[38] "Again, women who are deformed, women whose lives are made one constant and heavy burden by pregnancy so often repeated that they seem never able to have an end, women who are made miserable by the so-called 'habit' of abortion, and women whose former

[35] *Ibid.*, p. 614.
[36] *Ibid.*, p. 615.
[37] *Ibid.*
[38] *Ibid.*

gestation and delivery have brought them almost to the door of eternity"—all these women should receive knowledge of prevention.[39]   There is no other way; for men will not abstain from sexual relations even at the danger of the wife's health.   Recognizing the fact that prevention is imperative in certain cases, the author admits that he is

at a loss to know what are the means best suited to accomplish this and how to apply them.   The number of preventive measures which have been proposed is not small, but the selection of one which we can control and its restriction to those alone who really need it are not easy.   Let it become generally known that the medical profession countenances a preventive even in a few cases, and there is reason to fear [that] this will be stretched to a license which will work much mischief to women who are already experimenting in this direction, who have no reason why they should not fulfill the God-given function which makes happy homes, and who are now only held in check by the judgment of the world [sic].   Will it not also place in the hands of men a ready argument with which to destroy the purity of loving, trusting girls?[40]

This is the reason why the author has "for so long given the old woman's advice [!], 'to take a glass of cold water before going to bed and *nothing else.*' "[41]   Deceptive counsel, indeed; and one calculated to injure the confidence of the public in the medical profession.

Dr. Ernest C. Helm of Beloit, Wisconsin, anticipated many modern physicians in declaring that the prevention of conception "should be thoroughly understood by the physician;" that it should be discussed in the journals in a calm, clear, clean manner.   Upon a careful consideration of this subject depends in a large measure the welfare of the community.[42]   There is anticipation of a view much stressed by Margaret Sanger in Helm's statement that the young woman who marries prematurely, especially if she is in frail health, should use preventives in the first years of married life.

She will then have become more mature, and can better bear and rear children· Child-mothers do not make the best mothers, and child-bearing often wrecks their physical systems . . . The first few years of . . . married life [would] be far happier if they could be devoted to understanding each other, and securing and making a real home, so that when babies should come they could the better be cared for.[43]

Though it is doubtful whether contraceptive knowledge should be given to healthy women who married very early, it is the plain duty of the physician to advise contraceptively an exceedingly young wife who is "feeble and puny."

[39] *Ibid.*
[40] *Ibid.*, p. 616.
[41] *Ibid.*
[42] *Ibid.*, p. 643.
[43] *Ibid.*, p. 644.   For "could be devoted" original reads "could devote it."

Helm cites the case of a famous professor who, in commenting upon the case of a young mother, aged 22, who, though undernourished and anaemic, had three parturitions and thirteen miscarriages in seven years, could only say with a shrug of his shoulders: "The only thing to do with this case is to chain up the husband." Should this physician, asks Helm, have been content to give advice which he knew would be disregarded? It would be futile to refuse preventive instruction in such cases because women would only seek the professional abortionist. He adds: "When I hear men gravely denouncing the prevention of conception as a crime, I only wish that they could bear and rear one child. . . ." The physician should put himself in the place of heavily-burdened women. "Their wishes and interests are too often ignored, either from selfish or puritanical motives or from sheer carelessness on our part."[44] Physicians shrink unduly from this question lest their opinions should become public, and lest the diffusion of contraceptive knowledge should open the floodgates of immorality. These fears are groundless, for most women are not chaste for fear of impregnation. Motherhood is a noble function, but

to spend life from eighteen to forty-five bearing and rearing children is not unlikely to sap the vitality of any woman, and [to] prevent that development of mind and body, that improvement of children and of the home-life which should be the aim of every true wife and mother. Furthermore, too frequent conceptions and pregnancies are not good for the mental and physical well-being of the children. The mother with too many children has insufficient time to devote to their rearing and culture; . . . her entire time is occupied with a baby just born, or about to be born. She is shut out, to a great degree, from . . . social intercourse . . . ; all her chances for mental improvement are cut off; the cares and worries of her condition make her irritable and petulant, and the real pleasure she takes in the society of her husband, and in the neatness and home-like atmosphere of their home is greatly lessened.[45]

Women should not be mere childbearing machines having children so rapidly that it is necessary for the older children to spend most of their time in caring for the smaller ones. Moreover, economic conditions require family limitation. So long as there is a limit to the family income, there must be a limit to the responsibilities of parents toward reproduction. Many otherwise happy homes are wrecked because of too frequent maternity. These views, likewise, have a very modern ring.

After such a strong defense of contraception, Helm makes a curious confession: He says "My invariable practice when approached by a husband or wife in regard to the means of preventing conception has been to say: 'There

[44] *Ibid.*, 644.
[45] *Ibid.*, p. 645. Phraseology slightly edited, while remaining faithful to the sense of the original.

is a sure way: do not marry; but if you are married, sleep apart and never have sexual intercourse.' [But, he adds] I fear, however, that this chaste advice has never been followed; and as long as human nature remains unchanged, I do not think it is likely to be. Until a very recent period, I thought that a physician was not justified in giving any other advice; but now I am looking for more light on the subject. It seems to me that, even if they were instructed in regard to the methods of preventing conception with which physicians are familiar, self-respecting women may become pregnant fully as often as the welfare of themselves or their children would permit."[46]

Helm thinks the methods of prevention described in a previous issue (condom, douche, withdrawal, hood) simple and harmless, and calculated to be less harmful than unspaced pregnancies.

The article by Dr. de Hart[47] is chiefly of interest for the unscientific nature of its deductions and for the utopian idealism expressed. She declares that the general adoption of continence would not only solve the Malthusian problem, and render unnecessary "recourse to those unnatural means which are considered by many as both unhealthy and immoral,"[48] but would "prevent" infanticide and foeticide, "eradicate" prostitution, diminish the diseases peculiar to women, reduce hereditary disease, the unfaithfulness of husbands, etc. Such a spiritual triumph might bring more good to the race than such material advance as railroads, a telegraph system, steamships, etc. She suggests that the attempts to subvert nature by considering sexual congress as having any other purpose than procreation is "always fraught with danger." Although the author seems to have some knowledge of the history of medicine, it is somewhat amazing to find her declaring that continence is "rarely mentioned as a cure for the evils which flow so surely from incontinence."[49] Surely this is an amazing confession of ignorance.

In the issue of December 1, 1888, Blackwood returns to the fray, points out the inadvisability of recommending *coitus interruptus* in a case of nervousness, and recommends the mid-period followed by "ablutions."[50]

Dr. H. B. Runnalls congratulated the editor upon initiating a discussion from which "nothing but good can result."[51] He had long been of the opinion that the law [sic] should make it a criminal offense for members of

---

[46] *Ibid.*, p. 645.
[47] Madana F. de Hart, "Continence: an Unpopular Prophylactic," *ibid.*, pp. 674–676.
[48] *Ibid.*, p. 675.
[49] *Ibid.*
[50] *Ibid.*, p. 698.
[51] *Ibid.*, p. 710.

either sex, suffering from constitutional diseases, which might be transmitted to offspring, to indulge in sexual intercourse—a splendid instance of naïveté. There are indeed cases in which the prevention of conception is called for:

I would always advise it where puerperal or uraemic convulsions accompanied pregnancy; where vomiting was severe during pregnancy; where any pelvic deformity existed, or any uterine or ovarian growth was present; where excessive hemorrhage accompanied labor; where the perineum or other parts had been lacerated much during labor; where any hernia of the intestines was present; and where any heart, kidney or lung mischief was present—in fact, in all cases in which the medical attendant was of the opinion that evil results would follow conception; but never merely for social or economic reasons.[52]

Considering the period, this is not a bad summary of medical indications. But in failing to support economic and social indications, Runnalls, though in agreement perhaps with modern American medical thought, ran counter to the most authoritative American medical thought and to European medical thought. Fact-facing practitioners of medicine realize today that it is no longer possible strictly to separate economic and social conditions from conditions giving rise to medical needs.

Dr. David E. Matteson of Warsaw, N. Y., recommends,[53] in the issue of December 15, 1888, the use of a sponge of silk or sheep's wool. About one and one-half cubic inches of either material should be shaped into a ball, and tied with a silk thread for easy extrication. Matteson, in the following passage, anticipates the advice of Dr. Norman Haire: "All that is needed for its use is that the wife shall bear in mind that it is just as much a part of her night attire as is her *robe-de-nuit*."[54] Removal may be made before morning, if convenient. The device is simple and inexpensive, and the results are satisfactory. The syringe is, however, in Matteson's view, the most commonly used preventive in Great Britain and America. It has a certain value provided it is resorted to immediately after the conjugal act, and if an astringent is added to destroy the spermatozoa (the author says a strong astringent).[55] He seems to accept the idea, as have numerous other physicians of the period, that there is a suction activity of the cervix during orgasm. Such a view is still held by Stopes, Talmey, and others. It is probably without foundation, like Stopes's "coital interlocking." Matteson mentions the inconvenience of rising from a warm bed to syringe. Conjugal onanism is not as a rule harmful, but has aesthetic objections. The author also dislikes the condom and various types of female veil. The

[52] *Ibid.*
[53] *Ibid.*, pp. 759–760.
[54] *Ibid.*
[55] *Ibid.*, p. 759.

degree of skill required for the adjustment of the latter "practically puts them out of the question."[56]

Until recent times the erroneous view was unfortunately quite prevalent that the rubber pessary is difficult or even impossible for the ordinary woman to use, even when competently fitted by a physician. This statement occurs in many journal articles; but clinical experience has disproved it so far as the average woman is concerned. The statement is never found in modern papers by informed authors with clinical experience.

(1c) Symposium in The Cincinnati Medical News (1890)

Another early medical-journal symposium was that appearing in 1890 in the *Cincinnati Medical News*.[57] There is here a secretarial report (by F. W. Mann, M.D.) of the proceedings of a discussion meeting held by the Detroit Medical and Literary Association. Those taking part in the discussion were Drs. C. B. Gilbert, Helen Warner, Frank W. Brown, T. A. McGraw, A. L. Worden, Mulheron, Hutton, Bonning, Gibson, Chittick, Webber, Banks, Stevens, Devendorf, and Carstens.

Like the symposium in the *Medical and Surgical Reporter*, this discussion is strikingly modern for America in the eighteen-nineties.

The prevention of conception seemed to C. B. Gilbert "a purely private affair"[58]—a view held by J. Bentham and J. S. Mill. It was commonly supposed that a woman should bear as many children as physiologically possible, however much suffering she might be called upon to undergo. This point of view Gilbert objected to on the score alone of inability to provide for the offspring. He implies that sexual instruction should be given in our schools. Contraception is not contrary to the moral law. This is a question of utilitarianism.[59] So long as the practice is not harmful, there can be no reason against it. It would not endanger our civilization, nor Christianity.

Helen Warner took a more conservative view, and thought Gilbert's opinions "radical." However, she occasionally gave contraceptive advice. This was justifiable where a woman could not bring forth a living child, or where patients were insane, or likely to become so. She was less confident of the harmlessness of contraceptives than Gilbert.

Frank W. Brown thought abstinence (i.e., "moral" means) the best; but where these were inexpedient, he would apply mechanical methods. He

---

[56] *Ibid.*

[57] C. B. Gilbert, *et al.*, "The Prevention of Conception," *Cincinnati Medical News*, xix, n.s. (1890), 303–8.

[58] *Ibid.*, p. 303.

[59] *Ibid.*

made allusions to Malthus's teachings, and seemed convinced that there was a close connection between the extent of pauperism and the rapidity with which people reproduced. Moreover, since the progress of medicine was prolonging the span of life, especially by the reduction of the seriousness of epidemics, we were left with the problem of controlling population increase. It was useless to urge abstinence. Statistics would not prove that prevention was injurious to the woman. Brown admits that he usually advised methods of prevention, when asked; he was mindful of the fact that if physicians refused information, methods more harmful might be used in the absence of a physician's consent. He avows that "The facts of everyday life show us that a majority of [the] people practise these methods, and [that] among educated classes population is regulated."[60]

T. A. McGraw could not see anything wrong in prevention. Advising abstention when the prevention of conception was indicated would only drive the husband to the brothel. This meant breaking up family ties. Far greater injury proceeds from excessively large families than from the prevention of conception. Inasmuch as the standard of comfort had risen, it was now much more difficult than formerly to rear a large family.

A. L. Worden admitted that prevention was sometimes proper and justifiable, but in many instances this was not the case. As a rule, it is not the poverty-stricken who come for advice. Great discrimination should be used in giving such advice; and physicians should beware of too much leniency.

Mulheron, like many others before and after him, could see no distinction between the right to prevent conception and to produce an illegal abortion. The practice was morally wrong. Gibson agreed.

Hutton agreed with McGraw. The manner of prevention was an individual and personal one. If it could be accomplished without physical injury, it was advantageous to society. He thought irrigations with a bichloride of mercury solution effective.[61]

Bonning also supported prevention, and referred to its advantages among the French. Chittick would leave each individual case to the conscience of the physician. To Webber contraceptive practices were "decidedly harmful,"[62] a thwarting of nature's laws. His view was that of the modern Catholic Church. Banks, a woman physician, believed that it was "right" to prevent conception.

Stevens held that prevention should be used wherever there was evidence

---

[60] *Ibid.*, p. 305.

[61] Such active poisons are certainly not to be recommended now. It is apt to get concentrated in the bottom of the douche bag.

[62] *Ibid.*, p. 307.

of hereditary mental incompetence or in cases where childbearing was dangerous either to the mother or to the child. But the method should be abstinence. "He did not believe that it was ever intended that the indulgence of sexual desires should be a pleasure [sic], or that it should be pursued for pleasurable motives [sic.]"[63]

Devendorf stated that "nine-tenths of the educated classes are using means to prevent conception;"[64] that a Dr. Van der Warker, professor of gynecology at Albany or Syracuse, had some time ago examined a community [Oneida] in which contraceptive practices were used, and found no harm resulting. It was advantageous for humanity in general to limit the number of children.

In Carstens's view, the state as well as individuals had an interest in human reproduction. Contraception was justified, however, where, for reasons of heredity, defective offspring would result. It was unfortunate that the insane and criminal classes perpetuated their kind. "He thought all insane and criminal individuals should be castrated."[65] One objection to prevention was that it was practised most by those who ought especially to propagate, least by the pauper classes.[66]

To summarize this symposium: Of the fifteen participants in the above discussion, eight may be said definitely to favor the prevention of conception by modern "artificial" methods; one other approved the idea of prevention, but said the method should be abstinence. Three were favorably inclined but cautious in their approval; while only three were definitely opposed, and these evidently not on scientific, so much as on moral and religious grounds. There is no reason to believe that there was any editorial selection of the points of view; the report was sent to the journal by the secretary of the group. If there was selection—and some there must have

[63] *Ibid.*

[64] *Ibid.*

[65] Sterilization without unsexing is, of course, the modern substitute for castration. It is unquestionably an extreme position to recommend the sterilization of "all insane and criminal persons," a view partly responsible for the extreme reaction of certain contemporary environmentalists in social work against sterilization as a therapeutic measure. A typical example of sentimental, environmentalistic reaction against the older indiscriminate recommendation of sterilization is to be found in Stanley P. Davies, *Social Control of the Mentally Deficient*, (New York: Crowell, 1930), a work of some authority, I gather, among social workers in America, and which, though characterized by much good judgment, contains also much shoddy reasoning against sterilization on environmentalistic grounds. However, it must be admitted that much of the earlier talk on heredity was nonsense. Genetic knowledge has advanced considerably in the past two decades, and fifty years from now we may know something about the subject. But this should not prevent us from acting in the interim according to our best lights.

[66] *Ibid.*, p. 308.

been—it was by the secretary who heard the proceedings, and thus the selection was presumably based upon his views of the relative significance of the statements made by various speakers. Outside of the support of conception control, the most striking feature of the viewpoints here expressed is the placing of eugenic indications on a plane with medical indications. Nor is mention of economic indications absent. Striking also is the recognition by Brown that since the medical profession has been largely responsible for the increase in population as a consequence of improvement in health conditions, it has likewise a responsibility in the matter of population control. Here is clear recognition of the fact of the inseparability of medical and economic indications—a view which is not open to dispute. There is recognition by the same author that if the medical profession does not recognize its responsibility in furnishing contraceptive information, there is grave danger that the public may resort to harmful methods. As a matter of fact, clinical statistics, gathered by the present writer and others, have demonstrated the validity of this observation. Noteworthy also is the presence here of the Bentham-J. S. Mill view that what married couples may do by way of prevention is essentially, if not exclusively, their private concern. This view was stressed by Drs. Gilbert and Chittick. There is much to be said for the view of Carstens, however, that the state, as well as parents, have an interest in human reproduction.

In conclusion, one may observe that, on the whole, this is a strikingly progressive series of viewpoints for the U. S. A. in 1890.

(1d) W. P. Chunn

A liberal and sound point of view was taken by Chunn in a paper published in the *Maryland Medical Journal*[67] for 1895, in which indications and methods were interestingly treated. Though it is not known that Chunn had any special influence upon his colleagues—particularly is there an absence of evidence that he propagandized in any way—he is definitely to be placed among the late nineteenth-century American advocates of conception control. He deplored the fact that medical textbooks discussed treatment for sterility, but omitted to mention methods of preventing conception. He argued that it was just as immoral and unnatural to treat sterility as to prevent conception when it was medically indicated.[68] Chunn mentions as indications fibroid of the cervix, pelvic deformity, pelvic tumors and cancer, and repeated pregnancies which endanger the life of the mother.

[67] William Pawson Chunn, "The Prevention of Conception. Its Practicability and Justifiability," *Maryland Medical Journal*, 32 (1894–95): 340–3. A paper read before the Gyn. & Obst. Soc. of Baltimore on Jan. 29, 1895.
[68] *Ibid.*, p. 340.

"Why allow," he asks, "the children already born to run the risk of becoming motherless if such a contingency may be avoided? Whom would it benefit if this woman's husband should become a widower?"[69] In the cases of women who have been subjected to repeated Caesarian sections, Chunn recommends ovariotomy. One need hardly remark that such radical interference is no longer recommended. When it is genuinely indicated, we would now recommend tying the fallopian tubes, which, indeed, Chunn himself mentioned.[70]

Curiously enough, Chunn considered the condom injurious,[71] but mentions the syringe as "one of the most certain and harmless preventives at our disposal."[72] He is careful to state that the vagina should be carefully distended in order to wash out all the semen. His recommendation of the use of a solution of bichloride of mercury added to warm water would probably not find support now.[73] Chunn states that he has had prepared for himself vaginal suppositories composed of cocoanut butter containing 10 per cent of boric acid. He recommends also suppositories medicated with tannic acid, bichloride of mercury or boracic acid. These he considered next in value to the vaginal douche, if not equal to it.[74] Chunn was also early in pointing out the difficulties of cocoa butter suppositories melting with sufficient rapidity. He recommends that in such instances, olive oil or glycerine may be used.[75] In view of the considerable emphasis which Stopes has recently placed on the use of olive oil, this early mention of it by an American physician is interesting. And Aristotle slightly preceded Chunn.

The cervical rubber cap is harmless and "doubtless effectual," but liable to be displaced during coitus. Chunn thought this the chief reason why the cap was not more widely used in the U. S. A. at the time. But general inaccessibility was the real reason. His final recommendation seems to be as follows:

In case a determined woman has decided

to prevent conception . . . for sufficient reasons, I should recommend a vaginal suppository before sexual relations and a vaginal douche immediately after, taken

[69] *Ibid.*, p. 342.
[70] *Ibid.*
[71] *Ibid.*
[72] *Ibid.*
[73] For a generation or two bichloride of mercury douching was popular in the U. S. A. This is shown, for example, in the K. B. Davis series of cases. Such douching is dangerous. The prevalence of such a harmful method is a good example of the stupidity of legal repression. Neglect of the profession to take a hand in reform of the laws is thus partially responsible for public injury.
[74] *Ibid.*
[75] *Ibid.*, p. 343.

in the dorsal position, as before mentioned. This would undoubtedly seem the safest plan outside the condum.

In these days when such clinics as the Walworth Women's Welfare Center of London and the Maternal Health Association of Cleveland arrange for special sessions for the husbands in order that they might be instructed in coöperating with their wives not only in properly executing the contraceptive technique taught, but in sexually adjusting one to another, there is special interest in the following report of Chunn, in which he mentions instruction of the husbands as well as of the wives:

Some four years ago I had occasion to advise another woman concerning the danger of future pregnancy; and in order that her husband might be as well instructed as herself in the matter, she accompanied him to my office. While making a vaginal examination it was demonstrated how easy it is to depress the perineum and slip a wad of cotton into the vagina, the woman being in the dorsal position, and the index finger pressing back the perineum. Mr. X was of the opinion that he could perform the necessary manipulation as well as I could. He therefore had [made] a number of borated cotton pledgets about the size of an English walnut, and tied a short string to each. After [sic] conjugal relations one of the pledgets was soaked in a bichloride solution and introduced into the vagina, the index finger of the left hand being used as a perineal depressor. This woman had had four children at short intervals. The husband met [me] a few days ago, and was profuse in his expressions of gratitude, three years having passed without further increase in his family.[76]

(1e)   Later Symposia and Surveys of Opinion

After the 'nineties, symposia and especially articles became more common in medical journals as a perusal of the Bibliography will show. Symposia have, however, never been numerous. Among them have been those in *La Chronique Médicale* (1905),[77] the *Medical Review of Reviews* (1918), the *Practitioner* (special number, July, 1923), *Medical Journal & Record* (New York, 1928 and later. See Open Forum).

Forty-seven physicians replied to the questionnaire which constitutes the symposium published in the *Medical Review of Reviews*. Despite the fact that the list contained the names of many leading figures in American medicine, the most conspicuous characteristic of the replies is a dogmatic judgment in an absence of knowledge of the subject. Twelve of the forty-seven confessed that they had not given the subject sufficient attention to warrant an expression of opinion. Twenty-one, nearly half, supported birth control, five making certain qualifications. Six approved present restrictive legislation, and ten voted for repeal. Twelve thought birth

---

[76] *Ibid.* Punctuation mine.

[77] *Chronique Médicale*, xii (1905), 97–138.

control would increase immorality; seven denied this. Evidently many were swayed more by theological and philosophical considerations than by scientific ones. Dr. A. L. Goldwater, who took a strongly progressive viewpoint, claimed that physicians not only believed in birth control but practised it. He cited statistics in rather feeble support of his thesis. He observed that those who voted at the New York County Medical Society against birth control were "the members whose children averaged one or less, while the chief supporters of the minority resolution, which asked for a repeal of these inequitable laws, came from physicians who had comparatively large families, i.e., two, three, or four children. . . ."[78] A professor of orthopedic surgery holding an important post said "I believe in it [birth control] for geniuses and for the feebleminded; for clergymen and habitual criminals; for total abstainers and habitual drunkards, and for all other degenerates. I do not believe in it for healthy men and women."[79]

The same confused state of medical opinion was shown in a symposium conducted by the *Practitioner* (London) in a special number published in July, 1923. Although many prominent physicians contributed to this symposium not one of the papers surpasses a mediocre level except that by Dr. Norman Haire. Symposia of this type certainly give scientists in other fields a very bad impression of the way in which the medical profession follows scientific method.

Latterly, however, there has been a stabilization of medical opinion in the direction of a more liberal viewpoint and in the realization that medicine has a definite responsibility in scientific research, in the development of better methods and in the proper guidance and protection of the public.

Several surveys have been made in recent years to ascertain the state of medical opinion. Dr. C. Killick Millard in England sent a questionnaire to physicians and the Committee on Maternal Health (now the National Committee on Maternal Health) has had since 1927 a standing committee on indications for contraception, sterilization and abortion. Dr. Louise Stevens Bryant prepared for one of my articles[80] a discussion of indications for contraception. It is the first published attempt in English to formulate indications. There is a more complete discussion in Dickinson and Bryant, *Control of Conception*, pp. 166–183. Gall published a pamphlet including indications in the title. Grotjahn and Fraenkel, among others, have discussed the subject. Several works treat indications superficially without attempting a systematic, ordered, complete account.

[78] *Med. Rev. of Rev.*, 1918, p. 142.

[79] *Ibid.*, p. 138.

[80] "Birth Control for the British Working Classes," *Hospital Social Service*, xix (1929), 578–617.

It was about 1919 that Dr. Millard made his survey of medical opinion in England. This he was prompted to do by the fact that the 1908 Lambeth Conference condemned birth control not only on ethical grounds but for medical reasons, citing Bergeret and a Birmingham obstetrician. Accordingly, Millard about 1919, sent questionnaires to medical men and women in provincial towns. One of the questions asked whether certain contraceptives in common use, for instance, the condom and the quinine suppositories, were injurious to health under ordinary circumstances. Of seventy-four replies, fifty-two answered in the negative, eleven in the affirmative; but of the latter, only two could say that they had personal experience with bad effects. Six replied indefinitely, and five failed to answer the question. Thus was Bergeret's "evidence" thrown out of court even before the collection of irrefragable statistics by the clinics.[81]

In 1922 Dr. Millard, in collaboration with Dr. Binnie Dunlop, sent out a second questionnaire. This was addressed primarily to eminent male gynecologists both in London and the provinces, though some women physicians of standing were also included. At the time of the report sixty-five replies had been received.[82] For the full returns the reader may refer to the published account. In a word, the results showed that those who approved the use of contraceptives outnumbered three to one those of a contrary view. The condom was outstandingly favored, being mentioned twenty-three times as opposed to twenty-five mentions of all other methods combined. The "check pessary" or cervical cap, despite its great advocacy by a prominent English lay writer, was mentioned only four times. One may hazard the guess that a survey on techniques preferred, if taken now, would show preference for the Mensinga diaphragm. That is the method now chiefly used in the English[83] and American clinics; and it is quite possible that private practitioners in England have followed their lead.

Until 1930 there was no way of knowing how many colleges or schools

---

[81] A great body of testimony could be presented, were it required here, on the harmlessness of the contraceptive methods clinically recommended. Almost all practitioners have now discarded intrauterine stems, "wishbones," "butterflies" etc. The Graefenburg ring is still suspect, and chemicals can be abused or used unintelligently. This is all there is to the volumes of nonsense that have been written on injuriousness. It is an interesting commentary on the rarity of critical intelligence that Bergeret—who thought "conjugal frauds" caused nearly every ill human flesh is heir to—should be quoted by the 1908 Lambeth Conference and by the Report (1904) of the Royal Commission in New South Wales investigating the declining birth rate. I believe some Catholic writers with an axe to grind still quote him. Some myths are long in dying.

[82] C. Killick Millard, "Birth Control and the Medical Profession," *Report of the Fifth International Neo-Malthusian and Birth Control Conference*, p. 231.

[83] Norman E. Himes, "Contraceptive Methods: The Types Recommended by Nine British Birth Control Clinics," *New Engl. Jour. Med.*, ccii (1930), 866–873.

taught the technique of contraception in regular medical courses. In that year Dr. S. A. Knopf reported on a questionnaire sent to seventy-five medical colleges in the U. S. A.[84] Of the sixty-four institutions replying, thirteen colleges gave regular instruction in contraception and sterilization, twenty-eight taught these subjects incidentally, ten taught neither, four taught sterilization but not contraception, and nine failed to consider the subjects because they had only two year courses, and hence did not take up gynecology and obstetrics.

This shows progress over a former state of affairs in which virtually no medical schools in the country included instruction in contraceptive technique.

A more recent survey, made by the National Committee on Maternal Health—on the initiative of Dr. Stuart Mudd of the University of Pennsylvania—shows some progress in teaching contraception and sterilization in the Class A medical schools in this country. By 1933 three out of five schools having clinical years, and not under control of the Roman Catholic Church, reported instruction in the indications and technique of contraception or sterilization or both. Such teaching is not limited to any section of the country, nor to the larger institutions, and is found in both rural and urban areas. The report is based on replies from seventy-six Grade A schools to a questionnaire sent out by the National Committee on Maternal Health in 1933.

The Medical Society of Michigan in 1933 appointed a "Committee to Study Birth Control" from the section on obstetrics and gynecology. The committee began its work by the compilation of a bibliography of 1,800 books, articles and pamphlets, and five members were delegated "to investigate and summarize in writing the main phases of birth control . . . medical, legal, religious, social and economic." A questionnaire was sent to each member of the state medical society; another to heads of departments of obstetrics and gynecology in medical schools throughout the country, including a question on teaching. I quote a summary[85] by Dr. Louise Stevens Bryant, formerly Executive Secretary of the National Committee on Maternal Health:

Among 1,846 replies from members of the Michigan Society, 1,745 reported their attitude toward birth control, with 1,538 or 88 per cent. in favor. This proportion varied surprisingly little according to the particular interest of the doctors, ranging from 100 per cent. of those in tuberculosis work, to 96 in pediatrics, 90 in

[84] *Med. Jour. and Rec.*, xx (1930), 456.

[85] To be published soon in *Amer. Jour. Obstr. & Gyn.* This text varies slightly both from the National Committee's unpublished manuscript draft and from the original report in the *Jour. Mich. St. Med. Soc.*, xxxiii (March, 1934), 140–145.

gynecology and obstetrics, 89 in surgery, with 88 in internal medicine, neurology and psychiatry, and the lowest, 87 per cent., in general medicine. . . .

The great majority of the doctors in all areas reported the *practice* of contraception. Among 1775 replying to the question "Do you prescribe contraceptives in your practice?" 522 said no, including many who were not opposed in principle; while 1,233 said yes, 988 without qualifications and 245 specifying "under control," or "when the patient asks," or "when advisable." Acceptable *indications* were stated by 1,346, of whom 460 or about one-third gave contraceptive care for "health reasons only," and the rest for social, economic and health reasons in various combinations.

Objections were specified by 144 of the 207 who were not in favor of birth control, and the great majority, 84, being on religious or ethical grounds, with a second group of 49 for various reasons of social expediency, and only seven on grounds of health.

The questionnaire to the teachers of obstetrics and gynecology throughout the country elicited much the same sort of replies, with 38 out of 41 expressing approval, and practicing contraception, 27 prescribing with qualification; and 32 reporting in addition some teaching of contraceptive technique and indications, five specifying that "only general principles are discussed."

[Among the conclusions of the committee after studying the returns the following points were stressed:]

(1) An intense interest in birth control was shown throughout the state, with a majority of the profession favorable in attitude.

(2) Indications for the use of contraceptives vary, but it is generally believed that by careful use of contraceptive procedures the health of certain individuals afflicted with disease can be maintained at a higher level; and also that by the proper spacing of children and limitation of their numbers that a higher health level can be maintained by society in general. A more general use of contraception may aid in decreasing the incidence of abortions with their attendant fetal and maternal mortality and morbidity.

(3) [The legal status of birth control in Michigan is indicated by the statement of the Attorney General that] there is no law preventing the giving of birth control information or materials by physicians as professional advice. The Federal Law concerning the transmission of contraceptive information and material through the mails by inter-state commerce has practically been annulled by recent decisions of the Federal Courts.

(4) Opposition to Birth Control when expressed by religious bodies appears to be more concerned with *method* than with principles; family regulation through "natural methods" (abstinence, observance of the so-called period of "physiological sterility") is considered permissible, whereas "unnatural methods" (contraceptives) are condemned by these groups.

(5) [Among the comments on the social and economic aspects of birth control were these:] There is no positive evidence that "race suicide" has resulted from the use of contraceptives. It has been suggested that eugenic aims can best be realized by extending the knowledge of contraception to, or by enforcing sterilization upon, undesirable elements of society whose rate of propagation is in excess of the apparently more desirable classes. A judicious birth control program must, however, also combat voluntary and involuntary sterility among the eugenically more desirable elements if the harmful effect of a differential birthrate is to be overcome . . . .

This report was accepted by the Michigan State Society, and a standing "Committee on Maternal Health" appointed to continue the study of birth control and related subjects and to sponsor the recommended program, with special stress upon: (a) postgraduate teaching so that practitioners may be informed upon the most modern and scientific methods; (b) the reduction in both criminal and therapeutic abortions; and (c) the protection of society from commercial exploitation by unscrupulous and unqualified persons.

The speaking tours of Dr. J. F. Cooper, former medical director for the American Birth Control League, have been an important educational force among physicians outside of the literature. Since his death this work has been carried on by Dr. Eric Matsner, who has lately issued an admirable brief treatise on technique.[86]

No proof is needed that almost every one of the standard medical texts, including those on gynecology and obstetrics, omit discussion of contraceptive technique. It is gratifying to observe, however, that the new edition of Dr. Milton J. Rosenau's *Preventive Medicine* (just issued, 1935), does justice to the subject by including a chapter on technique from the pen of Dr. Eric Matsner. That the temper of opinion has changed rapidly in the last decade is shown also by the fact that Dr. Victor Robinson could secure as contributors to his ably-edited *Encyclopedia Sexualis* such outstanding men as Thomas Hunt Morgan, F. H. A. Marshall, F. A. E. Crew, Robert Briffault, Robert T. Frank, Smith Ely Jelliffe, to mention only a few. As I write (December 18, 1935) the *Encyclopedia* has not yet come from the press. But the prospectus leads me to believe that it may well prove to be the best work of its type ever published. This work is, so far as I know, the first treatise of its kind ever published in the United States. Ten years ago it simply could not have been produced.

In Germany as well as in the Anglo-Saxon countries the medical profession is beginning to take more interest in contraception. The 1931 meetings of the German Gynaecological Society devoted itself to contraception and many were the papers read, some by leading figures in Germany.[87] Though some of these are of interest, no paper presented compares in scientific importance with the recent papers on chemistry by Baker and Voge. Voge's *Chemistry and Physics of Contraceptives* and Baker's *Chemical Control of Conception* are the two leading works in their field.[88]

---

[86] Eric M. Matsner, The Technique of Contraception. An Outline. Foreword by Robert L. Dickinson. Introduction by Foster Kennedy. Published for the American Birth Control League by Williams & Wilkins, Baltimore, 1933, pp. 38.

[87] *Archiv. f. Gynäk.*, xliv (1931).

[88] Cecil I. B. Voge, *The Chemistry and Physics of Contraceptives*. London: Jonathan Cape, 1933, pp. 288. In the series of the National Committee on Maternal Health. John R. Baker, *The Chemical Control of Conception*. London: Chapman Hall, 1935, pp. x, 173.

That there has been notable advance in liberalization of medical opinion in the U. S. A. is shown also by the long list of medical and other groups that have endorsed repeal of the restrictive legislation. Such a list of endorsing organizations is to be found in the published report[89] of a governmental hearing and on a large sheet (34 by 21 inches) recently issued (1935) by the National Committee for Federal Legislation on Birth Control. On this last list probably a thousand organizations are listed, among them national, state and county medical societies and clubs, deans of medical schools, public health and nursing organizations and officials, social, educational and labor groups, business and professional women's clubs, parent-teacher associations, Junior Leagues, American Legion Auxiliaries, Rotary groups and political societies.

For a summary of the modern legal situation in the U. S. A. as it affects the physician the reader should consult the works by Dickinson and Bryant, C. H. Robinson, M. W. Dennett, W. J. McWilliams, Gladys Gaylord, Robert Homans, *et al*, and an anonymous article in the *Harvard Law Review*.[90]

Many sources declare that birth-control clinics started in Holland. In the strict sense of the term clinic—a medical center staffed with physicians where medical students are instructed—they did not start in Holland. To be sure, Dr. Aletta Jacobs opened the first systematic office work in contraception in Holland about 1881. But until recently there was no dispensary or hospital work in contraception. Two out of fifty of the "clinics" were served by midwives, the rest by workingmen's wives especially instructed, mainly by Dr. Rutgers.

Workers in Holland, however, gave much inspiration to the workers in other countries, to Mrs. Sanger and Dr. Haire especially. Now clinics are spread all over the world, though many regions have far too few.

In the early days of the Dutch Neo-Malthusian League the propaganda stressed dangers of over-population; latterly more emphasis has been given health considerations. The English and American propaganda organizations went through the same change of emphasis, save perhaps Dr. Stopes' group in England and Mrs. Dennett's Voluntary Parenthood League in the United States. However, both of these have been late developments. Dr. S. Van Houten, Minister of the Interior and later Prime Minister, was one of the most active people in Holland in public instruction back in the 'eighties and 'nineties, as was Pierson, the well-known Dutch economist, who frankly discussed the subject of birth control in his *Principles*.

[89] Birth Control Hearings before a Subcommittee of the Committee on the Judiciary United States Senate Seventy-first Congress Third Session on S. 4582 . . . (Washington: Gov't Pr't'g Off., 1931), pp. 5–7.

[90] *Har. Law. Rev.*, xlv (1932), 723–729. See Bibliography for other items.

The Dutch League early issued a medical pamphlet in which techniques were rather well outlined.[91] It described the usual devices such as the condom, sponge, rubber pessary, etc. It is especially worthy of note in view of recent chemical researches by Baker and Voge on the highly spermicidal effect of soapy solutions, that Dr. Rutgers as early as the eighteen eighties, recommended a vaginal plug of soap. Large numbers of the medical pamphlets were distributed.

Data are not at hand to prepare an adequate account of the history of contraception in Holland. From one point of view the developments are recent rather than historical events. Moreover, Holland's significance in the history of contraceptive development seems much more social than medical. Accordingly, the history of the Dutch propaganda work will receive attention in another volume.

The Scandinavian countries, being highly civilized, have done relatively little talking and writing about birth control. They have simply practised it for decades. Knut Wicksell, the economist, was the Swedish counterpart of John Stuart Mill, who defended birth control as early as 1825.[92] Many have followed Wicksell in defending the social case for birth control. I know of no medical handbook on contraception originating in Sweden, though there are doubtless translations. There are no important developments in Norway known to me. But in Denmark new energy has been introduced into the movement by the lectures and writings of Dr. Leunbach. Professor Brandt of Stockholm and Professor Gammeltoft of Copenhagen are fine examples of foreigners outstanding in gynecology and university life who took conception control as a matter of course in their teaching long before England, the United States, or Germany did.

§2   TWENTIETH CENTURY AUTHORS

(2a)   William J. Robinson (1869–1936)

One of the most indefatigable workers for contraception has been Dr. William J. Robinson. About 1904 he began a vigorous educational campaign in his little book, *Limitation of Offspring*, with its blank pages to impress one with the illegality of furnishing contraceptive advice in printed books. His periodicals, the *Critic and Guide* and the *American Journal of Urology*, more especially the former, carried the same message month after month along with other interesting, thoughtful and iconoclastic ideas. Dr. Robinson was not content simply to hold advanced views on contraception. With considerable courage and in innumerable ways he ventured to drive

---

[91] See the second and seventh items in the Bibliography under J. Rutgers.
[92] I shall eventually edit Mill's articles on birth control.

home the need of a sensible, reasonable attitude. And his efforts have borne fruit, as have the efforts of his predecessors, in a more enlightened public opinion. Particularly did Robinson protest against legal interference with the right of the physician to furnish contraceptive information when he felt it economically and medically indicated. Many were the letters received from every state in the union requesting contraceptive advice; and in 1916, in the *Medical Review of Reviews*, several of these were quoted. This was not, however, the first time that such letters of appeal had been published. The first record of their appearance was, to my knowledge, in Owen's *Moral Physiology* (1830 or 1831); then appeared Robinson's letters, and finally a whole volume of them in Margaret Sanger's *Motherhood in Bondage*.[93] Dr. Stopes in England then followed Mrs. Sanger by publishing *Mother England*.[94] A fuller account of Robinson's career will be found in Dr. F. M. Vreeland's thesis.

Robinson's influence was not confined to journal editorials and to popular sexological treatises of which latter he published nearly thirty. For in 1905 he isued to physicians a leaflet describing contraceptive techniques, and more recently has published a medical handbook.[95] It was he who induced Dr. Jacobi to take up birth control in his presidential address before the American Medical Association in 1912; and he became Jacobi's literary executor. Few American physicians of our time, save perhaps Dr. J. F. Cooper and R. L. Dickinson, have had more influence in moulding opinion on contraception than Robinson. His son, Dr. Victor Robinson, the medical historian, has also been active to a lesser degree. Dickinson has done much to "educate" the more prominent figures in medicine, Cooper has worked more with general physicians and with a clinic population, while Robinson has influenced not only physicians, but through his popular books, the general public.

(2b) *Abraham Jacobi (1830–1919) and William A. Pusey*

Two ex-presidents of the American Medical Association, Abraham Jacobi and William A. Pusey, have been in the vanguard striving to convince their colleagues that the medical profession should recognize and discharge its solemn obligations to preserve and further the public health by a judicious use of contraception. Dr. Jacobi was the first president of the American

---

[93] Margaret Sanger, *Motherhood in Bondage*. New York: Brentano, 1928, pp. xix' 3–446.

[94] Marie C. Stopes [Ed.], *Mother England. A Contemporary History Self-written by those who have had no historian*. London: Bale, 1929, pp. vi, 1–206.

[95] W. J. Robinson, *Practical Prevenception*. Hoboken, N. J.: American Biological Society, 1929, pp. v, 1–170.

Medical Association who courageously approved the limitation of offspring in his presidential address. In 1912 he spoke unequivocably, though in guarded language, in favor of contraception. A man of penetrating mind and a sensitive social conscience,[96] he had intelligence enough to know that a physician who practised in ignorance of social conditions would be apt to function blindly. Accordingly, he protested against inequalities in the distribution of wealth, and declared that it seemed "almost impossible" to prevent unnecessary physical and mental illness "as long as the riches provided by this world are accessible to a part of the living only."

The resources for prevention or cure [he continues] are inaccessible to many—sometimes even to a majority. That is why it has become an indispensible suggestion that only a certain number of babies should be born into the world. As long as . . . the well-to-do limit the number of their offspring, the advice to the poor . . . to limit the number of their children . . . is perhaps more than merely excusable. I often hear that an American family has had ten children, but only three or four survived. Before the former succumbed, they were a source of expense, poverty, and morbidity to the few survivors. For the interests of the latter, and the health of the community at large, they had better not have been born.[97]

Jacobi also recommended a certificate of freedom from venereal and transmissible disease prior to matrimony; and declared that the propagation of degenerates, imbeciles, and criminals should be prevented, presumably by sterilization, though this was not mentioned by name. Altogether it was a

[96] Jacobi opened the first free clinic for diseases of children in the U. S. A. Trained in Germany, he took part in the revolution of 1848, was jailed, escaped, fled to America. Boston was inhospitable in giving him practice, but he achieved in New York not only a large practice but international renown. In 1862 he founded the *American Journal of Obstetrics* (now the *Amer. Jour. Obst. & Gyn.*). At the New York Medical College he became the first professor of diseases of children in the U. S. A. Twice president of the American Pediatric Society, he also led the Association of American Physicians (1896), the New York Academy of Medicine (1885–1889), finally the American Medical Association (1912–1913). The *Festschrift* presented on his seventieth birthday, to which many European physicians contributed, is testimony to the international influence of his voluminous literary output and to the warm affection with which he was regarded. W. J. Robinson assembled in eight volumes his papers as *Collectiana Jacobi*. So young was he in body and mind at eighty-eight that he attended the annual A. M. A. meeting and took part in the proceedings. The children and mothers of America lost him in 1919.

For more information on Jacobi see *Lancet Clinic* (Cincinnati), May 14, 1910; *Amer. Jour. Obst.*, May, 1913; Francis Huber, in *The Child* (London), Dec. 1913; *Med. Life*, Oct., 1926; Victor Robinson, "The Life of A. Jacobi," *Ibid.*, May–June, 1928; *Med. Record*, July 19, 1919, July 24, 1920; *N. Y. Med. Jour.*, July 19, 1919; *Jour. Amer. Med. Asso.*, July 19, 1919; F. H. Garrison, "Dr. Abraham Jacobi," *Science*, Aug. 1, 1919; *Scientific Monthly*, Aug. 1919; N. Y. *Times*, July 12, 1919.

[97] *Critic and Guide*, xv, 240. For a full account see *Jour. Amer. Med. Asso.*, lviii, 23, June 8, 1912.

memorable, historic address. At the time, however, it caused no little discussion, and some protest, in medical circles.

Jacobi supported economic and social indications as well as medical indications not only in his presidential address but also in several published papers, of which a *Critic and Guide* article is an example. Though he was ever sensitive to the opposition of professional sentiment, he was courageous enough never to flinch from publicly avowing his soberly-arrived-at conclusions. He well knew that even the most reasoned case for birth control usually met with opposition, but added "yet no valid argument can be presented against it. It benefits the parents, it is decidedly beneficial to society, and it is even more merciful toward the unborn and unconceived creature, which is frequently saved from a life of misery. If we have no right to demand a sacrifice of the mother for the sake of the child, neither have we the right to demand sacrifices which, tho stopping short of being immediately fatal, nevertheless shorten and cripple the woman's life."[98] Jacobi further revived an old argument of Place's when he said that diffused contraceptive knowledge would doubtless contribute toward more hygienic sexual relations.[99]

Though W. A. Pusey was perhaps not as outspoken for birth control as Jacobi, he supported contraception and eugenics in his 1924 presidential address on the "Social Problems of Medicine" delivered before the American Medical Association.[100] And at the Sixth International Neo-Malthusian and Birth Control Conference, when he spoke on "Medicine's Responsibilities in the Birth Control Movement" he did likewise.[101] In the first address he gained the ear of his audience by opposing socialized medicine; then went on to urge the medical profession to take the lead in guiding birth control and eugenics. His support of birth control, curiously enough, was not mainly on health grounds, but was built rather on the more vulnerable point that if population growth were not slowed down the pressure on existence would become so intense that the death rate, particularly infant mortality, would overtake the birth rate and the population become stationary.[102] We now know that the post-war Malthusian fears were based upon fallacious extrapolation of past rates of growth and therefore exaggerated. More

---

[98] *Critic and Guide*, xv (1912), 463.

[99] *Ibid.*, p. 464.

[100] William Allen Pusey, Social Problems of Medicine. Address Before the American Medical Association at Chicago, June 9th and 10th, 1924. Chicago: Amer. Med. Asso. Press, 1924, pp. 1–33. See also *Jour. Amer. Med. Asso.*, lxxxiii, 1905–1908; 1960–1964.

[101] See *Birth Control Review*, ix (1925), 134–136, 156–158. Reprint by American Birth Control League, [1925], pp. 14. Also in [*Proceedings*] *Sixth International Neo-Malthusian and Birth Control Conference* (New York: A.B.C. League, 1926), iii, 19–30.

[102] Pusey, Social Problems, pp. 8–9.

sound was the central purpose of Pusey's presidential address: to emphasize "that the subject is of vast importance to the welfare of man; that it is one which should have scientific guidance; that for this medicine must be looked to and that medicine should undertake to approach its responsibilities here by beginning to give the subject the continuous and serious thought that it justifies."[103]   Pusey went on to declare that we are likely to be deluged with the unfit if steps are not taken to control their reproduction.   He affirmed that "Society will, and should, make every effort to do its best for its weaker members, but there is no good reason why it should not try to stem the tendency to the peopling of the earth by the defective, the unfit and the incompetent."[104]   The address contained some logical errors, but on the whole it was sound and forward-looking.

(2c)   The Career of Margaret Sanger

Though there is no intention of bringing this historico-medical chronicle down to date by including numerous contemporary figures—that will be done in a subsequent volume—and no intention of going into the social and economic history of contraception, this account would be incomplete without some attention to the career of Margaret Sanger, leading lay advocate of contraception in America.   Though she has done more than any other American to make birth control popularly known as a result of her educational or propaganda campaigns, it is in the medical aspects of her career that we are interested in the present volume.

A woman of great vision, personal courage and organizing ability she has been the central figure in organizing the American birth-control movement into a conscious unity.   It was in 1912 that, at considerable personal risk, she began in earnest her work for birth control.   Her life as a nurse in the poor quarters of the lower East side in New York had convinced her that in many instances mothers who needed contraceptive advice, not only for social and economic reasons but on the most conservative medical indications, were being refused such advice by physicians.   Accordingly, she took the reins into her own hands and began giving advice.   There was a grand plan for flooding the country with copies of her pamphlet, *Family Limitation*,[105] by releasing them for distribution from several geographical points at a given signal.   Though this plan fell through, *Family Limitation* was surreptitiously issued through a printer whose name to this day is a wellguarded secret.   Court difficulties impended; and there was a flight to Europe.   While Mrs. Sanger was abroad gaining more knowledge regarding

---

[103] *Ibid.*, p. 9.
[104] *Ibid.*
[105] See Bibliography for editions.

the latest developments in contraceptive technique, *Family Limitation* was getting well launched in popularity.   Eventually several hundred thousand copies were to be published in the U. S. A. and England, not alone in English but in many foreign languages.   It was about this time also that Mrs. Sanger published her first radical periodical, *The Woman Rebel*, several numbers of which were suppressed.   It advocated not only contraception but other radical economic reforms concerning which Mrs. Sanger today holds much more modified opinions.

Not often are reformers willing to go to jail for their opinions or for the cause which they represent.   But Mrs. Sanger was an exception.   Clearly the fact that she opened the first contraceptive advice station[106] in the U. S. A. in the Brownsville section of Brooklyn, N. Y. in 1916, marks a milestone in American contraceptive history.   Here a fair number of poor women were advised before the police closed the clinic as a public nuisance. Mrs. Sanger was, however, influential in securing a decision in the Court of Appeals because of which it is now possible for medical men and women of New York State to give contraceptive advice legally for "the cure and prevention of disease"—a term now very broadly interpreted.

It was not until 1923, when Mrs. Sanger was still president of the American Birth Control League (founded in 1917 as the National Birth Control League), that the New York Birth Control Clinical Research Bureau was opened as a department of the American Birth Control League.[107]   This has paved the way for approximately two hundred and twenty-five other clinics in the U. S. A., a few of which are not extramural clinics as is the New York Clinical Research Bureau, but connected with hospitals and dispensaries.[108]

The story of Mrs. Sanger's struggle for amendment of American legislation, her organization of several international birth-control conferences is a part rather of the social history of the movement.   The same is true of her organization of the World Population Conference in Geneva in 1927, from which there developed an important volume of proceedings[109] and the

[106] For the full story see M. Sanger, *My Fight for Birth Control*.   New York: Farrar & Rinehart, 1931, pp. vii, 3–360.   The sociologist is not interested in whether the Brownsville and later "clinics" may be so classed or not, since his interest is in the diffusion of knowledge.   It is not necessary that there should be medical teaching in a station to have a clinic in the American sense.   It need only be under medical direction.

[107] For a summary of case records on 10,000 cases, see Dr. Marie E. Kopp. *Birth Control in Practice*.   New York: McBride, 1934.

[108] For a fairly up-to-date list, see M. Sanger, *My Fight for Birth Control*; Dickinson & Bryant, *Control of Conception*, Appendix C, and the files of the *Birth Control Review*.   The clinic movement is progressing so rapidly in the U. S. A. that a list is out of date before it can be published.

[109] Margaret Sanger [Ed.], *Proceedings of the World Population Conference. . . . Geneva*, 1927.   London: Arnold, 1927, pp. 383.

organization of the International Union for the Scientific Investigation of Population Problems. The Population Association of America is a child, legitimate or illegitimate, of the latter.

The International Medical Group for the Investigation of Birth Control and the Birth Control Investigation Committee, both having headquarters in London, grew out of interests forwarded at the Geneva Conference. Dr. C. P. Blacker, who is secretary of the former, has issued on behalf of the Group a number of interesting annual reports (See Bibliography under Blacker). These summarize a great deal of recently published medical material on contraception. They also contain material not available elsewhere. Accordingly, the reports are of great interest to medical students of this subject.

Mrs. Sanger also organized the first international clinical conference in Zürich in 1930.[110] The Geneva and Zürich conferences were especially valuable because of some of the papers presented. Hence it is beyond question that Mrs. Sanger's activity in this field will give her a permanent place not only in social but in medical history.

Since she resigned the presidency of the American Birth Control League Mrs. Sanger has devoted her main energy to securing the passage of the "doctors only bill" in Washington. In her earlier efforts to secure the liberalization of statutes restricting the dissemination of contraceptive information, Mrs. Sanger devoted herself exclusively to the repeal of state laws. Latterly she has become convinced that since the state laws were modelled in part on the national Comstock legislation of 1873 restricting the use of the mails, and since states without laws were still subject to the Federal laws, more rapid progress could be made by appealing first to Washington. It is not our purpose here to record the difficulties involved in that enormous task. But it may be pointed out that those physicians who are inclined to view the career of Mrs. Sanger as that of an interfering laywoman, should remember that if they secure a clarification of statutes it will be largely through her indefatigable efforts; if not directly through her efforts, then through the public opinion which she has been a central agent in creating.

Members of the medical profession should also remember that Mrs. Sanger has from the first attempted to operate through the medical profession; that it has been largely as a consequence of their unwillingness to assist and lead that she has been forced to take this function of education upon herself. I am personally acquainted with most of the lay leaders of

[110] Margaret Sanger and Hannah M. Stone [Eds.], *The Practice of Contraception. An International Symposium and Survey*. Foreword by Robert L. Dickinson. Baltimore: Williams & Wilkins, 1931, pp. xviii, 3–316.

the birth-control movement in the United States and England. It is my judgment that no one has given of her time, limited physical energy (Mrs. Sanger at one time had active pulmonary tuberculosis) and money more unselfishly than Mrs. Sanger. Only reforming zeal and a firm conviction of ultimate triumph could enable one to surmount the obstacles and abuse she has met. Always level-headed, she has frequently sought the advice of scientific men. In this respect she has been an able leader. She picked her advisers carefully; then she usually, but not always, took their advice.

Mrs. Eleanor Robertson-Jones and Mrs. Francis N. Bangs, Mrs. Sanger's successors as presidents of the League, have continued the latter's educational work, concentrating upon the organization of state leagues, and the encouragement of clinics. Many more physicians have come in recent years to the League's point of view and have even taken an active part, especially in the clearly medical activities. The League has a medical advisory board containing many prominent medical names. Mrs. Jones has also stressed the eugenic implications of birth control and has worked for closer coöperation with groups interested in eugenical education.

The form of the *Birth Control Review* has changed. Since October, 1933, it has been essentially a news bulletin. Space being severely restricted, it has since become of much less value to serious students, though perhaps fulfilling the needs of the League more effectively.

Mrs. Sanger has recently started a service to the medical world in the form of a new periodical, the *Journal of Contraception* (first issue November, 1935). This is being edited by Dr. Abraham Stone, assisted by an editorial board of prominent physicians. The journal is beginning very modestly as an eight page monthly, at a low subscription price (one dollar a year) the purpose being to assist physicians in keeping informed on the latest developments in the field of contraceptive medicine. Besides brief articles, it contains abstracts. The American Birth Control League began issuing at the same time its *National Clinic Courier*, designed to serve essentially the same purpose.

Marriage Hygiene, a scientific quarterly published in Bombay, but having editors in several countries, is the only international journal in this field having the necessary space for scientific articles, many of them of a pure science character. Its emphasis is upon discovery rather than upon the diffusion of what is already known. Its book reviews especially are of a very high order, equalled in fact by those of very few medical journals published anywhere. It also runs the usual editorials, abstracts, and a section on World News. It welcomes contributions of high merit from physicians and scholars all over the world. The main editorial office is at Kodak House, Hornby Road, Bombay, India.

§3 NATIONAL COMMITTEE ON MATERNAL HEALTH, INC.

There has been only one organization in the United States under complete medical leadership doing active work in the interests of control of conception, which has maintained full time offices and salaried secretarial staff, and laid its emphasis on research and publication rather than on clinical service, carrying on actively for a dozen years.

Starting in March, 1923, at the instigation of Mrs. Gertrude Minturn Pinchot, the Committee on Maternal Health insisted on tying birth control, the emergency measure, to marriage problems in general, to sterilization, abortion and sterility, to normal sex function and anatomical structure.

It has issued a large number of papers and reports and by 1936 will have in its series twelve volumes which are of basic importance in the study of medical aspects of sex life. Five of these are on birth control and the sterilization volume is under way.

In 1930 the committee was incorporated as the National Committee on Maternal Health, Inc. The offices for eight years have been in the New York Academy of Medicine (with the President of the Academy as Chairman of the Committee for five years). Its Secretary for eleven years was a full time volunteer, Dr. R. L. Dickinson, a former clinical professor of gynecology and obstetrics, ex-President of the American Gynecological Society. The Executive Secretaries were first, Gertrude Sturges, M.D., second, for eight years, Louise Stevens Bryant, Ph.D. in medical sciences, with invaluable experience in biology, statistics, publication and the law courts. The Medical Executive Secretary is now Raymond Squier, M.D., gynecologist and obstetrician at Bellevue and Lenox Hill Hospitals, formerly at Johns Hopkins.

The books above referred to are these: *Seventy Birth Control Clinics*, by Caroline H. Robinson; *Control of Conception*, by Robert L. Dickinson and Louise Stevens Bryant; *The Chemistry and Physics of Contraceptives*, by Cecil I. B. Voge; the present volume; *Time of Ovulation in Women*, by Carl G. Hartman; and another under way, *Sterilization*: *Medical Aspects of the Subject*, by Howard C. Taylor, Jr.

§4 GERMAN AND OTHER WRITERS

Before considering the modern German writers, which is the main purpose of this section, I shall devote special attention to the two most important German pioneers, Friedrich Adolph Wilde and Mensinga.

In 1838, in a gynecological treatise of considerable importance,[111] but now

---

[111] Friedrich Adolph Wilde, *Das weibliche Gebär-unvermögen. Eine medicinisch-juridische Abhandlung zum Gebrauch für practische Geburtshelfer, Aerzte und Juristen.* Berlin, 1838, pp. xvi, 1–413.

long since forgotten, Wilde describes a rubber cervical cap specially moulded to fit each individual case. Moll in 1912[112] and Stopes in 1931[113] have erred in concluding that Wilde anticipated Mensinga in recommending what is now known as the Mensinga or Dutch pessary. On the contrary, Wilde advised a rubber cervical cap similar to that now used in Dr. Stopes's clinic.

Wilde's gynecological treatise, which is notable for its preventive point of view and for a discussion of indications for contraception, treats not only of magical, ineffective measures (reported within on p. 113) but mentions the condom, withdrawal, sponge and rubber cap. He thinks the condom tears easily; and that both the condom and withdrawal are ineffective. Perhaps Wilde had experience with a poor grade of condom. In his day rubber ones were hardly available as yet.

Wilde scouts the idea that prevention is morally censurable especially when medically indicated, and declares that "a prophylactic procedure against pregnancy under such circumstances is not only completely justifiable, but might rather be approved on grounds of morality in preference to a dangerous Caesarian section."[114] He contends that the methods known in his time (1838), withdrawal, the condom and sponge, are insufficiently reliable. Hence many physicians advise continence; but this invariably falls on deaf ears. It is much better to use a rubber cervical cap specially moulded to fit each individual case:

On that account [inability to be continent in marriage] it would be highly desirable in such cases to become acquainted with a thoroughly reliable and practicable method for the prevention of pregnancy. For this reason the author counsels that such persons who are affected with an inability to bear should constantly wear a rubber pessary (ein Pessarium aus Resina elastica), which has no opening, which completely covers the os, fits snugly, and which is taken off only during the menses. In order that it may suit every individual case just right, it must be made from a special model made each time by taking a wax impression of the parts by use of a vaginal speculum. This rubber pessary (Cautschuk-Pessarium) would be less troublesome and uncomfortable than any other kind of cervical cap (Mutterkränze). That such a method can, in a limited way, effectively protect from conception is shown clearly and certainly by the example cited by von Hufeland: "A certain section of the rural area showed a striking decline in the number of children. Most of the farming families had only two or three children, and then no more. More thorough inquiry disclosed that a midwife possessed this secret. Unknown to the woman, she placed, at the end of delivery, a foreign body in front

---

[112] *Handbuch*, Leipzig, 1912, p. 452.

[113] Marie C. Stopes, "Zur Geschichte der vaginalen Kontrazeption," *Zbl. f. Gynäk.* (Leipzig), lv (1931), 2549–2551. Reprinted in English as "Early Vaginal Contraceptives," in *Clinical Med. and Surgery*, xxxviii (1931), 889–891.

[114] Wilde, *op. cit.*, p. 317.

of the os which occluded the entrance."[115]   Something similar must be the custom elsewhere in Germany because women, when they wish to avoid pregnancy, introduce a piece of sponge into the vagina before coitus, and, in so doing, occlude the os—a method which might very often fail of its purpose.[116]

C. A. Weinhold,[117] a contemporary of Wilde, recommended a male method genuinely bizarre: infibulation, which dates at least from Roman times.[118]   Weinhold, a staunch German Malthusian, urged that boys be required to wear, from the age of fourteen onward, until they had sufficient income to marry and found a family, a ring through the prepuce, inserted after it is pulled over the glans.   The lead wire perforating the prepuce is twisted, soldered and stamped with a seal which is retained so that the ring cannot be unfastened and the stamp duplicated.   Such was Weinhold's grand specific for preventing overpopulation!   It is just one more bit of evidence of the absurd extremes to which mankind will go in seeking to control sexual expression.[119]   Public authorities were to see to it that the young men did not set themselves free.   And there were to be fines, thrashings, and even imprisonment as punishment for doing so!   Those who never acquired sufficient wealth to maintain a family were to wear it throughout life.   Weinhold even worked out a system of gruesome punishments for

[115] *Journal der practischen Heilkunde*, lvi (Jan. 1823), 10.   [Hufeland's paper, "Von dem Rechte des Arztes über Leben und Tot," was mainly concerned with showing the harmfulness of *coitus interruptus* on the nervous system and as a cause of impotence.]

[116] *Op. cit.*, pp. 317–318.   It is interesting to note that Wilde also mentions sterilization by extirpation of the uterus and by excision of a portion of the Fallopian tubes.   Some physicians in his day must have held that extirpation of the clitoris prevented conception.   Wilde usefully pointed out that this was erroneous.

[117] For a good secondary account see Felix A. Theilhaber, "Ein deutscher Malthus. Vorschläge aus dem Jahre 1828 gegen die Übervölkerung Europas," *Ztschr. f. Sexualwissensch.*, xviii (1931), 45–50.   See Theilhaber for the titles to the original works which are too long to cite here.   The chief one is: *Über des menschliche Elend welches durch den Missbrauch der Zeugung herbeigefuhrt wird.*   Leipzig, 1828.

[118] Celsus said that the Romans infibulated as follows: the prepuce was drawn over the glans and two threads were drawn through the prepuce and moved mechanically backward and forward each day until two openings were made into which a ring could be placed. (See J. Heller, "Ein Beitrag zur Geschichte der Infibulation," *Archiv. f. Frauenkunde*, xiii, 276 ff.)   Heller describes an infibulation ring from East Turkestan which dates from 700 B.C.   Correspondingly the girdle of chastity was used in the Middle Ages.   See Eric John Dingwall, *The Girdle of Chastity; A Medico-Legal Study.*   London: Routledge, 1931, pp. x, 171.   For a short account see E. J. Dingwall, "The Girdle of Chastity" in *Proc. Sec. Int'l Cong. for Sex Research*, (A. W. Greenwood, ed.), pp. 586–591.   Hirschfeld's *Geschlechtskunde* must also discuss this subject; but it is not available as I write.   *Cf.*, *Encyclopedia Sexualis*.   New York: Dingwall-Rock, 1936.

[119] For more of them on the legal side see Geoffrey May, *The Social Control of Sex Expression*.   New York: Morrow.

those who would dare to break the seal.   Though Weinhold had no economic training (he was a physician) and though there is no evidence that he ever read Malthus, he wrote "Whoever cannot nourish a family is denied the enjoyments of marriage.   This principle must be considered, for heavily populated states, an iron rule; it cannot be given up, for without it the whole society cannot stand."   Weinhold had some sound ideas on population theory, but people would not listen to him because (partly) of his impractical support of infibulation.

While Weinhold's suggestion always remained a laughable, unapplied curiosity, Wilde's modest and forgotten recommendation of a cervical cap was ultimately to find wide usage in Europe and the United States during the nineteenth century and subsequent decades.   It was quite widely used until the Mensinga diaphragm came on the market.   As indicated previously, Stopes's clinic and her books champion the cap; and many were the references to it in medical literature published in the United States during the nineteenth century. Presumably the fact that it was made in few sizes facilitated self-fitting.   The Mensinga, which was ultimately to displace it in popularity, is now produced in many sizes making accurate fitting by skilled hands more imperative.

The Mensinga diaphragm which is not a cervical cap, but which fits longitudinally in the vagina, the forward end under the pubic bone, the back end in the posterior fornix, was ultimately destined to find most general favor in our time among clinic physicians.   It is used in nearly every clinic as the preferred method, the medication varying.   This instrument, sometimes known also as the Dutch pessary, because Dr. Rutgers and his followers in Holland did much to make it well known, was invented by Dr. Mensinga (pseudonym Karl Hasse or C. Hasse) formerly of Flensburg (near the Danish border), subsequently Professor of Anatomy at Breslau.   He not only described its use but in various publications,[120] he dealt in some detail with its medical indications accompanied by rather full contraceptive case histories.   These were much more systematic, more complete than any published previously.   In fact they are the first published ones worthy of the name.

Knowledge of the new device, first made known in the early eighteen eighties, spread especially to Holland, only several decades later to England, while in the U. S. A. it was hardly known until 1920, if we omit random exceptions.   I am thinking now of knowledge of physicians, especially birth-control clinic physicians.   Even today, fifty years after its invention, the Mensinga pessary is by no means the contraceptive most commonly employed by the general populace.   Certainly the condom is, *coitus interruptus*

---

[120] See Bibliography for titles.

exceeding it in frequency of use so far as non-mechanical measures are concerned.

More recent events will now receive summary consideration.

Modern German writers on the general theory of birth control, and especially on the declining birth rate and the ways to combat it or encourage it, are legion. Baum has recently published a doctoral thesis[121] (Leipzig) on Neo-Malthusianism; and he was preceded by many other writers, mostly non-academic.[122]

Inasmuch as the nineteenth-century German writers covered much the same ground as their American and English colleagues, there is no need to treat here in detail the technique recommended by these writers.[123] One might mention a few, mostly physicians, who have produced separate treatises, usually pamphlets of less than one hundred pages. A few are the authors of books. The following list does not include approximately a hundred contributors to medical journals; for these consult the Bibliography. Besides the authors of certain anonymous and pseudonymous pamphlets, we have works by Adolf, Albert, Baum, Bendix, Bock, M. Braun, R. Braun, Brupbacher, Damm, Ferch (really an Austrian), Ferdy (pseud.), Fraenkel, Freygang, Gall, Gerhard, Gerlach, Gerling, Gerson, Goldstein, Gräfenburg, Grotjahn, Haire (English), Hardy (French pseud. for Giroud), Harter, Hartmann, Hasse (i.e., Mensinga), Hellmuth, Henkel, Hettler, Hinz, Hirsch, Hirschfeld, Holländer, Holmes (trans. of English work), Hüfler, Justus, Kamp, Kramer, Krüger-Letau, Ladewig, Lesser, Leunbach (a Dane), Lewis, Levitt, McArdle (an American), Mack, Max Marcuse, Julian Marcuse, a writer using the pseudonym Matrisalus, Mensinga (pseud. K. Hasse), A. Müller, Heinrich Müller, Naujoks, Otto, Prager, Protz, Rossen, Ruben-Wolf, Rutgers (Dutch), Schadlitzer, Schröder, Schweitzer, Serson, Souveur, Stopes (English), Theilhaber, Treu, Wald, Werner, Wilde, Winkler, Wurzberger, Zadek, Zikel, and Zschommler.[124] There are many others.

This list includes a few non-Germans, some of whose works appear in

---

[121] Fritz Baum, *Über den praktischen Malthusianismus, Neo-Malthusianismus und Sozialdarwinismus*. Leipzig, 1928, pp. vii, 1–134. Plate. This is hardly a very substantial contribution; but it naturally contains some information of value.

[122] Olberg, *Über den Neo-Malthusianismus*, 1906, pp. 846. Fahlbeck, "Der Neo-Malthusianismus," *Zeitschr. f. Sozialwissenschaft*, vi (1913), 638. Stille, *Der Neo-Malthusianismus, das Heilmittel des Pauperismus*. Berlin, 1880. Kötzsche, *Die Gefahren des Neu-Malthusianismus*, Berlin, 1895.

[123] I know virtually nothing of the nineteenth century writers on technique publishing in Eastern Europe, especially Russia. But it would be odd if they did not cover much the same ground as the other Europeans. Probably also they were less numerous and less influential, as we might infer from the higher birth rate in Eastern and Southern Europe. Chief among the modern Russian writers are E. J. Kvater and C. A. Selitzky.

[124] See these names in the Bibliography.

German. As stated above, it is confined almost entirely to those who have produced separate treatises. At least several score more have discussed contraception in various technical and learned journals. The above are of peculiar interest to the sociologist in that they represent, with a few exceptions, popularization—an attempt to democratize this knowledge, and to bring it to the masses. With a few exceptions all the authors are physicians. Perhaps the most important figures in the list are Wilde, Fraenkel, Ferdy, Grotjahn, Gräfenburg, Hardy, Hirschfeld, Holländer, Mensinga, Marcuse; and, if we were to include foreigners publishing also in German, Haire, Stopes, and perhaps Leunbach.

In striking contrast to the prolific output of German physicians in this field, both in the form of popular pamphlets for sale directly to laymen and in the form of contributions to standard medical journals, stands that of the Italians. Though I have not made a thorough inquiry into the historical development of thought on birth control in Italy, a preliminary investigation suggests that little literature of value on contraceptive technique has been published there. Allbutt tells[125] us that Dr. Giovanni Tari of Naples published a Malthusian tract in 1880 entitled (in English) "The Way to Limit the Family in Accordance with the Teachings of Economical Science, Morality, and Sexual Hygiene;" but I have never seen a copy. Morghen published a popular, "practical" pamphlet in 1900,[126] and a woman physician, Ettorina Cecchi, followed about 1916.[127] Though these are the only Italian pamphlets on technique that have come to my attention, it would seem that a few must have been published in recent years.

About a score of articles on birth control have appeared since 1900 in the Italian medical journals by such authors as Castoro, Cristalli, De Camillis, Levi, Mazzeo, Nardi, Rizzacasa, Verney and Viglino,[128] but none meet the most ordinary standards. There has also been translated into Italian the altogether atrocious treatise on conjugal frauds originally published in French by Bergeret (See Bibliography). The Italian medical-journal articles on contraception are, in general, uninforming, verbose, illogical and invariably anti-birth control. These writers often give much lip-service to eugenics; yet none manifest even an elementary understanding of the relation between contraception and racial selection and improvement. If

[125] H. A. Allbutt, *Artificial Checks* (London, 1889), p. 20.

[126] Guglielmo Morghen, Mezzi preventivi per impedire il concepimento nelle donne deboli malate. Roma: Capaccini, 1900, pp. 61.

[127] Ettorina Cecchi, *Neo-Malthusianismo Pratico.* Quarta edizione. Florence: Istituto Editoriale "Il Pensiero," n.d. (c. 1916), pp. 120. Ch. vii (pp. 76–102) is on "Mezzi per regolare e impedire concepimento," while the last chapter gives much interesting material of an historical nature.

[128] See the literature cited under these names in the Bibliography.

this statement seems exaggerated, let the reader refer to the average Italian journal articles on the subject.

The fact, however, that the birth-rate in Italy continues to fall suggests that the inhabitants are gradually learning about contraceptive techniques somehow. One suspects that information is gradually being diffused even under the suppression of the Mussolini regime and the dominance of the Catholic Church. Injurious methods are probably more resorted to in Italy than in modern Germany or England. Superstitious methods are still tolerably general, and there is reason to believe that the diffusion of contraceptive instruction is more out of the control of the medical profession than in Germany, England, the Scandinavian countries, or the United States. On grounds of general social policy these circumstances are unfortunate.

No attempt is made in this work so much as to list and classify, much less to essay a critical interpretation of the relative values of, modern contraceptive practices. All this will be found in the works of Grotjahn,[129] Stopes,[130] Cooper,[131] Fielding (pseud.),[132] Konikow,[133] Dickinson and Byant,[134] Butterfield,[135] Haire,[136] Stone,[137] Holländer,[138] Hirschfeld,[139] Fraenkel,[143] W. J.

[129] Alfred Grotjahn, *Geburten-Rückgang und Geburten-Regelung im Lichte der individuellen und der sozialen Hygiene.* Berlin: Marcus, 1914, pp. xiv, 371.

[130] Marie C. Stopes, *Contraception: Its Theory, History, and Practice.* London: Bale, 1923, pp. xxiii, 1–417. New York: Putnam, 1931.

[131] James F. Cooper, *Technique of Contraception.* New York: Day-Nichols, 1928, pp. xvi, 1–271.

[132] Michael Fielding [Pseud. for a prominent English physician], *Parenthood: Design or Accident?* (Preface by H. G. Wells), London: Noel-Douglas, 1930, pp. 168. New York: Vanguard.

[133] Antoinette F. Konikow, *Physicians' Manual of Birth Control.* New York: Buchholz Publishing Co., 1931, pp. xiii, 3–245.

[134] Robert L. Dickinson and Louise Stevens Bryant, *The Control of Conception.* Baltimore: Williams & Wilkins, 1931, pp. xii, 1–290.

[135] Oliver M. Butterfield, Marriage. Some Practical Suggestions for Happy Married Living, pp. 48. With a special medical supplement: Some Suggestions Concerning Contraception, pp. 12. Obtainable from the author, Monterey Park, California.

[136] Norman Haire, "Contraceptive Technique: A Consideration of 1,400 Cases," *Practitioner*, cxi (1923), 74–90. "Hygienic Methods of Family Limitation," London: New Generation League, [1922], pp. 19. "The Comparative Value of Current Contraceptive Methods." Reprint of paper read before the Internationalen Kongress für Sexualforschung at Berlin, October, 10–16, 1926 Berlin u. Köln: A. Marcus & E. Weber, 1928, pp. 117–127.

[137] Hannah M. Stone, "Contraceptive Methods: A Clinical Survey." New York: Birth Control Clinical Research Bureau, [1927], pp. 16. "Therapeutic Contraception," *Med. Jour. & Rec.*, March 21, 1928. For other medical works see Bibliography.

[138] Michael Holländer, *Vorbeugung der Empfängnis und Verhütung der Schwangerschaft.* Leipzig u. Wien: Schneider, 1927 and later, pp. 128.

[139] Magnus Hirschfeld & Richard Linsert, *Empfängnis-Verhütung. Mittel und Methoden.* 6 Aufl. Berlin: Neuer Deutscher Verlag, 1930, pp. 48.

Robinson[140] and, for the latest chemical investigations, the works of J. R. Baker[141] Cecil I. B. Voge,[142] Poehlmann, Steinhäuser, Günther and Rodecurt.

Gräfenburg made famous the Gräfenburg intra-uterine silver ring, but uses it less often since he found that only twenty-five per cent of his cases adapt to it. Dr. Leunbach of Copenhagen, who had previously reported on it rather favorably, has also given it up. Haire, however, is still (1933) carrying on an experimental series in London. W. J. Robinson condemned it from the first and R. L. Dickinson early pointed out that, at best, the ring could be used in not over forty per cent of the uteri, the others being so shaped as to expel it or to be injured by it.

In the field of German medical manuals on contraceptive technique that by Julius Fraenkel of Breslau,[143] published in 1932, takes first rank. As has been shown above, it was preceded by about forty other treatises, mostly pamphlets addressed to laymen. Fraenkel's book is, however, a medical handbook. His high standing adds prestige to the subject.

No special investigation has been made by the writer on the diffusion of contraceptive information in Austria; but the fragmentary material possessed may be put on record here. In 1910 an anarchist paper, *Welfare for All*, published a series of frank Neo-Malthusian articles. Though these were confiscated, some reached subscribers. About this time a little green leaflet entitled *Directions for Mothers and Women*, which frankly gave contraceptive advice and instruction, was distributed gratuitously. Ramus informs us that one Joseph . . . . . [the surname has not been made public] published about this time the first Neo-Malthusian pamphlet appearing in Austria. It was confiscated. After the Revolution a "League Against Enforced Motherhood" was formed. In this decade certain anarchists published a pamphlet of which 20,000 copies were distributed, and a second issue of 20,000 was printed in 1920.

A layman, Johann Ferch, has been one of the most active workers in

[140] William J. Robinson, *Practical Prevenception*. Hoboken, N. J.: Amer. Biol. Soc., 1929, pp. v, 1–170.

[141] *Jour. Hyg.*, xxix (1930), 323–329; xxxi (1931), 189–214; 309–320; xxxii (1932), 171–183; 550–556. Also see Bibliography.

[142] Cecil I. B. Voge, *The Chemistry and Physics of Contraception*. London: Jonathan Cape, 1933, pp. 288. Compare also his "Future Research upon Sterilization and Contraception," in Sanger and Stone [Eds.], *Practice of Contraception*, pp. 76–90. "Natural Infertility. Factors Influencing the Results of Contraceptive Methods," *Eugenics Review*, xxxv (1933), 85–90. "Contraception," *Brit. Med. Jour.*, May 27, 1933. For later papers see Bibliography.

[143] Ludwig Fraenkel, *Die Empfängnisverhütung. Biologische Grundlagen, Technik und Indikationen, für Ärtze bearbeitet.* Stuttgart: Enke, 1932, pp. 212.

Austria in recent years. He has written not only upon contraceptive technique, but has been active in founding and supervising clinics.

The chief opposition to the spread of contraceptive knowledge in Austria has come from the Church and from the Communists and Socialists.

A sketch of recent developments would be incomplete without mention of a tendency new in contraceptive history at least so far as its extent and emphasis is concerned. This is diffusion of contraceptive knowledge commercially by medical pamphlets and by large-scale sale of numerous devices.

§5 COMMERCIALIZATION OF CONTRACEPTIVE INSTRUCTION

The failure of the medical profession to accept leadership in contraceptive instruction has undoubtedly played a part in the tremendous increase in recent years in the commercial and sometimes anti-social dissemination of such advice. Several of the English newspapers carry advertisements of wholesale and retail distributors of contraceptive supplies; and for a penny or two one can secure by mail descriptive medical literature and supply catalogues. The London *Daily Herald*, a labor newspaper, in 1927, for example, carried nearly half a column of such advertisements. I replied to them all, and received a considerable body of literature.[144] A popular almanac thrown annually on the doorsteps and down the areaways of London houses, the distribution of which must run into several millions, contained large numbers of advertisements of firms distributing contraceptive supplies and abortifacient pills. The traffic in this business must be very considerable; but to date I have not had the opportunity to compile statistics.[145] There is some doubt whether the confidential figures would be

[144] Among the commercial pamphlets on technique are the following: C. F. Wilson ("with the collaboration of experts"), *Practical Birth Control and Instructions for Working Mothers*. Bristol: Blake's Medical Stores [1926], pp. 32 [marked 6d., but actually free through post]. Annie Phelps, *Birth Control and What it Means*. Preface by Ahluwalia Gopalji. London: Kingsland Hygienic Co. [1926], pp. 23. Douglas Neal, *A Manual of Wisdom*. Dr. Oster Mann, *Birth Control*. London: Marble Arch Pharmacy, 1926, pp. 64. Dr. St.Clair Maurice, *Advice to Married Women*. London: Medical Publishing Co. [1926], pp. 16. "An Eminent London Physician," *A Practical Treatise on Birth Control*. London: S. Seymour [1926], pp. 16. Advertising copies of the following pamphlets are also distributed: Dr. A. H. Allbutt's *The Wife's Handbook*, Margaret Sanger's *Family Limitation*, M. C. Stopes's *A Letter to Working Mothers*. Margaret V. Graham, *A Common-Sense Treatise on Birth Control*. London: Bale, 1926, pp. 16.

[145] The Report of the *Royal Commission on the Decline in the Birth-Rate and on the Mortality of Infants in New South Wales* (Sydney, 1904, 2 vols.) contained a great deal of evidence on the commercial distribution of contraceptives. Under "Preventives" the index contains five folio pages of references, under "Limitation of Families" seven folio pages of references. Retail druggists ("chemists"), wholesalers, manufacturers and importers were subpoenaed to give testimony in 1903. There is more opinion than

forthcoming. At all events, it is clear that the commerical business in England, and recently in the U. S. A. is considerable.

The subject of the commercial dissemination of contraceptive knowledge has received almost no study in recent years; and such inquiry is highly desirable. Mr. Randolph Cautley, however, has done some able work in this field for the National Committee on Maternal Health. (See Chapter VIII, §§ 5 and 6, *infra* and "Commercialization" in the Index. *Cf.* also our joint article in the *Encyclopedia Sexualis*.) Control will be bungling until such time as we secure an adequate basis of fact for action.

This is not to suggest, however, that all this traffic, perhaps even the majority of it, is unethical. Increasingly, among the better manufacturers in England, there is growing up a certain *esprit de corps* designed to protect the legitimate interests of the business and the public. Some of the English firms have been in business for many years and are anxious to coöperate with the medical profession in standardizing products and in maintaining high ethical business standards.

On the other hand, London and undoubtedly many provincial towns have a large number of retail distributors of contraceptive supplies which are advertised in the windows in the most blatant fashion. The illustration below well illustrates the nature of this commercialization. Practically all of these "rubber shops" distribute free literature, and some distribute literature advertising pills for female illnesses and to restore regularity. They are, of course, by design abortifacient. Cases have been reported to me in which poor women have been charged ten shillings for a box of such

---

science in the verbose, bulky report, but it is of great interest for this subject. The Commission might have secured more information of great scientific and sociological value had it not been completely dominated by the fixed idea that prevention is invariably immoral, indecent and obscene. Many questions asked witnesses were leading questions designed to elicit the response desired. Even some of the statistical charts and inferences are absurd. For example, the negative correlation of the increase of insanity with the decline of the birth rate leads to the inference that the increased adoption of prevention is responsible for the increased insanity! Despite its unscientific procedure, the Commission learned something.

Legally, dissemination has been unrestricted in New South Wales, and in Australia generally, where English law and traditions prevail. Except for minor skirmishes the law in the case Ex Parte Collins, for distributing Annie Besant's *Law of Population*, has prevailed. According to testimony before the Commission the sale, and especially the importation, of contraceptives was not great, though nearly everyone agreed they were increasing. Sheaths and Rendell's quinine suppositories were the chief items imported. The figures of the Commission, though interesting, are no guide to retail consumption. Hence they are not used here.

The Commission *Report* is difficult to procure. It was ordered published but distribution restricted. The Surgeon General's Library has a copy.

pills, and told that if they did not operate satisfactorily to return for a box of stronger pills. For these a charge of fifteen shillings was made. The client was again told that if they did not prove satisfactory, she should return for another box. These were the strongest and sold for a pound.

A rather unique case of the commercial diffusion of contraceptive information in England is the publication and gratuitous distribution by Lambert & Co., of the *Wife's Adviser*.[146] This is given away at the Wives' Clinic, an institution commercially-owned and operated by that manufacturer. The clinic was first opened by Dr. Marie C. Stopes in 1921 as the first contracep-

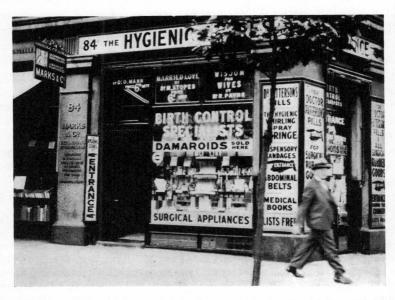

Fig. XX. Shop of a London Commercial Retailer of Contraceptives

tive clinic in England, and is located in the northern part of London. When Dr. Stopes wished to move to a more central location in London near the poor quarters, she sold the establishment to Lambert, the well-known manufacturer of contraceptive supplies, who uses it as a retail outlet for contraceptive supplies. The pamphlet, distributed in large numbers, contains up to page twenty reading matter on contraception; the rest is a catalogue of supplies. Though it is a commercial tract designed to advertise the

[146] Edward Joshua Lambert, *The Wife's Adviser. An up-to-date handbook . . . [containing] also a few notes on contraception.* London: Wives' Clinic, 1927, pp. 48.

clinic, it does not seem in bad taste.   The pamphlet has an excellent picture of the interior of the clinic.

Typical of the commercial distribution of contraceptive information are the advertisements in numerous women's magazines in the United States advertising literature on "feminine hygiene," that is, douching with anti-septics.   This type of advertisement thrives in the United States where the whole subject of birth control is more or less under cover, and operating under legal disabilities.   Not only the women's magazines but countless cheap magazines found on the public newsstands of large cities contain advertisements of such "feminine" procedures, the advertisements being interleaved with announcements of fake aphrodisiacs, secret love powders, perfumes, and potions.

The manufacturers of Lysol have been running a series of full-page adver-tisements on feminine hygiene in women's magazines of which the excerpt below is an example.   Under the following caption the advertisement quotes from a Lysol Co. booklet presumably prepared by a Parisian woman gyne-cologist:

> "The most frequent eternal triangle
> A HUSBAND . . . A WIFE
> and her
> F E A R S"

"Fewer marriages would flounder around in a maze of misunderstanding and unhappiness if more wives knew and practiced regular marriage hygiene.

"Without it, some minor physical irregularity plants in a woman's mind the fear of a major crisis.   Let so devastating a fear recur again and again, and the most charming and gracious wife turns into a nerve-ridden, irritable travesty of herself.   Bewildering, to say the least, to even the kindest husbands.   Fatal, inevitably, to the beauty of the marriage relation.

"It all sounds very dreadful, doesn't it?   But it needn't happen.   The proper technique of marriage hygiene, faithfully followed, replaces fear with peace of mind.   Makes what seems a grave problem no problem at all.

"What is the proper technique?   To my practice I recommend the 'Lysol' method.   I know that 'Lysol' destroys germs in the presence of organic matter, not just on a glass slide.   I know that it has high penetrating power, reaching into every fold and crevice.   And I further know that with all its power, it is very gen-tle.   Soothing and healing enough, for example, to be used in childbirth cases. You see there is no free caustic alkali, such as you find in chlorine compounds [such as Zonite], to inflame tender feminine tissue.

" 'Lysol' makes the whole ritual of feminine hygiene refreshing and agreeable. It contributes to a woman's sense of fastidiousness, as well as to her freedom from fear.   It's a dainty and cleanly habit . . . and a wise one, if health and harmony are to dwell with her throughout her married life."[147]

[147] *McCalls*, July, 1933, p. 85.

Such advertisements are good examples of the antisocial effects of the legislative disabilities under which contraception operates in the United States. They have tremendously increased douching with strong coal-tar disinfectants.   There are instances on record in the medical literature of such douching solutions having unfortunate effects especially when, either through ignorance or through ordinary mistakes, they are used in too strong concentration.   Both Dickinson and Haire distinctly warn against the use of such solutions.   Yet injury is being done because American women are hampered in free access to reliable medical knowledge and because practices are not always guided by competent medical advice.

The diffusion of contraceptive information through commercial and noncommercial channels has been supplemented in recent years by the work of numerous clinics.   It was inevitable that such diffusion should not be limited to the offices of private physicians, to printed pamphlets, to commercial prodding and encouragement, not even to putting patients in touch with physicians by mailing names and addresses from the office of a birth control league, but that a systematic attempt should be made to get this knowledge, through clinics, to the classes who needed it most—physicians to give advice even though the organizing and financing board was made up of laymen and lay women.   To the proof that the clinical work represents a diffusion downward of contraceptive knowledge, a democratizing process, we now turn.

PART SIX

DEMOCRATIZATION AND ITS
FUTURE EFFECTS

CHAPTER XIII

THE RESULT: DEMOCRATIZED BIRTH CONTROL

§1 INTRODUCTION

UP TO this point there has been an attempt to show that the desire to control conception is a well-nigh universal phenomenon; further that even the means of fulfilling the desire have been much more generally known than has commonly been assumed; that fragmentary knowledge of contraceptive means has existed in all major cultures throughout the entire range of social development.

To be sure, there is an important distinction between the desire for control, on the one hand, and its complete or partial achievement on the other. And though the actual methods have often been magical, with a gradual trend throughout history toward their rationalization and scientific improvement, we have seen that even in the very earliest days of man (as represented by contemporary societal fossils, primitive societies), rational, and theoretically effective techniques were by no means absent. Among the Egyptians, and, to a greater extent, among the Greeks, Persians and Arabians, there were notable steps forward. We have likewise traced the development of contraceptive knowledge in folk medicine, dealt with the development of the condom or sheath, and treated at some length the more formally organized birth-control agitation or movement beginning with Francis Place in England in 1822 or 1823. We then scanned the rather considerable medical literature published on this subject during the nineteenth century and in recent decades. Estimates of the circulation and influence of this literature were made when possible. We observed that millions of tracts furnishing medical instruction have been distributed in England, the United States, and Germany since 1800. Though contraceptive practices are very old, diffused knowledge of them is recent. We noticed commercialized diffusion as a recent trend. In fact the major portion of the democratizing, socializing process has taken place in Western societies in the last century and a quarter.

The question now naturally arises: What has been the result of all this? To exactly what extent does the population of the United States or of any other country practise preventive measures? This question cannot be answered with complete satisfaction in the present state of knowledge.

But it is quite possible to arrive at suggestive answers by the sampling method and to throw more light on the problem than it has yet received. Despite the difficulties, it seems worth while to venture upon a preliminary determination of the degree of democratization or diffusion of contraceptive knowledge as a result of all the afore-described publication, agitation and commercial instruction.

The series of data studied are, in the first place, data showing the use of contraceptives prior to visits to birth control clinics. The shorthand term for this is pre-clinical-visit or pre-clinical evidence. In the same category, for convenience, are included Pearl's preliminary data on a supposedly representative United States sample. In this case the data were collected not prior to a birth-control clinic visit but at the time certain women were delivered of a baby in selected hospitals. We want an estimate of what people know about contraceptive techniques, an estimate of how steadily and effectively they are used prior to special instruction at a clinic. These points are discussed in the subdivisions of §2.

The second line of evidence, proving increased socialization of this knowledge in recent years, is extracted from birth-control clinic records and from clinical reports. The shorthand term for this is "clinical evidence" (§3). The occupations of patients' husbands, the racial and nationality groups attending, the incomes of patients, the percentage dependent, the source of reference of patients, that is, the extent to which charitable and social service agencies refer them—all these data show conclusively that the middle and lower classes are either acquiring knowledge they never had before, or else are learning of more reliable methods. In most cases patients come for a workable method to replace one that has for some reason been unsatisfactory.

Since the clinics are relatively new, and since their data do not extend very far back—the first British clinic was opened in 1921, and the first continually effective American clinic in 1923—it will be desirable to present a third type of evidence. This will consist of a study of the fertility rates of native and foreign-born women in the New England states in the period 1852–1923 (§4). In this discussion it will be shown that while the fertility of the native-born New England stock began to decline shortly after the Civil War, and then reached a steady level until approximately 1914 (since when it has increased)[1] the fertility of foreign-born women, high at first, has, in this period, steadily declined. The chief explanation of the latter seems to be a gradual spread of contraceptive knowledge among the foreign-born, who, it should be noted, represent, in the main, the lower economic classes. No doubt, some of the decline was due to increased resort to abortion. But

---

[1] The increase is probably spurious. See below p. 372ff.

this cannot explain all of the decline, probably not even the major portion. This interpretation is supported by the tremendously varied racial groups served by American birth-control clinics, especially by those in the racially polyglot metropolitan districts like New York and Chicago. Such clinics receive in their clientele a cross-section of the nationalities residing in the community.

In the fourth place, certain evidence presented by E. Sydenstricker, seems to run counter to this thesis. But W. Willcox has explained away this apparent enigma.

Furthermore, in the fifth place, Notestein and others have contributed to our knowledge of differential fertility by social class. Such studies suggest that in the United States the lower classes practise contraception less effectively than the upper social classes, a conclusion which seems reasonable on other grounds.

§2 PRE-CLINICAL-VISIT EVIDENCE

(2a) *Percentage of Various Populations Using Contraceptive Methods Prior to Clinical Instruction.*

In 1928 I showed that of 164 patients attending the Liverpool Mothers' Clinic, 102, or 62 per cent used, and 62, or 38 per cent, did not admit the use of contraceptives prior to the clinical visit.[2] In M. H. Kahn's series (1917), 272, or 59 per cent of a total of 464 cases, had a knowledge of contraceptive technique.[3] Of 500 cases coming for all reasons to Polano (1917), German gynecologist, only 17 admitted no knowledge of contraception, and 483 admitted knowledge; but of these, 339 admitted use. Yet this is 68 per cent of all the cases.[4]

In J. J. Blair's series of 107 cases at a clinic in Philadelphia 65 cases, or 61 per cent, used contraceptives previously.[5]

In the investigation by K. B. Davis into the *Factors in the Sex Life of Twenty-two Hundred Women* (1929), 73 per cent of the 1000 women (mostly college and university graduates) replying to her questionnaire used contraceptives.[6] In G. V. Hamilton's *Research in Marriage* (1929) 90 per cent

---

[2] *Eugenics Rev.*, xx (1928), 159, Table VI. No record in 70 cases in the original series of 234.

[3] *New York Med. Jour.*, cv (1917), 790–791.

[4] *Zeitschr. f. Geburtshilfe*, lxxix (1916–17), 567–578.

[5] *Med. Jour. & Rec.*, February 1, 1933. The published report does not mention the name of the clinic, but I find by correspondence with the author that it is the Maternal Health Center at 69th and Market Streets, Philadelphia.

[6] Katharine Bement Davis, *Factors in the Sex Life of Twenty-two Hundred Women* (New York: Harper, 1929), p. 14.

of 200 men and women likewise reported use.[7]   In a somewhat later report by Dickinson and Beam 95 per cent of 532 cases used some technique besides abstinence.[8]   In each of these three studies the social and economic status of the patient is, on the average, probably considerably above that of clinic patients.

Two English reports on pre-clinical use may be given before considering three larger American series: those by Stone, Kopp, and Pearl.   Stopes found (1925) that 25 per cent of 4,834 women attending her Mothers' Clinic in London had used some measure prior to the first clinical visit.[9]   But she thinks this greatly underestimates the real situation; and so it must.   Mrs. Sargant Florence, who published in 1930 a follow-up report on a few hundred cases that had attended the Cambridge Women's Welfare Association in England, found that 72 per cent of 265 cases reported prior use.[10]

Up until the publication in 1934 of Kopp's series on nearly 10,000 cases at the New York Clinical Research Bureau, Dr. Hannah M. Stone's report (1933) on 1,987 cases at the Newark Maternal Health Center was one of the longest.[11]   Of these 1,987 cases, 1,809, or 91.5 per cent, had used some preventive measures, and only 169, or 8.5 per cent had never used any.

Over 80 per cent in Stone's series had tried several methods.   Sixteen different practices are recorded.   Says Stone: "It is obvious, then, that these patients came to the Centre not because they wanted to learn something about birth control, but rather because they wanted to obtain more adequate and scientific information than they had possessed heretofore."

Among 1,978 patients there are 4,178 instances of prior use of various techniques.   *Coitus interruptus* was most common with 1,267 instances, being employed at some time by 64 per cent of the patients.   The douche was next most frequently used.   There were 1,424 instances among 1,183 women.   At some time or other 60 per cent used a douche.   Several used more than one type.   The influence of "feminine hygiene" advertising is clear: 507 cases of Lysol use, 127 of Zonite as against 239 of plain water, 99 salt, 80 medicated tablets and powders, 75 boric acid, 50 sodium bicarbonate, 37 vinegar, 31 bichloride of mercury [!] and 22 soap.   No record of medication was given in 95.   Soap and vinegar appear more frequently than I would expect.   The condom was third in popularity in Stone's series: 956 patients, 48.3 per cent.   Yet only 111 used it exclusively.   Suppositories

[7] P. 120.

[8] R. L. Dickinson and Lura Beam, *A Thousand Marriages, a Medical Study of Sex Adjustment*, p. 248.

[9] Marie C. Stopes, *The First Five Thousand*, p. 41.

[10] Lella Secor Florence, *Birth Control on Trial* (London: Allen & Unwin, 1930), p. 91.

[11] *Med. Jour. & Rec.*, April 19 and May 3, 1933.

were next with 280 cases, or 14.2 per cent. Pessaries, chiefly cervical, were used by 88 patients.

To summarize: 91.5 per cent of all the Stone cases used some method or methods prior to the clinical visit. The techniques in order of importance ranked as follows: *coitus interruptus,* douching, condom, suppositories, other methods (pessaries, sponges, stems, jellies, sterile period, etc.).

Similar to the Newark pre-clinical-use figure of 91.5 per cent is Kopp's New York figure of 93.3 per cent (not counting abstinence) of 9,916 women

TABLE I

PRE-CLINICAL METHODS OF CONTRACEPTION EVER USED BY 9,250 PATIENTS AT THE BIRTH CONTROL CLINICAL RESEARCH BUREAU, NEW YORK[1]

Methods	Total		Success		Failure	
	Number	Per cent.	Number	Per cent.†	Number	Per cent.
Instances............	19438	100.0	8826	45.4	10612	54.6
Withdrawal............	5894	30.3	2406	40.8	3488	59.2
Condom............	4759	24.6	2617	55.0	2142	45.0
Douche............	4165	21.4	1225	29.4	2940	70.6
Jelly or suppository............	1751	9.0	952	54.4	799	46.6
Lactation............	884	4.5	384	43.4	500	56.6
Pessary............	748	3.8	538	71.9	210	28.1
Sponge and all other methods.....	377	1.9	188	50.0	189	50.0
Stem............	320	1.7	157	49.1	163	50.9
Safe period............	303	1.6	122	40.3	181	59.7
Abstinence............	237	1.2	237	100.0	—	—

* "Total" does not mean the number of occasions methods have been used, but the total number of cases recording the various types of methods previously employed. The total equals more than the 9,250 patients who have used more than one method.

† Percentages are based on the proportion of success and failure according to the type of method employed.

[1] Kopp, *op. cit.,* p. 134.

(i.e., 9,250 cases) at the Birth Control Clinical Research Bureau. Only 666 women, or 6.7 per cent, made no attempt whatever at prevention of conception.[12] Table I shows the distribution of pre-clinical methods employed, and also presents figures on success and failure to be discussed at the end of this section. Note that withdrawal, or *coitus interruptus,* the condom, and the douche, were, in that order, most frequently used, and that together they account for three-fourths (76.3 per cent) of the methods tried. Even

[12] Marie E. Kopp, *Birth Control in Practice. Analysis of Ten Thousand Case Histories of the Birth Control Clinical Research Bureau* (New York: McBride, 1934), p. 133.

though cases are counted who ultimately abandoned the method before coming to the clinic, observe the very infrequent resort to the so-called safe period and to abstinence. Exhortation to employ the latter has been especially prominent in the last century, and with what result the figure suggests. Likewise only 1.6 per cent ever used the safe period, advocated for two thousand years since Soranos' early mention.[13] Will our sex preachers never learn the futility of attempting to cajole the public into using methods that do violence to the decent demands of wholesome human nature? It is dangerous to attempt prediction; but it seems clear that many such preachers have learned little so far.

If the above figures are stated another way, it is seen that there are 1,424 instances, 7.3 per cent, of natural methods (lactation, safe period, abstinence); 5,894 instances, 30.3 per cent, of non-mechanical methods (withdrawal); 12,120 instances, 62.4 per cent, of mechanical methods.[14]

It will be recalled that the purpose of this section is to show the extent of the democratization of contraceptive knowledge by the use of contraceptives on the part of samples of the population prior to a clinical visit. Since there may be some selection operating on the Stone and Kopp series—perhaps the less successful tend to seek out the clinics—it is important to present here data recently collected by Pearl upon which this selective influence could not operate.

Pearl's attempt to determine the extent to which preventive measures, as applied, intelligently or unintelligently, precisely or carelessly, by a large sample of American married couples, white and Negro, in selected urban centers in the United States, have reduced pregnancies in relation to 100 ovulations, represents, undoubtedly the most careful, scientific and brilliant attack on this problem by any investigator in any country to date.[15] There is no room here to describe his method. Readers who wish to do so, should refer to the first[16] and second original reports, which may be supplemented by others before this is in print. In the hospitals of several large cities internes have collected data on a pre-arranged form, and queried patients on, among other things, their use of preventives. The number of preg-

---

[13] See p. 15 for a report of use by the Isleta Indians in New Mexico.

[14] Kopp, p. 136.

[15] Raymond Pearl, "Contraception and Fertility in 4945 Married Women. A Second Report on a Study in Family Limitation," *Human Biology*, vi, 355–401. Abstract in *Milbank Mem. Fund Quart.*, xii, 248–269 (July, 1934). Pearl estimates this problem of attempting to determine the extent to which contraceptive practices *as now used* have reduced fertility to be "nearly if not quite the most important still unresolved question connected with the problem of human population growth at this moment." *Human Biology*, vi, 386.

[16] *Human Biology*, iv, 363–407.

nancies per 100 ovulations was studied in a contraceptive-using and a non-contraceptive using group with further subdivisions according to economic status and according to whether or not the use of contraception was regular and steady, intermittent mainly because children were planned, or lastly, intermittent for other reasons, chiefly carelessness, indifference and the like. Consideration of the main results are postponed to §2b Degree of Success with Pre-clinical Methods. In this particular section we are concerned with the degree to which a sample[17] of 4,945 women, presumably representative, resorted to preventive measures. Pearl's figures show that 42.2 per cent admitted use. Of 4,166 white married women, 1,886, or 45.3 per cent, practiced contraception in some form regularly or intermittently; while of 766 Negro married women, 197, or 25.7 per cent, did likewise. The average for both whites and Negroes is 42.2 per cent.[18]

It is interesting to observe in Table II below the relation between the practice of contraception and economic status. This measures more accurately, what has been known for many years, namely, that there is an inverse correlation between economic status and the degree of practice of contraception. Figure XXI presents the same information graphically. Resort to contraception rises steadily as economic status rises, but not quite so fast owing to more deliberate planning for children in the upper classes.[19] This generalization applies to regular use. Where the practice is intermittent for reasons not involving deliberate planning, the rates of use do not change appreciably as economic status rises. In this connection it is interesting to note that a "hunch" I have long held is proved by Pearl's figures, namely, that "the percentage of women *not practicing* contraception is higher among the prima-gravidae than among those who have been pregnant two or more times. This is true for both whites and Negroes, and within each economic group."[20] This is graphically illustrated in Figure

[17] Seventy-five per cent of the whites in Pearl's study and 80 per cent of the Negroes reside in the four states of Illinois, Maryland, Pennsylvania and New York; the remainder live in nine other states. In religion 40 per cent of the whites are Catholics, and 15 per cent Jewish. Of the white women 61.6 per cent had never been educated beyond the elementary schools. The figure for Negro women is 69.9 per cent. It is estimated that less than 1 per cent of the women ever had any formal or scientific instruction in contraception, or contact with a birth-control clinic. The mean duration of marriage was 5.72 years for whites and 6.44 years for Negroes. "The white women in the sample had, on the average, spent 38.6 per cent of their whole married lives in the business of being pregnant and bearing children. The negro women had spent 42.5 per cent of their married lives in the same way." [*Human Biol.*, vi, 397.]

[18] *Human Biology*, vi, 371.

[19] I showed the same point on a small sample in 1928. See *Eugenics Review*, xx, 159, Table VI.

[20] *Human Biology*, vi, 375.

TABLE II

THE PRACTICE OF CONTRACEPTION IN RELATION TO ECONOMIC STATUS, PEARL SERIES[1]

A. Whites

Contraceptive Genus Group	Very Poor		Poor		Moderate Circumstances		Well-to-do and Rich		Totals	
	No.	Per cent.	No.	Per cent.	No.	Per cent.	No.	Per cent.	No.	Per cent.
A. No contraception..........	343	67.3	1191	61.2	669	49.4	77	21.7	2280	54.7
B. Regular and steady practice of contraception........	59	11.6	323	16.6	276	20.4	78	22.0	736	17.7
C. Contraceptive practice intermittent mainly for planned children........	68	13.4	262	13.4	325	24.0	169	47.6	824	19.8
D. Contraceptive practice intermittent for reasons other than planning......	39	7.7	172	8.8	84	6.2	31	8.7	326	7.8
Sub-totals (B + C + D). Contraception practiced.........	166	32.7	757	38.8	685	50.6	278	78.3	1886	45.3
Totals (A + B + C + D). All cases......................	509	100.0	1948	100.0	1354	100.0	355	100.0	4166	100.0

B. Negroes

Contraceptive Genus Group	Very Poor		Poor		Moderate Circumstances		Well-to-do and Rich		Totals	
A. No contraception..........	263	76.0	275	72.2	31	79.4	—	—	569	74.3
B. Regular and steady practice of contraception........	30	8.7	45	11.8	4	10.3	—	—	79	10.3
C. Contraceptive practice intermittent mainly for planned children........	8	2.3	20	5.2	3	7.7	—	—	31	4.0
D. Contraceptive practice intermittent for reasons other than planning......	45	13.0	41	10.8	1	2.6	—	—	87	11.4
Sub-totals (B + C + D). Contraception practiced.........	83	24.0	106	27.8	8	20.6	—	—	197	25.7
Totals (A + B + C + D). All cases......................	346	100.0	381	100.0	39	100.0	—	—	766	100.0

[1] *Human Biology*, vi, 372.

XXI. For all genera (lowest row of bar diagrams) the cross-hatched bar is higher than the solid bar. Of the white women who had two or more pregnancies 50 per cent used contraceptives; only 37.3 per cent when they had experienced one pregnancy. The corresponding figures for Negroes

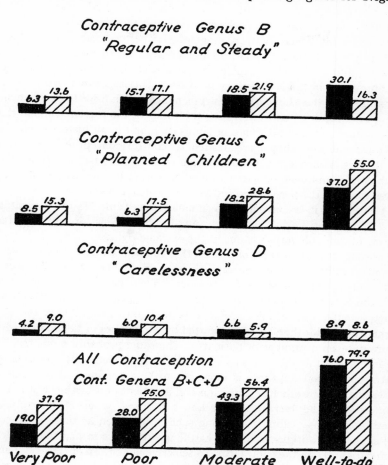

FIG. XXI. Precentages of White Women Practising Contraception in Relation to (1) Contraceptive Genus, (2) Economic Status, and (3) Number of Pregnancies ever Experienced. Pearl Series. *Human Biology*, vi, 378.

were 28.6 per cent and 17.5 per cent.   Pearl subdivides these figures further by social classes.   Among the white women who had experienced two or more pregnancies, contraception had been practiced among the very poor by 37.9 per cent, among the poor by 45.0 per cent, among those in moderate circumstances by 56.4 per cent, among the well-to-do and rich by 79.9 per cent, the average being 50.1 per cent.   Among the primapara the figures are considerably lower, as the average of 37.3 per cent indicates.   This is especially true of the very poor.   These figures tend to confirm my theory that poor and middle-class families, at least under the circumstances which have prevailed in the last century in Western societies, practice contraception more after they have had a few pregnancies than prior to experiencing any.   This theory squares well with the thesis of the present volume that while women have, in all stages of civilization and in all historical epochs, disdained sterility, they have desired to control conception.   How else can the persistence and general diffusion of sometimes painful, obnoxious, troublesome, and even dangerous expedients used by women be explained unless we posit the persistence and power of such a desire?

At this stage it is convenient to summarize in Table III the percentage using contraceptives in the twelve sample populations already reported. The significant column is the one at the extreme right.

The most striking feature of Table III is the wide range in percentage of patients admitting use of contraceptives: from 25 per cent of the Stopes series to 93.3 per cent of the Kopp series.   There can be little doubt that both the Stopes and Pearl figures, 25 and 42.2 per cent respectively, are underestimates and atypical.   There is reason to believe that the staff workers at the Mothers' Clinic operated by Dr. Stopes in London failed to secure data on a number of patients.   The same probably holds true for the internes gathering data in Dr. Pearl's series.   Generally speaking, on contraceptive matters there is more apt to be a confidential relationship between a social worker or physician and a patient at a birth control clinic than between the average interne and a hospital patient.   Probably internes are not as skillful in securing such information as those birth-control-clinic staff workers who have had long experience in prying such data from patients.   In the clinical cases a selective factor also operates.   Those who have tried several methods without notable success, and who wish urgently to control pregnancy have stronger incentives to attend a birth control clinic.   Another important factor is the different composition of the various groups studied by different investigators.   The Hamilton, Davis, Dickinson-Beam series contain a high proportion of upper-class women. The Stopes, Stone, Blair, and Kopp series contain, as far as we can determine, a fairly representative clinic population, which means that they contain a large proportion of working-class mothers. I believe that my own Liverpool figure, 62 per cent, is an underestimate. These data were among the first collected at Liverpool when the staff had little experience in getting "confessions" from the patients.

Another factor making the Pearl percentage of prior use unduly small is the large proportion (40 per cent) of Catholics. The average for the United States is only 15–20 per cent.[21] Even in clinics in large eastern cities, which are Catholic centers, nowhere near 40 per cent of the patients are Catholic.

TABLE III

SUMMARY OF STUDIES ON PRE-CLINICAL USE OF CONTRACEPTIVES

Investigator	Country of Data	Date of Publication	Number in Series	Number Stating Use of Contraceptives	Percentage Stating Use
Kahn	U. S.	1917	464	272	59
Polano	Germany	1917	500	339	68*
Stopes	England	1925	4834	1284	25
Himes	England and Scotland	1928	164	102	62
Davis	U. S.	1929	1000	730	73
Hamilton	U. S.	1929	200	180	90
Florence	England	1930	265	189	72
Dickinson-Beam	U. S.	1931	532	507	95
Stone	U. S.	1933	1987	1807	91.5
Blair	U. S.	1933	107	65	61
Kopp	U. S.	1933	9916	9250	93.3
Pearl	U. S.	1934	4932	2083	42.2
Total			24901	16808	67.5
Total except Stopes group			20067	15524	77
Total except Stopes and Pearl groups			15135	13441	89

* 96.5 per cent. stated possession of contraceptive knowledge.

From Table XXIX on page 415 it will be seen that at Baltimore 25 per cent of the clinical population were Catholics; 36 per cent of the general population. At Cleveland only 25 per cent of the clinic population were

[21] The lower figure is probably nearer the truth. The religious census is not accurate. Then again, different groups have different bases of estimate. The doctrine of "once a Catholic, always a Catholic" inflates Catholic figures of church membership. Protestants who drop church membership are presumably dropped from the rolls. But a person once baptized a Catholic is always considered as one by the Church. Such a person is only temporarily lost to heresy.

TABLE IV

FREQUENCY OF USE OF VARIOUS CONTRACEPTIVE METHODS IN THREE LARGE AMERICAN SERIES: NEWARK, NEW YORK, AND SEVERAL CITIES OF THE UNITED STATES

Stone Series*			Kopp Series†			Pearl Series§		
Method	No. of Instances of Use	Per Cent.	Method	No. of Instances of Use	Per Cent.	Methods‡	No. of Instances of Use	Per Cent.
Douche	1424	34.1	Coitus interruptus	5894	30.3	Douche (med. and water)	1333	41.9
Coitus interruptus	1267	30.2	Condom	4759	24.6	Condom	813	25.6
Condom	956	22.9	Douche	4165	21.4	Coitus interruptus	612	19.2
Suppositories	280	6.7	Jelly or suppository	1751	9.0	Med. vag. sup. or jellies	199	6.2
Pessaries	88	2.1	Lactation	884	4.5	Safe period	102	3.2
Sponges	64	1.5	Pessary	748	3.8	Pes. with med. jelly	47	1.5
Intrauterine stems	48	1.2	Sponge and all other methods	377	1.9	Other methods	36	1.1
Other	51	1.2	Stem	320	1.7	Pessary alone	21	0.7
			Safe period	303	1.6	Pes. with douche	17	0.5
			Abstinence	237	1.2	Intrauterine mech. device	5	0.2
All Methods	4178	99.9	All Methods	19438	100.0	All Methods	3185	100.1

* H. M. Stone, *Med. Jour. & Rec.*, April 19 and May 3, 1933.
† Kopp, *op. cit.*, p. 134.
§ *Human Biology*, vi, 383.   Abstracted From Table 13.
‡ Alone or in combination.

Catholic, while 51 per cent of the general population adhered to the same faith. At Newark the corresponding figures are 29 per cent and 53 per cent and at New York 26 and 25.4. At Newark 91.5 per cent of the patients used contraceptives prior to the clinical visit; but only 29 per cent were Catholic. With 40 per cent Catholic, as in Pearl's series, we would expect a lower rate of prior use of contraceptives, but not a rate as low as 42.2 per cent. When Pearl's final figures are published, it will be interesting to see whether 40 per cent of the contraceptive-using groups were Catholics.

Table IV compares the frequency of use of various contraceptive methods in three large series of 26,801 instances. Recall that in the Stone and Kopp series (Newark and New York) the data represent use prior to instruction

TABLE V

CONDENSED SUMMARY. FREQUENCY OF USE OF VARIOUS CONTRACEPTIVE METHODS. THREE SERIES, 26,801 INSTANCES

Method	Number of Instances	Per Cent.
Total	26801	100.0
Withdrawal	7773	29.0
Douche	6922	25.8
Condom	6528	24.4
Suppositories and jellies	2230	8.3
Pessaries (alone or with douche or jelly)	921	3.4
Stem	373	1.4
All others	2054	7.7

at a birth control clinic. In the Pearl series the use is prior to being delivered of a baby in selected large urban hospitals in the United States.

While, in the three series, there is some variation in the order of the three leading frequencies, *the condensed Summary (Table V) shows that in the entire 26,801 instances, withdrawal leads with nearly one-third of the cases, followed by the douche and condom, in that order, with about one-quarter each.* These three methods constitute nearly four-fifths of all instances. Other methods are used much less frequently. This quantitative elaboration squares pretty well with the subjective conclusions of the experienced observer. This is the first time these facts have been determined in a series anywhere near as large as this.

These figures, especially those on percentage using contraceptives, suggest the extent to which such knowledge has been diffused throughout the population even before special instruction at clinics. They do not, however, tell us anything about the effectiveness of such practices. To this brief attention will now be given.

(2b) *Degree of Success with Pre-clinical Methods*

Estimates of the effectiveness of various contraceptive measures used before application to a clinic are without high reliability because of the many unknown and uncontrollable factors influencing the tabulated data thus far made available. But inasmuch as they represent the best estimates we have, they are presented for what they may be worth.

It has not infrequently been said that the techniques generally used by women prior to special medical instruction are worthless, ineffective. This is an extreme position, and untenable if for no other reason than that many methods are used, some theoretically effective, others theoretically of very little reliability, by women of high, low and average fertility. The condom, for example, which, according to Havelock Ellis, Lord Dawson of Penn, L. S. Florence, Enid Charles[22] and others, is still our best contraceptive, hardly requires elaborate instructions. It is true, however, that if a few simple rules are known and followed, its effectiveness should increase.[23] Likewise, the effectiveness of douching, which has rather a poor record as generally used, will be increased if a few simple rules are known and followed.[24] The strain on the male with *coitus interruptus*, and consequent lapses into carelessness or lack of control, possibly account for its poor record at those birth control clinics which tabulate pre-clinical practices.

Moreover, the failure rate of all pre-clinical methods is doubtless overrated by selection. Those, for example, who are applying successfully what they know, are less likely to come to a clinic in search of a better method. Moreover, the clinic populations are more fertile than the general population; which suggests that, if other circumstances are equal, the clinic populations may be, *prior to clinical advice*, less successful in preventing births than the general population.

We shall first present estimates of success tabulated from clinic records but based on use before the clinical visit. Then we shall report the studies of Pearl, Notestein and Stix.

Data from Stone and Kopp will suffice for the clinical sources.

From Stone we have the following figures on success and failure with various methods prior to clinical advice and supervision. On *coitus interruptus:*

---

[22] That is, Mrs. Lancelot Hogben.

[23] See Dickinson and Bryant, *Control of Conception*, pp. 60–69.

[24] *Ibid.*, pp. 69–73.

Result	Number of Instances	Per cent.
Success (i.e., no pregnancy)............................	368	29
Failed (i.e., conception resulted)......................	761	60
Doubtful (Pt. using several methods. Not clear which failed)...	138	11

Success and failure with the douche (1424 cases) Stone records as follows:

Result	Number of Instances	Per cent.
Success..	139	10
Failure..	600	42
Doubtful...	685	48

The record of the condom follows:

Result	Number of Instances	Per cent.
Success..	442	46
Failure..	402	42
Doubtful...	112	12

Regarding the Kopp series of 19,438 instances, reference back to Table I (p. 337) will show that, if we except abstinence, success ranged from 40.3 to 55.0 per cent and this with a minimum—one might guess an almost entire absence of—competent medical instruction. Note that we are not now concerned with success of contraceptives *subsequent* to instruction at a clinic. Those interested in these data will find valuable information in the books by Kopp and Charles and in the reports (called issues) of the International Medical Group for the Investigation of Contraception.[25]

We now return to the Pearl series to find out the rate of pregnancy reduction found by that investigator in various social classes and Contraceptive Genus Groups.

The relevant data for whites and Negroes by economic classes is shown in Table VI. This looks complicated only at first glance. We first explain the meaning of the figures: The number in the upper-left-hand box, 14.02, means that among the "very poor" *who did not practice contraception*, the pregnancy rate was a trifle over 14 per 100 ovulations, that is, 14 per cent

[25] These reports are summarized in my paper on "New light on the Causes of the Declining Birth Rate," in Norman E. Himes [Ed.], *Economics, Sociology, and the Modern World*. Cambridge: Harvard University Press, 1935.

TABLE VI

MEAN PREGNANCY RATES PER 100 COMPUTED OVULATIONS IN ALL MARRIED WOMEN IN THE PEARL SAMPLE, BY CONTRACEPTIVE GENUS GROUP AND ECONOMIC STATUS[1]

A. Whites

Contraceptive Genus Group	Very Poor (Per Cent.)	Poor (Per Cent.)	Moderate Circumstances (Per Cent.)	Well-to-do and Rich (Per Cent.)	Totals All Women in Group (Per Cent.)
A. No contraception	14.02±0.62	16.00±0.38	13.59±0.46	16.97±1.89	15.03±0.26
B. Regular and steady practice of contraception	8.77± .92	10.56± .50	8.63± .46	9.71± .88	9.60± .31
C. Contraceptive practice intermittent mainly for planned children	6.32± .40	7.27± .32	6.55± .27	5.16± .28	6.48± .16
D. Contraceptive practice intermittent for reasons other than planning	8.59±1.25	10.41± .65	9.67± .84	8.87± .89	9.85± .44

B. Negroes

Contraceptive Genus Group	Very Poor (Per Cent.)	Poor (Per Cent.)	Moderate Circumstances (Per Cent.)	Well-to-do and Rich (Per Cent.)	Totals All Women in Group (Per Cent.)
A. No contraception	14.03±0.74	14.67±0.71	18.24±2.55	—	14.57±0.51
R. Regular and steady practice of contraception	10.42± .84	10.83±1.40	21.35±5.35	—	11.20± .92
C. Contraceptive practice intermittent mainly for planned children	5.63± .58	9.25± .64	9.17±1.84	—	8.30± .51
D. Contraceptive practice intermittent for reasons other than planning	9.22± .88	9.33± .86	—*	—	9.45± .62

* Only one woman in this class, with a pregnancy rate falling in the class 20.0–29.9 per cent.

[1] *Human Biology*, vi, 388.

of the ovulations resulted in pregnancy; whereas (two boxes below) the married couples of similar economic status who *practiced contraception intermittently mainly for planned children* had a pregnancy rate of only 6.32 per 100 ovulations (or, 6.32 per cent of their ovulations). Thus, those who planned their pregnancies with contraception had a pregnancy rate only 45 per cent of those in the same class who did not practice contraception.

Stated another way, this is a reduction of 55 per cent ($100 - \frac{6.32}{14.02} = 55$).

Pearl adds that "the white women who practiced contraception most intelligently and precisely, intermitting it only for planned and wanted pregnancies, exhibited a mean pregnancy rate only 43.1 per cent of that of the women not practicing contraception at all, a reduction of about 57 per cent. The corresponding reduction among women of the Well-to-do and Rich class is approximately 70 per cent."[26] We do not know what the average reduction in pregnancy rate is for all Contraceptive Genus Groups (B + C + D) for both whites and Negroes. This will doubtless appear in Pearl's final report. Preliminary rough estimates lead me to think the final figure will be in the neighborhood of 55 per cent.[27] This is a considerable reduction in the rate of pregnancy in view of the lack of medical control and the "back fence" source of much of the information.

The most striking reduction of fertility is among women of the well-to-do and rich class, whose fertility was reduced, when they practiced contraception regularly and steadily, by 70 per cent ($100 - \frac{5.16}{16.97} = 70$). Among white women not practicing contraception, the very-poor have nearly the lowest mean pregnancy rate and the well-to-do and rich class the highest mean pregnancy rate. The mean pregnancy rates for the white women in this sample are very similar in each economic class for the same type of contraceptive practice. This is shown by the similar height of the correspond-

---

[26] *Human Biology*, vi, 399.

[27] In his first preliminary report (*Human Biology*, iv, 363–407) Pearl, using a different method, concluded that the reduction was only 20 per cent, a figure manifestly too small. The figure was too small partly because of lack of certain refinement in statistical statement, a difficulty overcome in the second report; partly to fundamental defects in Pearl's method not capable of being overcome so long as this particular method is used (see below for details). Primipara, with which the series is over-loaded, resort less frequently to contraceptives, as the second report showed. There is another fundamental objection to Pearl's method not yet overcome: If a woman wants to avoid pregnancy and is successful, she could not possibly get into Pearl's series. Hence, the series is over-loaded with failures. This is a *very serious* defect in Pearl's method. Hence the question originally posed in his first report—to what extent has the pregnancy rate been reduced by resort to contraceptives in a defined sample of the population of the United States—is not capable of answer by his method. However, it is the best attempt yet made.

ing bars in each of the 5 groups in Figure XXII. Pearl concludes that this suggests "that the innate natural fertility of these women is about the same in the different economic classes here distinguished, and that the differences in average *expressed* fertility observed in the different economic classes are due mainly to different degrees of artificial alteration of the innate natural fertility. On the basis of the present material this conclusion seems clear and indubitable."[28]

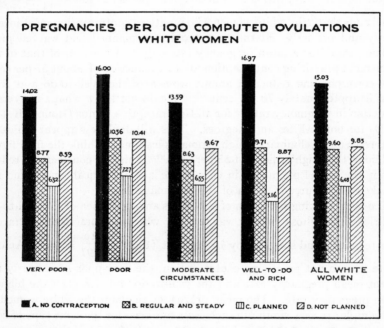

FIG. XXII. Pregnancy Rates per 100 Computed Ovulations. By Economic Class, Use, Non-use, and Kind of Use of Contraceptives. Pearl Series. *Human Biology*, vi, 390.

The lower half of Table VI, dealing with Negroes, shows much the same result, except that the lowering of the mean pregnancy rate among the contraceptive-using group is not quite so large in amount as among white women. Pearl thinks this result surprising,[29] probably because a larger proportion of Negroes than of whites belong to the lower economic classes, but also because Pearl seems to believe the Negro biologically inferior,[30] a view not accepted by the majority of sociologists.

[28] *Ibid.*, pp. 390–391.
[29] *Ibid.*, p. 391.
[30] Fifth Report Baltimore Bureau for Contraceptive Advice, *passim.*

The Negro and white groups who did not practice contraception have almost identical pregnancy rates, in fact, that for the Negroes is slightly lower.

Pearl's tables on mean live *birth* rates by Contraceptive Genus Groups and by social status show similar results, and need not be reviewed here.

Following the method in Pearl's first report, Stix and Notestein found[31] that, in a sample of 714 New York City women[32] who attended the chief clinic there, *the contraceptive practices when and as employed prior to clinic advice brought about, for a given exposure to the risk of conception, a 75 per cent reduction in pregnancies.* The rate for first pregnancies was seven times greater in the non-contraceptive-using than in the contraceptive-using group.[33] For second and later pregnancies the difference is only about half that for first pregnancies.[34] "We can therefore conclude," say the authors, "that in all durations of married life and for first, as well as for

---

[31] Frank W. Notestein, and Regine K. Stix, "Effectiveness of Birth Control. A Study of Contraceptive Practice in a Selected Group of New York Women," *Milbank Mem. Fund. Quart.*, vol. xii, no. 1 (January, 1934). References are to pages in reprint. See Bibliography under Stix for references to later studies.

[32] Dr. Stix, a physician, personally interviewed these former patients of the Birth Control Clinical Research Bureau, who came from the Bronx, still lived there after attending the clinic in 1931. Two-thirds of the women were Jewish, one-sixth Catholic, and only one-ninth Protestant. Married less than 10 years on the average, they had 3.23 pregnancies and 2.26 live births on the average. Median income was $2,300; in 1932 it had dropped to $1,200, and a fifth were either destitute or supported by relief. *Prior to the clinical visit 95 per cent had made some effort at family limitation.* Forty per cent used contraceptives immediately after marriage; an additional 40 per cent started such use immediately after the beginning of the second pregnancy. Each couple employed an average of 1.8 methods.

[33] *Ibid.*, p. 8. Curiously enough Stix and Notestein found that "the rate at which women became pregnant with the first child seems to be significantly higher [by two months for each pregnancy] *after they have used contraceptives and interrupted that practice in order to become pregnant* [italics mine] than in the rate for women who have never used contraceptives." The authors "are at a loss to explain this ... [except] that in many marriages a certain amount of time elapses before complete entry takes place." This is hardly a satisfactory explanation until it is shown that incomplete entry, to the extent of reducing the chances of conception, is common. On the contrary, it is probably not common. A more likely explanation seems to be this: there is probably some inheritance of fecundity (i.e., power to participate in procreation), and those coming from large families, and who are therefore more likely themselves to conceive, have, at the same time, been more than ordinarily impressed with the desirability of not repeating the maternal overburden of their mothers. Hence they are more likely than the average of their class to use contraceptives early in marriage. When they stop using them for the purpose of having children their greater fecundity naturally expresses itself in more prompt impregnation.

[34] *Ibid.*, p. 9.

later pregnancies, the pregnancy rate of this group of women is significantly reduced by their use of contraceptives."[35] The number of pregnancies actually experienced was only one-fourth the number expected. This reduction of 75 per cent is higher than Pearl's preliminary figure perhaps because the Stix-Notestein group is somewhat selected: those who came to the clinic meant business about limitation even before being advised there. It should be understood that, since the authors are comparing pregnancy rates for equal units of time during which conception is possible and not rates for equal units of married life,[36] "we cannot conclude from these results that women who habitually use contraceptives throughout their married life would average one-fourth as many pregnancies as those who did not practice contraception." Probably, however, the above figures are a rough measure of this. As with the Pearl figures, it is necessary to recall that we are dealing here mainly with "back-fence" and amateur contraception. Success with clinically-advised methods comes nearer 90–95 per cent. Kopp's figure is 93.3 per cent.

We now turn to the clinical evidence on democratization.

§3   CLINICAL EVIDENCE

The argument used to be commonly heard that the working classes would not use contraceptive information, or would not use it properly, even if it were given them. This last-resort argument against birth control is less frequently heard now. For clinical records in the United States and England prove it thoroughly false—as could have been determined inductively before the opening of clinics, if such critics had taken the pains to inform themselves on the real situation. Actually, there has been for many years great demand among the populace for reliable information.

(3a)   General Vital and Social Data

Table VII presents preliminary vital and social data on 3,296 cases advised at several British birth-control clinics. This is presented solely as background material, for it has no immediate bearing on the present thesis. The average number of pregnancies was 4.00, and the mean number of living children 3.17. Later studies have only supported these representative

---

[35] *Ibid.*, p. 10.

[36] The distinction is important, for a woman cannot conceive when she is pregnant. Moreover, successful prevention increases the time period when the contraceptive might fail. Thus, in a special sense, the paradox is true that the more successful a woman is at prevention the greater the chance at failure because the greater the exposure risk.

TABLE VII

VITAL AND SOCIAL DATA ON 3,296 CASES—BRITISH BIRTH CONTROL CLINICS

Location of Clinic	Series Total	Pregnancies Total	Pregnancies Arith. Mean	Pregnancies σ	Living Children Total	Living Children Arith. Mean	Living Children σ	Losses Total	Losses P.C. Pregs.	Losses Miscarriages P.C.	Years Married Arith. Mean	Years Married σ	r with Pregs.	r with L.C.	Ages Wife Mean	Ages Hus. Mean
North Kensington	1000	3855	3.86	2.83	3005	3.00	2.56	886	23.0	51.9	8.7	6.0	.73	.60	31.3	33.9
Manchester	600	2331	3.89	2.66	1783	2.98	1.79	548	23.5	47.5	8.8	5.4	.66	.66	31.0	33.5
Wolverhampton	498	1775	3.56	2.41	1450	2.91	1.83	338	19.0	41.5	8.2	8.2	.75	.70	30.8a	—
Cambridge	309	1202	3.89	2.72	1014	3.28	2.28	198	16.4	46.0	9.7	6.0	.72	.62	32.2f	34.9g
Liverpool	234	1178	5.05	3.16	911	3.89	2.27	284	24.2	31.0	9.8	5.8	.79	.75	31.8d	34.8e
Birmingham	165	604	3.66	2.98	479	2.90	2.55	130	20.7	45.4	9.5b	5.9	.68b	.55b	32.4	35.1
Glasgow—																
Adequate Series	150	691	4.60	2.97	520	3.46	2.10	179	25.8	39.6	9.5	5.9	.75	.74	31.3h	34.6h
Inadequate Series	89	366	4.15	—	324	3.64	—	—	—	—	—	—	—	—	—	—
Total	239	1057	4.38	—	844	3.55	—	—	—	—	—	—	—	—	—	—
Aberdeen	109	619	5.67	2.8	486	4.45	2.25	134	21.6	30.6	10.0	5.0	.78	.73	31.1	33.4
Cannock Miners	114c	465	4.08	2.4	386	3.39	1.96	—	—	—	8.6	8.6	.63	.68	—	—
Cannock Non-Miners	28	97	3.46	2.78	80	2.86	2.25	—	—	—	7.8	4.9	.73	.54	—	—
Grand Totals	3296	13183	4.00	—	10438	3.17	—	2697	—	—	9.1	—	—	—	31.5	34.3

a Based on 496 cases instead of 498.
b Based on 161 cases instead of 165.
c The records of 17 of these cases were kept at Wolverhampton, but are not included in the Wolverhampton series, since these miners are counted in this group.

d Based on 232 cases instead of 234.
e Based on 226 cases instead of 234.
f Based on 308 cases instead of 309.
g Based on 292 cases instead of 309.
h Based on 148 cases instead of 150.

figures.[37]　Even though the wages of the husbands of these women in the relatively prosperous days of 1925–27 averaged only $12.50–$15.00 per week, fertility was normal or above normal.　Moreover, most of the families studied are incomplete.　Had the women passed the child-bearing age they would not have come to the clinics for advice.

(3b)　Occupational Status of Husbands

Table VIII summarizes the occupational status of the husbands.　Omitting the extreme exceptions of Wolverhampton and Cannock, from one-third to one-half of the clinic husbands were unskilled.　From 7.3 to 18 per cent were semi-skilled.　With the exception of Wolverhampton, and Birmingham, which had an extraordinarily high proportion of skilled workers,

TABLE VIII

SUMMARY OF OCCUPATIONAL STATUS OF HUSBANDS OF BRITISH BIRTH-CONTROL CLINIC PATIENTS

Location of Clinic	Unskilled	Semi-skilled	Skilled	All Others
Liverpool	46.8	16.2	19.6	17.4
Aberdeen	38.5	7.3	20.2	34.0
North Kensington	37.9	(32.8)	*	29.3
Glasgow	34.6	18.0	24.6	22.8
Manchester	32.6	11.1	31.0	25.3
Cambridge	32.0	17.2	25.2	25.6
Birmingham	24.2	13.9	40.0	21.9
Wolverhampton	12.6	5.6	77.9	3.9
Cannock	—	100.0†	—	—

* No distinction between skilled and semi-skilled.

† Miners exclusively.

the skilled group ranged (in round numbers) from 20–30 per cent.　For the entire group (2,915 cases) one-half of the patients' husbands (51 per cent) fall either in the unskilled or semi-skilled groups.　It is the aim of the clinics to deal almost exclusively with the working classes, and a predominant proportion come from that source.　While a few wives of professional men have attended clinics rather than private practitioners, as a rule they seek the

[37] Even in a recent Chinese sample the averages ran only a little over one higher.　In 99 cases mentioned in the first report of the Peiping Committee on Maternal Health there was an average of 5.6 pregnancies and 4.3 births.　The mean interval was 1.7 years.　See Marion Yang, "Birth Control in Peiping.　First Report of the Peiping Committee on Maternal Health," *Chinese Med. Jour.*, xlviii, 786–791 (August, 1934).　However, this small Chinese sample was weighted with upper-class patients, as one might expect where good contraceptive facilities are not generally available.

private office. The attitude toward socialized medicine is such among the general populace of Great Britain that all save the well-to-do tend to seek medical information through the public or semi-public agencies (e.g., the panel doctor). In the case of contraceptive advice it is often the birth-control clinic; but many also depend on printed matter and the commercial shops. This latter is possible because there is no legal restriction on the distribution of printed material on contraception in England provided it does not run counter to the common law interpretation of decency (e.g. distributing medical handbills promiscuously on a street corner).

The somewhat unreliable data on wage incomes corroborate the trend of occupational figures in supporting the view that the clinics serve predominantly the working classes. In the present state of fact-collecting by the English clinics, estimates of wage incomes by the sampling process are more accurate probably than elaborate tabulations. In 1927 I personally examined a few thousand of these records; and I concluded that roughly 90 per cent of the clinic husbands then earned from two to three pounds per week. The arithmetical mean for Glasgow, for instance, was £2–15–8. At Cambridge the highest weekly income was £5. It is true that a few wives of Cambridge University teachers visited the Cambridge clinic, but their incomes were invariably not recorded on the clinic case sheets. Such exceptions, however, only prove the rule.

Mrs. C. H. Robinson, using my published data on the occupations of British clinic husbands, has usefully compared the occupational distribution of the husbands of English clinic clientele with the general occupational distribution of the total population of England and Wales. These latter data are presented in Table IX. In Figure XXIII the data are presented graphically.

The most striking feature of Figure XXIII is the large proportion of unskilled husbands in the clinic group as compared with the general population (34 versus 13). Of the two upper classes the clinic has only half the proportion of the general population (12 vs. 23). The so-called intermediate and skilled groups are a trifle smaller in the clinical than in the general population.

From these and other data Robinson concludes that the English clinics are operating eugenically. Though there are numerous difficulties involved in the interpretation of such data, and though we need a greater accumulation of facts, this position may be tentatively accepted as sound. There are numerous problems of interpretation involved the discussion of which would take us too far afield. For instance, it is by no means clear that Robinson has, in every instance, allocated the clinic husbands to the proper social class. Moreover, there are questions connected with the extent to

TABLE IX

OCCUPATIONAL DISTRIBUTION IN BRITISH BIRTH-CONTROL CLINICS COMPARED WITH GENERAL
POPULATION IN ENGLAND AND WALES[1]

Based on occupations reported for 2915 husbands in nine British clinics

Location of Clinic	Total Cases	V Unskilled	IV Inter-mediate	III Skilled	II and I Two Highest Classes
Distribution in Occupational Classes					
Wolverhampton.......................	479	63	28	(368)?	(20)?
Birmingham..........................	150	40	23	66	21
Manchester...........................	531	196	86*	186	63*
Glasgow.............................	139	52	27	37	23
Cambridge...........................	263	99	53	78	33
North Kensington...................	898	379	94*	281*	144
Aberdeen............................	98	42	8	22	26
Liverpool............................	215	109	38	46	22
Cannock.............................	142	—	142	—	—
Clinic Total......................	2,915	980	499	1,084	352
Per Cent. Distribution					
Wolverhampton.......................	100	13	6	(77)	(4)
Birmingham..........................	100	27	15	44	14
Manchester...........................	100	37	16*	35	12*
Glasgow.............................	100	37	19	27	17
Cambridge...........................	100	38	20	30	12
North Kensington...................	100	42	10*	31*	16
Aberdeen............................	100	43	8	22	27
Liverpool............................	100	51	18	21	10
Cannock.............................	100	—	100	—	—
Total Clinic Per Cent..............	100	34	17	37	12
Percentile Division in 1921 Census England and Wales..............	100	13	20	43	23

* Figures for two categories originally combined are here redistributed according to average proportion in remaining clinics.

[1] Revised from C. H. Robinson, *Seventy Birth Control Clinics*, p. 324.   Original sources: For clinic data, Himes, *Eugenics Review*, xx, 157–165.   For census data, *Occupational Mortality, Fertility and Infant Mortality. Registrar General's Decennial Supplement, England and Wales*, 1921, *Part II*, London, 1927.

which we should accept completely even the classification made by the British census.   Into these matters it is not possible to enter here.   One of the difficulties is well illustrated by a personal experience.   When these data were first published in the *Eugenics Review*, I was of the opinion that miners should be classed as unskilled laborers. Though I have long been a student of labor problems, at the time I considered this classification sound. I have since, however, been convinced by an authority on labor problems, that miners should be classified as semi-skilled laborers as the very lowest grade. Some consider them skilled. Similar problems of interpretation arise in connection with classifying each of the occupations. It is difficult to find a series of objective tests, but perhaps that of the length of training involved is one of the best. Recently, however, Pearl has very usefully classified occupations in a paper in *Human Biology*.

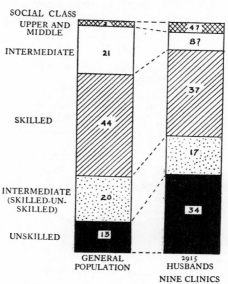

Fig. XXIII. Percentage of Distribution by Social Classes of Clientele of Nine British Birth-control Clinics as Compared with the Percentage Distribution of Social Classes in the General Population.

It seems clear from the above that the English clinics, all of which have been founded since 1921, have been influential in disseminating contraceptive advice to the lower social classes. This, then, seems an established fact.

Is the situation similar in America? Yes. It may be stated dogmatically that the American birth-control clinics serve primarily the working classes. In the absence of a full analysis of the occupational, wage, and social statistics, samples of which can alone be presented, it may be said that this thesis finds support in the partial reports already issued by many American birth-control clinics, and that the judgment is confirmed by those best acquainted with their operation.

(3c)   Age Distribution, Duration of Marriage, and Reproductive History.

Tables X and XI present preliminary evidence on the age distribution and duration of marriage, respectively, of patients at Baltimore and Cleveland clinics.   Likewise Tables XII, XIII and XIV deal with the reproductive life of the patients at these clinics.   These and similar data show that American birth-control clinic patients are well along in their reproductive and married life.   The typical patient is about thirty years of age, has been married ten years, has had about four pregnancies and has three living children.   This is also the situation among British clinic patients.

TABLE X

AGE DISTRIBUTION OF PATIENTS.   BALTIMORE AND CLEVELAND[1]

Age Group	Total		Baltimore		Cleveland	
	No.	Per Cent.	No.	Per Cent.	No.	Per Cent.
	4269	100	1152	100	3117	100
15–19	118	3	34	3	84	3
20–24	954	22	200	17	754	24
25–29	1240	29	317	27	923	30
30–34	1022	24	307	27	715	23
35–39	665	16	215	19	450	15
40–44	230	5	67	6	163	5
45–49	33	1	12	1	21	*
50 or over	1	*	—	—	1	*
Unknown	6	*	—	—	6	*

[1] Sources: Baltimore, *Fifth Report Bureau for Contraceptive Advice*, p. 7.   Cleveland, unpublished report.

Occupational statistics suggest that the lower and middle social classes are mainly served.   In 4,269 cases at Baltimore and Cleveland (Table XV), 30 per cent are unskilled laborers, 30 per cent skilled or semi-skilled workers, 11 per cent tradesmen.   The percentage in domestic and personal service is naturally small since the marriage rate in this group is low.   Professional men represented only 6 per cent of the cases, and probably this small group would not be present were adequate contraceptive skill more generally available in the United States.   Wives of such men, through their contacts, get acquainted readily with such a source of advice.   At Newark (Table XVI) one-tenth are professional men, yet one-third are unskilled workers, and one-quarter skilled and semi-skilled workers.

TABLE XI

DURATION OF MARRIAGE OF PATIENTS. BALTIMORE AND CLEVELAND[1]

Years married	Total		Baltimore		Cleveland	
	No.	Per Cent.	No.	Per Cent.	No.	Per Cent.
	4269	100	1152	100	3117	100
Premarital	31	1	—	—	31	1
0–4	1161†	27	204	18	957†	31
5–9	1320	31	339	29	981	32
10–14	1002	24	330	29	672	21
15–19	526	12	197	17	329	11
20–24	181	4	63	5	118	4
25–29	42	1	19	2	23	*
30–35	2	*	—	—	2	*
Unknown	4	*	—	—	4	*

* Less than 0.5 per cent.

† Includes also an unknown number of premarital patients.

[1] Sources: Baltimore, *Fifth Report Bureau for Contraceptive Advice*, p. 7. Cleveland, unpublished report.

TABLE XII

REPRODUCTIVE LIFE OF PATIENTS. BALTIMORE. SERIES FOR FIRST FIVE YEARS[1]

Number	Number of Patients Having the Specified Number of		Number	Number of Patients Having the Specified Number of	
	Pregnancies	Children		Pregnancies	Children
0	21	31	11	30	20
1	82	119	12	27	6
2	127	146	13	21	8
3	136	161	14	8	4
4	140	154	15	12	4
5	136	137	16	2	—
6	114	112	17	4	1
7	91	84	18	2	—
8	75	66	22	1	—
9	71	67			
10	52	32	Totals	1152	1152

[1] Source: *Fifth Report of the [Baltimore] Bureau for Contraceptive Advice*. Baltimore, 1933, p. 8.

(3d) *Source of Reference of Patients*

The source of reference of patients supports the view that the clinics are reaching the lower economic and social classes. At Cleveland 44 per cent of the patients were sent by health and other social agencies. Approximately 7 per cent are referred by private physicians.   Ministers send a small but rapidly growing number.   Now that the clinic has been operating for a few years there has been an increase in the number of patients referred by older patients.   In 1928–29 this figure was only 2.2 per cent; but in 1931–33 it was 14.9 per cent.   In the same period the percentage of patients

TABLE XIII

PREGNANCIES, CHILDREN, AND ABORTIONS AND/OR MISCARRIAGES.   BALTIMORE[1]

From the Total Number of Women	Who Have *Each* Had the Number of Pregnancies Indicated in This Column	And Who Have *All Together* Had the Total Number of Pregnancies Indicated in This Column	The Reproductive Results Have Been			
			The Number of Children Indicated in This Column		And Also the Number of Abortions and/or Miscarriages Indicated in This Column	
			Absolute	Per Cent. of Pregnancies	Absolute	Per Cent. of Pregnancies
21	0	0	0	—	0	—
82	1	82	74	90.2	8	9.8
127	2	254	221	87.0	33	13.0
136	3	408	369	90.4	39	9.6
140	4	560	493	88.0	67	12.0
136	5	680	580	85.3	100	14.7
114	6	684	611	89.3	73	10.7
91	7	637	556	87.3	81	12.7
75	8	600	513	85.5	87	14.5
71	9	639	556	87.0	83	13.0
52	10	520	436	83.8	84	16.2
30	11	330	255	77.3	75	22.7
27	12	324	252	77.8	72	22.2
21	13	273	213	78.0	60	22.0
8	14	112	89	79.5	23	20.5
12	15	180	140	77.8	40	22.2
2	16	32	20	62.5	12	37.5
4	17	68	36	52.9	32	47.1
2	18	36	14	38.9	22	61.1
1	22	22	7	31.8	15	68.2
1152	—	6441	5435	84.4	1006	15.6

[1] *Fifth Report*, p. 9.

referred by other interested individuals rose from 6.2 per cent to 24.5 per cent.   At the English clinics one of the chief sources of reference is former patients.   Evidently the situation at Cleveland suggests that this may now be true of the older clinics in the United States.

Baltimore reports that 336 patients advised during its fifth year of operation were sent by 119 different physicians in Baltimore, 18 different physi-

TABLE XIV

REPRODUCTIVE LIFE OF PATIENTS. CLEVELAND[1]

No. of Known Pregnancies	Total Pregnancies	Per Cent of Total Pregnancies	Patients with Each Number of Children Born Alive															
Total No. of children.....			0	1	2	3	4	5	6	7	8	9	10	11	12	13	14
	1045	100	128	177	233	185	112	68	43	35	26	14	12	4	5	1	2
0	103	10	103														
1	155	15	19	135	1												
2	206	20	3	28	170	5											
3	156	15	1	7	35	111	2										
4	120	12	1	3	14	41	60	1									
5	78	8	1	3	4	10	27	33									
6	71	7			5	11	13	13	28	1							
7	51	5			1	4	8	15	9	14							
8	30	3					1	4	4	7	13	1					
9	22	2			1	1	1	1	2	4	5	7					
10	15	1		1	2	1		1		3	1		6				
11	14	1				1				4	4		2	1	2		
12	9	1								1	2	3	1	1	1		
13	6	1								1	1	1	1	1	1		
14	5	—										2	1	1	1		
15	1	—											1				
16	1	—															1
17	1	—														1	
18	1	—													1		

[1] Unpublished report from Maternal Health Association, Cleveland.

TABLE XV

OCCUPATIONS OF PATIENTS' HUSBANDS.[1] BALTIMORE AND CLEVELAND. FIVE YEARS[2]

Occupational Class	Total		Baltimore		Cleveland	
	No.	Per Cent.	No.	Per Cent.	No.	Per Cent.
	4269	99.7	1152	100	3117	100
Unskilled laborers........................	1277	30.0	305	27	972	31
Skilled and semi-skilled...................	1271	29.8	356	31	915	29
Tradesmen.............................	468	11.0	96	8	372	12
Transportation.........................	391	9.2	124	11	267	9
Professional men.......................	252	5.9	54	5	198	6
Clerical occupations.....................	193	4.5	47	4	146	5
Domestic and personal service............	193	4.5	60	5	133	4
Farmers and fishermen..................	91	2.1	58	5	33†	1
Public service..........................	82	1.9	36	3	46	2
Miners................................	3	*	3	*	—	
No occupation (student)................	11	*	—	—	11	*
Occupation unknown....................	34	0.8	13	1	21	1
Out of work (temporary)................	3	*	—	—	3	*

* Less than 0.5 per cent.

† Farmers only.

§ Approximate, calculated by slide rule.

[1] Source: *Fifth Report of the* [*Baltimore*] *Bureau for Contraceptive Advice.* Baltimore, 1933. Unpublished data for Cleveland from Gladys Gaylord, Secretary, Cleveland Maternal Health Clinic. Owing to financial conditions Cleveland has been unable to publish its fifth report.

[2] Baltimore, Nov. 2, 1927 to Oct. 31, 1932 inclusive. Cleveland from opening to April 1, 1933.

TABLE XVI

OCCUPATIONS OF PATIENTS' HUSBANDS. NEWARK[1]

Occupation	Number	Per Cent.
	2000	100.0
Unskilled.................................	649	32.5
Skilled and semi-skilled................................	488	24.4
Business.................................	342	17.3
Professions.................................	196	9.8
Clerical.................................	171	8.5
Executives.................................	84	4.2
Civil Service.................................	37	1.9
No record.................................	29	1.4

[1] Hannah M. Stone and Henriette Hart, *Maternal Health and Contraception ... Part I, Social Data,* p. 13.

cians in Maryland, outside of Baltimore, and 3 different physicians in neighboring states.[38] Up until the end of the fifth year the Baltimore Bureau for Contraceptive Advice received patients only on medical indications.

At Chicago, of 1,329 patients received at four centers during the first two years of operation, 504, or 37.9 per cent, heard of the clinic through newspapers; 235, or 17.7 per cent, were referred by friends; 91, or 6.9 per cent, came from medical sources such as physicians and hospitals; and 392, or 29.5 per cent, from social agencies. The remainder (8 per cent) were directed to the clinic from miscellaneous sources. During 1929 the corresponding figures for 1,340 patients at Chicago was 46.5 per cent referred by friends and former patients, 23.4 per cent from social agencies, 21.9 per cent from medical sources, and 8.2 per cent from miscellaneous sources.

At Newark, New Jersey, in a series of 2,000 cases, 778, or 39 per cent, were referred by friends or former patients, 344, or 17 per cent, by social agencies and nurses, and 744, or 37 per cent, by such medical sources as hospitals, clinics, physicians, the board of health, etc.[39]

A survey made in May, 1929 by the Los Angeles Mothers' Clinic Association shows that, of the first 3,000 cases, 40.5 per cent were referred by various departments of the Board of Health, 32.5 per cent by friends and former patients, and 10 per cent by the County Charities. Less than 1 per cent were referred by private physicians; but since that time the percentage of patients so referred has increased steadily. The association is a member of the California Conference of Social Workers, and coöperates with all the social service and charitable organizations of the city and surrounding country.

At the Mothers' Health Clinic of Alameda County, California, 58 per cent of the cases were referred by the social agencies of one kind or another.[40]

Table XVII, from Kopp's report on 10,000 cases at New York, is the most complete single series of data we have on the agencies prompting women to apply for contraceptive advice at that clinic. Nearly half of all applicants were referred by former patients and friends; one-third by welfare groups, if we include physicians; one-fifth as a result of publicity, the incentive coming twice as frequently as a result of contact with the League as of reading newspapers. Individual physicians referred 10 per cent of the cases, hospital social services 6 per cent.

Generally speaking, it requires a few years after the founding of a clinic

---

[38] *Fifth Report*, p. 17.

[39] Stone and Hart, *op. cit.*, p. 10.

[40] Mabel Gregg Boyden, "The Mothers' Health Clinic of Alameda County, California," *Birth Control Review*, xv, 286–288 (October, 1931).

before the social agencies in a given community appreciate its function sufficiently to coöperate with it in full. Hence in the early years relatively few patients are sent by "recognized" agencies; but as time passes, the percentage invariably increases. An analysis by Dr. Max Wershow[41] of the source of reference of patients at the Detroit Mothers' Clinic shows that 73 per cent of the cases came from the Visiting Nurses Association, private physicians, and the Detroit Board of Health. Even the Police Department and the Red Cross sent at least one client. Despite the fact that contra-

TABLE XVII

AGENCIES RESPONSIBLE FOR THE APPLICATION OF PATIENTS FOR CONTRACEPTIVE ADVICE
AT THE BIRTH CONTROL CLINICAL RESEARCH BUREAU, NEW YORK

Total Cases	Number 10000	Per Cent.
No report...	44	
Cases reporting source of reference.......................	9956	
Cases reporting source of reference.......................	**9956**	100.0
Patients and friends.................................	**4809**	**48.3**
Patients..	3547	
Friends..	1262	
Welfare groups......................................	**3197**	**32.1**
Social agencies.....................................	1211	
Physicians..	1003	
Hospitals...	615	
Nurses...	368	
Public Activities....................................	**1950**	**19.6**
American Birth Control League......................	604	
Birth Control Review...............................	482	
Books..	369	
Newspapers...	351	
Birth control meetings..............................	144	

[1] Marie E. Kopp, *Birth Control in Practice*, p. 37.

ceptive service was not offered by any hospital in Detroit at the time Dr. Wershow wrote, only 103 patients out of the 1,000 were referred to the Mothers' Clinic in a period of three and one half years from the entire group of twelve leading hospital units in the city.

(3e) *Income Status of Patients*

Statistics on the income status of patients point in the same direction as the occupational statistics and the figures on source of reference of patients.

[41] Max Wershow, M.D., "A Social Experiment in Birth Control. An analysis of over 1,000 cases from the records of the Mothers' Clinic of Detroit." Detroit: Mothers' Clinic, [1931].

TABLE XVIII

INCOME STATUS OF PATIENTS. CLEVELAND, 1928–1933[1]

Weekly Family Income	No. of Cases	Per Cent.	
		Each Group	Cumulative
Total....................................	3120	100	
Dependent.............................	892	29	29
Income Irregular......................	237	8	37
Less than $10.00......................	252	8	45
$10.00–14.00..........................	231	8	53
15.00–19.00..........................	223	7	60
20.00–24.00..........................	301	9	69
25.00–29.00..........................	292	9	78
30.00–34.00..........................	186	6	84
35.00–39.00..........................	117	4	88
40.00–44.00..........................	75	2	90
45.00–49.00..........................	33	1	91
50.00 plus............................	213	7	98
Unknown..............................	65	2	100

[1] Data from Maternal Health Association, Cleveland.

TABLE XIX

INCOME STATUS OF PATIENTS. NEWARK[1]

Weekly Family Income	No. of Families	Per cent.	Cumulative Per Cent.
	2000	100.0	100.0
No income.............................	47	2.4	2.4
$1–10.................................	9	0.4	2.8
11–20.................................	144	7.2	10.0
21–30.................................	628	31.4	41.4
31–40.................................	474	23.7	65.1
41–50.................................	266	13.3	78.4
51–60.................................	116	5.8	84.2
61–75.................................	94	4.7	88.9
76–100................................	87	4.4	93.3
101–150...............................	40	2.0	95.3
151 and over..........................	49	2.4	97.7
No record.............................	46	2.3	100.0

[1] Hannah M. Stone and Henriette Hart, *Maternal Health and Contraception . . . Part I, Social Data*, p. 14.

Baltimore does not publish this information, but the data for Cleveland and Newark appear in Tables XVIII, XIX and XX. Of 3,120 cases seen at Cleveland in the first five years of operation (to April 1, 1933) 892, or 29 per cent, were dependent; 237, or 8 per cent, had an irregular income. Sixty-nine per cent of the cases had a *family* income of less than $25 a week. Seven per cent had a family income in excess of $50 weekly. Consult column 4 in Table XVIII for the cumulative percentages.

The situation is similar at Newark (Table XIX), though here there are more in the higher income brackets. Still, 41 per cent of the 2,000 families had a weekly *family* income of less than $30. Wage rates tend to be higher

TABLE XX

DISTRIBUTION OF AVERAGE WEEKLY INCOME OF HUSBANDS ACCORDING TO INCOME PER YEAR.
BIRTH CONTROL CLINICAL RESEARCH BUREAU, NEW YORK[1]

	Number	Per cent.
Total Cases...	10000	
No report...	222	
Total reports on income.............................	**9778**	**100.0**
Amounts not recorded...............................	619	6.3
No income from husband's earnings....................	252	
Amount unknown, unemployed at present.............	222	
Amount unknown, income adequate...................	145	
Reports on income, amounts recorded.................	**9159**	93.7
Total cases reporting weekly earnings....................	**9159**	**100.0**
Less than $10..	16	0.2
$10–19..	468	5.1
$20–29..	2279	24.9
$30–39..	2962	32.3
$40–49..	1410	15.4
$50–59..	760	8.3
$60–69..	361	3.9
$70–79..	246	2.7
$80–89..	83	0.9
$90–99..	60	0.7
$100 and over.......................................	514	5.6

[1] Marie E. Kopp, *Birth Control in Practice*, p. 60.

in or near a metropolitan center. The chief explanation of a higher wage income in Newark than at Cleveland is probably selection of patients: Newark has more patients in higher occupational levels. This situation also reflects the limited clinical facilities available for giving contraceptive advice. When more private physicians take up the work, the percentage of cases from the higher income groups may be expected to drop at Newark. There was a general inaccessibility of the best contraceptive advice until recent years for many patients. Five or ten years ago many private physicians had difficulty in getting supplies, especially those of good quality. This, together with the unsympathetic attitude of many physicians, drove well-to-do patients to the clinics. Those opposed to all moves in the direction of socialized medicine might note this.

In the Kopp series on 10,000 cases in New York we have data on the distribution of average weekly income of the husbands in 9,159 cases (see Table XX). Dr. Kopp reports that the typical patient, nearly two out of three, is a wage-earner's wife with an income of less than $40 a week.[42] The group contains a relatively small number of families in extreme poverty at one end of the scale, and a still smaller group at the other end, whose husbands average $100 per week or more. Inasmuch as these figures were gathered in a period of business prosperity, the amount of unemployment recorded, and the number of instances of husbands having no income are small. More than three-fourths of the cases received incomes below $50; two-thirds below $40; one-third below $30. The first quartile falls on $25, the median on $30, the third quartile on $45 weekly.[43]

The following table, also extracted from Dr. Kopp's able study, compares the distribution of annual income of clinic husbands with the corresponding figures for the general population of New York City in 1926 taken from the State Housing Bureau Report:[44]

| | Clinic Cases | | Per cent. in State Housing Bureau Report |
	Number	Per cent.	
Below $1000	488	5.3	5.4
$1000 to 2000	5243	57.2	45.9
$2000 to 3000	2172	23.7	29.4
$3000 to 5000	751	8.2	11.8
$5000 and over	511	5.6	7.5

Thus the distribution of incomes of the clinic husbands is seen to be lower than that for the population as a whole.

(3f) Housing Conditions and Unemployment

The housing conditions of the Cleveland patients (Table XXI) support the view that a goodly proportion come from the lower classes. Fifty-three per cent are crowded or over-crowded, 1 per cent "greatly overcrowded," 34 per cent are described as living under spacious conditions, and only 11 per

---

[42] Kopp, p. 59.
[43] *Ibid.*, p. 61.
[44] *Ibid.*

TABLE XXI

HOUSING CONDITIONS OF PATIENTS. CLEVELAND, 1928–1933[1]

Degree of Spaciousness or Crowding	Cases	
	Number	Per cent.
Total..	2955†	100
Very spacious..	328	11
Spacious...	993	34
Crowded...	1353	46
Overcrowded...	202	7
Greatly overcrowded.................................	48	1
Premarital (unknown)................................	28	1
Home broken...	1	*
Unknown...	2	*

* Less than 0.5 per cent.

† Omits 155 cases of the years 1928–30 entered before information was secured on this point and 7 premarital cases of the year 1930–31.

[1] Data from Maternal Health Association.

TABLE XXII

PERIOD AND CAUSES OF UNEMPLOYMENT OF 332 DEPENDENT FAMILIES. CLEVELAND, 1932–1933

Period of Unemployment	Total		Causes of Unemployment		
	No.	Per Cent.	Man's Health	Depression	Other
	519	100	49	461	9
Less than 6 mos......................	88	17	4	82	2
6 mos. to 1 yr........................	99	19	11	85	3
1 yr. to 1½ yrs........................	109	21	10	98	1
1½ yrs. and more.....................	223	43	24	196	3

TABLE XXIII

RACES OF PATIENTS. BALTIMORE AND CLEVELAND[1]

Race	Total		Baltimore		Cleveland	
	Number	Per Cent.	Number	Per cent.	Number	Per cent.
	1662	100	1152	100.0	510	100.0
White.....................	1323	80	944	81.9	379	74.4
Negro.....................	339	20	208	18.1†	131	25.6*

* 8 per cent. in the general population of 1930.

† 17.7 per cent. of the general population in 1930.

[1] Sources: Baltimore, *Fifth Report of the Bureau for Contraceptive Advice*, p. 6. Cleveland, unpublished data from Maternal Health Association.

cent have very spacious accommodations. A clinic official has very carefully defined these terms.[45]

Table XXII deals with the causes and period of unemployment among 332 dependent families advised at Cleveland during the year preceding April 1, 1933. Since there were 397 dependent families in the series of that year, the 332 dependent having unemployed breadwinners, constituted 84 per cent of the total of that group. It is difficult to record causes accurately. Health was tabulated when this was an obvious factor. Those tabulated under "depression" omitted cases in which the man's health was good. It thus underestimates unemployment resulting from the business cycle.

(3g) Racial and National Diversity of Clinic Populations in U. S. A.

Racial and nationality statistics, when gathered by the clinics, point also toward democratization. Few clinics in the United States gather or tabulate this information; but it is clear from the few reports available that the clinics tend to serve a cross-section racially, and occupationally, but not religiously, of the communities they serve. Occupationally, however, they serve the lower groups in greater percentage. The clinic population at New York and Chicago is racially most diverse, many nationalities being represented, and with some variation, in due proportion. The patients at the Harlem clinic in New York are virtually all Negroes. Reference to Table XXIII shows that at Baltimore Negroes were 18.1 per cent of the clinic population, 17.7 per cent of the general population in 1930; at Cleveland 25.6 per cent in the clinic population and 8 per cent of the 1930 general population. Since Negroes generally have a lower economic and social status than whites, these figures show the percolation downward of contraceptive information of a more reliable sort than has heretofore been generally available.

Several settlement houses and social agencies have in recent years either started clinics or arranged for contraceptive service. Their patients are, of course, selected; social agencies reach the classes most in need of such service. For example, of the first fifty women advised through the Maternal Aid Society of New York, a Jewish organization doing prenatal work with mothers, only four were financially able to pay anything.

If it were possible to present statistics on the percentage of patients able to pay fees, the same general story would be told. Large numbers of the

---

[45] "Very spacious: 2 rooms more than number of persons.

"Spacious: 1 room per person or more than 1 and less than 2 rooms in excess.

"Crowded: More than 1 and not more than 2 persons per room.

"Overcrowded: More than 2 and not more than 3 persons per room.

"Greatly overcrowded: More than three persons per room."

poor are helped.   In many cases these women could not pay for the services of private physicians even were they generally known and accessible to such women.

Having reviewed the use of contraceptives in samples of the general population prior to clinical visits, and having considered the evidence from British and American clinical statistics pointing toward the socialization of birth control; and having found little or no contrary evidence therein which could not be explainable by special circumstances, I shall now survey certain non-clinical evidence.

§4   NON-CLINICAL EVIDENCE

(4a)   Access to Contraceptive Knowledge Accounts for Distinguished American Physicians Achieving a Low Birth Rate Early.

The birth rate of distinguished American physicians, low compared with the rates of other distinguished Americans, was low even before 1850, suggesting the availability of contraceptives as an important cause.   Huntington and Whitney have studied the size of families of the members of different occupational groups represented in *Who's Who?*   The data are plotted in Figure XXIV.   Though the birth rate of these physicians has oscillated somewhat, the most striking feature of the diagram is the prevalence of smaller families among distinguished physicians as compared with the distinguished members of other occupational groups.   It is true that other occupational-group birth rates have declined for several decades, but the rate for physicians was low even before 1850.   The causes are doubtless complex; but can there be any doubt that access to contraceptives was the "catalytic agent" in the whole process?   So say the makers of the chart:

It represents the way in which the birth rate has tended to become stabilized by means of knowledge.   During the four decades represented in the diagram, the size of physicians' families has suffered no real change.   It has fluctuated, to be sure, but the mild irregularities now apparent would probably disappear if we had records of 10,000 physicians instead of only 645.   The uniform size of physicians' families from decade to decade seems to mean that doctors, by reason of their professional knowledge, began to practise contraceptive measures long before this happened with other professions.[46]

What the physicians first possessed and applied, other higher professional and upper-class groups then adopted.   Presently the information percolated downward by popular literature (Chapters IX, X and XI) and then with the assistance of specially-founded clinics (this chapter).

[46] *The Builders of America*, p. 186.

(4b) *Fertility of Foreign Born Declining*

The fact that the fertility of the foreign-born women of the United States is approaching the fertility of native women further supports the thesis that contraceptive knowledge is rapidly becoming diffused. The rate of diffu-

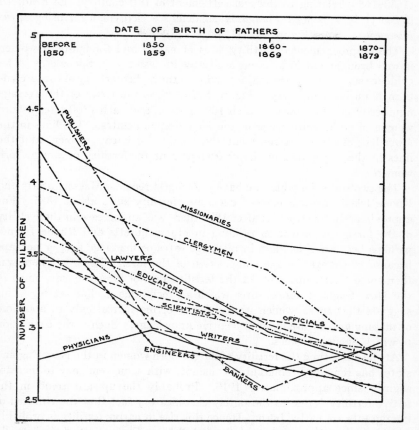

Fig. XXIV. Chart Showing Small Families Among a Group of American Physicians Early in the Nineteenth Century. Source: Huntington and Whitney, *Builders of America*, p. 187. Redrawn by Martin Van Stappen.

sion is, in fact, a special characteristic of the past century and a third. The birth rate of the United States began to decline as early as 1810 as has been shown by W. F. Willcox[47] and by numerous genealogical studies showing variations in the size of families since that period. It was not long after

[47] *Publ. Amer. Statis. Asso.*, xii, 490–499 (March, 1911).

1810 that Owen and Knowlton wrote (c. 1830). We know, however, that
birth-control practices were known here before Owen and Knowlton, for
there was an American edition of Carlile's *Every Woman's Book* published
in Philadelphia about 1827. Moreover, one of the oldest manuscripts
(1630–1650) relating to the first settlement of this country, the Bradford
[*History*] *Of Plimmoth Plantation* condemns a clergyman for using *coitus
interruptus*. (See Figure XVIII, page 225).

The rapprochement of fertility rates of native and foreign-born women
is well brought out in a recent study by Professor J. J. Spengler.[48] The
evidence suggests that the major portion of the higher fertility of the foreign-
born is purely temporary. Figure XXV shows the trend of the average
number of children born to each 1000 native, and each 1000 foreign-born
women of child-bearing age in the New England states. The lines in the
lower half of the chart represent the fertility of native women, and the
lines in the upper half of the chart represent the fertility of foreign-born
women.

The two states for which we have the longest records, Massachusetts and
Rhode Island, show a marked decline in fertility since about 1855. For
approximately two decades after 1875 there was an increase in the fertility
of the foreign-born women residing in Massachusetts and Rhode Island,
perhaps because of changes in marriage rates or marriage age, or perhaps
because of changes in age composition of the foreign born.[49] There was
then some "flattening out" of the fertility rate of foreign-born women in
the New England states, after which a precipitous decline set in. This
suggests that these women were either resorting increasingly to abortion,
or making greater use of contraceptive knowledge. Such is the conclusion
to which Spengler comes.

At the same time the fertility of native-born women in the New England
states has remained remarkably constant, with some tendency to increase
slightly since approximately 1910. Probably the upward trend in the
native fertility is due to the purely classificatory fact that the children of
immigrants are native born. Hence this rise in native fertility is probably
spurious when it implies that the "old" New England stock is actually
increasing. It is probably decreasing, this fact being covered up by the

---

[48] Joseph J. Spengler, "The Decline in Birth-Rate of the Foreign Born," *Scientific
Monthly*, xxxii (1931), 54–59. See also "The Comparative Fertility of the Native and the
Foreign-Born Women in New York, Indiana, and Michigan," *Quar. Jour. Econ.*, May,
1931. "Has the Native Population of New England Been Dying Out?" *Quar. Jour.
Econ.*, August, 1930. *The Fecundity of Native and Foreign-Born Women in New England.*
Washington: Brookings Institution, 1930, pp. 63.

[49] It is possible that the suppression of birth-control literature with the passage of the
Comstock law (1873) may have been a factor.

circumstance that the children of immigrants (natives) have been more fertile than the "old" native stock. Indeed the steady rate of the figures for "natives" after 1860 is probably due in part to the offset in a decline among the "old" New England stock by the higher fertility of "native" children of immigrants. With the cessation of net immigration, and with

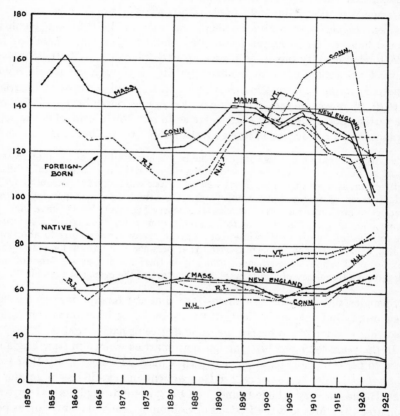

Fig. XXV. Fertility of Native-born and Foreign-born Women in New England. Source: J. J. Spengler in *Scientific Monthly*, xxxii (1931), 56. Redrawn by Martin Van Stappen.

the enormous additions to our "native" element owing to the large families of the immigrants coming here in 1898 to 1914, the native rate should hold its own or even increase slightly for a while. Spengler has not given attention to the factors just mentioned. But it seems that they have a direct bearing on so-called "native" increase in fertility. That the circumstances are relevant is suggested also by Willcox's reply to Sydenstricker (see p. 375 ff.).

Moreover, Spengler contends that the fertility of the foreign-born women of New England exceeds that of native-born women mainly because a much larger percentage of foreign-born women of child-bearing age are living in the married state. Spengler calculates that on the ground of a higher marriage rate alone, the 1890 foreign-born fertility should have been 15 per cent higher than native fertility; and that by 1920 foreign fertility should have exceeded native fertility by about 50 per cent. Whereas in 1890 foreign fertility was twice as great as native fertility, by 1921–25 it was only 44 per cent greater than native fertility. Though we should have expected, on the basis of a higher marriage ratio, a 35 per cent differential in 1920, there was, in fact, a sharp decrease of one-fourth in the fertility of the foreign born. Spengler goes so far as to say "birth control is the sole explanation of the decline in foreign fertility."[50]   He further says:

The only explanation of this sharp decline in foreign fertility lies in an increased resort to birth control on the part of foreign-born women. Advocates of birth control can, as a reading of the *Birth Control Review* will indicate, offer many individual cases of foreign-born women who unfortunately know nothing of the practice of birth control. Nevertheless the figures I present clearly prove that an increasingly larger proportion of foreign-born women are voluntarily restricting the number of children. Possibly, too, a great many are resorting to abortion. It has, in fact, frequently been asserted that between one half million and two millions of abortions are performed annually in the United States. Proof of this alleged high frequency of abortion is, in the nature of the case, not possible.[51]

Spengler then goes on to demonstrate that the foreign-born women of New York, Indiana, and Michigan "are [now] practising birth control or resorting to abortion in nearly the same degree as native women."[52]

In the years 1919 and 1920 foreign-born married women in New England bore 26 per cent more children than native married women. By 1922 this average had fallen to 18 per cent in Connecticut and to still less in Vermont, New Hampshire and Rhode Island. In 1922, in the United States registration area (27 states and the District of Columbia), the number of births per 1000 native married women aged 15–44 years was 155; and 159 per 1000

---

[50] This statement is a little strong.   Spengler modifies it in other passages to allow for a possibly increased abortion rate.

[51] *Scientific Monthly*, xxxii, 57.

[52] *Ibid.*   Considerable emphasis should be placed on the "nearly."   Clinical data show that foreign-born women use abortion more and contraception less than native women of comparable social status. The proof of this cannot now be marshalled here; but an analysis of the clinical data from American birth control clinics would prove it.   Here is a subject worthy of further investigation.

foreign-born women of corresponding ages. This shows that the fertility of foreign-born women is approaching that of native women. From this, says Spengler, "it follows that in a number of states foreign-born women practise birth control and resort to abortion as frequently as do native women."[53] There can be no doubt that there is a tendency in this country towards an equality of fertility rates of foreign-born and native women.

For the United States as a whole the birth rate of native-white women aged 15–44 years declined about one-third from 1900 to 1930. It declined over one-fifth between 1920 and 1930, compared with almost two-fifths for foreign-born white women and one-fifth for negro women. Whelpton, who furnishes these figures,[54] thinks that though it is possible that specific birth rates may continue to decline at this rapid rate, it is more probable that future decreases will become smaller relatively as well as absolutely.

Now, inasmuch as the foreign born represent, on the whole, the lower occupational groups, these data go a long way toward demonstrating that contraception is rapidly becoming democratized in America.

(4c) Rise in Native-White Fertility Spurious. Result of Influx of Foreign Born

Dr. Edgar Sydenstricker in "A Study of the Fertility of Native White Women in a Rural Area of Western New York"[55] argued that the fertility of native women living in five rural townships in Cattaraugus County, New York, showed no significant downward trend when the period 1920–1930 was compared with corresponding census records of the native white farmers' wives living on Cattaraugus County farms in 1900 and 1910.

Willcox considered this conclusion improbable on account of the general downward trend of the birth rate in the United States and in foreign countries, and because of the question of the adequacy of the sample. When he arranged the states in a rank order according to the percentage living in rural districts, he found that seven states along the northern border of the United States showed an actual increase in fertility (Figure XXVI).[56] Several others showed a decrease less than the average for the United States. The southern states were all below the average in fertility, in some instances the decrease being more than twice that of the average of the United States. Comparison of Figures XXVI and XXVII shows a high correlation between high fertility and high percentage foreign born.

[53] *Ibid.*, p. 58.

[54] *Amer. Jour. Soc.*, xxxviii, 832.

[55] *Quart. Bull. Milbank Memorial Fund*, x, 17–32 (Jan. 1932).

[56] Walter F. Willcox, "Changes Since 1900 in the Fertility of Native White Wives," *Ibid.*, x, 191–202 (July, 1932).

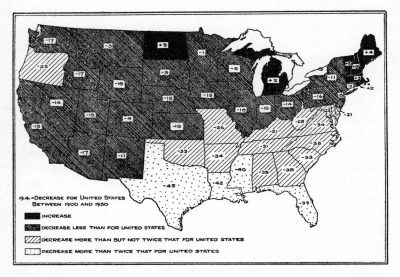

FIG. XXVI. Changes Between 1900 and 1930 in the Number of Children Under 5 Years of Age of Native-white Parents per 100 Native-white Married Women from 15 to 44 Years of Age.   Source: Willcox, *op. cit.*

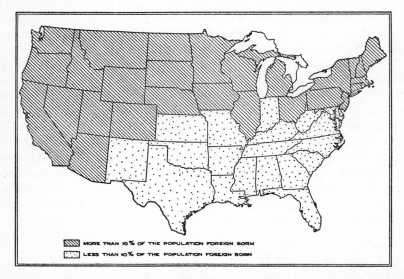

FIG. XXVII. States in Which More Than 10 Per Cent of the Population was Foreign-born in 1900.   Source: Willcox, *op. cit.*

Willcox accordingly concludes that the lack of fall found by Sydenstricker in a small northern section of the United States has been due to the influx of foreign-born stock, and of the consequently higher fertility of their immediate descendants. He says: "All this evidence seems to show that an important, if not indeed the main cause of rising fertility of native-white women since 1900, both in seven states along the Canadian frontier and in Cattaraugus County, if it has risen there as Mr. Sydenstricker's study suggests, has been the slow permeation of the class of native-white women within the present century by American-born daughters of foreigners carrying some part of the high fertility of their stock, and thus counterbalancing the tendency to a fall in the birth rate of native-white women, which has been traced in all other parts of the country."[57]   Incidentally, it ought to be noted that it is incorrect to imply that the temporary padding of the fertility of the native born is a result only of the influence of "American-born *daughters* of foreigners," since the *sons* of foreigners likewise transmit the mores of higher fertility.   It would be interesting if we knew—but we do not—which married partner has the greater influence in determining the size of family.   If neither has preponderant influence, it is important to know that.

Thus we see that Sydenstricker's evidence which was apparently not in harmony with my thesis of increasing democratization of birth-control knowledge, so harmonizes when set in its proper light by Willcox's able analysis.   For it is a well-established fact that the foreign-born inhabitants have been slower to adopt prevention than the older stocks.   Willcox's data show prettily the process of socialization in operation.

(4d)   *International Convergence of Birth Rates*

Not only is there a tendency for the fertility rates of the native and foreign born in the United States to approach one another, but fertility rates in various nations are converging as shown in Figure XXVIII.[58]   The differences in national birth rates are now much smaller than a few decades ago. Probably this is true also of occupational and religious groups.   While it is not suggested that the diffusion of contraceptive knowledge is the only immediate cause, there can be no doubt that it is the most important one.

[57] *Ibid.*, x, 202.   Punctuation mine.

[58] See R. M. MacIver, "Trend of Population with Respect to Future Equilibrium [Between Classes]," in L. I. Dublin [Ed.], *Population Problems*, pp. 287–310.   *Cf.*, also the charts of the Population Reference Bureau, Washington Square East, New York City. The same tendency has been noted by R. R. Kuczynski in his *Balance of Births and Deaths*, and by other writers.   The tendency was noted as early as 1890 by Levasseur. Note the recent rise in German birth rate.   For discussion see Whelpton in *Amer. Jour. Soc.*, xli, 299–313 (Nov. 1935).

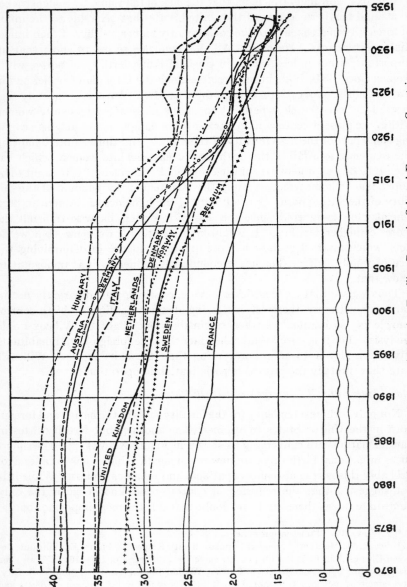

FIG. XXVIII. Convergence of Effective Fertility Rates in Selected European Countries

(4e) Differential Fertility. Its Existence Proves Democratization Incomplete

The existence of a differential birth rate between social classes in the United States has been more or less established for some time as a fact. Questions have arisen mainly about interpretation. Several studies have been made showing that the graduates of leading colleges are hardly, if at all, reproducing themselves; while studies of the size of families of the dependent and of the feebleminded have shown sometimes large families, almost always families more than adequate to replace the stock. More recently there have been able studies of differential fertility by Baber and Ross,[59] Sydenstricker,[60] Ogburn and Tibbitts[61] and Pearl,[62] while Moore[63] has issued a bibliography. However, until recently we have lacked a study half-way comparable to that published in 1911 as part of the Census Report for England and Wales.[64]

Though Notestein's papers[65] report the situation not for the whole country but for a sample taken from states north of the Mason and Dixie line, it was numerically large, and certainly the most inclusive study of data for

[59] Ray E. Baber and E. A. Ross, *Changes in the Size of American Families in One Generation.* Univ. Wisconsin Studies in the Social Sciences and History, No. 10. Madison, Wisconsin, 1924, pp. 99.

[60] Edgar Sydenstricker, "Differential Fertility According to Economic Status," *Public Health Reports*, xliv, 2101–2106 (August 30, 1929). Edgar Sydenstricker and G. St. J. Perrott, "Sickness, Unemployment, and Differential Fertility," *Milbank Mem. Fund Quart.*, vol. xii, no. 2, (April, 1934).

[61] W. F. Ogburn and Clark Tibbitts, "Birth Rates and Social Classes," *Social Forces*, September, 1929.

[62] Raymond Pearl, "Differential Fertility," *Quart. Rev. Biol.*, ii, 102–108 (March, 1927). "Some Data on Fertility and Economic Status," *Human Biol.*, iv, 525–553 (December, 1932).

[63] *Bibliography of Differential Fertility in English, French, and German.* Edited by Eldon Moore on behalf of Commission II of the International Union for the Scientific Investigation of Population Problems. Edinburgh, 1933, pp. vi, 1–97. Still more titles will be found in *Social Science Abstracts*.

[64] *Census of England and Wales*, 1911, vol. xiii.

[65] Frank W. Notestein, The Relation of Social Status to the Fertility of Native-born Married Women in the United States. In *Problems of Population*, Edited by G. H. L. F. Pitt-Rivers. London: Allen & Unwin. The above summarizes the following former papers by Notestein and others: Edgar Sydenstricker and Frank W. Notestein, "Differential Fertility According to Social Class," *Jour. Amer. Statis. Asso.*, March, 1930; Frank W. Notestein, "Social Classes and the Birth-rate," *Survey Graphic*, April, 1931; "Differential Age at Marriage According to Social Class," *Amer. Jour. Soc.*, July, 1931; Xarifa Sallume and Frank W. Notestein, "Trends in the Size of Families Completed Prior to 1910 in Various Social Classes," *Proc. Amer. Soc. Soc.*, 1931.

the United States that has yet been published.   There are other studies by Kiser[66] and Berry.[67]

Notestein's studies were based upon special tabulations, financed by the Milbank Memorial Fund, of portions of the original U. S. Census for 1910. The fertility of 99,226 native-white married women was studied according to their social class.   The conclusions are confirmatory and refining rather than new: (1) that "Women of the rural population were more fertile than those of the urban;" (2) that "in both the urban and rural populations there was a definite inverse relation between the net fertility of the classes and their social status as conventionally ranked."   Studies of smaller samples by others had shown the same results.   Notestein concludes further that (3) "This inverse association between fertility and social status is *in part* [italics mine] accounted for by a direct relation between marriage age and social status. . . . The proportion of childless marriages varied directly with social status in both the country and city, but was distinctly higher in the urban than the rural classes.   The trends in the birth-rates for women over 45 years of age in 1910 seem to indicate that in all classes for which the data are adequate, the size of completed families had been declining at least since 1870, but that this decline was less rapid in rural than in urban areas, and probably somewhat less rapid in the 'lower' than in the 'upper' urban classes."[68]

Kiser presents a useful chart (shown in Figure XXIX) and then concludes: "In general, the changes of fertility which took place were in the direction of lower rates and added differentiations according to social class. The fertility of the professional class became dissociated from the other white collar workers although even in 1910 the difference between the professional and business classes was less than that observed between other social classes.   The urban unskilled laborers fell below the rural classes. There were also increasing differentiations within the rural group.   At all ages and especially among women 25 years of age and over the age-specific rates for the farm laborers were higher than those for farm renters and farm owners.   The age-specific rates for the farm owners and farm renters were practically identical for women under 35 years of age, but among women 35 and over the rates of the farm owners were quite lower."[69]

[66] Clyde V. Kiser, "Trends in the Fertility of Social Classes from 1900 to 1910," *Human Biol.*, vol. v, no. 2, (May, 1933).   "Fertility of Social Classes in Various Types of Communities of the East North Central States in 1900," *Jour. Amer. Statis. Asso.*, December, 1932.

[67] Katharine Berry, "Differential Fertility According to Geographic Areas in the United States," *Quart. Bull. Milbank Memorial Fund*, vol. ix, no. 3, (July, 1931).

[68] F. W. Notestein in Pitt-Rivers [Ed.], *op. cit.*   Reprint, pp. 18–19.

[69] *Human Biol.*, v (1933), 272.

These data seem to square pretty well with the fact of increasing diffusion of contraceptive knowledge since 1800, with a more rapid rate of diffusion in the cities than in the rural areas, with the view that the upper social classes have first used contraceptives most effectively, and that gradually the lower classes have imitated them. These principles of diffusion are quite general.

The same point of lag in use of contraceptives by the lower classes may be inferred from a recent preliminary report by Sydenstricker and Perrott.[70]

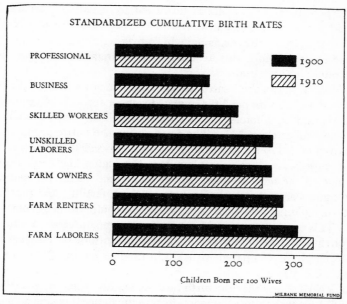

STANDARDIZED CUMULATIVE BIRTH RATES

Fig. XXIX. Standardized Cumulative Birth Rates for Each Social Class in 1900 and 1910. Data for East North Central States. Native-white Women Only. Source: Kiser.

House-to-house-canvas records of 8,000 families of unskilled and skilled laborers and of white-collar workers in eight cities collected during the current depression show not only the expected class differentials in birth rates (elaborated below), but that "the birth rate was highest during the depression in families which were without employment or on part-time work in 1932;" "that high fertility was associated with inability to succeed in the

[70] Edgar Sydenstricker and G. St. J. Perrott, "Sickness, Unemployment, and Differential Fertility," *Milbank Mem. Fund Quart.*, vol. xii, No. 2, (April, 1934). Page references are to the reprint.

severe competition for jobs brought about by the depression;" that those families "which had dropped from comparative comfort in 1929 to poverty in 1932 were families having a higher birth rate than those which did not suffer a drop in income."[71]

"Low social status, unemployment, and low income in 1932 went hand in hand with a high illness rate and increased malnutrition among children. It was in these same groups of families that a high birth rate prevailed. . . it is evident that a high birth rate during the depression prevailed in families which could least afford, from any point of view, to assume this added responsibility."[72] There is no intent to disparage this unusually competent research by Sydenstricker and Perrott when the observation is made that the Neo-Malthusians have been making much the same points, though of course without this accuracy of measurement, for nearly a century, certainly for fifty years.

Table XXIV shows the birth rate and employment status of the group. Note that the birth rate per 1,000 married women aged 15–44 years was, in families of unskilled laborers, 182; in families of skilled laborers 150; in those of the white-collar class, 134. The average for the entire group was 152 as compared with 126 for the United States birth-registration area. Note that the more severe the unemployment, the higher the birth rate. Of course, not all the more frequent births took place during the depression; but the figures show a correlation between high fertility and inability to compete in holding jobs at a time when the competition becomes most severe. This is what one would expect from common observation.

The birth rate in families receiving an annual income of less than $1,200 in 1929 was 176 as compared with 115 in families having $2,500 or more. (See Table XXV).

Table XXVI shows that the birth rate was higher when the poor[73] stayed poor (178) than when those in moderate[74] circumstances became poor during the depression (157). In fact it was highest of all groups. It was next to lowest among those whose comfortable[75] position continued throughout the depression (107), and lowest among those who went from comfortable to moderate circumstances.

The birth rate in families without employed workers in 1932 was 197; with part-time workers 154, with one or more full-time workers 134, lowest of all. "Thus, the families without any employed workers in 1932 had a

[71] *Ibid.*, p. 8.
[72] *Ibid.*
[73] Less than $1,000 annual income.
[74] $1,200–$2,000 annual income.
[75] $2,000 or more annual income.

TABLE XXIV

BIRTH RATE AND SOCIAL AND EMPLOYMENT STATUS, 1929–1932.* SYDENSTRICKER AND PERROTT SAMPLE[1]

Social and Employment Status	Birth Rate† per 1000 Married Women Aged 15–44	Births 1929–1932	No. Years Recorded 1929–1932. Women Aged 15–44
Unskilled Labor	182	586	3792
No employed workers	234	154	702
Part-time workers	166	263	1775
Full-time workers	169	169	1315
Skilled Labor	150	2173	14436
No employed workers	188	318	1655
Part-time workers	152	1183	7374
Full-time workers	134	672	5407
Salaried Workers	134	559	4312
No employed workers	167	59	337
Part-time workers	153	173	1142
Full-time workers	120	327	2833
Total	152	3318	22540

* For population groups canvassed in Birmingham, Baltimore, Cleveland, Detroit, Greenville, New York City, Pittsburgh and Syracuse.

† Adjusted for age.

[1] Source: Sydenstricker and Perrott, *op. cit.*, reprint, p. 5.

TABLE XXV

BIRTH RATE AND INCOME.* SYDENSTRICKER AND PERROTT SAMPLE[1]

Income	Birth Rate per 1000 Married Women Aged 15–44†	Births 1929–1932	No. Years Recorded 1929–1932 Women Aged 15–44
Under $1200	176	428	2526
$1200–$1999	145	572	4198
$2000–$2499	124	140	1484
$2500 and over	115	102	1171

* For population groups canvassed in Baltimore, Cleveland, New York, and Syracuse.

† Adjusted for age.

[1] Source: Sydenstricker and Perrott, *op. cit.*, reprint, p. 6.

birth rate *during the depression* 48 per cent higher than those which had one or more full-time workers in 1932."[76]

In connection with relief, data are available for families with less than $1,200 annual income in 1932 in four of the eight cities studied. The birth rate in families receiving relief in 1932 was 210 as compared with 137 in families not receiving relief, an annual average rate 53 per cent higher than that of those not on relief.[77] Doubtless those with more dependents were more likely to receive relief. None the less, the correlation is clear, and while correlation does not always mean causation, it seems reasonable to suppose that the higher rate was one of the causes of relief need. This again is a common enough observation, and has been made since the days of Francis Place, in fact, many savages saw as clearly as many people now-

TABLE XXVI

BIRTH RATE AND CHANGE IN ECONOMIC STATUS, 1929–1932.*   SYDENSTRICKER AND PERROTT
SAMPLE[1]

Economic Status in		Birth Rate† per 1000 Married Women 15–44 Years of Age	Births 1929–1932	No. Years Recorded 1929–1932 Women Aged 15–44
1929	1932			
Poor	Poor	178	406	2404
Moderate	Poor	157	448	2994
Moderate	Moderate	113	118	1152
Comfortable	Poor	133	143	1287
Comfortable	Moderate	104	75	831
Comfortable	Comfortable	107	37	537

* For population groups canvassed in Baltimore, Cleveland, New York, and Syracuse.
† Adjusted for age.
[1] Source: Sydenstricker and Perrott, *op. cit.*, reprint p. 7.

adays—and more clearly than some—that too many babies or babies born too frequently spell poverty not prosperity.

These figures are recent and convincing proof not only of the reality of the differential birth rate, but of the still-extant maldistribution of contraceptive knowledge. The information is percolating downward, but the process is by no means complete.

(4f)   Is Differential Fertility Tending to Reverse Itself?

Some writers have tried to show, and they perhaps have shown in small, limited samples, that there has been some modification or alleviation recently of differential fertility by social classes.

[76] *Ibid.*, p. 7.
[77] *Ibid.*

Edin shows that higher income classes of Stockholm are now having larger families than the working classes.[78] This suggests that birth control is being used more extensively than ever by the working population of that city. Recent research by Julius Wolf likewise suggests some tendency toward a modification of the differential birth rate by social class.[79] Huntington is inclined to think that in the United States we are at a turning point; that several lines of evidence suggest that the differential birth rate is being modified slightly. He finds that the more successful Yale graduates in given graduating classes have larger families than the less successful. But this is only a reversal (if, indeed, it is such) within a given social class, and within a numerically restricted class at that. *As yet there is no reason to believe that there has been a very material reversal of the differential birth rate in any country. Until several trends become more marked, the differential birth rate will still be a subject of concern.*

§5 SUMMARY AND CONCLUSION

We have argued that contraceptive knowledge has been enormously diffused and democratized especially in the last one hundred years. This has, perhaps, been generally suspected; but we have attempted to prove it by documentary evidence. We have tried to examine the result of the extensive diffusion of literature and discussion of birth control in the last century. What was once more or less a monopoly of physicians and midwives has now been generally extended even to the layman. Accordingly, the problem is not, shall we have conception control or no conception control, but rather shall we diffuse the latest knowledge on scientific contraception or encourage by indifference and laissez-faire the use of quasi-unreliable, quasi-harmful methods with which many, including not a few of the otherwise enlightened, are in the habit of worrying along.

In presenting evidence in this chapter on the percentage of various populations using contraceptives in the English-speaking world it has not been thought necessary to prove an absence of general diffusion before 1800. This seems to me clear. The burden of proof is on the doubter. A study of 25,000 cases in twelve series ranging in date from 1917 to 1934 showed that *two-thirds admitted use; and, if certain series believed atypical, are omitted, over nine-tenths. In 26,801 instances in two large series it was found that the*

[78] *Proceedings World Population Conference*, 205–207. *Cf.*, *Eugenics Review*, xx, 258–266 (January, 1929). Enid Charles argues in her able *Twilight of Parenthood* that differential fertility has been disappearing since 1891. I find her case unconvincing.

[79] Julius Wolf, *Das neue Sexualmoral und das Geburtenproblem unserer Tage*. Jena, 1928, pp. 182. "Rollentausch zwischen Berlin und Paris in Geburt und Sterblichkeit," *Deutsch-Französische Rundschau*, ii, 744–752.

most popular methods were withdrawal (one-third), the douche, and condom in that order with about one-quarter each. Among the general population, prior to special medical instruction, other methods are used much less frequently.

The degree of success of methods as at present practiced is difficult to estimate owing to a large number of uncontrolled factors. In the Stone series, success percentages for the three leading methods ranged from 10 to 46 (*coitus interruptus* 29, douche 10, condom 46); whereas in one Kopp series the range for eight methods was, if we except abstinence, 40 to 55 per cent.

Pearl's preliminary but carefully-arrived-at figures show that, even among the very poor white women, those who practiced contraception intermittently for planned children reduced their pregnancy rate 55 per cent below that of the very poor who did not practice contraception. Among the well-to-do and rich white women the reduction was 70 per cent. I have estimated the average—a figure not yet presented in the second preliminary report—at 55 per cent. This is a considerable reduction. In Stix's pre-clinic sample pregnancies were reduced 75 per cent.

It should be clearly understood that these figures represent estimates of success with methods as now employed by samples of the married population prior to competent medical instruction. It is a result of what I call, for want of a better term, "back-fence" contraception. It is contraceptive technique learned from friends, neighbors, childhood or adulthood acquaintances, contraception, in a few instances, learned by reading books. It is amateur contraception.

Success after clinical advice approaches more nearly 90 to 95 per cent with a range from 70 to 98 per cent. In her large New York series Kopp concluded that when the clinically-advised methods were regularly used 93.3 per cent of the women were successfully protected.[80]

Democratization of contraceptive knowledge is further shown by the social and economic data in §3. Data on occupations of the patients' husbands show that from one-third to one-half in my British series were unskilled. The skilled group ranged from 20 to 30 per cent. For the entire group (2,915 cases) one-half of the patients' husbands (51 per cent) fall either in the unskilled or semi-skilled groups. A comparison of percentage distribution of occupations in the clinic sample with that for the general population of England and Wales shows that the working classes are being reached with contraceptive advice by the clinics in more than due proportion. At Baltimore and Cleveland (4,269 cases) 30 per cent were unskilled, 30 per cent skilled or semi-skilled, 11 per cent tradesmen. Professional men represented only 6 per cent of the cases, and even this proportion is doubtless a reflection of the legal ban actually or supposedly existing in

[80] *Op. cit.*, p. 211.

certain regions. At Newark one-third were unskilled, one-quarter skilled or semi-skilled, one-tenth professional men. At New York (Kopp) four-fifths of the husbands belong to the industrial and clerical groups. Professional men, high executives, owners and skilled workers together comprise one-fifth.

It is, of course, impossible for me to go behind these data. One who has never tried to classify men occupationally has no idea of the difficulty involved, especially in this day of widespread mechanization. Doubtless clinic officials—and I include myself, of course—have made countless errors. Many will cancel out; many will not. There is no hope of improving this situation unless and until we can persuade all clinics to adopt a standard occupational classification such as that recently published by Pearl in *Human Biology* and to make still more careful inquiries than they have in the past into the exact classification of each husband.

Data on wage or family income, as the case may be, corroborate the occupational data. Though there is a scattering of people from the higher income groups (again a reflection of special social facts)[81] the overwhelming majority are either poor or in moderate circumstances. What little information we have on over-crowding, unemployment, source of reference of patients, supports the thesis of democratization so far as the present work of the clinics is concerned.

Let us review first some of the more outstanding facts on the source of patients. At Cleveland's Maternal Health Center, up to April 1, 1933, 44 per cent were referred by health or social agencies, 7 per cent by private physicians. More recently, as the clinic has become known and has established itself, friends and former patients are playing a more important rôle. I am inclined to believe, though I have not made the necessary statistical investigations, that this is a general pattern typical of all clinics: after a center gets established for a few years patients referred by former clients increase relatively until an unknown maximum is reached. It would be interesting to know—yet we do not know—just how much the proportion changes with time. I found in 1928 that at the English clinics former patients were one of the chief sources of new patients.

During its fifth year the Baltimore Bureau for Contraceptive Advice, which originally accepted patients only on medical indications, received 336

[81] I think the chief causes are as follows: (1) Some higher-income-class women came to the clinics because they are more likely to find sympathetic guidance, more certain to get what they want there than from the general run of private practitioners, who are often too prone to moralize. (2) It is now becoming "the thing to do" for many society women to take up birth control, especially the organization and financing of clinics. Thus a certain fringe of their class drift to the clinics. (3) Some physicians still withhold information.

new patients sent by 119 different physicians in Baltimore, and by 21 different physicians outside of Baltimore. In a series of 1,329 cases at Chicago the newspapers stood out with 38 per cent, friends[82] 18 per cent, medical sources 7 per cent, social agencies 30 per cent. During 1929 in 1,340 cases we have: friends and former patients 47 per cent, social agencies 23 per cent, medical 22 per cent. There was thus an increase from friends and former patients and from medical sources. The facts at Newark and Los Angeles are roughly similar. Dr. Kopp's data on New York are of more than ordinary reliability: patients and friends 48.3 per cent, welfare groups (including physicians and hospitals), 32.1 per cent, public activities 19.6 per cent. Dr. Wershows' analysis of 1000 cases at Detroit showed that 73 per cent of all patients came from the Visiting Nurses Association, private physicians, and the Detroit Board of Health.

At Cleveland in five years up to April 1, 1933, 30 per cent of the patients were dependent. The *family* income in 69 per cent of the cases was under $25 weekly. At Newark over 41 per cent had less than $30 weekly as a *family* income. At New York, in 9,159 cases, three-fourths received incomes below $50; two-thirds below $40; one-third below $30. The typical patient at New York (two out of three) has less than $40 per week. The income of the clinic group is slightly below that of the general population of New York in 1926 as shown in the State Housing Bureau Report.

Cleveland alone reports housing conditions. There 53 per cent were "crowded" or "over-crowded" as defined, 10 per cent "greatly over-crowded."

Racial and nationality statistics show, in a word, that the "old-timers," generally speaking those of higher social status, are educating in contraception the "newcomers," or more recent immigrants. In the main, nearly all the racial and nationality groups are being reached by the large clinics in the metropolitan centers, and this apparently in due proportion.[83] Certainly one is impressed by the great diversity of nationalities served, for example, by the chief clinics in New York and Chicago. In more homogeneous communities one would not expect such diversity. Another factor making for diversity is the location of several clinics in settlement and neighborhood houses. Kopp, for instance, found[84] that the New York women she studied were predominantly of foreign birth and extraction (45 and 28 per cent), southeastern Europe and Semitic Russia contributing the largest

[82] This term is usually undefined and one cannot always be certain whether friends of the patient or of the clinic organization or birth control league are meant. Probably the first—friend of the client—is meant.

[83] This is a tentative judgment. It needs much more quantitative study than I have been able to give it to date.

[84] *Op. cit.*, p. 204.

number. North European groups come next, with the Germans and Irish predominating. Latin peoples appear in a ratio of 1 to 6, Negroes 1 to 33. Hence it is not surprising, as Kopp remarks, that "four-fifths of the husbands belong to the industrial and clerical groups."

It is a fact well-known to clinic staff officers that many patients are unable to pay even a small fee for contraceptive advice and supplies, a circumstance suggesting that contraceptive knowledge is percolating downward, that is, being democratized. Since most clinics do not publish information on this subject, it is not at present possible to present quantitative data.

Just as the pre-clinical-visit and clinical evidence point to democratization, so does the non-clinical evidence on the declining birth rates of various groups. Even for their class, distinguished American physicians have a low birth rate, a situation which dates before 1850, suggesting the influence not only of accessibility to contraceptive information but accessibility antedating that of any other professional group in the United States. This is what one would theoretically expect.

The fact that the fertility of the foreign born is gradually approaching that of the natives of the United States likewise illustrates the process of social diffusion. The high fertility of the foreign born is a purely temporary phenomenon. It has declined markedly with tighter and tighter immigration restrictions. The slight increase in native fertility shown in Figure XXV is probably spurious due to the purely statistical fact that the children of immigrants are native born and that they carry over into the native group the mores of high fertility. Professor J. J. Spengler, whose data are used in this connection, ventures the opinion that the overwhelming proportion of the decline in foreign-born fertility is a consequence of increased birth control and abortion (more contraception than abortion), a view clearly in accord with the weight of authority. He concludes that the foreign-born women of New York, Indiana and Michigan "are [now] practicing birth control or resorting to abortion in nearly the same degree as native women."

For the United States as a whole the birth rate of native-white women aged 15–44 years declined about one-third in three decades alone (1900–1930); one-fifth in a single decade (1920–1930); two-fifths for foreign-born white women in a single decade (1920–1930). The decline will be much less rapid in the immediately-following decades. Since the foreign born represent the less privileged classes, such evidence is certainly relevant to our discussion of the democratization process.

It was seen that Sydenstricker's apparent exception to the fall in fertility of native-white women in a small northern section of the United States (5 rural townships of New York) was satisfactorily explained by Willcox as due to an influx of foreign born, padding the "native" category with their children, who, in turn, tend to have a fertility in between that of the native and foreign born.

Just as it has been shown that in the United States the fertility of the native and foreign born is equalizing itself, so we noted that *there has been going on in recent decades an international convergence of birth rates. All are approaching, or tending to approach with some delay* (as in the case of Russia and southeastern Europe) *what might be called the level of controlled fertility. Thus the democratization process is not culture-bound; it is not applicable only to one or two Western societies. With the exceptions already noted, it is characteristic of all important Western civilizations.* I predict that within fifty years, certainly within a century, the exceptions in Europe will fall into line, and it is only a question of time before the process will be repeated in Oriental societies. This seems to me one of the most certain of sociological predictions.

The data on differential birth rates by social classes fit well into the thesis that the socially-privileged groups have been the first to adopt this new economizer of human energy. Notestein showed in nearly 100,000 cases in the United States that "in both urban and rural populations there was a definite inverse relation between the net fertility of the classes and their social status as conventionally conceived." This conclusion is not new; but such competent proof of it is. As one would indeed expect, childless and small families were found more frequently in the upper and urban classes. Kiser's chart (Figure XXIX) shows similar results for various social classes.

Such a differential is what one would expect. The upper classes are, on the whole, more intelligent. They have more foresight and probably more personal ambition. As with mechanical improvements newly placed on the market, the lower classes ape the upper classes. In the masses, stronghold of the mores, there are more impediments to the prompt adoption of improved contraceptive methods. To the rich nothing is radical which serves their interests—which is one, but by no means (fortunately) the sole reason why many of the rich will support birth-control propaganda but not many other reform movements equally important, for example, the more equitable distribution of wealth.

So much then, for the case that *democratized* contraception is an ultra-modern phenomenon even though contraception as a practice is as old as civilization itself. In earlier chapters we attempted to show that the *desire to control conception has been a constant characteristic of civilizations throughout the entire range of social development.* The great, and sometimes absurd lengths to which human ingenuity has gone to devise control methods witness the bold determination of humankind to master the reproductive process. If results did not always correspond with desires it was due to an absence of modern technical knowledge. The Vital Revolution[85] now going on, which has been going on since 1800, would probably have come centuries ago had accumulated knowledge made it possible. Therefore, those who view the spread of modern birth control with horror ought to realize that our age harbors no special tribe of devils; they have merely seized their "opportunities." There can be no doubt that throughout the ages there has been not only a steady accumulation of knowledge of contraception but a decided improvement in reliability, the most noteworthy stages being the invention of the rubber condom and Mensinga pessary—both accomplishments of the mid-nineteenth century.

In preceding chapters we have traced not only the practice of contraception but the development of accumulated knowledge on this subject. In this chapter especially we traced its diffusion socially throughout the population.

It has not been within the province of this book to discuss modern aspects of such measures as vasectomy and salpingectomy. There are over eighty papers on spermatoxins. The research has, however, been performed almost entirely on animals. It is now clear that much additional thorough and costly study will have to be made, first in laboratories, before a relatively simple vaccine method can furnish safety for women for several months at a time. Such a method would be especially valuable in those over-crowded, poor regions of the world as India, parts of China, and Puerto Rico. There is urgent need to develop and diffuse simple methods for the poor of such regions. The average annual income of a large sample of Chinese farmers is about $300 (Chinese). Modern clinical methods are far too costly for such people. We need to develop household contraceptives of the simple type: wads of cotton, douches of salt or vinegar, etc. Dr. Dickinson has discussed this subject in an article in the November, 1935, issue of *Marriage Hygiene*.

The next chapter considers briefly some of the probable economic and social results of diffusion or democratization of contraceptive knowledge.

§6 A METHODOLOGICAL NOTE: IMMEDIATE VS. LONG-RUN CAUSES OF THE VITAL REVOLUTION

In order to consider the future, it is necessary to clarify our position on a matter of social causation. Some might have assumed from what preceded in this and other chapters that I felt that mere agitation, publication,

---

[85] Stabilization of population at a more economic level, i.e., with low birth and death rates instead of high birth and death rates. I intend to clarify the concept further in a special paper; but this is precise enough for present purposes.

etc., was sufficient to "cause" the diffusion already reported and measured. Of course, I hold no such sociologically-naïve view. It has been said, and with no little justification, that not birth control but social and economic forces have been the cause of the declining birth rate. In the main this is true. But I think a sounder insight into recent trends is afforded by the view that *while social and economic forces are the ultimate causative influences, democratized birth control is the immediate causative factor, the catalytic agent, without which the whole reaction could not have taken place.* It is bad chemistry to omit or overlook the catalytic agent. Likewise it is bad sociology to overlook the means or mechanism by which the Vital Revolution has been, and is being achieved. Economics has been guilty of this error[86] in emphasizing almost exclusively the rising standard of living to account for small families. But sociology need not fall into the same trap. And lest it be charged that I have devoted too much attention to authors, to the quantitative distribution and influence of their works, to agitators, etc., and not enough to broad social forces, I shall anticipate briefly an analysis which belongs more properly in my social and economic history of birth control, a work to follow the present one. The discussion below recapitulates an analysis of the social and economic forces which, in my judgment, have been mainly responsible for the democratizing process, a movement post-dating 1800 for the most part, and traced in some detail in recent chapters.

All the following social, economic and intellectual changes have paved the way for widespread adoption of contraceptive practices: the growth of hedonism, utilitarianism, materialism; the declining hold of orthodox religion and the rise of rationalism and the scientific spirit; growing emancipation or independence of women and feminism, including careers for women outside the home and their industrial employment; urbanism, the automatic development of a controlled death rate consequent upon the progress of general and preventive medicine, a change necessitating socially a controlled birth rate; fear, in the early stages of the Industrial Revolution, of over-population, a fear not totally unfounded before the opening of our agricultural West and before the mechanization of agriculture and of ocean and land transport;[87] a certain fear of land scarcity following the gradual settlement of the major habitable vacant spaces of the globe as a consequence of one of the most phenomenal human migrations that the annals of history record—

---

[86] Aside from the legitimate charge of one-sided causation, the process could not have taken place without diffused knowledge of contraception. Nine-tenths of modern neo-Classical economists have fallen, either expressly or implicitly, into this error.

[87] Even today the chief "cause" of repeated Chinese famines is poor, unmechanized transport and hand rather than modern, mechanized methods of agriculture. These factors, especially lack of transport, still play a rôle in Russian famines.

a migration caused basically by population pressure.[88] To these should be added other social forces, a few newly accelerated: urbanism, making a large family costly and inconvenient, social mobility and social ambition likewise promoting family restriction; army instruction in sexual prophylaxis during the war; above all, improved means of communicating knowledge, especially the technical factors which have cheapened printing and brought people into closer contact or caused them to exchange ideas with greater facility and frankness. The widespread desire for self-advancement economically,[89] which is such an outstanding characteristic of capitalistic civilization is no doubt fundamental. Most of the other forces mentioned have dovetailed well with personal ambition; hence the unique thoroughness and sweep of the Vital Revolution.

Only two forces of any account have tended to combat it: the metaphysics, doctrine and sophistry of the Catholic Church, and the revival of nationalism since the World War, especially in the forms of fascism and Hitlerism. Prophecy is always dangerous; but I venture the opinion that neither Catholicism nor fascism will be successful. This is not a mere projection of personal wishes; it is based upon facts and analyses which can find no place here.

These are, in the main, the chief forces promoting or retarding the increased practice of contraception since 1800. Most all are likely to continue for an indefinite period in the future. Even in the United States it will require several decades for the democratizing forces to work themselves out. That they will go further than socially necessary is another safe sociological prediction. This will happen for much the same reason that a pendulum, when drawn far to one side, will, upon being released, swing too far in the other direction. The same is true of the use and misuse of birth control. Those who understand the processes involved will not permit themselves to make the extreme public pronouncements so commonly met with in the press, especially in the Catholic press and in tirades by priests in general newspapers. There is every historical and theoretical reason to believe that the common sense of the masses will assert itself and that birth control will, if we can only keep the hot-heads in check, eventually find its proper extent of use. It will be such an extent as will give us reasonably sized families, well-distributed by social class, promoting maternal,

[88] The higher standard of living in the United States was largely, though not exclusively, a result of a sparse population not causing diminishing returns in agricultural production. A greater efficiency of labor, and perhaps also better managerial supervision were related important factors.

[89] Who knows but this tendency, carried to excess, will be the noose that capitalism has constructed for its own neck?

infant and family health, economy in human reproduction, checking irresponsible automatic spawning. It implies for the immediate future of most Western societies a stationary rather than a rapidly increasing population—a situation historically most typical and, in my judgment at least, socially most desirable, all present circumstances considered.[90]

[90] See the paper by Professor A. B. Wolfe on "The Rationalization of Production and Reproduction," in Himes [Ed.], *Economics, Sociology and the Modern World. Essays in Honor of T. N. Carver.* Cambridge: Harvard University Press, 1935, pp. 226–244.

CHAPTER XIV

PROBABLE EFFECTS OF DEMOCRATIZED CONTRACEPTION

§1   THE ADVENT OF STATIONARY POPULATIONS

So FAR as is known Edwin Cannan was the first (in 1895) to predict a stationary population for England.[1]   Some years later Bowley predicted a stationary population by 1941.[2]   Using the United States data the chief writers have been Dublin and Lotka,[3] Thompson and Whelpton[4] and more

---

[1] See *Econ. Jour.*, 1895; *Fortnightly Review*, March, 1902.   "Population and Production," *Nature*, cxxviii, 658–661 (Oct. 17, 1931).   *Economic Scares.*   London: P. S. King, 1933, pp. vii, 135.

[2] A. L. Bowley, "Estimates of the Working Population of Certain Countries in 1931 and 1941."   Geneva: League of Nations (Economic and Financial Section.   Submitted to the Preparatory Committee for the International Economic Conference), 1926, pp. 19.

[3] Louis I. Dublin and Alfred J. Lotka, "On the True Rate of Natural Increase," *Jour. Amer. Statis. Asso.*, September, 1925.   "Present Outlook for Population Increase," *Pub. Amer. Soc. Soc.* xxiv (1930), 106–114.   Louis I. Dublin, "America Approaching Stabilized Population," New York *Times*, May 4, 1930.   "Our Population Again," New York *Times*, January 4, 1931.   "The American People: A Census Portrait," New York *Times*, October 11, 1931.

Some of the following works by Dublin, or by Dublin collaborating with Lotka, touch upon the idea of future stabilization and stress the point that the diffusion of birth control has already gone too far for the welfare of the country.   L. I. Dublin [Ed.], *Population Problems*, Houghton Mifflin, 1926, pp. xi, 318.   *Health and Wealth.*   See ch. vii on "The Problem of Old Age;" ch. ix on "On the True Rate of Natural Increase;" ch. x on "Birth Control and the Population Question."   "American Population and the Future World Leadership," *Forum*, November, 1931.   "True Rate of Natural Increase," (with Dr. Lotka), *Metron*, viii (June 1930), 107–119.   "Evolution of the American Population," *Proc. of the Third Race Betterment Conf.*, Jan. 1928.   "Old Age and What it Means to the Community," *Bull. of the N. Y. Acad. of Med.*, iv, 1928.   "Old Age: An Increasing Problem," *Survey*, August 15, 1926.   "Excesses of Birth Control," Reprint of address before the Sixth Neo-Malthusian Conference, March 26, 1925.   "Birth Control," *Social Hygiene*, January, 1920.   "Birth Control—What it is Doing to America's Population," *Forum & Century*, lxviii (Nov. 1931), 270–275.   "Shift from Farm to City Goes Steadily on," New York *Times*, June 15, 1930.   "Population Changes Shifting Balance of Power in Europe," New York *Times*, September 14, 1930.   "Danger Spots on Europe's Population Map," New York *Times*, February 22, 1931.   "Italy's Population Surplus Cause of Friction in Europe," New York *Times*, May 3, 1931.   "Changing New York: The Census Analyzed," New York *Times*, November 8, 1931.

[4] Warren S. Thompson and P. K. Whelpton, ch. i in *Recent Social Trends*.   New York:

recently Spengler.[5]   Pearl's logistic curve studies have implied a stationary population eventually.[6]   The predicted dates have varied from 1950 to 2100; but later estimates based upon a steadily declining birth rate have set the date early rather than late.   In estimating the date, much depends on the assumptions used.   Probably 1950 or 1960 is approximately accurate.

R. R. Kuczynski preceded even Dublin and Lotka in the field of prediction.[7]   His recent studies show that in Northern and Western Europe one-hundred mothers are producing only ninety-three future mothers.   If present conditions persist or continue to develop in the same direction, there is implied not only stabilization but a very slight decline in absolute numbers. Though Ernst Kahn, a later worker on German data, has been cautious about naming a date for stabilization of the population of Germany, his research[8] clearly shows it to be not far off.

Table XXVII gives the latest estimates of the future population of the

McGraw Hill, 1933, 2 vols.   Ch. i in *Population Trends in the United States*, a monograph in the *Recent Social Trends* Series.   New York: McGraw Hill, 1933, pp. x, 1–415.   Warren S. Thompson, "Population Trends and Some Probable Effects upon Industry," paper read before the Amer. Statis. Asso., December, 1931, published in *Annalist*, January 15, 1932. See also the conclusion (ch. ix) to *Ratio of Children to Women* 1920.   *A Study in the Differential Rate of Natural Increase in the United States*.   Census Monograph XI.   Washington: Gov. Prtg. Off., 1931, pp. ix, 1–242.   P. K. Whelpton, "Increase and Distribution of Elders in Our Population," *Proc. Amer. Statis. Asso.*, March, 1932.   "Population: Trends in Age Composition and in Specific Birth-Rates, 1920–30," *Amer. Jour. Soc.*, xxxviii, 855–861 (May, 1932).   "Calculation of Future Development of Population," Reprint from *Proceedings* Rome Population Conference, (1931), Roma: Instituto Poligraphico dello Stato, 1932, pp. 31–41.   "Trends in Population Increase and Distribution during 1920 to 1930," *Amer. Jour. Soc.*, xxxvi, 865–879, (May, 1931).   "Population," *Amer. Jour. Soc.*, xxxviii, 825–834.   For an earlier estimate see "Population of The United States, 1925–1975," *Amer. Jour. Soc.*, xxxiv, 253–270 (September, 1928).

[5] Joseph J. Spengler, "The Social and Economic Consequences of Cessation in Population Growth," *Proceedings* Rome Population Conference, 1931.   Reprint pp. 3–29.

[6] Raymond Pearl, *Biology of Population Growth*, New York: Knopf, 1925, pp. xiv, 260.

[7] R. R. Kuczynski, *The Balance of Births and Deaths*.   Vol. i, *Western and Northern Europe*, New York: Macmillan, 1928, pp. ix, 140.   Vol. ii, *Eastern and Southern Europe*, New York: Macmillan, 1931, pp. xii, 3–170.   *Fertility and Reproduction: Methods of Measuring the Balance of Births and Deaths*.   Washington: Brookings Institution.   "The World's Population," *Foreign Affairs*, vii, 30–40 (October, 1928).   "The World's Future Population," in *Population* (Harris Foundation Lectures) (Chicago: Univ. of Chicago, 1929), pp. 283–302.   See also an early volume, *Der Zug nach der Stadt*.   "The World's Future Population," *New Republic*, lxii, 315–319 (May 17, 1930).

[8] Ernst Kahn, *Der Internationale Geburtenstreik. Umfang, Ursachen, Wirkungen, Gegenmassnahmen.*   Frankfort-am-Main: Societäts-Verlag, 1930, pp. 218.   "Keinkindersystem," *Wirtschaftskurve*, x (1931), 167–173.   "Der Geburtenrückgang in Stadt und Land," *Wirtschaftskurve*, x (1931), 80–83.   Dr. Kahn is also an eminent authority on housing.

United States published by P. K. Whelpton in May, 1933.[9] If birth rates, immigration, and expectation of life follow the low trend outlined, the population of the United States will increase to a maximum of about 136,500,000 between 1955 and 1960 and then decline. If the medium trends are followed, there will be a gradual increase to 155,200,000 in 1980. If net immigration should amount to 100,000 per year more than the medium assumption, the 1950 population would be increased by about 2,000,000 and the 1980 population by about 7,000,000. Thompson believes that the medium

TABLE XXVII

FUTURE POPULATION OF THE UNITED STATES ACCORDING TO ESTIMATED TRENDS[1]

	1900	1910	1920	1930	1940	1950	1960	1970	1980
	Expectation of Life at Birth of White Persons								
Low	51.0	53.3	56.6	61.2	62	62	62	62	62
Medium					63	65	66	66	66
High					63	66	69	71	72
	Births per 1000 Native White Women 15–44								
Low	116	105	98	78	65	59	55	55	55
Medium					70	64	60	60	60
High					75	73	72	72	72
	Arrivals of Aliens and Citizens Less Departures (Thousands per Year)*								
Low	375	450	144	60	None	None	None	None	None
Medium					120	150	150	150	150
High					260	300	300	300	300
	Population, April 1 (Millions)								
Low	75.8	91.9	106.3†	122.8	130.9	135.6	136.0	132.5	126.5
Medium					133.1	142.9	149.8	153.8	155.2
High					135.1	150.8	167.3	184.2	202.0

* Five-year average centered on year indicated.

† Includes 150,000 allowance for underenumeration of Negroes.

[1] Source: P. K. Whelpton in *Amer. Jour. Soc.*, xxxviii, 833.

or low assumptions are more likely to represent actual future trends than the high assumptions. The high, but somewhat improbable, assumptions are that the expectation of life of whites will increase to 72 years by 1980, that the birth rate of native-white women aged 15–44 will decline to only 72 per 1000 in 1980, and that net immigration will rise from its present 0 level to 200,000 annually during 1935–39 and to 300,000 thereafter. If these improbable assumptions should become a reality, the population

[9] P. K. Whelpton, "Population," *Amer. Jour. Soc.*, xxxviii, 825–834 (May, 1933).

would increase by about 10 or 11 per cent a decade, and pass the 200,000,000 mark before 1980.   But it is much safer to assume that we shall have a population of 136,000,000 to 155,000,000 between 1955 and 1980.

(1a)   Alarms Unjustified.   False Assumptions of Dublin and Kuczynski

It should be clearly noted that there is an important distinction between a stationary population actually achieved and a population which, though still increasing, exhibits characteristics, which if they persist, will inevitably bring about a stationary population.   Thus a population can be "failing to reproduce itself" and yet be temporarily increasing in numbers.   For example, by 1930 the United States had achieved the conditions which, if unaltered, would give us a stationary population a few decades hence.   Yet natural increase in 1932, as in 1931, amounted to about 1,000,000.[10]   This shows that there can be substantial natural increase in a population manifesting conditions which will soon bring about a stationary population.

Much of the quasi-alarmist literature by Dublin and Kuczynski refers to such populations.   There is much nonsensical talk abroad about populations "doomed to die out."   This is the able Kuczynski's phrase.   It is true that the population of the countries of Northern and Western Europe will be stationary in a few decades; true also that after that there may be a very slow decline, provided demographic conditions do not adapt themselves to the changed situation.

In talking thus about the "doom" of populations, Kuczynski assumes that conditions will not adapt themselves.   He assumes that tendencies now operating will persist without end.   Now if there is anything certain in demographic history it is that demographic conditions have a way of shifting faster than students of demography.   The Dublin-Lotka-Kuczynski school has done brilliant and original research.   But many students of demography have erred in accepting too uncritically the conclusions of Dublin and Kuczynski without examining the validity of their assumptions.   At best the assumption of this school is not proved valid for the reason that we cannot forecast conditions so far in the future.   The assumption is also unwise because it presupposes demographic rigidity and an absence of tendencies toward new equilibria, which tendencies have always been characteristic of demographic phenomena.

§2 SOME POSSIBLE CONSEQUENCES OF THE ADVENT OF STATIONARY POPULATIONS

What are likely to be some of the major social consequences of the advent of a stationary population?   It should be clearly understood that in the

---

[10] P. K. Whelpton in *Amer. Jour. Soc.*, xxxviii, 826–827.

speculations which follow there is an attempt to determine what would be the theoretical effect of one factor (population stabilization), other circumstances remaining the same. Of course this is purely a logical device. Economists are too prone to forget that circumstances never do remain the same. But to arrive at first steps in reasoning the method is defensible. It will not be possible to allow for all the modifying circumstances as no one knows what they will be.

Many are the social effects likely to follow from the aging of the population as natural increase falls to zero. Other things being equal (this phrase is always implied), there will be a heavier drain on the social income devoted to care of the aged—still largely an unsolved problem in America. On the other hand, that portion of the life span of individuals devoted to economic productivity should be, other factors remaining the same, somewhat lengthened. This should make possible greater savings during the period of gainful employment; but, human beings being what they are, one may doubt whether savings corresponding to the increased need will be made. We may expect rather a greater burden on relatives, or enhanced demands for old age insurance systems whether private or state-subsidized.

Since the above was written Spengler has also concluded that "The decrease in the proportion of unproductive youth more than counterbalances the increase in the proportion of unproductive aged." He cites the estimates of Dublin and Lotka in *The Money Value of a Man* in support of the proposition that per capita earning capacity, which is a fair measure of productivity "will be eight per cent higher [in a stationary population] than in a growing population of the age composition of the American population in 1920."[11]

So far as changes in the demand for commodities are concerned we may expect, in a word, a demand for fewer toys and more footwarmers. A larger proportion of the national income will go to satisfy the desires of adults, a smaller proportion to satisfy the desires of the young. For there will be a decreased proportion of the latter. These changes take place so slowly, however, that there is no reason to expect that they will be as disrupting industrially as sudden changes in fashion. Certainly they will not be as catastrophic as technical change.

How will the advent of a stationary population affect the market for American goods? There can be no doubt that the cessation of population growth will slow up the expanding market for agricultural products, industrial equipment and certain raw materials. We may, other factors remaining the same, expect in the next half-dozen decades a slower rate of

[11] J. J. Spengler, "The Social and Economic Consequences of Cessation in Population Growth," *Proceedings* of the Rome Population Conference (1931).

expansion of our basic industries.   Doubtless there will be exceptions, as in the instance of new products not heretofore marketed; but as a general proposition the above statement seems sound.   Certain business leaders of otherwise unusual acumen and foresight have been led, by a statistical fallacy, the extrapolation of past population trends, to make false deductions regarding the future domestic market.   This extrapolation has been made without due allowance for factors causing a decline in the natural rate of increase.   If entrepreneurs over-expand plant capacity on the basis of such false inferences, they will meet unexpected difficulties.   The return on capital thus unwisely over-invested will necessarily be low.   It may also aggravate the employment situation.

What will be the effect upon the demand for capital?   Other things being equal, there will be less demand for funds for investment and accordingly a decline in interest rates.   It is highly probable, however, that this tendency will be neutralized by other factors.   The remarkable steadiness of interest rates for several centuries suggests that it would require more than the advent of a stationary population in the United States to have any appreciable and noticeable effect on the rates for loanable funds.

Will the demand for gold as a basis for media of exchange slacken?   Yes. Other conditions remaining the same, there will be a less rapid increase in exchanges, less need for money, less need for an ever-increasing amount of gold to back it.   What effect this may or may not have upon world prices we can not say as yet.

What effect will a stationary population and changed age composition have upon the labor market?   If present tendencies continue, and barring the development of a keener social conscience among employers,[12] we may expect increasing difficulty in placing older men, but probably not an increase in general unemployment from this cause.   Already we have something of a problem.   Unemployment for those in middle and advanced years may be aggravated in the future by the presence of a greater proportion of older men and women still able to, and still willing to earn a living; by increasing mechanization, each increment of which causes at least temporary occupational dislocation.   Training workers for several jobs may be a practical way out.   If an increasing proportion of the rising generations should enter the professions, this would be an offsetting factor, since one can, in the professions, ordinarily work at full capacity for a longer period.   Productivity may in fact actually increase with advancing years up to a certain point at least.   But skilled and especially unskilled workers are likely to face a different situation.

[12] That there are some tendencies in this direction lately is suggested in a recent bulletin issued by the Metropolitan Life Insurance Company and reported in the New York *Times*, August 2, 1933.

It may be doubted, however, whether stabilization will increase total unemployment. This phenomenon proceeds primarily from causes associated with changes in business activity, not from the growth of population itself. For it is present in periods of declining population. Probably jobs expand about as rapidly as population under "normal" conditions in Western, industrialized societies. Yet the view of Cassel, the Swedish economist, seems reasonable that, upon the advent of a stationary state, business cycles will, other things being equal, be less violent. If so, one would expect some decrease in unemployment. If, with the advent of a stationary state, there should be increased difficulty in finding jobs for older workers in a mechanized society demanding motor-coördination and agility, this might offset some of the gains following a reduced violence in cyclical variations of business activity.

Will wage rates for the older workers tend to go down and for the younger workers in their prime to go up? This seems a theoretical possibility, if the factors above mentioned are not offset, as they well may be, by other factors.

This leads to the important question of the effect of democratized birth control and of a future stationary population upon the relief of occupational congestion. This is a condition of relative over supply of labor in certain occupations or levels of occupation and an under supply in others, whereby a lack of balance in relation to needs is created. Over supply, usually characteristic of the lower levels, leads to low rates; under supply, usually characteristic of the higher levels, to high wages.

Because poor labor balance has always been a characteristic of modern industrialized societies, we have taken its extent for granted. A dynamic society will always show lag in adjustment, but that imbalance need persist in present proportions is untrue.[13] Professor T. N. Carver, who has given more thought to this fundamental problem than any other economist, has shown[14] that occupational redistribution, or the restoration (or creation) of

[13] The well-known report of ex-President Hoover's Committee on *Recent Economic Changes* made repeated mention of the idea of economic balance without, as far as I know, giving any credit to Carver. In mitigation of this it may be said that the whole idea of balance or equilibrium is implicit in the mode of thought of neo-Classical economists. But Carver applied it to the labor problem and especially to the population problem with originality.

[14] See especially chs. x and xiv in *Essays in Social Justice* (Cambridge: Harvard Univ. Press, 1915 and later); ch. ix on "Some Consequences of a Balanced Economic System" in *The Present Economic Revolution in the United States* (Boston: Little Brown, 1925). [With Hugh W. Lester] *This Economic World and How It may be Improved.* Chicago & New York: A. W. Shaw. London: A. W. Shaw, 1928, pp. vi, 432. The subject of occupational congestion is also touched upon in *The Economy of Human Energy* (New York: Macmillan, 1924), p. 61 ff. Consult also the following papers: "Occupational Distribution of the Labor Supply," *Bull. Amer. Econ. Asso.*, 4th Series, i (April, 1911), 20–45. "A Construc-

occupational balance must be the solution for this type of congestion; that, in fact, it is the only solution that will go to the root of the matter. Most other suggestions that have been presented by thinkers of various schools the world over either will not work[15] at all, or are mere palliatives.[16]

Readers should refer to the literature by Professor Carver for a full exposition of the importance of occupational congestion. Professor Carver has discussed this subject so thoroughly that little remains to be said, save to stress, in connection with one of the theses of this book, that diffused contraception is the most economical method of achieving that control over human reproduction which the theory of occupational balance presupposes. Professor Carver has demonstrated, as no economist or sociologist here or abroad has ever demonstrated, that *approximate economic equality*[17] *under liberty is impossible without democratized contraception.* I venture to suggest that some day this demonstration will be recognized as one of the most valuable contributions to social and economic theory made by anyone for a century.

The problem of securing better wages for the working class and of relieving occupational congestion by balancing the labor supply of various non-competing groups, reducing the birth rate where it is high, doing what little can be done to raise it where it has been unduly low, is intimately connected with migration from abroad. The stabilization of population abroad, had it come sooner, would have done much to reduce the pressure of immigration to the United States, if there had been no restrictive legislation. Under all the circumstances, the latter was socially necessary.

Stabilization abroad and in the United States under conditions of restricted immigration in the United States ought to do much to alleviate many problems aggravated by mass immigration. There are scores of

---

tive Labor Program," *Harvard Alumni Bulletin*, xxi (April 17, 1919), 556–560. "Four Labor Programs," *Quart. Jour. Econ.*, Feb., 1919. "Some Probable Results of a Balanced Industrial System," *Amer. Econ. Rev. Supp.*, x (1920), No. 1. "The Problem of Occupational Congestion," *Chinese Students' Monthly*, Columbia University, Jan., 1926. "Occupational Congestion," *Birth Control Review*, xii (1928), 275–277.

[15] Cases in point are the Single Tax, Communism and Socialism. At least it may be said that Socialism has yet to demonstrate that it can give us economic equality or democratized prosperity under liberty.

[16] Palliatives of this kind are, for example, the various programs now commonly heard for curing unemployment, especially "made-work" programs. Others are trade unionism, various programs for limiting the output of goods, especially raw materials and agricultural products. One might go on to enumerate these—but hardly to effective purpose.

[17] The term "economic equality" does not mean equal incomes. It means approximately equal incomes after allowance has been made for such factors as skill, productivity, cost of training, reward for exceptional ability (a rent-like income), etc.

problems. Two important ones are the worst type of slum[18] and the disruption of national unity by a conflict of cultures. Stabilization ought to enable us to catch our breath in tackling the problem of housing our citizens by applying mass-production methods on a national scale with adequate land-use planning. This is difficult, but not impossible, under very dynamic population conditions.

Likewise it is reasonable to suppose that national unity and cultural and social integration ought to be promoted. This is not to suggest that immigrant stocks have not made notable contributions to the enrichment of our national culture. Nor does it imply that the aim of Americanization should be standardization of personality and of habits. But it does imply that stabilization here and abroad should render easier that degree of unity which makes for effective industrial team-work and for a pattern of cultural life, which, while retaining desirable but non-conflicting variations, makes possible agreement on fundamentals. Such fundamentals are the separation of church and state, government by democratic, parliamentary procedure, settlement of disputes by counting heads instead of breaking heads, respect for the heritage of Anglo-Saxon common and statute law, etc. Only the one-hundred per cent Americans want everyone alike. Sensible men want unity on essentials, diversity for enrichment, diversity in order that the forces of social selection may have a free hand to winnow for survival those habits, customs, techniques and values that may prove superior to our own. Though the cessation of immigration into the United States will imply certain cultural losses, probably the gains will be greater considering the fact that we have passed the mushroom stage of growth. At all events, it is clear that it will reduce the severity of those problems which were aggravated by the addition of many million immigrants in a few decades. Mr. Harold Fields, executive director of the National League for American Citizenship, is of the opinion that the cessation of net immigration has already speeded up assimilation.[19] Immigrants are now more evenly distributed geographically. This has facilitated slum clearance and assimilation. Since 1932 more foreign-born residents have left the United States annually for permanent residence abroad than have come to this country.

[18] Poorly-housed areas existed, of course, before mass immigration; but the latter aggravated the problem. So it is with nearly all the problems aggravated rather than caused by mass immigration. Since the slums of our great cities have had a floating population, one immigrant group displacing another with successive waves of immigration, we may expect alleviation of the congestion in an absence of immigration. The radical remedy is, of course, condemnation, clearance and rebuilding, if accompanied by a rising standard of living of the group affected.

[19] So. Atl. Quart., August, 1933. Cf., New York Times, August 6, 1933, Second News Sec.

Historically this is an altogether novel situation. Its social effects are already being felt since the absence of net immigration was preceded in recent decades by a steady decline under restrictive legislation.

Stabilization and changing age composition will materially affect many problems of educational administration. Local migration has always affected this problem; now there is a relatively new factor: an increased average age of the population. Already in some cities there are free desks in the lower grades of the public schools. The reduced proportion of children will gradually advance to the higher grades, to the high schools and eventually to the colleges. This factor alone will tend to reduce the demand for teachers. However, a rising standard of living and an increased demand for education may somewhat mitigate the tendency. But there are definite limits to such mitigation, and it is difficult to see how it can materially alter the situation. P. K. Whelpton has touched upon this problem and Professor Harold F. Clark of Teachers College, Columbia University, has written a pamphlet[20] on population phenomena as they affect education, and a book[21] on education's responsibility for bringing about a better occupational distribution of the labor supply. Whelpton says:

School facilities and teaching staffs will be affected by this age shift. In some parts of the country the number of children under school age was much higher in 1930 than in 1920—in Detroit, Los Angeles, Hammond, White Plains, Newton, and part of rural Massachusetts, for example. Here, the problem of how to build schools and hire teachers fast enough may continue for some time, since there will be more children entering school from 1931 to 1936 than there were from 1921 to 1926. A more common situation, however, will be that of Boston, Chicago, Bay City, and most of the farming areas of the United States where the number of children below school age is declining. These places should soon be able to abandon certain obsolete buildings or ease crowded conditions, and to weed out some of the less able teachers. A complicating factor in some cities, however, is that while there may be fewer children to enter school now than ten years ago, they are quite differently distributed within the city boundaries. New York furnishes a striking example, children under 5 in Manhattan decreasing 45.8 per cent from 1920 to 1930, while in the Bronx they increased 35.2 per cent.[22]

Up to this point we have traced some of the effects of the democratization of contraceptive knowledge as it will probably operate through the nexus of a stationary population and through a changed age composition more heavily weighted on the upper end. We shall now consider certain possible

---

[20] The Effect of Population upon Ability to Support Education. Bloomington, Indiana: Univ. Book Store. Bull. School Educ., Indiana Univ., vol. ii, no. 1.

[21] *Economic Theory and Correct Occupational Distribution....* New York: Teacher's College, Columbia Univ., 1931, pp. viii, 176.

[22] *Amer. Jour. Soc.*, xxxvii, 857–858 (May, 1932).

social changes which may be more direct consequences of this democratization than those mentioned above.

§3 MORE DIRECT CONSEQUENCES OF DEMOCRATIZED CONTRACEPTIVE KNOWLEDGE

We may expect an increase in the liberty of men and women. Women will, for the first time in human history, be emancipated from the slavery of uncontrolled reproduction. I say slavery advisedly. For, while even uncontrolled motherhood is not usually to be so described, there are undoubted instances on record of high rates bringing unendurable distress—so much so that suicide is the preferred way out. But fortunately such cases are not typical. How well this greater liberty afforded by diffused contraceptive knowledge will be used, time alone will tell. Those who oppose birth control often assert that it is likely to be abused. Others have faith that it will be used properly. My own view is that past experience leads us to have some confidence in the intelligence and adaptive power of human beings. In the last analysis it is up to the masses and their leaders to create such instruments of social control as will guard society from the more serious consequences of man's inventive ability.

The diffusion of contraceptive information will tend to equalize the costs (i.e., sacrifices) of child-bearing. These are now very inequitably distributed among social classes, the so-called upper classes by no means bearing their due share of the sacrifices involved in producing succeeding generations. And there is reason to believe that this has not always been so.

As children become scarcer, they will probably increase in "value."[23] They are likely to be more esteemed, cared for, protected. Here again, whether they will be over-protected and coddled the future alone can tell. There is much erroneous thinking current in our time regarding the coddling, and therefore the inferiority of character, of only children. There is a very considerable body of evidence that only children are, on the whole, not only as regards intelligence but as regards character, superior to children from large families. This leads to the suggestion that the character of succeeding generations will not necessarily suffer as a consequence of being born into smaller families.[24]

[23] This is the view also of the Hoover Research Committee on *Recent Social Trends*. See the "Review of Findings" as published in vol. i, p. lxiv, or in the special supplement (Sec. 2) to the New York *Times*, January 2, 1933, p. 5, col. 2.

[24] On the other hand, part of the superiority of only children or of children from small families is a consequence of many circumstances correlated with small families or only children: high intelligence, high occupational status, large incomes and many environmental advantages. With democratization of contraceptive knowledge only children will probably lose some of their superiority, especially in intelligence, because many of them will come from the lower classes.

The advent of the smaller family is likely to reduce somewhat the problem of child labor. Having large families as a form of old-age insurance is passing. It is being replaced by other forms of insurance. As families among the laboring classes become smaller, there will be less need for the gifted children born in such surroundings to earn a living early. The sum total of social gain accruing under the newer system will, it seems reasonable to infer, exceed that under the older system, according to which gifted children began earning a pittance early in industry, unable later in life to return to society the full benefit of their native endowments. The legal ban on child labor in the recently-adopted emergency codes of the Roosevelt administration is merely a recognition of these changed social circumstances.

In so far as maternal mortality is a consequence of short-interval births, we may expect it to decline with the increase of child-spacing. With improved methods of child care diffused, we may expect infant mortality to decline somewhat; though Neo-Malthusians have made altogether too much of the argument that low birth rates and low infant mortality rates necessarily accompany one another. A number of studies have, however, conclusively proved that there is an intimate and direct relationship between too rapid child-bearing and infant mortality.[25]

In the field of marital adjustment, it is a reasonable inference that the diffusion of contraceptive information will promote better relations. In recent years many data have been collected on this subject by the German marriage advice stations.[26] These data show that rational sex instruction, together with a knowledge of contraception, promote sexual adjustment in marriage. It is probable that a considerable proportion—no one knows exactly what proportion—of divorces and separations are a consequence of sexual maladjustments. If this reasoning is sound, the gradual diffusion of contraceptive information may be expected to promote marital adjustment, and to cause a decline, other things being equal, in the divorce rate. Whether or not this decline will be offset by other factors, no one can now predict.

Curiously enough, very little psychiatric investigation of genuine scientific

[25] Some of the evidence is reviewed in my paper "The Relation of Birth Control to Infant Mortality and Pregnancy Waste," *Jewish Social Service Quarterly*, June, 1928.

[26] For the best survey of the work of the Eheberatungsstelle see M. Kopp in *J. Obst. & Gyn.*, July, 1933; also occasional brief reports to the *Jour. Amer. Med. Asso.* from foreign correspondents. *Cf.*, citations in Bibliography for Lurie and Charles. Dr. Robert L. Dickinson is soon to publish *The Doctor as Marriage Counsellor*. Baltimore, Williams & Wilkins, 1936. A useful handbook for the general reader is Hannah M. Stone and Abraham Stone, *A Marriage Manual. A Practical Guide-Book to Sex and Marriage*. New York: Simon and Schuster, 1935, pp. 334.

value has been carried on into the mental hygiene aspects of contraception.[27] But the evidence that has come to my attention suggests that such knowledge of contraception has a tendency to reduce sexual and mental conflicts. There are some instances on record, however, of mental conflict being promoted by a desire to control conception in the presence of orthodox religious mores opposed to such practices. Dr. Bowman, assistant director of the Boston Psychopathic Hospital, and a former colleague of mine on the staff of the Simmons School of Social Work, has personally reported cases to me of this nature. These were Catholic women already over-burdened with large families, of somewhat unstable personality, perhaps bordering on the psychopathic. In a few such instances the need of control of conception was obvious even to a borderline psychopathic patient; but the mores of her group have been so impressed upon her in childhood and adolescence that there was created, for a number of years, a deeply-rooted conflict of long duration. The adjustments necessary to remove such conflicts are time-consuming and few psychiatrists are prepared to conduct such mental retraining and re-orientation even when they see fit to run counter to the group mores.

Will stabilization in the United States and in Northern and Eastern Europe reduce the likelihood of war by mitigating or eliminating one of its actual or supposed causes? The answer depends upon the extent to which population pressure has been a cause of past wars. It would be naïve and unfounded to claim that it is the sole cause of war, or even that it has been its chief cause. A survey of the literature, however, suggests that population pressure has not been a negligible factor in at least some wars and acts of military aggression. The best recent example has been the aggression of Japan in Manchuria and China. While there is reason to believe that Japan is at present governed by a cabinet possessed of military propensities, there can be no doubt that the peculiar demographic and economic circumstances there existing have been influential in prompting Japanese statesmen to embark upon the course recently adopted. Many economic surveys of Japan have clearly demonstrated that its population is increasing rapidly. They have shown further that Japan lacks the necessary coal, iron, and other raw materials for the expansion of her basic industries; that Manchuria not only possesses these raw materials in great abundance but has a sparse population. This situation has naturally been a great temptation to nationalistic Japanese statesmen. Military aggression, initiated no doubt as a consequence of more superficial "causes," such as the lack of a stable government in Manchuria, the desire of Japan to

[27] For an exception see Hannah Stone, "Contraception and Mental Hygiene," *Mental Hygiene*, xvii, 417–423 (July, 1933).

protect investments there, etc., has naturally followed.   But whatever the superficial causes of the conflict, there can be no doubt that the demographic situation is a primary cause.

Should the opinion become universally widespread that each nation should be held responsible—but to whom?—for its own collective acts, including responsibility for a lack of control of population, one might reasonably expect to see in the future a decline in the danger of war from that cause alone.   But that day seems very far off as yet.   Moreover, even should such a public opinion be built up, we cannot be certain that it might not be counteracted by other new influences making for international misunderstanding and military aggression.

Just as the weight of economic authority teaches that population pressure is and has been a cause of military aggression, so, in my judgment, the weight of authority also teaches that a control of population growth is necessary to protect a standard of living, whatever that standard may be.   It is a proposition pretty well accepted by American, English, and German economists and sociologists—less so by French, Belgian and Italian thinkers— that it is in the social interest that population should cease growing at that mystical point usually called the "optimum."   The optimum point is that point in the growth of the population of any given large area (usually a nation) where, given a certain level of productive arts and of social organization, there will result the highest per capita income in economic goods and services.   This point has never yet been determined in actual figures for the population of any nation of the globe.   It is as yet a purely theoretical point.   W. S. Thompson has suggested that there are many optima,[28] provided we do not accept the standard of living test, but prefer some other. Other tests, however, have not found much favor, at least among economists.   Such factors are generally less measurable.   And no one has yet suggested an adequate substitute for, or amplification of, the standard of living test for the optimum.

Probably the optimum should be measured in terms of what people want most.   Is it leisure?   No.   Learning and cultivation?   No.   Wealth and material enjoyments?   Yes.   The proof of this is in the materialism of our age.

The validity of the standard of living test of the demographic optimum is shown further by the theory that the character of any age is determined (i.e., colored) by its dominant urge.   When fear of the supernatural and unseen ruled men, the religious leader and the shaman or medicine man was dominant.   When need for protection was the ruling passion, the military

---

[28] *Population Problems*, ch. xxiv.   Thompson objects to what he calls the subordination of personal and spiritual values in the economic optimum.

class ruled the roost.   In the Middle Ages the priest had his innings.   Now the business entrepreneur is taking his turn.   Only the Chinese have done more than the Greeks to make philosophers kings.   In a nationalistic age it is too much to expect that the test of population density should be other than national.   Even if swarming in New York City be unaesthetic, it is useless to tell the residents so.   Correspondingly, perhaps the populace should care more for well-used leisure, for learning and genuine self-development; perhaps they should care less for new and more things.   But it is well-nigh useless to tell them this.   This has been preached to the rabble for two thousand years.   People are materialistic whether certain intellectuals like it or not.   Hence the test for population will be based on reality not on wishes; the test will be materialistic.   And rightly so, for observation of the conduct of the world shows that its chief worry since medieval times has been to increase prosperity, material well-being.   And who shall say that this ideal is necessarily lower than many others that have dominated civilizations in the past?

There seems to be a growing feeling among demographers in the United States that the population of the U. S. A. is not, in point of time, very far at present from the optimum.   It may even be that the optimum point for any nation is located at the mid-point in Pearl's logistic or flattened S curve at the point marked X in the sketch below.

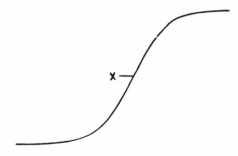

The fact that at this point it is possible for population to grow most rapidly suggests that at this stage in the cycle of growth there is a maximum of free energy.   Above and below this point the rate of natural increase is slower.

With a stationary population there will be less excuse for the wasteful consumption of irreplaceable natural resources.   The conservation movement may be expected to grow.   Few people realize that there is no substitute for oil in a mechanized civilization.   Yet it may well become the great limiting factor in mechanical production of the future.   Our coal resources are by no means unlimited.   A stationary population will provide a margin of safety until we learn how to harness effectively the winds, tides, sun, the heat stored in tropical ocean water, etc.   Without sources of cheap power and cheap lubrication a mechanized civilization cannot endure.   The threat of shortage is a long way off from the standpoint of the duration of a single lifetime; but it is very near from the standpoint of the history of social development (say 500 years).

This discussion of the optimum may be summed up by concluding that, though no one has yet been able to define and clarify the concept, it may be of some tentative use in formulating public policy.   It is at least better than no guide at all.   It has a fairly definite theoretical, if not practical meaning.   Furthermore, American, English, and German demographic thinkers are pretty well agreed upon it as a test of the desirability of further growth; speaking generally, the demographers of France, Belgium and Italy are less inclined to accept it.   The reasons are often political and religious rather than scientific.

There can be no doubt that population control is indispensable to the creation and maintenance of a reasonably high standard of living.   In fact, it may be dogmatically asserted that a high standard of living is impossible without some form of population control.   If this can take place by rational and harmless methods so much the more fortunate.   There can be no doubt that the Orient would be better off economically were a system of rational population control generally prevalent.   This is denied even in our day by some romanticists and sentimentalists; but it is no longer doubted by the informed.

As suggested in another section of this work, the increasing prevalence of small families is likely to mitigate many of the minor and some of the major causes of poverty.   The advent of a stationary state, therefore, works both indirectly and directly: indirectly by forestalling the operation of diminishing returns in the extractive and elaborative industries and by relieving occupational congestion; directly by promoting individual and family welfare, and by reducing the force of certain causes of poverty.

Democratized contraception thus becomes a tool of social adaptation, an instrument which, if intelligently used, may promote national strength and group survival.   This conclusion is so sound that it is rapidly finding acceptance.

Public health conditions will improve, barring again counteracting forces. Many unnecessary deaths will be prevented and mothers will have a chance to care properly for small rather than excessive families.   We may expect improved prevention of morbidity and mortality especially in those cases in which contraception is clearly indicated.   Hundreds of thousands of such cases are not now being adequately cared for.

The social and economic implications of differential rates of adoption of contraception by various social classes is a wide and difficult subject. It is so difficult and important as to merit a special volume. Here I wish merely to recognize the importance of investigation in this field. Thoughtful observers—though there are exceptions—are pretty well agreed that, inasmuch as the genetically better-endowed classes were the first to adopt contraception, birth control has, on the whole, operated dysgenically. Now that it is reaching those less well-endowed genetically, the same thinkers are coming to believe that birth control is operating eugenically. Stated as a general proposition this view seems sound; but we really know little about the subject. There is much silly anti-eugenic criticism abroad nowadays much of which will not stand logical examination. Many critics of eugenics lack a sound grounding in the eugenical and social theory involved in the problem of differential fertility and its probable consequences. Not a few of these critics view with indifference the prevalence of ultra-small families among the well-endowed, and of large families among those less well-endowed genetically. They hold that those who do survive are necessarily the fit, regardless of the mechanism of selection. This may be doubted. It may well be that society has relatively suddenly discovered in *effective* contraception a tool which it has not yet learned most wisely to employ. Still other writers, those of greater penetration, I believe, are much impressed with the serious nature of the differential birth rate. Probably it makes a great deal of difference which social classes employ most thoroughly contraceptive practices. Here is an area of investigation that has been all too little covered.[29] The qualitative implications of differential rates of adoption of contraceptive practices by various social classes in America is one of the most fundamental, important and least-understood aspects of population theory. This field needs much more research than has heretofore been devoted to it. Its implications for the future of all that is desirable in American group life are far-reaching.

§4 ARE CATHOLIC STOCKS OUTBREEDING NON-CATHOLIC STOCKS?

It is interesting, if not always scientifically fruitful, to speculate on the possible effects of differential rates of reproduction between religious groups essentially authoritarian on the one hand and those that are libertarian on the other. It is about time that systematic fact gathering began in this field. Is there a tendency for Catholic stocks to outbreed non-Catholic stocks in the U. S. A.? We do not know. The subject is much disputed

[29] Since this was written Lorimer and Osborn have given us an excellent summary of current knowledge in their valuable reference work: Frank Lorimer and Frederick Osborn, *Dynamics of Population. Social and Biological Significance of Changing Birth Rates in the United States*. New York: Macmillan, 1934, pp. xiii, 461.

and merits inquiry.   If Catholic stocks are outbreeding non-Catholic stocks what are its implications for the future of American education, politics, the relation between Church and State, and, more important than any of these, what are its implications for the freedom of scientific inquiry?   Upon freedom of inquiry, more than upon almost any other factor, the progress of science probably depends.

Is it a fact that Catholics in the United States have a higher net reproductive rate than non-Catholics?   The few figures we have suggest that they do, even after allowance has been made for the lower standard of living of Catholics.   Catholicism is strong in immigrant groups where incomes are low and where many are in the lower occupational levels.   It seems highly probable that accurate fact collecting would show that not only a lower standard of living but also Catholic religious mores have had an influence in making for large families.[30]   Fragmentary clinic figures point to this conclusion as probably valid.

That such is the fact is corroborated also by a very able study just published (two or three years after this section was written) by Professor Samuel A. Stouffer of the University of Chicago.   His analysis of the confinement rates of 40,766 urban families in Wisconsin showed that, even for given occupational groups, the fertility of Catholics was consistently higher than that of non-Catholics; that between 1919 and 1933 the fertility of Catholics declined much more rapidly than that of non-Catholics.   Moreover, Professor Stouffer believes that the more rapid decline in Catholic

---

[30] Warren S. Thompson and John Moore in *Will America Become Catholic?* have come to a contrary view.   Thompson declares [*Ratio of Children to Women 1920*.   Census Monograph, xi, p. 184] that he has been able to find "but one clear case of the influence of religion on the size of the family."   This is among the Utah Mormons.   But even in this case there are urban-rural differences.   Thompson continues: "Religion seems to have but little influence in preventing the decrease of the size of the family when it comes into competition with urban influences making for the limitation of the family.   There is reason to think that this is true among the Catholics as well as among Protestants.   In Catholic communities the ratios of children are often quite high but how much of this ratio can be attributed to the influence of religion, how much to foreign birth, how much to low economic status, and how much to essential rural-mindedness no one can decide.   Our study, then, contributes little to the determination of the influence of religion on the size of the family.   But it does seem to indicate that even in closely-knit religious groups the birth rate is on the decline."   Thompson's study was hardly designed to bring out differences in fertility due to religious influences.   There can be no doubt that religion has tended to keep the birth rate high in the past not only in Eastern but in Western societies.   Probably Thompson would be the first to admit this.   Probably he would admit further that the lessened hold of orthodox religion on people since the rise of science has caused the birth rate to decline.   If these principles be generally conceded, there is certainly a strong presumption that orthodox family mores and attitudes still operate to some extent among certain groups in our population whether Thompson's ratios bring out this fact or not.

fertility than in non-Catholic fertility is characteristic also of northern and western cities of the United States, inasmuch as a partial correlation analysis, with several factors held constant, shows this. Though Professor Stouffer does not point out the fact, it is quite clear that the main reason why Catholic fertility is falling more rapidly arises from the fact that it has farther to fall; because there has been, in fact, a cultural lag here. Dr. Stouffer adds this significant statement: "It is not within the scope of the present study to investigate the mechanisms by which this decline in the fertility rate was brought about. It cannot be proved from these data that contraception actually was used, although scattered evidence from birth-control clinics in Wisconsin, as in other American cities, has indicated a desire on the part of some professed Catholics for birth-control information. However, if contraception (including *coitus interruptus*) was not used extensively, the only other explanation would be an increase in continence, since age has been for all practical purposes a constant throughout the period, since no biological change could account for such a sharp decline in fertility, and since the Ogino-Knaus 'rhythm' method of birth control, which has ecclesiastical approbation, appeared too late to have an appreciable influence during the time period covered by this study."[31]

Are Catholic stocks in the United States, taken as a whole, genetically inferior to such non-Catholic libertarian stocks as Unitarians and Universalists, Ethical Culturists, Freethinkers? Inferior to non-Catholic stocks in general? No one really knows. One is entitled to his hunches, however, and my guess is that the answer will some day be made in the affirmative. If there are no material group differences there is no eugenical problem raised by a supposed differential in net reproductive rates. On the other hand, if the differences in genetic endowment should prove to be real, and if the supposed differentials in net productivity are also genuine, the situation is anti-social, perhaps gravely so.

There is a view naïvely held by many economists that the population growth of any particular class is exclusively determined by its standard of living. Next to the mythical *homo oeconomicus* this is probably the most widely held error—at least when the statement is thus baldly declared—in the whole history of the development of Classical economics. It is, of course, sound up to a certain point; but when stated to imply that it is the sole or even the chief determiner of different rates of class growth, it is false. Even though contraception is more a means of control than a motive, access to contraceptive information is just as important. If the means are not at hand, how can a class control its birth rate, much less its rate of

---

[31] Samuel A. Stouffer, "Trends in the Fertility of Catholics and Non-Catholics," *Amer. Jour. Soc.*, xli, 143–166 (September, 1935).

reproduction (which includes eliminative factors, etc., over which there is little control)?   The view that the standard of living is the sole determiner of the birth rate of a class is largely a consequence of the fact that Classical economics developed in England during an abnormal demographic period, i.e., a period of phenomenal population growth.

Religious faith as well as the standard of living has a direct influence on the birth rate.   It seems difficult to believe that the Catholic Church has purely a religious and no numerical motive in taking a stand against effective contraception.   The present pope is the first of his line to honor the subject with special condemnation in an encyclical.   The historical significance of this is that the leaders of the Church grasp the import of the swift spread of contraceptive information and its widely increasing availability for their own people.

Still, preliminary clinic figures suggest that there is a lag; that Catholics are not attending birth-control clinics at the same rate as Protestants.   It is well known that Catholics, as compared with Protestants, have a larger number of pregnancies; further, that they have larger families of living children despite a somewhat higher mortality in the young age groups.   It is not so generally known that the abortion rate among Catholic mothers is lower.[32]   This is clearly a reflection of religious influences.   There is also reason to believe that Catholics, when they use contraceptive methods, tend to use the less reliable ones.   Here again religion is an influence.

Not only do the priests have a good deal to say publicly against the sin of practicing birth control, but the lay organizations, membership in which is increasing, are more active than ever in combating birth control by all the means which lie in their power.   Nor is organization confined to Church officers directly in contact with the public and to lay organizations.   The Church has an official Division of Pastoral Medicine whose function it is to pass finally on the content of medical books.   It supervises the instruction in Catholic medical colleges.   In fact we have in the Catholic Church the only modern organized opposition to birth control on any scale worth mention.   Small wonder, then, that Catholics, contrary to a widely held opinion, are not attending our birth-control clinics in due proportion.

That this is the case, figures in Table XXVIII will show.   At Baltimore, Cleveland, and Newark there is a much higher proportion of Protestants than Catholics, the smallest differential being at Baltimore where women have been accepted only on conservative medical indications.   Contracep-

---

[32] This is true as an average.   The average, however, obscures the fact that while Catholic mothers have fewer abortions when they have had up to three or four children— which covers the majority of cases—those Catholic mothers having large families have a very high abortion rate.

tive information has not, until after this series was completed, been freely given there. Though Catholics are 36 per cent of the population of Balti-

TABLE XXVIII

RELIGIOUS AFFILIATIONS OF PATIENTS. BALTIMORE, CLEVELAND, AND NEWARK[1]

Affiliations	Total		Baltimore		Cleveland		Newark	
	No.	Pct.	No.	Pct.	No.	Pct.	No.	Pct.
	6259	100	1142	100	3117	100	2000	100
Protestant..............	3620	58	766	67	1764	57	1090	55
Catholic {Roman.......... / Greek..........	}1621	}26	}258	}23	728 / 62	23 / 2	}573	29
Jewish.................	716	11	112	10	274	9	330	16
Mixed.................	270	4	—	—	270	9	—	—
Others.................	10	}	—	—	3	*	7	*
None..................	15	} 1	6	*	9	*	—	—
Unknown..............	7		—	—	7	*	—	—

* Less than 0.5 per cent.

[1] Sources: Cleveland data from secretary of the Association. Baltimore data from Fifth Report, Table 9. Newark data from Stone and Hart, *op. cit.*, Table 11, p. 21.

TABLE XXIX

COMPARISON OF RELIGIOUS AFFILIATIONS BY PERCENTAGES OF GENERAL POPULATION AND CLINIC POPULATION. BALTIMORE, CLEVELAND AND NEWARK[1]

	Baltimore		Cleveland		Newark		New York City	
	General Population	Clinic Population	General Population	Clinic Population	General Population	Clinic Population	General Population	Clinic Population
All denominations..............	100	100	100	100	100	100	100	100
Roman Catholic..........	36	25	51	25*	53	29	25.4†	26
Protestant..............	31	59	17	57	24	55	49.2§	30
Jewish..................	15	9	23	9	16	16	25.4	42
Other..................	18	7	9	9	7	—	§	—

* Includes 2 per cent Greek Catholics.

† Includes very small percentage of Catholics other than Roman.

§ "Other" group included with Protestants.

[1] Sources: Clinic populations: Baltimore, *Fifth Report*, p. 16. Cleveland, data for 1928–1933 from Secretary, Maternal Health Association. Newark, Stone and Hart, *op. cit.*, 21. New York, Kopp, p. 204. General population: U. S. Religious Census, 1926.

more, being the largest denomination in that city, they are represented in the clinic population by only 25 per cent. This is a differential of 11 per cent.   At Cleveland there is the largest differential, 26 per cent (51 − 25 = 26); while at Newark there is also a substantial differential, 24 per cent (53 − 29 = 24); at New York, the basis of Mrs. Sanger's generalizations, none.   These differentials between proportion in clinic attendance and proportion in the general population is, for Catholics, best brought out in the bar diagram (Figure XXX).   There is clearly a religious deterrent here.   For since Catholics tend to represent the immigrant groups of lower standard of living and lower occupational status, and since the clinics reach these classes in greater proportion than they exist in the general population, we ought to find a *larger* not a smaller proportion of Catholics than Protestants in the clinic population.   Actually we find the reverse.   Hence the

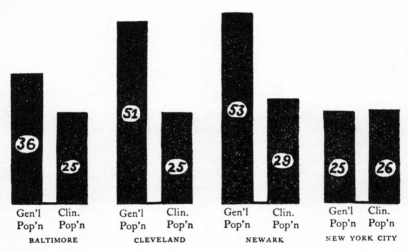

FIG. XXX. Percentage Catholic in Total City Populations and Clinic Populations at Baltimore, Cleveland, Newark, and New York.

explanation of a religious deterrent seems to be the only one capable of explaining the facts.

Beginning to realize that they cannot effectively prevent Catholics from adopting birth control, the leaders are renewing and widely emphasizing their sanction of the so-called "sterile" period,[33] although its safety is

[33] L. J. Latz, M.D., for example, hails this as a "new" scientific discovery lately made known by Knaus and Ogino (Leo. J. Latz, M.D., *The Rhythm of Sterility and Fertility in Women*.   Chicago: Latz Foundation, 1932, pp. vii, 1–108.   For Ogino and Knaus see Bibliog.), evidently quite oblivious of the fact that Soranos and Aëtios made mention of a similar practice, though without some of the modern embellishments of marking calendars and other calculations which run for a year before the method is to be used

insufficiently attested, being based on limited reports that run counter to the extensive evidence to be found in all previously published records of experience.

Every woman has a sterile period, but research has not yet developed any simple test to detect it, nor is there assurance that a woman holds to a reasonably steady habit as to her exact time of high and low fertility. In extensive statistics from well accredited sources, pregnancy is reported as starting on every day of the month but with a low rate in the week preceding the period. All the older published records show *more than half the pregnancies starting in the days called sterile or safe in the new Catholic claims*. Much research by unbiased observers is in order to straighten out this serious contradiction. Meanwhile danger hovers over those who experiment.

§5 CONCLUSION

In this chapter we have traced some of the possible consequences of democratized contraception. Perhaps the most certain is the advent of stationary populations in the United States and most of the countries of Northern and Western Europe in the next few decades. Cannan and Bowley, and later Kuczynski, Lotka, Dublin, Thompson, Whelpton, Pearl, E. Kahn, Charles and others have made contributions to this subject. Thompson's latest estimates suggest a stationary population of 136 to 155 million to be achieved between 1955 and 1980 in the United States, according to the assumptions adopted.

This situation, so different from the historically atypical rapid growth of the nineteenth century, has been dramatized and wept over to more than the logical limit, and has formed the basis for dire predictions and new, emotional, nationalistic appeals. I think I have shown that there are good grounds for discounting these predictions and appeals. Populations in the West are not "doomed to die out," and to assume that present conditions will persist is to commit a fallacy of extrapolation—into which one might reasonably expect competent statisticians not to fall. The whole history of population thought shows that populations adjust to conditions more promptly than do writers on population. The present instance is by no means the only one on record. Thinking never will be straight on this

---

or trusted. This class of publication largely ignores the elaborate medical output on the subject antedating Ogino and Knaus, some forty papers. These are summarized in Dr. R. L Dickinson's "The Safe Period as a Birth Control Measure," [*Amer. Jour. Obst. & Gyn.*, xiv (1927), 718–730], and in the forthcoming book by Carl G. Hartman, *Time of Ovulation in Women. A Study of the Fertile Period in the Menstrual Cycle* (Baltimore: Williams & Wilkins, 1936).

subject until it is generally realized that demographic phenomena are equilibria phenomena.

What, in turn, are some of the possible social and economic consequences of the advent of stationary populations in the West and eventually in the East, assuming that other circumstances remain the same? Since age composition is changing, giving us a larger proportion of elders and a smaller proportion of children, there are implications, as we have seen, for care in old age. We may expect a greater burden either on the relatives or the state. Probably individual savings will be inadequate in the future as in the past.

There will be effects also on the demand for commodities (fewer toys and more foot-warmers). At the moment, food is pressing on population rather than the reverse. Industry, other factors remaining equal, will expand more cautiously, less riotously. But this will help us in the next depression, though, of course, it will not be sufficient to prevent a recurrence of depressions. But there will be a levelling effect of stationary population on the business cycle. Demand for capital will, other things being equal, be less active and interest rates decline. In the labor market, industry will need to adjust by taking on a larger proportion of older men. The effect upon unemployment will probably be neutral, some factors operating either side of the norm (neutrality). The strongest influence of stationary population will be through the effect on the business cycle, which it should help to smooth.

Democratized contraception should substantially relieve occupational congestion and the low wages of the unskilled, thus alleviating many social problems caused by, or associated with, poverty. It is axiomatic that no economic system can achieve maximum productive and social efficiency with the notorious imbalance that has always been characteristic of capitalism.

Stabilization of population abroad means less immigration pressure on the United States. We shall have a chance to absorb, to unify, and economically and socially to elevate the thirty odd millions who came here in the decades preceding 1920. This implies more cultural unity of the right sort: agreement on essentials (e.g., settling disputes by law rather than by the vendetta), respect for differences on non-essentials (e.g., food habits). Stabilization here and abroad will give us the necessary breathing spell to enable us for the first time to house the masses properly. Education will be profoundly affected. So much for the effects of democratized contraception operating through stabilization and changed age composition.

But there are several, more direct effects possible: increased liberty for men and women, increased value placed on the child with its increasing scarcity, lowered infant and maternal mortality and morbidity. There will be a greater equalization by social classes of the sacrifices involved in producing the next generation. Child labor will be reduced. The gifted children of the poor will have greater social advantages. Marital adjustment will be promoted, some forms of mental conflict in marriage alleviated. We might even catch up with Malinowski's Melanesian savages. Then we would know the world had "progressed." Divorce and separation, in so far as they are promoted by sexual ignorance, may be expected to decline. (Actually, they may increase for other reasons.)

Above all, democratization is a eugenic trend. The wide gap now existing between high reproduction and high genetic endowment will be somewhat closed. This will be all to the good not only genetically but socially. But personally I expect that the intelligence of the American population will decline five to eight per cent in the next two hundred years before the process of reversal of differential fertility is complete. And it is quite conceivable that, even when given two hundred years, societies will not prove rational enough socially to direct and speed up the process of reversal by appropriate social measures. After that, we will not have brains enough left to worry much about the biological quality of future generations. It is even doubtful if we have brains enough now, considering how many misleaders of the people are loose in the world preaching unalloyed environmentalism.[34]

[34] This blast—for such I recognize it to be—is directed essentially at my colleagues, the sociologists; secondarily at the doctors; thirdly, at a few biologists, still widely esteemed, who are responsible for much fallacious reasoning on eugenics; fourthly, at naïve environmentalists generally. I grant the great importance of social environment and of social conditioning in moulding and developing human character, attitudes, abilities. No sociologist could be unaware of the case for social conditioning. Nor could he fail to admit that much ability now born goes to waste owing to our irrational social arrangements. I grant all this. But I do not grant, and never have granted, that environmental improvement is a substitute for the improvement of the genetic endowment. That it is a substitute is, indeed, the classic superstitition of our age. Some day it may well be classed with the naïve confidence of the savage rain-maker who thinks his ritualistic manipulations will coerce nature. Some will think these blasts based on pure sentiment and quite unscientific. If so, I think I may be granted the liberty, having devoted five hundred pages to fact reporting and cautious comment. My own judgment is that these insights are among the most valuable in this book, based as they are on fifteen years of specialized, objective study of population problems. That these opinions do not square with received opinions does not concern me in the least. I am concerned only whether further scientific research finds them true or false. The worst that can be said against the above is that it represents an orgy of sentiment; that it is opinion, not science; that the weight of evidence is against the views expressed. To reply to these would take me too far afield. With these allegations I intend to deal in other writings. For the present, critics may make the most of them. On the decline of intelligence and on environmental determinism I have had to content myself here with presenting conclusions rather than evidence.

Whether population pressure causes war is much debated by experts. It seems to be a cause at least in some instances, especially when it buttresses nationalistic sentiments. Clearly, it is socially desirable for the League of Nations to operate on the principle that irresponsible spawning does not give a nation a right to commit international thievery without the application of sanctions.

Democratized contraception should do much to protect standards of living and to enable us to stabilize at an optimum point, if we ever develop an accurate measure of it and agree upon it. I have suggested that a material test, at least in our age, is likely to meet with more favor than one based on leisure or personality development.

Stabilization should promote the conservation of national resources, promote the public health, and ameliorate a major cause of poverty, low incomes.

Lastly, it has been argued that differential increase by religious class, of which we have not been aware, has significant implications for the future struggle between liberty and authoritarianism, for freedom of inquiry, and hence for the whole future of science. Whether or not we enter upon a new Dark Age depends enormously upon the events of the next two centuries, especially on events of the next half century. Can we acquire no control over social processes, or can man modify and direct them, at least in a minor measure? It seems to me that to accept the first is to turn the future of civilization over to obscurantism and fatalism. But the society that operates on the second assumption will have a modest chance of "coming out on top" in the evitable struggle ahead between intelligently-directed freedom, on the one hand, and blind authoritarianism, on the other.

CONCLUSION

CHAPTER XV

Several generalizations, standing out in the author's mind as a result of his historical and social investigation of conception control, may usefully be mentioned in closing. It should be clearly understood, however, that this brief chapter is not intended to be a substitute for the summaries of preceding chapters. To these, also, the reader should turn who desires a rapid review of the main points.

The *desire* to control conception is a well-nigh universal culture-trait, universal, that is, in time and space. The *desire*, often unconscious, is much more universal and general than the *practice*. There has been desire for both release and control, each at its appointed time or place. Even when the physiology of conception was not understood—that is a recent achievement, and, in fact, is by no means complete—and even when pre-literates held magical theories of conception, there was often the suspicion that coitus played a part. This dim realization led to trial and error types of interference, some of which happened to be rational, more frequently irrational, magical. Man, then, has learned in this field as he has in all others—by trial and error, by observing what would and would not work.

One is impressed, I think, with the enormous amount of time it has taken man to winnow the rational from the magical. And the process is still going on. The sieve of time operates slowly. (Most of us are not even aware that it operates.) The time required is all the more impressive since the desire for control is old, though it has been accentuated in the past century.

We have found the contraceptive knowledge of Greek, Roman and Is-lamic physicians far more extensive than has heretofore even been suspected. Note that it was the geniuses of the healing art who forwarded the subject. Note, also, the conspicuous absence (with a few exceptions) of demagogical moralizing on the subject. These physicians had more sense of humor than many of their present followers: they rarely set themselves up as arbiters of public morals. This is not the business of the healing art.

Techniques are older than formulated, recorded indications. Man usually *acts*; then *justifies*. Contraception is no exception. The same, incidentally, goes for social systems. Even the early indications, however, manifest substantial traces of preventive points of view (see Index to Subjects, Indications). We find preventive indications among preliterate peoples, among the Greeks, Romans, Arabians, Persians, etc.

Contraception, therefore, is both old and new (see index); old in the sense that the *desire* dates back half a million years, and some *practice* nearly as long; it is virtually as old as the sexual life of man; new in the sense that democratized knowledge is an ultra-modern phenomenon; new in the sense that we have been able, more effectively than our ancestors (because we have more experience), to winnow out the reliable, the harmless. Contra-traception, therefore, has been refined, improved as a body of knowledge; but as a practice it is not new. This is not to suggest that all is old. New discoveries are, of course, being made, especially in the chemical field, which is quite new.

In view of the attitudes of the ancient physicians, modern support of contraception by physicians is not radical. It is a return to the Classical outlook. It is progress by reversion to a nobler tradition than that recently prevelant. The immediate task of medical science is to improve our knowledge by more research. To improve techniques is more important than to refine indications. There will be a failure to see problems whole, if medical indications are accepted, and social, economic, and eugenic indications rejected.

Equilibrium analysis of social phenomena, which often change in cycles, suggests that as contraceptive knowledge becomes democratized, its application may at first go too far. To say that we have to learn to use wisely our freedom in this as in other departments of human activity would be to utter a platitude, if it did not need emphasis. We must expect the movement to go beyond the equilibrium point—its location is uncertain—until new forces check it, and restore equilibrium. I predict that this situation will raise up its own crowd of panicky observers; in fact, their heads are already poking over the horizon. But if they steal our emotional gyroscope and induce us to lose our historical perspective, we shall most certainly adopt unwise policies. Every new invention is open to abuse; but we do not advocate illiteracy because some people forge checks. Increasingly, in the future, it will be desirable that our population policies should be based on a full knowledge of the facts rather than on patriotism, religion, racial mysticism, pseudo-science and naïve environmentalism.

Opposition to contraception and the democratization of such knowledge never has been successful whether repression came through religion or law. Will it be any more successful in the future? As Lippert said years ago, the power in history of an idea or desire is determined in no small degree by its universality.

There has thus been a general drift, whatever the occasional recessions, throughout history toward the acceptance of conception control. At least knowledge on the subject has been cumulative. And I think belief in it has been cumulative. Those who have strong sentimental attachments to ideas, values, etc., like to talk about their inevitability. Thus convinced socialists and communists, and ardent Catholics sincerely believe that it is only a question of time before the world will lie at their feet. Ardent believers in democracy, fascism, etc., have the same tendency. But the cycle of history has a most uncanny way of fooling the "ardent believers," just as it has fooled statesmen, economists and sociologists, times beyond number in the past. If I can help it, I have no desire to fall into this trap. But, on the other hand, if desire for conception control were a mere sentimental wish not requiring a certain technical knowledge for its skillful execution, it might, despite its long past and its cultural universality, at some time and for some period, go the way of most ideologies—out the window, at least temporarily. But mankind has been struggling for its reliable achievement for so long, it is now so institutionalized, it is so tied up with the hedonistic and materialistic impulses of mankind, and it so promotes economy of effort in reproduction, that it seems impossible to contemplate that man will ever give it up *completely* and turn the clock back to a situation that antedates even the infancy of group life. And after ten years of historical investigation I think I am entitled to that judgment without being accused of being a slave to my sentiments and wishes (and hence a poor social scientist). This book will be dust by several thousand years before the final verdict on that judgment is in. It will be the judgment of history. Apart from learning nature's laws, I know no other way of divining the future except by studying the past; and the historical method is one substitute, however inferior, for natural science techniques.

The medical history of conception control is much older than the social movement. A summary will be found elsewhere (pp. 391–394) of the reasons why the social agitation broke out when it did. There seem to have been definite reasons for the time and place. Correspondingly, the medical case for contraception is much older than the economic, social, psychiatric and eugenic indications. There are qualifications, of course, but as a general proposition that statement is true.

In view of the determination, deeply-rooted and increasingly widespread, on the part of the populace to achieve a knowledge of effective, harmless aesthetic prevention; and in view of the fact that opposition in the past or present never has been successful, it may be inferred that the determination can best be guided. Since the problem is essentially medical, instruction ought to be in the hands of the medical profession.

Recent symposia and recent summaries of questionnaires received from medical-school staffs show that medical opinion has been tremendously liberalized in the U. S. A. in the past decade or two; that we in the United States are now catching up with medical opinion in Western Europe. The change has been nothing less than revolutionary, especially in its rapidity. The American Medical Association, under strong pressure from prominent members, from local medical bodies, and from national specialist groups, has at last recognized the existence of contraception—now that it has revolutionized sexual conduct—by appointing a committee "to study the subject." The Associations Council on Pharmacy and Chemistry is just beginning to recognize its responsibility to the active practioner of medicine who needs to know without delay whether any of the hundreds of proprietary contraceptive products on the market are worthy of prescription by him. These moves are in the right direction; even if they have been unduly delayed. We may yet catch up with Soranos, Aëtios and the Arabians and Persians. Who knows? A little more courage and devotion to science and less pious obscurantism will take us a long way. Whether the curve of history will be projected into the future now depends on the physicians and on the kind of support they get from the general public and especially from legislatures.

BIBLIOGRAPHY

NOTE ON BIBLIOGRAPHY

THIS bibliography aims to mention most of the important papers on conception control contributed to medical periodicals as well as pamphlets separately published dealing with the medical aspects of the subject whether produced by medical men or laymen. It omits some three thousand titles chiefly of social and economic interest; these will appear in the bibliographies of succeeding volumes. Often there is, of course, overlapping between medical titles and those which are chiefly economic and social in nature.

The titles below, especially the medical-journal articles, were originally classified into five roughly-defined groups[1] with the intention of including it here. This idea was finally abandoned, however, lest it cause misunderstanding or even ill-feeling among writers still living. If this grouping had been made it would have had the advantage, in a rather full bibliography, of separating the chaff from the wheat. As a partial substitute I have starred valuable contributions, doubly-starred especially valuable contributions, whether judged from the historical or theoretical standpoints. Virtually all the items in Class IV and all those in Class V have been omitted unless produced by a man of standing. There are a few such instances. For medical periodicals the citations run to January 1, 1935, except that between June, 1933 and January, 1935 only the most important papers are listed. Much of the recent "safe period" literature has been omitted.

Pains have been taken to cite the place of publication of certain journals because there are sometimes two of the same name. The place cited is the place of publication at the time the journal article in question appeared.

[1] Class I: Brilliant, original contribution likely to be of enduring value. A definite step forward in scientific progress.

Class II: Presenting new material in a sound, logical manner, or else summarizing extant knowledge in a better than average manner.

Class III: An average performance. Usually a rehash of what is known with occasional, but not too frequent logical slips; or else simple news reporting not of unusual, permanent interest. Characterized by fairly sound reasoning as a rule, but manifesting no unusually shrewd insights.

Class IV: Material below the average, characterized by poor reporting and rather frequent logical errors. Apt to show rather strong admixture of prejudice whether for or against birth control.

Class V: Material so bad it never should have been published. Thoroughly unsound and unscientific; inaccurate reporting of facts; frequent *non sequitur* reasoning.

In many cases it is not the present place of publication.   In perhaps less than one per cent of the instances the place has been omitted either because it could not be traced or because it was well-known.

In order to facilitate the work of others in finding certain historically important or scarce titles, there is appended a list of the editions known to the compiler, together with a code symbol or symbols stating the location or locations of the item.   In the case of scarce, but not rare items, no attempt is made to list all locations.   For examples of the method, see the listings for the known editions of Robert Dale Owen's *Moral Physiology* and Dr. Charles Knowlton's *Fruits of Philosophy*.   In each instance where it is used the symbol appears after the corresponding title and reference in round brackets, thus: (B.M., Yale).   The code follows:

KEY TO LOCATION OF RARE ITEMS

A.A.S.	American Antiquarian Society, Worcester, Mass.
A.C.	Author's Collection
B.M.	British Museum
B.M.L.	Boston Medical Library, 8 The Fenway, Boston, Mass.
B.P.L.	Boston Public Library, Boston, Mass.
F.C.	Professor James A. Field Collection, Chicago, Ill.
G.L.	Goldsmith's Library, University of London.
H.M.S.	Harvard Medical School, Boston, Mass.
H.L.	Widener Library, Harvard University, Cambridge, Mass.
Ind.	Indiana State Library, Indianapolis, Ind.
J.C.	John Crerar Library, Chicago, Ill.
L.C.	Library of Congress, Washington, D. C.
N.Y.P.L.	New York Public Library, New York, N. Y.
N.Y.A.M.	New York Academy of Medicine, New York, N. Y.
P.H.	Private Hands. Address obtainable from author.
Phil.	Coll. Phys. & Surg., Philadelphia.
S.C.	Seligman Collection, Columbia University, New York City.
S.G.	Surgeon General's Office, Army Medical Library, Washington, D. C.
U.C.	University of Chicago, Chicago, Ill.
W.I.	Workingmen's Institute, New Harmony, Ind.
Yale	Yale University, New Haven, Conn.

It is hoped that the use of this code may further research by aiding workers to locate rare items.   If a title is mentioned as unique, I would be glad to be apprised of the whereabouts of other copies.

In citing titles the following is, in general, the system: Titles of journal articles appear in quotation marks, titles of books in italics; titles of contributions to edited volumes and of pamphlets are in regular type without quotation marks (a pamphlet is here defined as a title of less than one hundred pages, whether in cloth or paper binding).   An exception has been made in the instance of a few, early, rare pamphlets of historical interest which have been placed in italics. These usually have long, eighteenth-century-style titles. Also, in the instance of some of the long titles, lower-case type has been used throughout on account of the difficulties well-known to any bibliographer.

Not every title mentioned in footnotes is included in the Bibliography; and, of course, not every title in the Bibliography was used in the text. The main reason for the former is that in Chapters XIII and XIV, and to a lesser extent in some other chapters, references have been made to social and economic literature because it illumined special points in the medical history. Since this literature is not narrowly or essentially medical, it is omitted from this Bibliography. On the other hand, the Bibliography contains a few stray titles not strictly medical in content because they were published in medical journals.

With regard to the starring in the Bibliography it should be clearly understood that my judgments must be subjective and that others may well disagree. At all events, it should be clearly understood that certain works may be excellent treatises in their special line but not significant works on contraception (e.g., Carr-Saunders, *Population Problems*). Accordingly, failure to star a book does not necessarily imply that the present writer has a low opinion of it.

With some exceptions, articles appearing in the following birth-control propaganda periodicals have been omitted. They are, in general, of little interest to the physician, though a few of them are important to sociologists, economists, and social historians who wish to trace changes in public opinion, methods of moulding and influencing opinion, etc. These journals are:

Birth Control Herald, Birth Control News, Birth Control Review, Critic & Guide, Gelukkig Huisgezin, Malthusian, Neue Generation, New Generation, and Sozial Harmonie.

The journals themselves have, however, been mentioned in the Bibliography. While the news reporting on birth control appearing in very recent years in the *Lancet, British Medical Journal,* and the *Journal of the American Medical Association* has been tolerably good, no one wishing to follow contemporary events in this field, especially on the social side, can afford to overlook the propaganda journals. The best one was the old series of the *Birth Control Review.* Not infrequently it published more intelligent articles than the poor or mediocre medical journals. But since July, 1933 the *Review* has become hardly more than a brief news sheet. Though some of the old series *Review* articles have been good reports, they are not separately listed here. Readers should refer to the files of the journal. A great deal of news will also be found in the *Eugenics Review* and in the new journal, *Marriage Hygiene.*

Lastly, it ought to be said that not every title below has been seen by the writer. A few journals were inaccessible, either wholly or in part. Others in the possession of the Boston Medical Library were stored, owing to a present lack of funds for the construction of stack space, or even for indexing. Certain unique pamphlets, supposedly in the possession of the Library of Congress, are temporarily lost. And so the story goes. But such circumstances seemed no good reason why such titles should be omitted altogether. On the other hand, I have no desire to "fly under false colors." The percentage not seen, however, is small.

I cannot hope that this Bibliography is without error, but efforts have been made to make it accurate. Notice of errors or omissions will be gratefully acknowledged.

BIBLIOGRAPHY OF BIBLIOGRAPHY

DICKINSON, R. L. and BRYANT, L. S., *see* citation within bibliography on *Control of Conception*.

[Has the best bibliography of any of the English medical handbooks on contraception.]

FIELD, JAMES ALFRED, *Essays on Population and Other Papers*. [Edited by Helen Fisher Hohman]. Chicago: University of Chicago Press, 1931, pp. xxix, 1–440.

[See pp. 403–424 entitled "Books and Pamphlets on Population [and Birth Control] in the Library of James A. Field." Field's bibliography is disappointingly small, and does not draw sufficiently on the Continental literature.]

FRAENKEL, LUDWIG, *Die Empfängnisverhütung. Biologische Grundlagen, Technik und Indikationen, für Ärzte bearbeitet.* Stuttgart: Enke, 1932, pp. 212.

[The outstanding German text. Excellent bibliography.]

HANKINS, FRANK H., *see* citation in bibliography.

[This able article runs a short, but critically selected bibliography.]

HIMES, NORMAN E., *A Guide to Birth Control Literature. A Selected Bibliography on the Technique of Contraception and on the Social Aspects of Birth Control.* London: Noel Douglas, 1931, pp. 46.

[Short, but makes a beginning at critically evaluating the literature on technique.]

HIRSCHFELD, MAGNUS, *see* citation for *Geschlechtskunde* in bibliography.

——— and LINSERT, RICHARD, Empfängnisverhütung. Mittel und Methoden. Berlin: Neuer Deutscher Verlag, 1929, pp. 48.

[This is only a pamphlet, but it has a good small bibliography. The citations are not, however, always accurate.]

HOLMES, SAMUEL JACKSON, *A Bibliography of Eugenics*. Berkeley, California: University of California Press, 1924.

[See pp. 341–354. While this is a good start for a bibliography of eugenics, it is quite incomplete on conception control.]

JOHNSEN, JULIA E., *Selected Articles on Birth Control*. New York: H. W. Wilson, 1925, pp. lxxxiii, 1–369.

[This reprints mostly popular articles of the sort listed in the *Readers' Guide to Periodical Literature*. The uncritical bibliography is, however, of some use to the sociologist if sufficiently sifted.]

A London bibliography of the social sciences, being the subject catalogue of the British library of political and economic science at the School of Economics, the Goldsmiths' Library of London . . . [Edited by B. M. Headicar . . . and C. Fuller.] London: London School of Economics & Political Science, 4 vols.

[See i, 244 for about a score of references. This bibliography is exceedingly incomplete on our subject.]

ROBINSON, WM. J., "Birth Control Bibliography," *Amer. Jour. Urol.*, xiii (April, May, June, July, 1917), 185–192; 233–240; 281–286; 329–336.

[Probably the earliest American bibliography on contraception. Includes several general titles on population that do not in any way discuss birth control.

All of Wm. J. Robinson's papers to date of appearance of this bibliography are here. Now out of date.]

SCHROEDER, THEODORE [ALBERT], *Free Speech Bibliography* ... New York: H. W. Wilson, 1922, pp. 247.

[See pp. 188–193. Valuable chiefly for articles published in the second decade of the present century in the more inaccessible, radical journals. Hardly more than scratches the surface. But still it is valuable.]

——— List of References on Birth Control. New York: H. W. Wilson, 1918, pp. 52. [Useful, but the citations are of very unequal value (which is no criticism of the compiler). Now out of date. Of no use for the period before 1870. Some general works on population, which do not discuss contraception, are included.]

SOCIAL SCIENCE ABSTRACTS, *see* index to all volumes.

BIBLIOGRAPHY

ABBOT-ANDERSON, SIR MAURICE, "Birth Control as Seen by an Open Mind," *Practitioner* (London), cxi (1923): 6–13.

ABBOTT, F. W., "Limitation of the Family," *Mass. Med. Jour.* (Boston), x (1890): 337–347.

ABE, ISOO, "The Birth Control Movement in Japan," *Rpt. Fifth Int'l Conf.*, 192–196.

ABERLE, S. B. D., "Frequency of Pregnancies and Birth Interval among Pueblo Indians," *Amer. Jour. Phys. Anthrop.* (Phila.), xvi (1931): 63–80.

ADAMS, FRANCIS, *The Seven Books of Paulus Aegineta.* London: Sydenham Society, 1844–57, 3 vols.

ADAMSON, RHODA B., Methods of Conception Control.
[An English pamphlet I have not seen. By a Lecturer in Obstetrics at Leeds University.]

ADOLF, G., Die Gefahren der künstlichen Sterilität besonders in ihrer Beziehung zum Nervensystem. Eine Studie für Aerzte und Laien. 5 Aufl. Leipzig: Krüger, 1899, pp. 5–63.

———, ——— 6 Aufl. Leipzig: Krüger, 1899, pp. 5–63.
[L. C. has a Leipzig, 1889 edition.]

AEGINITA, PAULUS, *see* ADAMS.

AËTIOS [OF AMIDA], *see* ZERVOS.

AHLUWALIA, GOPALJI, "Indian Population Problem," *Rpt. Fifth Int'l Conf.*, pp. 86–95.

AIGREMONT, *Volkserotik und Pflanzenwelt.* Halle, 2 vols. Vol. i, 1908, pp. 1–165; vol. ii, pp. 1–121.

AIYER, M. S. KRISHNAMURTHI, Approved methods of family limitation compiled by a committee of the Madras Neo-Malthusian League with the assistance of Dr. M. S. Krishnamurthi Aiyer, M. B., & C. M., Madras: Madras Neo-Malthusian League, 1928, pp. 8.

[AIYER, M. S. KRISHNAMURTHI], Selected methods of family limitation compiled by a committee of the Madras Neo-Malthusian League. Second edition. Madras: Madras Neo-Malthusian League, 1929, pp. 16.

ALBERT, G., Die Regulierung der Kinderzahl, ihre Mittel und moralische Berechtigung. 4 Aufl. Hamburg, 1930, pp. 62.

ALBERT, GRAND, *Les secrets admirables du Grand Albert . . . suivi du trésor des merveilleux sacrets du Petit Albert.* Réédition par Marius Decrespe. Paris Guyot, n.d., pp. 190.

ALBRECHT, HANS, "Über Konzeptions Verhütung," *Münch. Med. Wchnschr.* (München), lxxviii (1931): 347–350.

*ALLBUTT, H[ENRY] ARTHUR, The Wife's Handbook: how a woman should order herself during pregnancy, in the lying-in room, and after delivery. With hints on the management of the baby, and on other matters of importance, necessary to be known by married women. Third edition. London: W. J. Ramsey, 1886, pp. 46 + adverts. (A.C.)

———, ——— Fourth edition. London: Forder, 1887, pp. 58. (A.C., H.L.)

———, ——— 41 edition (390th thous.). London: George Standring, 1907, pp. 5–59, advts. (A.C.)

434   BIBLIOGRAPHY

ALLBUTT, H[ENRY] ARTHUR, The Wife's Handbook: How a woman should order herself
    during pregnancy and after delivery with hints on the management of the baby, and
    on other matters of importance to married women. 50 edition (500th thous.).
    London: George Standring, n.d. [1926], pp. 5–59, advts. (A.C.)
    [Note modernization of title and large circulation.]
——— Le Livre de l'Épouse.
*——— The Trial of Dr. Henry Arthur Allbutt, of Leeds, by the General Medical
    Council of Great Britain and Ireland, at 299, Oxford Street, London, on November
    23rd, 24th, and 25th, 1887, for the Publication of "The Wife's Handbook" at so Low
    a Price; with Press Criticisms on the Same and Letter from Mr. Joseph Latchmore,
    of Leeds, to Sir Henry W. Acland. Stanningley: J. W. Birdsall, [1888], pp. 31.
    (A.C.)
*——— Artificial Checks to Population: Is the popular teaching of them infamous? A
    history of medical persecution; an address, delivered at Leeds, Bradford, Pudsey, and
    Morley, February, March, and April, 1888, by Henry Arthur Allbutt . . . Printed by
    request. [First edition.] London: R. Forder, 1889, pp. 31. (A.C.)
———, ——— 14 edition. London, 1909, pp. 35. (A.C.)
——— Sur le mortalité infantile et la mort prématurée.
    [Paper read before the Public Health Section of the International Medical
    Congress, Amsterdam, (1879).]
——— Evils Produced by Over-Childbearing and Excessive Lactation. London:
    Malthusian League, Malthusian [Propaganda] Tract, No. 4, [c. 1887–8], pp. 4. (A.C.)
——— Too Frequent Childbearing. San Diego: Neo-Malthusian Pub. Co., 1893, 16°.
    (S.G.)
ALMKVIST, J., "Inför frågan om födelse-kontroll [Concerning the Question of Birth Con-
    trol], Svenska Läkart. (Stockholm) xxvi (1929): 313–322; 352–361; 389–400.
ALPERT, N. A., "Birth Control and the Physician," Jour. Med. Asso. Ga. (Atlanta), xii
    (1923): 185–188.
[American Birth Control League], One Hundred Years of Birth Control. An Outline of
    its History. New York: Amer. Birth Control League, (various printings 1921 and
    later), pp. 8.
ANDERES, "Welche Mittel können wir Aerzte zur Verhütung der Konzeption empfehlen?"
    Schweiz. Med. Wchnschr. (Basel), n.s. vii (1926): 1132–1133.
ANDERSON, CYRUS W., "Natural Avoidance of Conception," Col. Med., xxx (June,
    1933): 223–227.
ANDREWS, HENRY RUSSELL, "Birth Control," Practitioner (London), cxi (1923): 14–16.
ANONYMOUS, Know thyself or nature's secrets revealed. . . . Marietta [Ohio?], 1910, pp.
    540.
    [L. C. copy "lost."]
——— The Book of nature containing information for young people who think of getting
    married on the philosophy of procreation and sexual intercourse showing also how to
    prevent conception and to avoid childbearing. James Ashton, M.D. [Author?]
    (F.C. Photostat A.C.)
——— A Few Words (to Men Only) on Over-population and Disease, and their Preven-
    tion by the Use of "Letters." Issued for Private Circulation Only. N.p., n.d.,
    pp. 8.
——— "Die Entwürfe der Gesetze zur Bekämpfung der Geschlechtskrankheiten und
    gegen die Verhinderung der Geburten," Deutsche Med. Wchnschr. (Leipzig), xliv
    (1918): 246–248.

ANONYMOUS, *Love without Danger. A Study in Social Science.* Paris: Privately issued, 1904, pp. 179. (A.C.)

——— [Ed. MARIE C. STOPES?], *Medical Help on Birth Control.* London: Putnam, 1928, pp. xii, 2–225.

——— The Power and duty of parents to limit the number of their children. London, 1868, pp. 11.

——— Medical views on birth control; being a short essay by a practising physician, together with some opinions on birth control by the following eminent doctors:... London: Workers' Birth Control Group, n.d. [1926], pp. 8.

——— Birth Control and Some of Its Simplest Methods. [*see* TYRER, A.H.]

——— "Some Legislative Aspects of the Birth Control Problem," *Harv. Law Rev.* (Cambridge), xlv (1932): 723–729.

——— Zur antikonzeptionellen Frage. N.d., n.p., pp. 7.

——— "Die ärztlichen Erfahrungen über medizinisch indizierte Konzeptions-verhütung," *Med. Welt.* (Berlin), (1931): No. 26.

——— Hygienisches Eheleben. Leipzig: Ficker, n.d., pp. 15.

——— Die Einschränkung der Familie aus Ehenot. Leipzig: Ficker, n.d., pp. 48.

——— Die Verhütung der Gravidität als ärztliches Problem. München: Luitpold-Werk, (*c.* 1928), pp. 28.

——— The Way to be rich and respectable addressed to men of small fortune. Second edition. London: R. Baldwin, n.d. (F.C.)

ANTI-MARCUS, Notes on the Population Question. London: J. Watson, 1841, pp. viii, 8–44. (B.M., A.C., F.C.)

APTEKAR, HERBERT, "In Anthropological Perspective," *Birth Control Rev.* (New York), xiv (1930): 202–203, 218.

——— "Primitive Psychology and Birth Control," *Birth Control Rev.* (New York), xv (1931): 112–114; 127.

——— *Anjea. Infanticide, Abortion and Contraception in Savage Society.* New York: William Godwin, 1931, pp. xv, 17–192.

ARENDT, E., "Bemerkungen zur operativen Konceptionsverhinderung," *Cbl. f. Gynäk.* (Leipzig), xxi (1897): 1318–23.

ARISTOTLE, *Historia Animalium.* [Vol. IV in the Works of Aristotle translated into English under the editorship of J. A. Smith and W. D. Ross. This vol. edited by D'Arcy Wentworth Thompson.] Oxford, 1910.

ARMSTRONG, GILBERT R. A., A General Practitioner's Views, in *Medical Help*, pp. 47–60.

ASHE, THOMAS, *Travels in America, Performed in 1806, for the Purpose of Exploring the Rivers Alleghany, Monongahela, Ohio, and Mississippi, and Ascertaining the Produce and Condition of their Banks and Vicinity.* London & Newburyport: 1808, pp. 366.

ASTRUC, JOHANNES, *De morbis venereis.* Paris, 1738.

ATHENAEUS [of Naucrates, 2nd century], *The Deipnosophists or Banquet of the Learned of Athenaeus. Literally translated by C. D. Yonge, B. A., with an appendix of poetical fragments, rendered into English verse by various authors, and a general index.* London: Bohn, 1854, 3 vols.

AYYAR, MURARI S. KRISHNAMURTHI, *Population and Birth-Control in India.* Madras, [1930–31?], pp. xv, 1–115.

——— *See* AIYER.

BABADAGLY, A. VON, ["Immune-biological Contraceptive Methods,"] *Odessky Med. J.* (Odessa), ii (1927): 65–71.

——— "Espermoinmunidad como metodo anticoncepcional," (Trans. by C. de San Antonio) *Siglo Med.* (Madrid), lxxxii (1928): 456–458.

BAIṬĀR, IBN AL-. See BEĪTHAR, IBN EL-.

**BAKER, JOHN R., "The Spermicidal Powers of Chemical Contraceptives. I. Introduction, and Experiments on Guinea-pig Sperms," *Jour. Hyg.* (Camb. Engl.), xxix (1930): 323–329. "II. Pure Substances," xxxi (1931): 189–214. "III. Pessaries," xxxi (1931): 309–320. "IV. More Pure Substances," xxxii (1932): 171–183. "V. A Comparison of Human Sperms with those of the Guinea-pig," xxxii (1932): 550–556. "VI. [with R. M. Ranson] An Improved Test for Suppositories," xxxiv (1934): 474–485.

———— "Chemical Contraceptives," *Proc. Sec. Int'l Cong.* [*1930*] *for Sex Research*, London: Oliver & Boyd, 1931, pp. 555–558.

———— Chemical Contraception. In Sanger & Stone, *Practice of Contraception*, pp. 72–76.

————, *The Chemical Control of Conception*, London: Chapman & Hall, 1935, pp. x, 173.

BALTHAZARD, "Provocation à l'avortement et propagande néo-malthusienne (loi du 1er Août 1920)," *Progrès Méd.* (Paris), 3 s., xxxvi (1921): 137–139.

————, ———— *Trans. New York Acad. Med. 1892*, 2 s., ix (1893): 119–124.

BARR, SIR JAMES, *see* ch. 2 in HAIRE [Ed.], *Some More Medical Views*.

———— The Question of Population, with Special Reference to Heredity and Birth Control. In *Medical Help*, pp. 73–104.

BARRETT, LADY FLORENCE ELIZABETH PERRY, Conception Control and its Effects on the Individual and the Nation. Foreword by His Grace, the Archbishop of Canterbury. London: J. Murray, 1922, pp. 48, 12°. New York: Dutton, 1922, pp. 5–52.

———— "Conception Control," *Practitioner* (London), cxi (1923): 17–24.

*BARTELS, MAX, *Die Medicin d. Naturvölker. Ethnologische Beiträge zur Urgeschichte der Medicin*. Leipzig: Th. Grieben, 1893.

———— *see* PLOSS.

BARTON, E. A., "The Ethics of Birth Control," *Practitioner* (London), cxxxi (Sept., 1933): 229–246.

BASKIN, M. J., "Contraceptive Methods and Their Indications," *Colorado Med.* (Denver), xxvi (1929): 186–188.

*BAUER, A. W., "Kritik der Konzeptionsverhütungsmittel," *Med. Klin.* (Berlin), xxvi (1930): 961–964, 1002–1006.

BAUM, FRITZ, *Über den praktischen Malthusianismus, Neo-Malthusianismus und Sozialdarwinismus*. Leipzig: Max Schmersow, [1928], pp. viii, 1–134. (Inaug. diss. Univ. of Leipzig.)

BAUM, MAX, Die künstliche Beschränkung der Kinderzahl; ein Mittel zur Verhütung der Conception (Empfängniss). Berlin: Hermann Schmidt, [1892], pp. 3–63.

BAUMANN, E. D., "Primitive Voorstellingen aangaande de Ontvangenis" [Primitive Conceptions of Conception], *Mensch en Maatsch.* (Gröningen), vi (1930): 252–268.

BEAM, LURA, *see* DICKINSON, R. L.

BEHM, H., "Geburtenrückgang und Volkssittlichkeit," *Ztschr. f. Bevölkrngspolit.* (Leipzig), x (1917): 65–85.

BEĪTHAR, IBN EL-, *Traité des Simples*. In *Notices et Extraits des Manuscrits de la Bibliothèque Nationale et autres Bibliothèques*, vol. 23 (1877), vol. 25 (1881), vol. 26 (1883).

BELL, T., *Kalogynomia or the Laws of Female Beauty: being the elementary principles of that Science*. London: Walpole, 1899, pp. xvi, 1–331. (B.P.L.)
    [Rubbish. There is also a London, 1821 ed.]

BELOT, J. and LEPENNELIER, "Le pessaire anti-conceptionnel de la vertueuse Amérique," *Hôpital* (Paris), xii (1924): 350.

BELOT, J., "Pessaire anticonceptionnel," *Bull. et mém. Soc. de radiol. méd. de France* (Paris), xii (1924): 129.

*BENDIX, KURT, *Geburtenregelung. Vorträge und Verhandlungen des Ärztekurses vom 28–30 Dezember, 1928.* Berlin: Selbstverlag, [1929], pp. 131.

——— Die Praxis der Berliner Beratungsstellen für Geburtenregelung. In Bendix, *Geburtenregelung,* pp. 43–50.

BERENDES, J., *Des Pedanios Dioskurides aus Anazarbos Arzneimittellehre in fünf Büchern. Übersetzt und mit Erklärungen versehen von Prof. Dr. J. Berendes.* Stuttgart: Enke, 1902, pp. 572.

BERGERET, L. F. E., Des fraudes dans l'accomplissement des fonctions génératrices, causes, dangers, et inconvénients pour les individus, la famille, et la société; remèdes. 5 ed. Paris, 1877, 16°.

——— Le frodi nell' esercizio delle funzioni generatrici. 9 ed. Italiana, eseguita sulla 6 francese. Rome, 1897, roy. 8°.

BERGL, K., "Ein neues Okklusivpessar," *Deutsche Med. Wchnschr.* (Leipzig), 50 (1924): 763–4.

BERKUSKY, H., "Volksvermehrung und Volksverminderung bei den Naturvölkern und ihre Ursachen," *Zeitschr. f. Socialwissensch.* (Berlin), n.f., i (1910): 657–666; 731–736; 789–795.

BERTA, L., "Beiträge zum Problem des Neomalthusianismus," *Arch. f. Sozialwissensch.* (Tübing.), xxxviii (1914): 425–459.

*BESANT, ANNIE, The Law of Population: its consequences, and its bearing upon human conduct and morals. London: Freethought Pub. Co., n.d. [Jan. 1879 or possibly late 1878], pp. 3–48, adverts. (A.C.)

[Probably first issue]

———, ——— 10th thousand, n.d., pp. 3–48, adverts. (A.C., F.C.)

———, ——— 70th thousand, n.d. [1882], pp. [1–2], 3–48, App. 49. (A.C.)

———, ——— 90th thousand, 1884, pp. iv, 5–47, App. 48, adverts. on cover (A.C.).

———, ——— 110th thousand, 1887, pp. 3–46, adverts. (A.C.)

———, ——— 135th thousand, 1887, pp. 3–46, adverts. (A.C.)

———, ——— 155th thousand, 1889, pp. [3], 5–46, adverts. (A.C.)

[All above editions printed by Charles Bradlaugh and Annie Besant. The 155th thousand has a special preface. Text varies from some of earlier editions both as regards methods and last chapter on "Answers to Objections." Here Mrs. Besant tries to pacify the opposition among her socialist friends.

Incidentally, this shows the importance of collecting and studying different editions of such influential works, if we would really understand the development of, and changes in, the author's thought.]

———, ——— 175th thousand. London: Freethought Publishing Co., 1891, pp. [3], 5–46, adverts. (A.C.)

———, ——— Authorized American from the 25th thousandth English edition. New York, 1878, pp. 47, 12°. [L.C., B.M.L., copy temporarily lost.]

———, ——— New York: Butts [c. 188-]. (L.C., H.L.)

———, ——— San Francisco, 1893, pp. 73, Readers' Library, (P.H.) pp. 73, viii.

BEST, ELSDON, "Ceremonial Performances Pertaining to Birth, as Performed by the Maori of New Zealand in Past Times," *Jour. Roy. Anthrop. Inst.* (London), xliv (1914): 127–162.

BIEBER, J., "Geschlechtsleben in Äthiopen," *Anthropophyteia* (Leipzig), v: (1908) 45–99.

BIKOFF, S., ["New Method of Prevention of Pregnancy,"] *Vrach. Delo* (Kharkov), x (1927): 1539–1541.

BILLUPS, H. B., The General Practitioner and Birth Control. In *Medical Help*, pp. 125–142.

BIRTH CONTROL. Hearings before a Subcommittee of the Committee on the Judiciary, United States Senate, Seventy-first Congress, Third Session on S. 4582. A Bill to Amend Section 305 (A) of the Tariff Act of 1922, as Amended, and Sections 211, 245, and 312 of the Criminal Code, as Amended. February 13 and 14, 1931. Washington: United States Government Printing Office, pp. 84.

"BIRTH CONTROL CLINIC IN CHICAGO," *Med.-Leg. Jour.* (New York), xl (1923): 122–128.

BIRTH CONTROL LIBEL ACTION. "Stopes v. Sutherland," *Brit. Med. Jour.* (London), ii (1924): 1028.

"BIRTH CONTROL LIBEL ACTION; STOPES V. SUTHERLAND and ANOTHER," *Cath. Med. Guard.* (Middlesex, Eng.), i (1923): 36–43.

*BLACKER, C. P., [Ed.] International Medical Group for the Investigation of Birth Control. (Five annual "issues" or reports published at London beginning in 1928. First issue, 1928. Second issue, June, 1929, pp. 35. Third issue, September 1930, pp. 43. Fourth issue, 1931, pp. 76. Obtainable from Hon. Mrs. Marjorie Farrer, 416 Clanricarde Gardens, London, W. 2. Sixpence each.)
[Good progress reports]

—— "Birth Control," *Guy's Hosp. Gaz.* (London), xxxviii (1924): 559; 577.

—— "A Critical Review of Some Medical Views on Birth Control," *Lancet* (London), i, (1927): 1165–1167.

—— The Need for Research in Birth Control. In Sanger & Stone, *Practice of Contraception*, pp. 154–164.

—— "The Choice of a Contraceptive," *Practitioner* (London), cxxxi (Sept., 1933): 257–267.

BLACKMAN, WINIFRED S., *The Fellahin of Upper Egypt*. London, 1927.

BLACKWOOD, W. R. D., "The Prevention of Conception," *Med. and Surg. Rep.* (Phila.), lix (1888): 394–396; 698.

BLAIKIE, TINA M., The Poor and Birth Control. In *Medical Help*, pp. 157–169.

BLAIR, JACOB J., "The Public Health Value of Contraceptives," Open Forum, *Med. Jour. and Rec.* (New York), cxxxvii: 7–9 (Feb. 1, 1933).

BLOCH, IWAN, *The Sexual Life of Our Time in Its Relations to Modern Civilization*. (Trans. by M. Eden Paul.) New York: Rebman, 1908; London: William Heinemann, Ltd.

—— *Die Prostitution*. Berlin: Marcus, 1912. Two volumes: i, xxxvi, 1–870; ii, vi, 1–728.

BLOCK, I. J., "Observations from Work of Birth Control Clinic," *South African Med. Jour.*, viii (1934): 490–492.

BLOUNT, ANNA A., A Talk to Mothers. By a doctor who is herself a mother. N.d., [c. 1915] n.p., pp. 7. (F.C.)

BLUMBERG, FLORA, The Manchester, Salford and District Mothers' Clinic. In Sanger & Stone, *Practice of Contraception*, pp. 222–225.

BLYTH, DAVID, "Notes on the Traditions and Customs of the Natives of Fiji in Relation to Conception, Pregnancy, and Parturition," *Glasgow Med. Jour.* (Glasgow), xxviii (1887): 176–186.

BOCK, P. V., Kleine Familie. Die Beschränkung allzureichen Kindersegens ohne Verletzung der Sittengesetze. Ein Beitrag zur Lösung der sozialen Frage. Leipzig: Klötzsch, 1898, pp. 18 and advt's.

BOCKER, DOROTHY, Birth Control Methods. New York: Birth Control League, 1924, pp. 31.

BOGELOT, P., "Produits anticonceptionnels," *Bull. d. Soc. Pharmacol.* (Paris), xxxiii (1926): 158–161 (Annexe.)

BOSTOCK, JOHN and RILEY, H. T., *The Natural History of Pliny.* London, 1855–57. 6 vols. Bohn's Classical Library.

BOUDEWYNS, M., *"Ventilabrum medico-theologicum.* Antwerp: 1666. Contains two papers as follows: An medicus possit impedire generationem seminis, vel genitum annihilare et destruere? (pp. 125–129). An medicus aliquando possit impedire conceptionem. (pp. 152–158).

BOUGHTON, ALICE, "First Report of the Committee on Maternal Health: Organization and Operating Policies," *Jour. Med.* (Cincinnati), ix (Jan. 1931): 576–579. Reprint, pp. 4.

BOURDEILLE, PIERRE DE, *see* BRANTÔMÉ, ABBÉ DE.

BOURNE, ALECK W., *see* ch. 3 in HAIRE [Ed.], *Some More Medical Views.*

BOWMAN, W. M., "Modern Methods of Birth Control," *Virginia Med. Monthly,* lxi (1934): 21–24.

BRADLAUGH, CHARLES, *see* p. 236, note 113.

BRANTÔME, ABBÉ DE, [PIERRE DE BOURDEILLE, ABBÉ DE BRANTÔME, d. 1614], *Les Dames Galantes.* Paris: Flammarion, 1930.

——— *Das Leben der Galanten Damen (La Vie des Dames Galantes).* (Trans. by Willy Alexander Kastner.) Leipzig: Deutsche Verlagsactiengesellschaft, 1904.

BRAUN, M., Die künstliche Beschränkung der Kinderzahl. Berlin: Hermann Schmidt, 1892.

——— Die willkürliche Beschränkung der Kinderzahl. Ein Mittel zur Vorbeugung der Empfängnis. Budapest, 1895, pp. 74.

BRAUN, R. und WINTERBERG, J., Kritische Bemerkungen über die verschiedenen antikonzeptionellen Massnahmen, *Monatschr. f. Harnkr. und Sex. Hyg.* (Leipzig), iv (1907): 494–506.

BREDIS, *Die künstliche Unfruchtbarkeit vor dem Gericht, der Wissenschaft und der Gesellschaft.* St. Petersburg, 1911, pp. 109.

BREED, MARY, *see* HOW-MARTYN, EDITH.

BROWN, GEORGE, *Melanesians and Polynesians; Their Life-Histories Described and Compared.* London: Macmillan, 1910, pp. xv, 451.

BROWNE, F. W. STELLA, "Die Geburtenregelung im heutigen England," *Neue Generation* (Leipzig), xxii (1926): 46–52.

——— "The Feminine Aspect of Birth Control," *Rpt. Fifth Int'l Conf.,* pp. 40–43.

BROWNLEE, JOHN, "Restriction of Birth in Relation to National Weal," *Lancet* (London), ii (1922): 223–225.

——— "On the Question of Birth Control in Some of Its Statistical Aspects," *Lancet* (London), ii (1924): 925–927.

BRUNING, H., "Geburtenrückgang und Volksgesundheit," *Ztschr. f. Bevölkrngspolit.* (Leipzig), x (1917–18): 1–19.

BRUNNER, F. R., "Is Onanism Justifiable?" *Med. Reg.* (Phila.), iii (1888): 78–79.

BRUPBACHER, FRITZ, Kindersegen, Fruchtverhütung, Fruchtabtreibung. 5 Auf. Berlin: Neuer Deutscher Verlag, 1929, pp. 5–46.

——— Liebe, Geschlechtsbeziehungen und Geschlechtspolitik. Mit einem Anhang von Dr. Med. J. Meyer (Berlin). Berlin: Neuer Deutscher Verlag, 1930, pp. 5–53.

BRYANT, LOUISE STEVENS, Medical Aspects of Human Fertility. A Survey and Report of the National Committee on Maternal Health, Inc. New York: National Committee on Maternal Health (Acad. of Med. Bldg., 2 E. 103 St., N. Y. C.), 1932, pp. 45.

*BRYANT, LOUISE STEVENS, with DICKINSON, R. L., see DICKINSON.

BUDGE, S., "Zum Malthus-Problem. Eine Antikritik," *Arch. f. Sozialwissensch.* (Tübing.), xxxvii (1913): 930–941.

BUIST, R. C., The Doctor in Relation to "Birth Control" for the Individual and for the Community. In Marchant [Ed.], *Medical Views*, pp. 89–103.

BULFFI, LUIS, Huelga de Vientres! Medios prácticos para evitar las familias numerosas. Barcelona: Biblioteca Editorial Salud y Fuerza, 1913, pp. 32.

BURG, C[ORNELIUS] L[EENDERT] VAN DER, *De Geneesheer in Nederlandsch-Indië.* Batavia: Ernst & Co., 1883–1885, 3 vols.

BUSCHAN, GEORG, Contributor to ALBERT MOLL's *Handbuch der Sexualwissenschaften.* Leipzig: Vogel, 1912. See Part III entitled "Das Sexuelle in der Völkerkunde."

BUSSEMAKER [Ed.], see ORIBASIUS.

BUTLER, LILY C., The Walworth and East London Centres. In Sanger & Stone, *Practice of Contraception*, pp. 216–218.

––––– A Students Manual of Birth Control. London: Noel Douglas, 1933, pp. 39.
[A brief account by a physician at two English clinics.]

*BUTTERFIELD, OLIVER, Marriage. Some Practical Suggestions for Happy Married Living. Medical supplement: (Some Suggestions Concerning Contraceptives. Birth Control Information, pp. 3–11). N.p., n.d. [1929 ?], pp. 48. (L.C., A.C.)
[Probably published by the author at Monterey Park, California.]

––––– Marriage and Sexual Harmony. New York: Emerson Books, 1934, pp. 40.

BYLOFF, FRITZ, "Die Arsenmorde in Steiermark." *Monatsschr. f. Kriminalpsychol. u. Strafrechtsreform* (Heidelberg), xxi (1930): 1–14.

BYRK, FELIX, *Die Beschneidung bei Mann und Weib. Ihre Geschichte, Psychologie und Ethnologie.* Neubrandenburg: Gustav Feller, 1931, pp. x, 1–319.

CABOT, R. C., "Are Sanitary Prophylaxis and Moral Prophylaxis Natural Allies?" *Jour. Soc. San.* (Lyons, N. Y.), v (1914): 20–44.

DE CAILHOL, E. A., "Conception," *South. Clinic* (Richmond), xiii (1890): 1–12.

DE CAMILLIS, BASILIO, "Concezioni fondamentali del problema demografico," *Annali di Nevreolgia* (Napoli), xliii (1929): 1–23.

CANADIAN BIRTH CONTROL LEAGUE, see TYRER, A. H.

CAPELLMANN-NIEDERMEYER, *Fakultative Sterilität.* Limburg a.d. Lahn: Gebr. Steffon, 1931.

CARLETON, H. M. and PHELPS, H. J., "Experimental Observations on the Gräfenburg Ring Contraceptive Methods." *Jour. Obst. & Gyn. Brit. Emp.*, xl (1933): 81–98.

CARLETON, H. M., see BAKER, JOHN R.

*CARLILE, RICHARD, What is Love? in R. Carlile's *Republican*, xi, No. 18 (May 6, 1825). (A.C.)
[Historically important]

––––– Every Woman's Book; or, What is Love? Fourth ed. London: Printed and Published by Richard Carlile, 62 Fleet Street, 1826, pp. iv, 48. (G.L., F.C., photostat at H.L.)
[Historically important]

––––– Every Woman's Book or, What is Love? abridged [by Godfrey Higgins], for more extensive circulation from No. 18 Vol. XI of 'The Republican.' Price three pence. Pp. 16. (S.C. unique.)

––––– Every Woman's Book. [With introduction by Robert Forder.] London: Robert Forder, 1892, pp. 24. (A.C., P.H.)
[Quite different in phraseology from the earlier authorized editions.]

[CARLILE, RICHARD], The Philosophy of the Sexes: or, EVERY WOMAN'S BOOK; a treatise on love in its Various Forms, Phrases [sic] and Results, including Practical Hints How to Enjoy Life and Pleasure without Harm to either Sex. By Dr. Waters. London: Printed and Published by R. Carlile, 62 Fleet Street, 1826. Preface iii–iv; 5–38 pp. duodecimo, 6⅝ x 4⅔. (B.M., A.C., P.H.)

[Rare. Based upon the authentic fourth edition. So far as one can determine without an exceedingly detailed collation, this is exactly like the fourth edition, save for the eccentric title page. Though it bears the date of 1826 it was probably published about 1880. The "Dr. Waters" remains a mystery.]

CARR-SAUNDERS, A. M., The Population Problem. A Study in Human Evolution. Oxford: Clarendon Press, 1922, pp. 516.

CASANOVA, J. DE SEINGALT, Mémoires ... Paris: Libraire Garnier Frères, n.d., 6 vols.

CASTORO, ROCCO, "Intorno alla sterilizzazione biologica temporanea della femmina con iniezioni di liquido seminale," Arch. d. Ostet. e. Ginec. (Napoli), 2 s. xii (1926): 558–569.

CECCHI, ETTORINA, Neo-Malthusianismo Pratico. Quarta edizione. Florence: Instituto Editoriale "Il Pensiero," n.d., (c. 1916), pp. 120.

CHACHUAT, MAURICE, Le Mouvement du "Birth Control" dans les pays Anglo-Saxons (avec un appendice sur la stérilisation et le contrôle des naissances en Allemagne). Paris: Marcel Girard, 1934, pp. lxxx, 553.

[A law thesis at the University of Lyons]

CHAPPLE, HAROLD, A Gynaecologist's Experience. In Medical Help, pp. 25–40.

*CHARLES, ENID [i.e., MRS. LANCELOT HOGBEN], The Practice of Birth Control. An Analysis of the Birth-Control Experiences of Nine Hundred Women. London: Williams & Norgate, 1932, pp. 190.

———— The Twilight of Parenthood. New York: W. W. Norton, 1934, vi, 226.

[An able, thought-provoking but somewhat alarmist summary of many recent population studies. Shows original insights and combinations of ideas.]

CHAVIGNY, "Appareils anticonceptionnels," Ann. de Méd. Lég. (Paris), iv (1924): 42–44.

CHIZH, V. F., "Coitus reservatus, kak prichina neĭrastenii" ["Coitus Reservatus as a Cause of Neurasthenia,"] Meditsina (St. Petersb.), viii (1896): 277–280.

CHUDARKOWSKI, W. J., "Über die Bedeutung in bezug auf die Schwangerschaft immunisierenden Serums. (Vorläufige Mitteilung)," Zbl. f. Gynäk. (Leipzig) xlix (1925): 383–384.

CHUNN, WILLIAM P., "The prevention of Conception; its Practicability and Justifiability," Maryland Med. Jour. (Balt.), xxxii (1894–5): 340–343.

CLAPP, C. R., see HOMANS, ROBERT.

COCKBURN, JOHN (THE HON. SIR), The View of an ex-Prime Minister of South Australia. In Medical Help, pp. 43–44.

COMMITTEE ON FEDERAL LEGISLATION FOR BIRTH CONTROL, Laws Concerning Birth Control in the United States. New York: Comm. on Fed. Leg. for B.C., 1929, pp. 39.

[COMMITTEE ON MATERNAL HEALTH], Biennial Report, 1928, "Medical Aspects of Human Fertility." New York: Committee on Maternal Health, n.d. [1928], pp. 32. See also BRYANT, L. S.

CONFERENCE, Report of the Conference on the Giving of Information on Birth Control by Public Health Authorities held on Friday, April 4, 1930 at the Central Hall, Westminster. [London, 1930] n.p., pp. 36.

COON, CARLETON STEVENS, Tribes of the Rif. Cambridge, Massachusetts: Peabody Museum (In Harvard African Studies No. IX), 1931, pp. xviii, 417 + plates.

*COOPER, JAMES F., *Technique of Contraception. The Principles and Practice of Anti-Conceptional Methods.* New York: Day-Nichols, 1928, pp. xvi, 1–271.

  [First medical book of our generation in the United States. Sale 46,000 copies by 1932.]

——— Tested Methods of Contraception. New York: American Birth Control League [1928 ?], pp. 3–7.

——— "An Effective Contraceptive Method," *Indianapolis Med. Jour.* (Indianapolis, Ind.) xxxii (1929): 123–126. Reprint pp. 4.

——— "An Outline of Contraceptive Methods." New York: American Birth Control League [1930], pp. 23.

CORBY, HENRY, "Birth Control and Economy," *Practitioner* (London), cxi (1923): 62–73.

CORMACK, J. G., "Contraception or Birth Control," *China Med. Jour.* (Shanghai), xl (1926): 973–985.

COWAN, JOHN, *The Science of a New Life.* New York: Cowan & Co., 1869, pp. 9–405. (B.M.L.)

  [Popular medicine. Much nonsense.]

———, ——— New York: Cowan & Co., 1870, pp. 9–405. (B.P.L.)

———, ——— New York: Cowan & Co., 1871, pp. 9–405. (B.M.L.)

———, ——— New York: J. S. Ogilvie, 1915, pp. 415. (N.Y.A.M.)

  [Omits chap. on prevention]

———, ——— Revised and largely rewritten by Arthur Rose Guerard. New York: J. S. Ogilvie, 1925, pp. 310. (N.Y.A.M.)

——— *What All Married People Should Know.* Chicago: Ogilvie, 1903, pp. 173.

  [No copy located. Please report.]

COX, GLADYS M., *Clinical Contraception.* London: Heinemann, 1933.

COX, H., "The Reduction of the Birth Rate as a Necessary Instrument for the Improvement of the Race," *Eugenics Rev.* (London), xiv (1922–23): 83–92.

CREW, F. A. E., *see* ch. 4 in Haire [Ed.], *Some More Medical Views.*

CRICHTON-MILLER, H., The Psychological Aspect of Contraception. In Marchant [Ed.], *Medical Views*, pp. 1–24.

CRISTALLI, G., "Indice demografico e idea imperiale. A proposito del controllo sulle nascite," *Med. Soc.* (Napoli), xvi (1926): no. 6, 1–8; no. 7, 5–10.

CROCKER, WALTER RUSSELL, *The Japanese Population Problem.* London: Allen & Unwin, 1931, pp. 240.

CRUVEILHIER, L., "Répression de la Propagande anti-conceptionelle," *Rév. d'Hyg.* (Paris), xlvi (1924): 156–160.

CUMMINS-VAILE BILL, *Joint Hearings before the Subcommittees of the Committees on the Judiciary. Congress of the United States. Sixty-Eighth Congress, First Session on H. R. 6542 and S. 2290, April 8 and May 9, 1924 Serial 38.* Washington: Gov't Printing Office, 1924, pp. 79.

CUREAU, ADOLPHE L., *Les sociétés primitives de l'Afrique équatoriale.* Paris: A. Colin, 1912, pp. xii, 420.

——— *Savage Man in Central Africa; a Study of Primitive Races in the French Congo* (Tr. by E. Andrews). London: T. F. Unwin, [1915], pp. 351.

CURRIER, ANDREW F., "A Study Relative to the Functions of the Reproductive Apparatus in American Indian Women," *Trans. Amer. Gyn. Soc.* (Phila.), xvi (1891): 264–294; (Also in *Med. News* (Phila.), lix (1891): 390–393, portion of same article).

CUTNER, HERBERT (translator), *see* HARDY, PROF. (pseudonym).

CZEMPIN, A., "Über Konzeptionsverhütung," *Ztschr. f. ärztl. Fortb.* (Jena), ii (1905): 572–574.

DAHL, H. B., ["Anticonceptional Methods,"] *Ugesk. f. Laeger* (København), lxxxvi (1924): 928–929.

DAMM, ALFRED, Die gesundheitsschädliche Wirkung der Mittel zur Vermeidung der Conception, Contra H. Ferdy und Andere. Für Aerzte und Nichtärzte. München, 1887.

—— *Die Ehe. Die Mittel zur Verhütung der Befruchtung in ihrer Schädlichkeit und in ihren Ersatz.* Berlin: Selbstverlag, 1898, pp. 207.

DANIELS, ANNA K., A Comparative Study of Birth Control Methods with Special Reference to Spermatoxins. In Sanger & Stone, *Practice of Contraception*, pp. 104–111.

DANIELS, NURSE [E. S.], An Enquiry into the value of the Mensinga or Dutch Pessary. In Sanger & Stone, *Practice of Contraception*, pp. 225–229.

—— The Children of Desire. A book on practical knowledge of family limitation. Second edition. London: By the author (George Standring, printer), [1927], pp. 24.

—— *see* material collected by Nurse Daniels reported in CHARLES, ENID, *The Practice of Birth Control.*

DAREMBERG [Ed.], *see* ORIBASIUS.

DAVIS, C. HENRY, "Birth Control and Sterility," *Surg., Gyn. & Obst.* (Chicago), xxxvi (1923): 435–439.

DAVIS, JOHN MOORE, *see* SMITH, BROUGH.

*DAVIS, KATHARINE BEMENT, *Factors in the Sex Life Of Twenty-two Hundred Women.* New York & London: Harper, 1929, pp. xx, 1–430.

DAWSON, WARREN R., Early Ideas Concerning Conception and Contraception. In *Medical Help*, pp. 189–200.

DENNETT, MARY WARE, *Birth Control Laws. Shall We Keep Them, Change Them, or Abolish Them* [?] New York: Frederick H. Hitchcock, 1926, pp. ix, 309.

*DENNETT, MARY W. and ROBINSON, F. H. [Eds.], "A Symposium on Birth Control, *Med. Rev. of Rev.* (New York), xxv (1919): 131–157.

DEWEES, A. Lovett, "Contraception in General Practice," *Med. Jour. & Rec.* (New York), February 3, 1932.

**DICKINSON, ROBERT L., "Contraception: A Medical Review of the Situation," *Amer. Jour. Obst. & Gyn.* (St. Louis), viii (1924): 583–604. Discussion, 654–5. (Also *Trans. Amer. Gyn. Soc.* (Phila.), xlix (1924): 95–119.

[Pioneer publication in the U. S. A. from any gynecologist and obstetrical authority, giving details of methods and evaluation. It was a deliberate challenge to the Federal Postal Laws both as a journal article and a pamphlet, but was never questioned.]

—— "The Birth Control Movement," *Med. Jour. & Rec.* (New York), cxxv (1927): 653–657.

——, —— Reprint by Comm. on Maternal Health [1927], pp. 14.

—— "The 'Safe Period' as a Birth Control Measure. A Study and Evaluation of Available Data," *Amer. Jour. Obst. & Gyn.* (St. Louis), xiv (1927): 718–730.

—— "Control of Conception, Present and Future," *New York State Jour. Med.* (New York), xxix (1929): 596–602.

—— "Control of Conception, Present and Future," *Bull. New York Acad. Med.* (New York), 2s., v (1929): 413–434.

——, —— [Reprint by] New York: Committee on Maternal Health, [1929], pp. 29.

—— "State Law, the Doctor and Conception Control," *Med. Jour. & Rec.* (New York) cxxix (1929): 592–593.

—— *see* SANGER and STONE.

—— *Human Sex Anatomy: A Topographical Atlas.* Baltimore: Williams & Wilkins, 1933.

DICKINSON, ROBERT L., Household Conceptives, *Marriage Hygiene*, ii (Nov. 1935): 133–138.
[In preparation.]
―――― *The Doctor as Marriage Counsellor*. Baltimore: Williams & Wilkins, 1936.
**DICKINSON, ROBERT L. and BRYANT, LOUISE STEVENS, *Control of Conception. An Illustrated Medical Manual*. Baltimore: Williams & Wilkins, 1931, pp. xii, 1–290.
[The authoritative manual on the subject. Contains original studies and first-class medical analyses. Includes, besides discussion of contraceptive techniques, sterilization, abortion, laws, clinical researches, program.]
DICKINSON, ROBERT L., and BEAM, LURA, *A Thousand Marriages*. Baltimore: Williams & Wilkins, 1931, pp. xxiii, 482.
DIOSCORIDES, *see* BERENDES, J.
DOCTOR OF MEDICINE, *see* DRYSDALE, GEORGE.
DOLAN, T. M., "Demographic Consideration of the Evils of Artificial Methods of Preventing Fecundation, and of Abortion Production in Modern Times," *Trans. Ninth Int'l Med. Cong.* (Washington, D. C.), v (1887): 210–218. [Also appears in *Med. Reg.* (Phila.), ii (1887): 393–398. *New Engl. Med. Monthly* (Bridgeport, Conn.), vii (1887–8): 181–189. *Prov. Med. Jour.* (Leicester), vi (1887): 434–438.]
[Rubbish]
DRYSDALE, CHARLES R. [Ed.], "Debate on Infanticide, in the Harveian Medical Society of London, May 17, 1866." Reprinted from *Med. Press and Circular*, June 13, 1866, London, 1866, pp. 12.
*―――― *The Population Question According to T. R. Malthus and J. S. Mill. Giving The Malthusian Theory of Over-population*. London: William Bell, 1878, pp. 94. (A.C.)
[Probably first edition.]
――――, ―――― London: Standring, 1892, pp. [1] 94. (A.C.)
―――― [Ed.] "The Population Question at the Medical Society of London; or the mortality of the rich and poor. A paper read at the society with the debate." London: Standring, 1879, pp. 12.
―――― "Presidential Address," *National Secular Society Almanack*, 1879, pp. 46–49. Also Malthusian Tract No. 6. London: Malthusian League, [1879], pp. 8.
―――― "The Principle of Population." Malthusian Tract No. 1, London: Malthusian League [1879], pp. 4.
―――― "Large Families and Over-Population, being the substance of a presidential address delivered at the second annual meeting of the Malthusian League ... " Malthusian Tract No. 9. London: Malthusian League, 1879, pp. 12.
*―――― *The Life and Writings of Thomas R. Malthus*. London: George Standring, 1887, pp. 120. (A.C., B.M.)
[First edition? See Standring's *Radical*, ii, 21 (Nov., 1887) and ii, 15 (Oct., 1887).]
――――, ―――― Second edition. London: Standring, 1892, pp. 120. (A.C., B.M.)
―――― "The Cause of Poverty. A paper read at the National Liberal Club, on 21st October, 1890." London: Standring, 1891.
―――― [Ed.] "Medical Opinions on the Population Question." London: Standring, 1901, pp. 32.
―――― [Ed.] "Clerical Opinions on the Population Question." London: Standring, 1904, pp. 19.
―――― Biographical Sketch in Standring's *Republican*, xii, 25–26. *Cf.*, 1904 or 1905 edition of George Drysdale, *Elements of Social Science*.
*DRYSDALE, C. V., "Birth Control and Eugenics in Holland," *Eugenics Rev.* (London), xv (1923–24): 472–479.

DRYSDALE, C. V., "The Birth Control Movement; Its Scientific and Ethical Bases," *Eugenics Rev.* (London), xx (1928–29): 173–178.

——— "The Criterion of Over-population," *Rpt. Fifth Int'l. Conf.*, 60–64.

——— "Neo-Malthusian Morality and Religion," *Rpt. Fifth Int'l. Conf.*, 100–106.

——— "The Personal and Family Aspect of Birth Control," *Rpt. Fifth Int'l. Conf.*, 54–59.

——— "Der Standpunkt des Contraceptionisten," *Verhandl. d. int'l. Kong. f. Sexualforsch.* (Berlin u. Köln), iv (1928): 80–82.

——— "The Birth Control Movement after a Century's Agitation," *Current Hist.*, xxx (1929): 381–386.

*[DRYSDALE, GEORGE], *The Elements of Social Science; or Physical, Sexual and Natural Religion. An Exposition of the True Cause and Only Cure of the Three Primary Social Evils: Poverty, Prostitution, and Celibacy.* By A Doctor of Medicine. Twenty-sixth edition, enlarged. Sixty-fifth Thousand. London: E. Truelove, 1887, pp. ix, 1–604.

DUBLIN, L. I., "Birth Control," *Soc. Hyg.* (Balt.), vi (1920): 5–16.

——— "The Excesses of Birth Control," *Chicago Med. Rec.*, xlviii (1926): 12–18.

——— see page 395, n. 3.

DUEHREN, "Le médecin Condom a-t-il existé?" *Méd. Int'l.* (Paris), April and May, 1901.

DUFFEY, ELIZABETH BISBEE, What Women Should Know. A woman's book about women containing practical information for wives and mothers. Philadelphia, 1873. Also 1882. (1882 ed. at N.Y.A.M.)

——— The Relations of the Sexes.

DUMAS, H. RIBADEAU, "Propagande anticonceptionnelle par la voie des journaux," *Gaz. d. Hôp.* (Paris), xciv (1921): 866.

DUNCAN, HANNIBAL G., *Race and Population Problems.* New York: Longmans, 1929, pp. xv, 1–424.

DUNLOP, BINNIE, "Contraception Is Necessary for the Elimination of Poverty, and Is Therefore Moral," *Rpt. Fifth Int'l. Conf.*, 111–115.

*——— Hygienic Methods of Family Limitation. Compiled by a Committee of the Malthusian League with the Assistance of Binnie Dunlop. M.B., Ch.B. 71st. Thous. [London: Malthusian League], n.d. [c. 1922], pp. 18.

E.B., A Private Letter from E. B. to J. S., on the Birth-Rate Question. London: George Standring, 1905, pp. 23 [2].

EBERS, GEORGE MORITZ [Ed.], *Papyros Ebers. Das hermetische Buch über die Arzneimittel der alten Ägypter in hieratischer Schrift. Herausgegeben, mit Inhaltsangabe und Einleitung versehen von George Ebers. Mit einem hieroglyphisch-lateinischem Glossar von Ludwig Stern.* Leipzig: W. Engelman, 1875, 2 vols.

EDDY, SHERWOOD, *Sex and Youth.* Tentative edition. New York: Doubleday, Doran, 1928, pp. 101.

EDER, M. D., see ch. 5 in HAIRE [Ed.], *Some More Medical Views.*

EDGAR, THOMAS WEBSTER and SANGER, MARGARET, "The Physician and Birth Control," *Med. Times* (New York), li (1923): 73–74; 77.

EERLAND, L. D., "De ligging van den uterus bij de Javaansche vrouw," ["The Position of the Uterus Among Javanese Women,"] *Geneesk. Tijdschr. v. Nederl.-Indië* (Batavia, Java), lxx (1930): 1239–1246.

EHRENBERG, "Geburtenrückgang und Volkswirtschaft," *Ztschr. f. Bevölkrnsgspolit.* (Leipzig), x (1917): 33–47.

EHRLICH, MARG., "Der männliche Anteil an der Bevölkerungs-Abnahme," *Neue Generation* (Berlin), xiii (1917): 31–34.

ELBERSKIRCHEN, JOHANNA, "Zur Frage des sexuellen Präventivverkehres," *Heilkunde* (Berlin), xiv (1910): 160–163.

ELIOT, THOMAS D., "The Policies of the Neo-Malthusian Movement: Criticisms and Appraisals," *Jour. Soc. Hyg.* (New York), xiii (1927): 129–138.

ELKAN, R., The German League for Birth Control and Sex Hygiene. In Sanger & Stone, *Practice of Contraception*, pp. 248–249.

———— "Die Konzeptionsverhütung als Gegenstand des klinischen Unterrichts. Einige Bemerkungen zu dem Artikel von W. Stoeckel in Zbl. Gynäk. 1931, Nr. 17," *Zbl. f. Gynäk* (Leipzig), lv (1931): 2555–2557.

**ELLIS, HAVELOCK, *Studies in the Psychology of Sex*. Philadelphia: F. A. Davis, 1923, etc. Especially vol. vi, *Sex in Relation to Society*.

———— "Birth Control in Relation to Morality and Eugenics," *Birth Control Rev.* (New York), iii (1919): 7–9.

———— "Birth Control," *Practitioner* (London), cxxxi (Sept., 1933): 228–238.

ELLISON, JOHN, GOODWIN, AUBREY, READ, CHARLES, D., RIVETT, L. CARNAC, *Sex Ethics: The Principles and Practice of Contraception, Abortion, and Sterilization*. London: Bailliere, Tindall & Cox, 1934, pp. xi, 281.

ENGELMANN, F., "Gibt es eine empfängnisfreie Zeit im Sexualzyklus der Frau? Ein kritischer Beitrag zur Frage der Geburtenregelung," *Deutsche Med. Wchnschr.*, lviii (Dec. 9, 1932): 1969–1972.

ERDWEG, P. MATHIAS JOSEPH, "Die Bewohner der Insel Tumleo, Berlinhafen, Deutsch-Neu-Guinea," *Mitt. d. Anthrop. Ges. in Wien*, xxxii (1902): 274–310; 317–399.

ERMAN, ADOLPH, *Die Ägyptische Religion*. Berlin, 1905. Trans. by A. S. Griffith as *A Handbook of Egyptian Religion*. London, 1907, pp. xvi, 262. Also New York: Dutton, 1907.

EULENBURG, A., "Über coitus reservatus als Ursache sexualer Neurasthenie bei Männern," *Internat. Centralbl. f. d. Physiol. u. Path. der Harn. u. Sex. Org.* (Leipzig), iv (1893): 3–7.

*EVERETT, MILLARD S., *The Hygiene of Marriage. A Detailed Consideration of Sex and Marriage*. Foreword by Clara M. Davis, M.D. Introduction by T. V. Smith, Ph.D. Physicians' Edition. New York: Vanguard Press, 1932, pp. xvii, 21–262. [A good general treatise.]

EYRE, EDWARD J., *Journals of Expeditions of Discovery into Central Australia, and Overland from Adelaide to King George's Sound, in the years 1840–41.* . . . London: Boone, 1845. 2 vols.

FAHLBECK, P., "Der Neo-Malthusianismus in seinen Beziehungen zur Rassenbiologie und Rassenhygiene," *Arch. f. Rassen-u. Gesellsch.-Biol.* (Leipzig), ix (1912): 30–48.

FAIRBAIRN, J. S., "Birth Control—Medical Advice," *Practitioner* (London), cxi (1923): 36–42.

FAIRFIELD, LETITIA D., The State and Birth Control. In Marchant [Ed.], *Medical Views*, pp. 104–131.

FALLOPIO, GABRIELLE, *De Morbo Gallico: Liber Absolutissimus*. Batavia, 1564.

FASBENDER, H., *Entwickelungslehre, Geburtshülfe und Gynäkologie in den Hippokratischen Schriften*. Stuttgart, Enke 1897, pp. xviii, 300.

FAWCETT, HUGH A., "Contraceptives; Methods in Common Use Compared," *Lancet* (London), i (1927): 515–516.

FEDERSCHMIDT, "Lamentationen über Geburtenrückgang im griechischen und römischen Altertum," *Bl. f. Volksgsndhtspfl.* (Berlin), xviii (1918): 111–112.

FEHLINGER, H., "Vom Sexualleben der Australier," *Ztschr. f. Sexualwissensch.* (Bonn), ii (1915–16): 137–141.

FEHLINGER, H., Das Geschlechtsleben der Naturvölker. Nr.I. In *Monographien zur Frauenkunde und Eugenetik, Sexual-biologie und Vererbungslehre* [Max Hirsch, Ed.]. Leipzig: Curt Kabitsch, 1921, pp. 93. (Tr. by S. Herbert and Mrs. Herbert as *Sexual Life of Primitive People*. London, 1921.)

FERCH, BETTI, The Birth Control Association of Austria. In Sanger & Stone, *Practice of Contraception*, pp. 268–270.

FERCH, JOH., *Geburtenbeschränkung*. Dresden: Aurora Verlag, 1923, pp. 103.

———— Neo-Malthusianism as a Necessity of Civilization, *Rpt. Fifth Int'l Conf.*, pp. 43–54.

———— *Birth Control*. (Translated with a Biographical Foreword by Christian Roland. Edited, with an Introduction, by A. Maude Royden.) London: Rider, 1932, pp. viii + 124.

[By the Austrian popular leader. One of seven chapters on contraception; balance on abortion.]

*FERDY, HANS (Pseud. for A. MEYERHOF), *Die Mittel zur Verhütung der Conception*. Berlin, 1887, 8°. (S.G.)

[Sub-titles changed rapidly. Hence omitted here. There were many editions of the above pamphlet, of which the following account does not pretend to be complete. Its purpose is rather to indicate the relatively early, sound, and considerable influence of Ferdy, who is an important figure in late nineteenth-century German thought on this subject. His contributions were much above the average in quality.]

————, ———— 3 Aufl., Berlin u. Neuwied: Heuser, 1889, 1–46. (S.G., A.C.)

————, ———— 6 Aufl., Berlin: Ludwig Heuser, 1895. (P.H.)

————, ———— 7 Aufl., Leipzig: Spohr, 1899, pp. 5–100, advts. (S.G., A.C.)

————, ———— 8 Aufl., Leipzig: Spohr, 1907, Part I, pp. 122; Part II, pp. 52. (S.G., A.C.)

———— "Contribution à l'étude historique du 'Coecal-Condom,' " *Chron. Méd.* (Paris), xii (1905): 535–537.

———— "Zur Geschichte des Coecal-Condoms," *Ztschr. f. Bekämpf. d. Geschlechtskr.* (Leipzig), iii (1904–1905): 144–147.

———— Sittliche Selbstbeschränkung. Behagliche Zeitbetrachtungen eines Malthusianers über die begriffliche Wandlung des "moral restraint" in dem Jahrhundert 1803–1903 und die Ausbreitung des Malthusianismus. Hildesheim: Bude, 1903. (S.G.)

————, ———— Hildesheim: Verfasser, 1904. (P.H.)

———— Der Congressus interruptus als ätiologische Basis nervöser Störungen der Genitalsphäre. Berlin u. Leipzig: Heuser, 1891.

———— *Die künstliche Beschränkung der Kinderzahl als sittliche Pflicht.* 5 Aufl., Leipzig: Spohe, 1897, pp. 141.

[Nothing on methods.]

————, ———— 7 Aufl., Leipzig, 1899.

FETSCHER, R., "Zur Frage des Konzeptionstermines," *Deutsche Med. Wchnschr.*, lix (May 26, 1933): 812.

*FIELD, JAMES A., "The Early Propagandist Movement in English Population Theory," *Bull. Amer. Econ. Assoc.*, 4th s., i (1911): 207–236.

———— "Publicity by Prosecution: A Commentary on the Birth Control Propaganda," *Survey* (New York), xxxv (1915): 599–601.

———— "The Beginnings of the Birth-Control Movement," *Surg. Gyn. & Obst.* (Chicago), xxiii (1916): 185–188. Disc. p. 234.

FIELD, JAMES A., "Problems of Population after the War," *Amer. Econ. Rev.*, vii (1917): 233–237.

———— *Essays on Population and Other Papers.* [Ed. by Helen Fisher Hohman.] Chicago: University of Chicago Press, 1931, pp. xxix, 1–440.

*FIELDING, MICHAEL (pseud. for prominent English physician), *Parenthood: Design or Accident? A Manual of Birth-Control.* Preface by H. G. Wells. London: Labour Publishing Co., 1928, pp. 96.

————, ———— Revised and enlarged edition. London: Noel Douglas, 1930, pp. 168.

————, ———— New York: Vanguard Press, 1935, pp. 239.
[By the editor of the *Eugenics Review*, Dr. Maurice Newfield, formerly an editor of the *British Medical Journal.* An able well-balanced book.]

FINK, LOTTE, The Frankfurt A. M. Advice Bureau. In Sanger & Stone, *Practice of Contraception*, pp. 246–247.

———— Birth Control by Sterilization. In Sanger & Stone, *Practice of Contraception*, pp. 122–126.

———— "Wirkung der Verhütungsmittel. Erfahrungen aus der Ehe- und Sexualberatungs Frankfurt a. M.," *Arch. f. Gynäk* (Berlin), cxliv (1931): 2777–8. [Abstr. in *Zbl. f. Gynäk.* (Leipzig), lv (1931): 2777–2778.]

*FISCHER, ISIDOR, *Die Gynäkologie bei Dioskurides und Plinius.* Wien, 1927.

FLESCH, MAX, "Probleme der sexuellen Hygiene. I. Die willkürliche Beschränkung der Zeugung," *Monatschr. f. Harnkr. u. sex. Hyg.* (Stuttgart), i (1927): 175–181.

*FLORENCE, LELLA SECOR, *Birth Control on Trial.* With a Foreword by Sir Humphrey Rolleston, Bart . . . and an Introduction Note by F. H. A. Marshall . . . London: Allen & Unwin, 1930, pp. 160.

FLYNN, T. E., "Birth Control," *Cath. Med. Guard.* (Middlesex, Engl.), iv (1926): 155–160.

*FOOTE, EDWARD BLISS, *Words in Pearl.*
[This is the exceedingly rare pamphlet (*c.* 1860 or later), set in pearl type, giving practical contraceptive information, for distributing which Foote was prosecuted. No copy in B.M., L.C., S.G., N.Y.P.L., H.L., etc. Will anyone knowing of the whereabouts of a copy advise the compiler?]

———— *Medical Common Sense; Applied to the causes, prevention and cure of chronic diseases and unhappiness in marriage.* Rev. and enl. edition. New York: Published by the author, 1863, pp. xviii, 390.

———— *Medical Common Sense applied to the causes, prevention, and cure of chronic diseases; and plain home talk about the sexual organs; the natural relation of the sexes; society civilization; and marriage.* Third rev. and enl. edition. New York: Published by the author, 1870, pp. xxiv, [25]–912.

———— . . . A Step Backward. Written by Dr. E. B. Foote . . . in reviewing inconsiderate legislation, concerning articles and things for the prevention of conception. New York: Issued by the author [Murray Hill Pub. Co.], 1875, pp. 16.

———— The Physical Improvement of Humanity: A Plea for the Welfare of the Unborn. New York: Murry Hill Pub. Co., 1876, pp. 16.

———— Physiological Marriage. An Essay Designed to Set People Thinking. New York: Murray Hill Pub. Co., 1876, pp. 13. (Also another copy, n.d.)

———— Reply to the Alphites, giving some cogent reasons for believing that sexual continence is not conducive to health. New York: Murray Hill Pub. Co., 1882, pp. 39.

———— *Plain Home Talk About the Human System—the habits of men and women . . . embracing medical common sense applied to causes, prevention, and cure of chronic diseases* . . . New York: Wells & Coffin; San Francisco: H. H. Bancroft & Co.; [etc., etc.] 1870, pp. xxiv, [25] 912.

FOOTE, EDWARD BLISS, *Plain Home Talk—Embracing Medical Common Sense.* . . . New York: Murray Hill Pub. Co., 1881, pp. xxiv, 909 and advts.

―――― *Plain Home Talk About the Human System—the habits of men and women—the causes and prevention of disease—our sexual relations and social natures. Embracing medical common sense applied to causes, prevention and cure of chronic diseases.* . . . New York: Murray Hill Pub. Co.; [etc.] 1896, pp. xxiv, 959.

―――― *Dr. Foote's New Plain Home Talk on Love, Marriage and Parentage. A fair and earnest discussion of human social, and marital relations* . . . Rev. and enl. by the author. *Embracing also Tocology for mothers.* By A. Westland . . . New York: Murray Hill Pub. Co., 1901, pp. 292. [Part of Foote's *Home Cyclopedia.*]

―――― *Dr. Foote's Home Cyclopedia of Popular Medical, Social and Sexual Science, Embracing his New Book on Health and Disease* . . . *also embracing Plain home talk on love, marriage and parentage* . . . Twentieth century rev. and enl. ed. . . . New York: Murray Hill Pub. Co.; London: L. N. Fowler & Co., 1901, pp. xiv, 75–1248.

―――― Dr. Foote's New Book on Health and Disease, with Recipes, Including Sexology . . . Rev. and enl. by the author . . . New York: Murray Hill Pub. Co., 1901, pp. 1198–1248.
[Also published in the author's *Home Cyclopedia*, New York, 1901.]

*FOOTE, EDWARD BOND, *The Radical Remedy in Social Science; or Borning Better Babies through Regulating Reproduction by Controlling Conception. An Ernest Essay on Pressing Problems.* New York: Murray Hill Pub. Co. 1886, pp. 122 + proem and bibliography. (Phil.)

――――, ―――― New York: Murray Hill Pub. Co., 1889, pp. 134 + Bibliography. (Phil.)

―――― "A Summary of My Views on the Prevention of Conception," *Med. Pharm. Critic* [i.e., Critic & Guide], (New York), xiii (1910): 408.

FORD, WILLIAM K., "Drug Eruption Due to Quinine: Recurrence Following Use of a Contraceptive," *Jour. Amer. Med. Asso.*, ciii (1934): 483.
[A case of dermatitis venata in a patient known to be sensitive to quinine, following use 2½ days previously by his wife of a suppository containing quinine bisulphate.]

FORSTMANN, F. and AUSEMS, A. W., *Het Neomalthusianisme.* Utrecht, 1911.

FORT, GEORGE, F., *Medical Economy during the Middle Ages: A Contributon to the History of European Morals, from the Time of the Roman Empire to the Close of the Fourteenth Century.* New York: Bouton; London: Quaritch, 1883, pp. xii, 1–488.

FOSSEL, VIKTOR, *Volksmedicin und medicinischer Aberglaube in Steiermark. Ein Beitrag zur Landeskunde.* 2 Aufl. Graz: Leuschner & Lubensky, 1886, pp. 172.

FOTHERGILL, W. E., "Birth Control—Medical and Sociological Aspects," *Practitioner* (London), cxi (1923): 49–55.

*FRAENKEL, LUDWIG, "Sterilisierung und Konzeptionsverhütung," *Arch. f. Gynäk.* (Berlin), xliv (1931): 86–132.

**―――― *Die Empfängnisverhütung. Biologische Grundlagen, Technik und Indikationen, für Ärzte bearbeitet.* Stuttgart: Enke, 1932, pp. 212.
[The outstanding German medical text. Includes full consideration of sterilization, operative and hormonal. Elaborate bibliography.]

VON FRANQUÉ [of Bonn], "Die Geburtenverhütung und die Deutsche Gesellschaft für Gynäkologie," *Arch. f. Gynäk.* cxliv (1931): 353–354.

FRANZ, ADOLPH, "Des Frater Rudolphus Buch *De officio cherubyn*," *Theologische Quartalschrift*, lxxxviii (1906): 411–436.

FREE, JAMES E., "Prevention of Conception," *Med. & Surg. Rep.* (Phila.), lix (1888): 726.

FREETHINKER, Fruits of Philosophy. An Essay on the [sic] Over Population. A New and Revised Edition. London: International Depot, 34, Bookseller's Row, Strand, W. C. [1880?], pp. 16. (A. C.)
  [Unique copy. Not by Knowlton. Someone evidently traded on the demand for Knowlton's pamphlet.]

FRENCH ARMY SURGEON, by A, Untrodden Fields of Anthropology. Observations on the esoteric manners and customs of the semi-civilized peoples; being a record of thirty years' experience in Asia, Africa, America and Oceania. Second edition. Paris: Librairie de Médecin, Folklore et Anthropologie, 1898. Vol. 1, pp. 1–343; vol. 2, pp. xxiv, 1–502.
  [Not of much scientific value.]

FREYGANG, C., Die Einschränkung der weiblichen Fruchtbarkeit durch Verhütung der Empfängnis. Leipzig, 1898 and later.

FRIEND TO FREE INQUIRY, A, A Review of "Fruits of Philosophy; or, Private Companion of Young Married People," by Charles Knowlton, author of "Modern Materialism." [Boston: Abner Kneeland, 1833–34, pp. 32.]
  [Known to the compiler through a contemporary newspaper report only. Would anyone locating a copy kindly communicate the fact to the author?]

FÜRBRINGER, P., "Präventivverkehr," in Handwörterb. d. Sexualwissensch. Bonn: Marcuse, 1923, pp. 359–361.

FÜRTH, HENRIETTE, Die Regelung der Nachkommenschaft als eugenisches Problem. Stuttgart: Püttmann, 1929, pp. 143.

——— "Ist der Geburtenrückgang eine bevölkerungspolitische Gefahr?" Hippokrates (Stuttgart), i (1928): 254–264.

FULLER, EDWARD, "Eugenic Aspects of the Walworth Women's Welfare Centre," Eugenics Rev. (London), xv (1923–24): 597–599.

FULLER, EVELYN, On the Management of a Birth Control Centre. London: Society for the Provision of Birth Control Clinics, 1926, pp. 17.

———, ——— Second edition—Revised and enlarged. London: Noel Douglas, 1931, pp. 38 [2].

——— A Note on the Work of the Society for the Provision of Birth Control Clinics. In Sanger & Stone, Practice of Contraception, pp. 209–215.

GÄNSSBAUER, HANS, "Ist der Arzt für die Schädigung durch intrauterinpessare haftbar?" Deutsche Med. Wchnschr., lix (June 2, 1933): 858–9.

GALL, R., Ein neues Ballon-Occlusiv-Pessar. Die Indikationen zur Verhütung der Schwangerschaft und meine Verbesserung des Occlusiv-Pessars mit bildlicher Darstellung. München: Seitz & Schauer, 1895, pp. 21

GAMGEE, KATHERINE M. L., "Some Modern Aspects of Birth Control," Cath. Med. Guard. (Middlesex, Eng.), iv (1926): 18–26.

GAMMELTOFT, S. A., ["Anticonceptive Measures,"] Ugesk. f. Laeger (København), lxxxvi (1924): 1078–1082.

——— ["Birth Control Question,"] Ugesk f. Laeger (København), lxxxvii (1925): 15–20.

GARSON, JOHN GEORGE, "Notes on the Deformations of the Genital Organs, Practised by the Natives of Australia," Med. Press (London), lvii (1894): 189–190.

*GAYLORD, GLADYS, "Restrictions in Regard to Regulation of Birth Imposed by Laws of Various Civilized Nations," Nat'l Conf. Soc. Work, 1931: 136–142.

GEISTLICHER, EIN (Pseudonym), Die Beschränkung der Bevölkerungszunahme. Leipzig, 1883.

GELUKKIG HUISGEZIN. Orgaan van den Nieuw-Malthusiaanschen Bond.

GERHARD, P., Die Mittel zur Vorbeugung der Empfängnis, nebst einer Beleuchtung der durch die überaus grosse Kinderzahl hervorgerufenen sozialen Misstände. 4 Aufl., Berlin, 1906, 12°.

GERLACH, H., Die Einschränkung der Kinderzahl durch Verhütung der Empfängnis. Berlin: Cassirer & Danziger, 1893.

GERLING, REINHOLD, Das goldene Buch des Weibes. Berlin: Verlag Wilhelm Pilz, 1909, pp. 157.

GERSON, HANS, Die Verhütung der Schwangerschaft. Berlin: Enck, 1920, pp. 131.

GILBERT, C. B. et al. [Discussion], "The Prevention of Conception," Cincin. Med. News (Cincin.), n.s., xix (1890): 303–308.

GILES, ARTHUR E., Birth Control. In Marchant [Ed.], Medical Views, pp. 69–88.

——— "The Need for Medical Teaching on Birth Control," Lancet (London), i (1927): 165–167.

GINI, C., "Sul controllo delle nascite," Difesa Sociale (Roma), iv (1925): 83–87.

GLASER, GERHARD, "Die Gefahr intrauteriner Fremdkörper," Deutsche Med. Wchnschr. lix (June 30, 1933): 994–996.

GLOVER, RALPH, see OWEN, ROBERT DALE.

GODDARD, CHARLES E., see ch. 6 in HAIRE [Ed.], Some More Medical Views.

GOENNER, ALFRED, "Die Berechtigung und die Indikationen der Konzeptionsverhinderung," Corr. Bl. f. Schweiz. Aerzte (Basel), xxxiv (1904): 265–270.

GÖTT, THEODOR, "Kann misslungene Empfängnisverhütung die Frucht schädigen?" München. Med. Wchnschr. (München), lxxviii (1931): 1329–1330.

*GOLDBERG, ERICH, "Darf der Arzt Beratung über Konzeptionsverhütung ablehnen?" Zbl. f. Gynäk. (Leipzig), lv (1931): 2557–2559.

——— "Empfängnisverhütung bei ledigen Frauen," Med. Welt (Berlin), 1929, Nr. 11.

——— "Über Empfängnisverhütung," Ztschr. f. Sexualwissensch. (Berlin), xvii (1930): 273–286.

——— "Sollen Entbindungsanstalten Empfängnisverhütung treiben?" Ztschr. f. Sexualwissensch. (Berlin), xvii (1930): 96–98.

GOLDSTEIN, FERDINAND, Geburtenschränkung. Staatsruin oder Wiederherstellung? Berlin: E. Berger, 1924.

GOODELL, W., "The Dangers and the Duty of the Hour; [the Faulty System of Female Education; the Decay of Home Life and the Unwillingness of Our Women to Become Mothers,"] Trans. Med. & Chir. Fac. Maryland (Balt.), lxxxviii (1881): 71–87.
    [A specimen of the mire from which we have mainly emerged.]

*GRÄFENBERG, ERNST, "Einfluss der intrauterinen Konzeptionsverhütung auf die Schleimhaut," Arch. f. Gynäk. xliv (1931): 345. [Abstr. in Zbl. f. Gynäk. (Leipzig), lv (1931): 2781.]

——— An Intrauterine Contraceptive Method. In Sanger & Stone, Practice of Contraception, pp. 33–47.

——— Silk als Antikonzipiens. In Bendix, Geburtenregelung, pp. 50–64.

——— The Intrauterine Silver Ring. In [C. P. Blacker, Ed.] Report of International Medical Group for the Investigation of Contraception, 1930, pp. 12–14.

——— Die Intrauterine Methode der Konzeptionsverhütung. In Proc. Third Congress World League for Sexual Reform. London: Kegan Paul, 1930, p. 116. (English translation, p. 610.)

GRANDESSO, M., ["Opinions of Various Authors (on Birth Control)]," Difesa Sociale (Roma), xi (Nov. 1932): 474–477.

GRANET, MARCEL, Chinese Civilization. (Translated by Chavannes.) London: Kegan Paul, 1930, pp. 435.

GRASSL, "Neomalthusianismus und das königl. bayerische Statistische Landesamt," *Ztschr. f. Med.-Beamte* (Berlin), xxv (1912): 637–49.

———— "Das Sterilisierungs- und Abtreibungsproblem mit besonderer Berücksichtigung Bayerns," *Ztschr. f. Sexualwissensch.* (Bonn), xii (1925–26): 367–377.

GREENWOOD, A. W. [Ed.], *Proceedings of the Second International Congress for Sex Research London 1930.* Edinburgh & London: Oliver & Boyd, 1931, xi, 3–637.

*GRIFFITH, EDWARD F., *Modern Marriage and Birth Control.* London: Victor Gollancz, 1935, pp. 221.

GRIFFITH, EDWARD F., and WRIGHT, HELENA, "Birth Control in Practice (I) General Practice (II) The National Movement," *Practitioner* (London), cxxxi (Sept., 1933): 278–285.

GRIFFITH, F[RANCIS] L[LEWELLYN], *The Petrie Papyri. Hieratic Papyri from Kahun and Gurob (Principally of the Middle Kingdom).* London: Bernard Quaritch, 1898, 2 vols.

GRIFFITH-JONES, E., MILLARD, C. KILLICK, *et al.*, "Birth Control," *Pub. Health* (London), xliii (1929): 5–12.

GROSE, FRANCIS, *A Guide to Health, Beauty, Riches and Honour.* 2nd. ed. London: Hooper & Wigstead, 1796, pp. viii, 1–64.

———— *A Classical Dictionary of the Vulgar Tongue.* (Ed. with a biographical and critical sketch and an extensive commentary by Eric Partridge.) London: Issued for Private Subscribers by Scholartis Press at XXX Museum Street, 1931, pp. lx, 396.

GROSSER, F. See GUREWITSCH.

**GROTJAHN, ALFRED, *Geburten-Rückgang und Geburten-Regelung im Lichte der individuellen und der sozialen Hygiene.* Berlin: Marcus, 1914, pp. xiv, 371.

[By the late pioneer professor of hygiene in the University of Berlin.]

———— "Eheberatungsstellen und Geburtenprävention," *Ergebn. d. soz. Hyg. u. Gesundhtsfurs.* (Leipzig), i (1929): 64–84. *Deutsche Ztschr. f. off. Gsndhtspflg.* (Berlin u. Wien), v (1929): 51–60.

GRÜNHAUT-FRIED, EMILIE, "Experimentelle oder praktische Prüfung von Anticonzipentien? Aus der Ehe- und Sexualberatungspraxis," *Zbl. f. Gynäk.* (Leipzig), lv (1931): 2560–2561.

GUREWITSCH, Z. A. and WOROSCHBIT, A. J., "Das Sexualleben der Bäuerin in Russland," *Ztschr. f. Sexualwissensch.* (Berlin), xviii (1931): 51–74; 81–110.

GUREWITSCH, Z. and GROSSER, F., *Probleme des Geschlechtslebens.* Staatsverlag der Ukraine, 1930, pp. 259 (in Russian).

H., M. G., *Poverty: its cause and cure. Pointing out a means by which the working classes may raise themselves from their present state of low wages and ceaseless toil to one of comfort, dignity and independence; and which is capable of entirely removing, in course of time, the other principal social evils.* London: E. Truelove, n.d. [1861 and later], pp. 16.

HADDON, ALFRED CORT, "Birth and Childhood Customs, and Limitation of Children." In Camb. Anthrop. Exp. to Torres Straits, Reports . . . Camb. Eng., 1901–12. Vol. VI on *Sociology, Magic, Religion of the Eastern Islanders*, 1908, pp. 105–111.

HAESER, HEINRICH, *Lehrbuch der Geschichte der Medizin und der epidemischen Krankheiten.*, Dritte Bearbeit. Jena: Dufft, 1875–82, 2 vols.

HAIRE NORMAN, Hygienic Methods of Family Limitation. 55th thousand. [London: New Generation League], n.d., [c. 1922], pp. 19.

———— "Contraceptive Technique," *Rpt. Fifth Int'l Conf.*, pp. 268–295.

———— "Contraceptive Technique: A Consideration of 1,400 Cases," *Practitioner* (London), cxi (1923): 74–90.

HAIRE, NORMAN, [Ed.], *Some More Medical Views on Birth Control*. London: Cecil Palmer, 1928, pp. 239. New York: Dutton, pp. 216.

———— *see* ch. 1 in HAIRE [Ed.], *Some More Medical Views*.

———— [Ed.], *Proceedings of the Third Congress of World League for Sexual Reform*. London: Kegan Paul, 1930.

———— Sterilization, Abortion and Birth Control. In *Proc. Third Int'l Cong. World League for Sexual Reform*. Reprint, pp. 8.

———— "The Comparative Value of Current Contraceptive Methods," *Verhandl. d. I. internat. Kong. f. Sexualforsch.* (Berlin u. Köln), 1928, iv, 117–127. Later published as reprint by London: Cromer Welfare Centre, 1928, pp. 12.

———— How I Run My Birth Control Clinic. London: Cromer Welfare Centre, 1929, pp. 11.

[Reprint from Proc. Sec. Int'l Cong. Wld. League for Sexual Reform.]

———— Vorläufiger Bericht über das Haire-Pessar und den intrauterinen Silberring. Wien: Elbemühl, 1931, pp. 12. Reprint from *Sexualnot u. Sexualreform. Verhandlungen des IV Kongresses der Weltliga für Sexualreform*, Wien, 1930.

———— A Preliminary Note on the Intrauterine Silver Ring. In Sanger & Stone, *Practice of Contraception*, pp. 47–56.

———— The Cromer Welfare Centre. In Sanger & Stone, *Practice of Contraception*, pp. 218–221.

———— "Zehnjährige intensive Erfahrungen über Präventivverkehr," *Arch. f. Gynäk.* (Berlin), cxliv (1931): 342–345.

———— *see* International Medical Group . . . Report, 1930.

———— *see* International Medical Group . . . Report, 1931.

———— Art. on "Contraception" in *Concise Home Doctor*. London: Amalgamated Press. Ltd., Fleetway House, 1932.

HAMANT, A. and CUÉNOT, "État actuel de la médecine anticonceptionelle en U. R. S. S.," *Gynéc. et Obst.*, xxvi (1932): 327–336.

HAMILTON-MUNCIE, ELIZABETH, "Family Limitation." Address before the American Institute of Homeopathy. June 25, 1918. Ms., pp. 8.

HAMMER, WILHELM, Das Liebesleid der Frau und die Mittel zu seiner Einschränkung. Leipzig: Verlag der Monatschr. f. Harnkr. u. sexuelle Hyg., pp. 90.

*HANKINS, FRANK H., Art. on "Birth Control" in *Encyclopaedia of the Social Sciences*, (New York), ii, 559–565.

[One of the ablest short accounts on the subject.]

HARDCASTLE, D. N., "Some Psychological Causes of Nervous Disorder Associated with the Use of Contraceptive Methods and Suggestions for Treatment," *Rpt. Fifth Int'l Conf.*, pp. 247–254.

**HARDY, G. (Pseud. for GIROUD, G.), *Moyens d'Éviter la Grossesse*. Nouvelle édition revue et augmentée. Paris, n.d., pp. 108, 39 figs.

[The pioneering French treatise.]

———— *Mittel zur Schwangerschafts-Verhütung*. Paris: Printed by the author, n.d., [c. 1900], pp. 104.

———— *How to Prevent Pregnancy* (Trans. [by H. Cutner] from the 120th French edition). Paris: By the author, n.d., [c. 1920], pp. 94, 39 illus.

———— Essay sur la Vasectomie. Stérilization de l'homme indolore et sans diminution des facultés viriles. Paris: Chez l'Auteur, 1913, pp. 13.

HARMSEN, HANS, Critical Survey of Contraception and Contraceptive Methods in Germany. In Sanger & Stone, *Practice of Contraception*, pp. 149–154.

HART, H., *see* STONE, HANNAH and HART H.

DE HART, MADANA, F., "Continence: An Unpopular Prophylactic," *Med. & Surg. Rep.* (Phila.), lix (1888): 674–676.

HARTER, RUD., Verhütung der Schwangerschaft aus Ehe-Not. Die Regulierung der Kinderzahl bei Eheleuten auf Grund moralischer Berechtigung. 8 Aufl. Stuttgart: Wilhelm Digel, n.d., pp. 80.

HARTMANN, Die Mittel zur Verhütung der Empfängnis auf ihren Wert geprüft und ihre moralische Berechtigung. 2 Aufl. Hagen (Westf.): Hermann Risel, [1896].

HASSE, *see* MENSINGA.

HAWTHORNE, JANIE LORIMER, *see* ch. 7 in HAIRE [Ed.], *Some More Medical Views.*

HEIMANN, F., "Präventivmassnahmen," *Med. Kl.* (Berlin), xxiv (1928): 1743–1744.

HELBIG, C. E., "Zur Geschichte der mechanischen Vorbeugemittel gegen Schwängerung und geschlechtliche Ansteckung," Krauss' *Anthropophyteia*, (Leipzig), x (1913): 3–12.

———— "Zu dem Schrifttume über den Condom," *Reichs.-Med.-Anz.* (Leipzig), xxxii (1907): 405–407; 424–426.

*HELBIG, CARL FRIEDRICH, "Ein Condom im Altertume," *Reichs-Med.-Anz.* (Leipzig), xxv (1900): 3.

HELLER, JULIUS, "Ein Beitrag zur Geschichte der Infibulation," *Arch. f. Frauenkunde* (Leipzig), xiii (1927): 277–280.

HELLMUTH, THEODOR, Aus der Praxis des Neo-Malthusianismus. Die neuesten und einfachsten Mittel zur Verhütung der Empfängnis. Konstanz: R. Oschmann, 1896, pp. 52.

HELM, ERNEST C., "The Prevention of Conception," *Med. & Surg. Rep.* (Phila.), lix (1888): 643–646.

HENKEL, OSKAR, Ehe und Liebe ohne Kinder. 4 Aufl., Dresden: H. L. Diegmann, n.d., pp. 32.

HERRICK, O. E., "Abortion and Its Lesson," *Mich. Med. News* (Detroit), v. (1882): 7–10.

HERS, F., "Beschouwingen naar Aanleiding van het Congres gehouden tegen het Nieuw-Malthusianisme te Amheim in 1919," ["The 1919 Anti Birth Control Congress,"] *Nederl. Tijdschr. v. Geneesk.*, (Amsterdam) lxiii (1919): 1344–1353.

HETTLER, Dr. Die Regelung der Kinderzahl. 2nd Aufl., Stuttgart: Wilhelm Digel, pp. 62.

HEYNES-WOOD, MERCIA, *Eugenics and Birth Control.* Lahore [India]: Times Publishing Company, 1931, pp. 119.

    [Handbook for social workers with section on contraceptive methods.]

HIGGINS, GODFREY [Ed.], *see* CARLILE, R.

HILL, LEONARD, Fertility and Its Control. In Marchant [Ed.], *Medical Views*, pp. 25–47.

HIMES, N. E., "The Birth Control Handbills of 1823," *Lancet* (London), ii (1927): 313–316.

———— "Birth Control Must Be Discussed," *Jewish Soc. Serv. Quart.* (Phila.), iii (1927): 61–63.

———— "The Place of John Stuart Mill and of Robert Owen in the History of English Neo-Malthusianism," *Quart. Jour. Econ.* (Cambridge, Mass.), xlii (1928): 627–640.

———— "British Birth Control Clinics: Some Results and [Some] Eugenic Aspects of Their Work," *Eugenics Rev.* (London), xx (1928): 157–166.

———— "Charles Knowlton's Revolutionary Influence on the English Birth-Rate," *New. Engl. Jour. Med.* (Boston), cxcix (1928): 461–465.

———— "The Relation of Birth Control to Infant Mortality and Pregnancy Waste," *Jewish Soc. Serv. Quart.* (Phila.), iv (1928): 309–316.

HIMES, NORMAN E. and VERA C., "Birth Control for the British Working Classes: A Study of the First Thousand Cases to Visit an English Birth Control Clinic," *Hosp. Soc. Serv.* (New York), xix (1929): 578–617.

HIMES, NORMAN E., "A Critical Review of 'Medical Aspects of Contraception'," *New Engl. Jour. Med.* (Boston), cc (1929): 13–17.

—— "A [Detailed] Critical Review of James F. Cooper's 'Technique of Contraception'," *Med. Jour. & Rec.* (New York), cxxix (1929): 291–294.

—— "McCulloch's Relation to the Neo-Malthusian Propaganda of His Time: An Episode in the History of English Neo-Malthusianism," *Jour. Pol. Econ.* (Chicago), xxxvii (1929): 73–86.

—— "John Stuart Mill's Attitude Toward Neo-Malthusianism," *Econ. Jour., Econ. Hist. Supp.* (London), i, No. 4 (1929): 457–484.

—— "Eugenic Thought in the American Birth Control Movement a Century Ago," *Eugenics* (New Haven, Conn.), ii (May, 1929): 3–8.

—— "Some Untouched Birth Control Research Problems," *Eugenics* (New Haven, Conn.), iii (1930): 64–71.

—— "Contraceptive Methods: The Types Recommended by Nine British Birth Control Clinics," *New Engl. Jour. Med.* (Boston), ccii (1930): 866–873.

—— "Robert Dale Owen, the Pioneer of American Neo-Malthusianism," *Amer. Jour. Soc.* (Chicago), xxxv (1930): 529–547.

—— [Ed.], Francis Place's *Illustrations and Proofs of the Principle of Population.* . . . London: Allen & Unwin, 1930. Boston: Houghton, Mifflin, 1930, pp. 62 (editor's introd.); (original text) xv, 1–280; (new appendices) 283–355.

—— "Soranus on Birth Control," (Second Century A.D.), *New Engl. Jour. Med.* (Boston), ccv (1931): 490–491.

—— "Note on the Early History of Contraception in America," *New Engl. Jour. Med.* (Boston), ccv (1931): 438–440.

—— "Birth Control in Earlier Days," *Birth Control Rev.* (New York), xv (1931): 280–282.

—— "The Coöperation of Social Agencies and Physicians with Representative American Birth Control Clinics," *Hosp. Soc. Serv.* (New York), xxv (1932): 17–30.

—— "Birth Control in Historical and Clinical Perspective," *Annals Amer. Acad. Pol. & Soc. Sc.* (Phila.), clx (March, 1932): 49–65.

—— "Note on the Origin of the Terms Contraception, Birth Control, Neo-Malthusianism, Etc.," *Med. Jour. & Rec.* (New York), cxxxv (1932): 495–496.

—— *John Stuart Mill and the Birth Control Controversy.* [In preparation.]

—— "Bibliography on Birth Control Clinics," *Birth Control Review,* June, 1934.

—— "The Rarissima of Birth Control," *Colophon.* Part XX, April, 1935.

—— "The Vital Revolution," *Survey Graphic,* April, 1935.

—— "Benjamin Franklin on Population: A Re-examination with Special Reference to the Influence of Franklin on Francis Place." Accepted for the *Economic Journal, Historical Supplement.* Probably will appear in January, 1937 issue.

—— Article on "Birth Control" in *Social Work Yearbook, 1935.* New York: Russell Sage Foundation, 1935.

—— Articles in the *Encyclopedia Sexualis:* "Birth Control, History of;" "Condom, History of;" "Condom;" Biographical articles on Owen, Robert Dale; Carlile, Richard; Knowlton, Charles; Place, Francis; Besant, Annie; Bradlaugh, Charles.

—— "The Birth Rate of Families on Relief: A Summary of Recent Studies in the U. S. A.," *Marriage Hygiene,* ii, 59–63 (August, 1935).

—— "Jeremy Bentham and the Genesis of English Neo-Malthusianism," *Economic Journal, Historical Supplement* (London). Probably will appear in the January, 1936 issue.

—— [Ed.] *Economics, Sociology and the Modern World. Essays in Honor of T. N. Carver.* Cambridge: Harvard Univ. Press, 1935, pp. xii, 3–327 [3].

HINZ, FRIEDRICH, "Der Wert der antikonzeptionellen Mittel," *Frauenarzt*, xiii, (1898), 349–358. Also reprint.

HIPPOCRATES, *see* LITTRÉ.

HIRSCH, M., "Empfängnisverhütung und Sittengesetz," *Zbl. f. Gynäk.* (Leipzig), lv (1931): 2992–3003.

—— *Fruchtabtreibung und Präventivverkehr im Zusammenhang mit dem Geburtenrückgang. Eine medizinische, juristische und sozialpolitische Betrachtung.* Würzburg: C. Kabitsch, 1914, pp. viii, 267.

*HIRSCHFELD, MAGNUS, *Geschlechtskunde auf Grund dreissigjähriger Forschung und Erfahrung.* Stuttgart: Püttmann, 1930, 5 vols.
  [Learned but diffuse.]

*HIRSCHFELD, MAGNUS and LINSERT, RICHARD, Empfängnisverhütung. Mittel und Methoden. Berlin: Neuer Deutscher Verlag, 1929, pp. 48.

HIRST, BARTON COOKE, "The Four Major Problems of Gynecology," *Jour. Amer. Med. Asso.*, ci (Sept. 16, 1933): 897–900.

HODANN, MAX, Birth Control and the Krankenkassen. In Sanger & Stone, *Practice of Contraception*, pp. 239–241.

—— Gesundheitliche und gesellschaftliche Voraussetzungen der Geburtenregelung. In Bendix, *Geburtenregelung*, pp. 25–29.

—— Methoden der Zunkunft. In Bendix, *Geburtenregelung*, pp. 84–89.

*HÖFLER, M[AX], *Volksmedizin und Aberglaube in Oberbayerns Gegenwart und Vergangenheit.* München: Ernst Stahl, 1888, pp. xii, 243 + plates.

*HOHMAN, HELEN FISHER [Ed.], *see* FIELD, JAMES A., *Essays.*

HOLDEN, F. C, Why Women Die in Childbirth. Some Reasons and Remedies, *Penna. Med. Jour.*, xxxviii (1934): 157–160.

HOLITSCHER, A., "Methoden der Geburtenkontrolle in England," *Neue Generation* (Leipzig), xx (1924): 295.

HOLLAND, EARDLEY, "Is the Practice of Contraception Injurious to Health?" *Practitioner* (London), cxxxi (Sept., 1933): 247–255.

*HOLLÄNDER, MICHAEL, *Vorbeugung der Empfängnis und Verhütung der Schwangerschaft.* Leipzig u. Wien: Schneider, 1927 and later, pp. 128.

HOLLIS, A. C., *The Nandi. Their Language and Folk-lore.* Oxford: Clarendon Press, 1909, pp. xl, 1–328.

HOLMAN, JEROME E., "Birth Control," *Nat. Eclect. Med. Asso. Quart.* (Cincin.), xx (1928–1929): 42–50.

HOLMES, J. R., Die wahre Moral oder Theorie und Praxis des Neomalthusianismus. Leipzig: Spohr. [Original English title: True Morality. Many eds.]

*HOMANS, ROBERT *et al.*, "Legal Opinions Concerning the Right of Doctors to Give Contraceptive Advice," *New Engl. Jour. Med.* (Boston), ccii (1930): 192–197. Reprinted as "Contraceptive Advice and the Massachusetts Law" by Mass. B. C. L., [1930], pp. 21.

HORDER, LORD, "Birth Control: An Introduction," *Practitioner* (London), cxxxi (Sept., 1933): 221–227.

*HOROWITZ, RABBI J., "Prevention of Conception According to the Jews's Religious Law," Contribution in Hebrew to *Festschrift für Jacob Rosenheim*, Frankfort a. Main, 1931, pp. 87–119.

*HOVORKA, O. V. and KRONFELD, A., *Vergleichende Volksmedizin. Eine Darstellung volksmedizinischer Sitten und Gebräuche, Anschauungen und Heilfaktoren, des Aberglaubens und der Zaubermedizin.* Stuttgart: Strecker & Schröder, 1908 & 1909, 2 vols. Vol. i, pp. v–xxiii, 3–459; vol. ii, pp. v–ix, 3–960.

How-Martyn, Edith and Beard, Mary, The Birth Control Movement in England. London: Bale, 1930, pp. 31. [A short history.]

Hrdlička, Ales, *Physiological and Medical Observations.* Washington: Bureau of American Ethnology, Bull. 34.

Huber, L., "The Prevention of Conception," *Med. & Surg. Rep.* (Phila.), lix (1888): 580–581.

*Huber, Rudolph, "Tränklein gegen Empfängnis im alten Rom," *Arch. f. Kriminalanthrop. und Kriminalistik.*, lviii (1914): 161. Also in *Ztschr. f. Sexualwissensch.* (Bonn), i (1914–15): 300.

Hüfler, Die Verhütung der Schwangerschaft. Berlin: Enck, (about 1920), pp. 80.

*Hufeland, C. W., "Von dem Rechte des Arztes über Leben und Tod," *Jour. Pract. Heilk.* (Berlin), lxvi (1823): I, 10.

*Hurgronje, Christian Snouck, *De Atjèhers.* Trans. as *The Achehnese* by the late A. W. S. O'Sullivan. London: Luzac & Co., 1906, 2 vols.

——— *Mekka in the latter part of the 19th century. Daily life, customs and learning. The Moslims of the East-Indian-Archipelago.* Trans. by J. H. Monahan. Leyden: Brill. London: Luzac & Co., 1931, pp. vi, 1–309 + errata and maps.

Ibn, see next word of name

Ihm, Hermann, see Krauss, Friedrich S.

Ill, Edward Joseph, "The Rights of the Unborn. The Prevention of Conception," *Amer. Jour. Obst. & Gyn.* (New York) xl (1899): 577–584.

Ingraham, Clarence B., "A Discussion of the Problem of Contraception," *Colorado Med.*, xxxii (1935): 26–30.

*International Medical Group for the Investigation of Birth Control, see Blacker, C. P. [Ed.]

Isma'il, Sayyid, of Jurjan, *Dhakhīra-i-Khārazmshāhī* [XII cent. Persian MS.]

*Jacobi, A., "Remarks on the Prevention of Conception," *Critic and Guide* (New York), vi (1906): 74–76.

——— "Infanticide, Abortion, and Prevention of Conception," *Critic and Guide* (New York), xv (1912): 451–64.

——— [News Report of the New York Academy of Med. Meeting, 1915], *Lancet Clinic* (Cincinnati), lxiii (1915): 618–619.

——— "My Position on Birth-Control," *Critic and Guide* (New York), xx (1917): 75–76.

Jacobs, Aletta, see ch. 8 in Haire [Ed.], *Some More Medical Views.*

*Jacobs, Julius, *Het Familie-en Kampongleven op Groot-Atjeh. Eene Bijdrage tot de Ethnographie van Noord-Sumatra. (Family and Village Life in Great Acheh. A Contribution to the Ethnography of North Sumatra.)* Leiden: Brill, 1894, 2 vols.

Jacobus X., Dr. [Sutor, J.?] see French Army Surgeon.

Jaworski, J., "Neomaltuzjanism ze stanowsika hygieny spolecznej i indywidualnej" ["Neomalthusianism from the viewpoint of public and private hygiene,"] *Now lek.* (Poznan), xxvi (1914): 340–348.

Johnson, I. V., "Profilaxia anti-natal," *Rev. med. veracruzana* (Veracruz), iii (1923): 37–40.

Joustra, M., *Hygienische Misstanden in het Karo-land.* Pub. by Bataksch Instituut, No. 1, 1909.

Junod, Henri A., *The Life of a South African Tribe.* London, 1912.

Justus, F. J., *Theorie und Praxis Neumalthusianismus.* 11 Aufl., Leipzig: Max Spohr, n.d., pp. 60. (A.C.)

Kaarsberg, H., ["New Ethics and Dangers of Birth Control Measures,"] *Ugesk. f. Laeger* (København), lxxxvi (1924): 206–216.

KÁCSER, MORY, *Original Beiträge über Volksmedizin in Ungarn.*

KAFEMANN, R., "Kann misslungene Empfängnisverhütung die Frucht schädigen?" *Münch Med. Wchnschr. (München)*, lxxviii (1931): 1918–1919.

KAHN, M. H., "A Municipal Birth Control Clinic," *New York Med. Jour.* [now *New York State Med. Jour.*], cv (1917): 790–791.

KAJI, TOKIJIRO, "Methods of Birth Control Known and Used in Japan," *Rpt. Fifth Int'l Conf.*, pp. 296–300.

KALYÁNAMALLA, *Ananga-ranga, traité hindou de l'amour conjugal rédigé en sanscrit par l'archipoète Kalyana Malla (XVIe siècle) traduit sur la première version anglaise (Cosmopoli 1885) par Isidore Liseux.*, Paris, 1886, pp. xvii, 196, 8°.

——— *Ananga-Ranga (Stage of the Bodiless One); or, the Hindu Art of Love. (Ars amoris indica.)* Translated from the Sanskrit, and Annotated by A. F. F. & B. F. R. Reprint: Cosmopoli 1885 for the Kama Shastra Society of London and Benares and for private circulation only.

KAMA SUTRA, *see* VĀTSYĀYANA.

KAMP, F. S., Die Mittel zur Verhütung der Conception. Auf praktische Anwendbarkheit, Sicherheit und gesundheitliche Einwirkungen untersucht. 2 Aufl., München, 1894, 8°. (S.G.)

——— Die Mittel zur Verhütung der Conception. Auf praktische Anwendbarkheit, Sicherheit und gesundheitliche Einwirkungen untersucht. Ein neues Mittel zur Verhütung der Schwangerschaft bei kranken und geschwächten Frauen. 5 Aufl., München, 1895, 8°. (S.G.)

KANTHER, H., Über Konzeptions-Verhinderung," *Fortschr. d. Therap.* (Berlin), i (1925): 318–325.

KANTOR, "Geburtenrückgang and Kurpfuscherei," *Therap. Monatschr.* (Berlin), xxx (1916): 513–520; 561–568.

KARSTEN, RAPHAEL, "Contributions to the Sociology of the Indian Tribes of Ecuador," *Acta Academiae Aboënsis. Humaniora*, Åbo Åkademi, 1920, No. 3.

KARVÉ, R. D., Morality and Birth-Control (Theory and Practice). Bombay, 1921, pp. i–iv, 82.

——— *Birth Control. Theory and Practice.* Fourth edition (in Marathi dialect). Bombay: Right Agency, 1931, pp. 123.

KARYSHEFF, K. A., ["Society for Prevention of Pregnancy in Germany,"] *Profilakt. Med.* (Kharkov), viii (1929): 68–69.

KATZENELSON, J. L., *Die normale und die pathologische Anatomie in der althebräischen Literatur und ihr Verhältniss zur altgriechischen Medizin.* Prepared from Russian by R. Kirschberg and published in *Historische Studien aus dem pharmocologische Institut zu Dorpat*, v (1896): 164–296.

KAVINOKY, NADINA R., California Public Health and Mothers' Clinics. In Sanger & Stone, *Practice of Contraception*, pp. 205–208.

KELLER, ALBERT G., "Birth Control," *Yale Rev.*, vii (1917): 129–139.

KELLY, HOWARD A., "The Biblical Side of Contraception," *Int'l Clin.* (Phila.), 40 s., iii (1930): 243–244.

KELLY, WEBB J., "One of the Abuses of Carbolic Acid," *Columbus Med. Jour.*, i (1882–3): 433–436.

KERSLAKE, MAUDE, Experience in Contraception. In *Medical Help*, pp. 107–122.

KING, E. L., "Medical Indications for Contraceptive Measures," *South. Med. Jour.*, xxvii (1934): 51–53.

KIRCHHOFF, AUGUSTE, The German League for the Protection of Motherhood. In Sanger & Stone, *Practice of Contraception*, pp. 230–234.

KIRSCHBERG, R., *see* KATZENELSON.

KISCH, E. H., "Artificial Sterility." In Eulenberg's *Real Enzyklopädie*, third ed., 1900, vol. xxiii, p. 372.

——— *The Sexual Life of Woman in Its Physiological, Biological and Hygienic Aspects* (Eng. trans. by M. Eden Paul). London and New York: Rebman, 1910, pp. xi, 686.

KISSENBERTH, WILHELM, "Über die hauptsächlichsten Ergebnisse der Araguaya-Reise," *Ztschr. f. Ethnol.* (Berlin) xliv (1912): 36–59.

KLARUS, Über künstliche Unfruchtbarkeit. Mittweida, 1893, pp. 85.

KLEIN, P., "Zur Frage der intrauterinen Konzeptions-verhütung," *Arch. f. Gynäk.* cxliv (1931): 345–347. [Ab. in *Zbl. f. Gynäk.* (Leipzig), lv (1931): 2781.]

KLEINWÄCHTER, LUDWIG, "Die wissenschaftlich berechtigte Conceptionsverhinderung," *Frauenarzt* (Berlin), vii (1892): 395–398.

*KLEIWEG DE ZWAAN, JOHANNES PIETER, *Bijdrage tot de Anthropologie der Menangkabau-Maleiers.* Amsterdam: Meulenhoff & Co., 1908, pp. xi, 1–206 + tables.

*KNAUS, HERMANN, *Die periodische Fruchtbarkeit und Unfruchtbarkeit des Weibes, der Weg zur natürlichen Geburtenregelung.* Vienna: Wilhelm Maudrich.

——— *Periodic Fertility and Sterility in Woman.* (Authorized English translation by D. H. Kitchen.) Hobart, Indiana: Concip Company, 1934.

——— "Sterilisierung und Konzeptionsverhütung," *Zbl. f. Gynäk.* (Leipzig), lv (1931): 2854–2857.

KNOCHE, W., "Einige Beobachtungen über Geschechtsleben und Niederkunft auf der Osterinsel," *Ztschr. f. Ethnol.* (Berlin), xliv (1912): 659–661.

*KNOPF, S. ADOLPHUS, "Legislation on Birth Control, with Special Reference to the Tuberculosis Problem in the United States," *Med. Woman's Jour.* (Cincin.), xxv (1915): 193–195. Also reprint.

——— "Birth Control, Its Medical, Social, Economic and Moral Aspects," *New York Med. Jour.*, civ (1916): 977–982. Also *Amer. Jour. Pub. Health* (New York), vii (1917): 152–172; *Pub. Health Jour.*, viii (1917): 117.

——— "Some Results of Birth Control," *New York Med. Jour.*, civ (1916): 1266.

——— "Preventive Medicine and Birth Control," *Med. Times* (New York), xlv (1917): 94–98.

——— "The Rights of the Wife and Mother," *Med. Woman's Jour.* (Cincin.), xxvii (1917): 25–32.

——— "The Problem of Birth Control and Tuberculosis After the World War," *Birth Control Rev.* (New York), iii (1919): No. 11, 5.

——— "Birth Control and the Rock Island and Scott County Medical Society of Illinois," *Amer. Med.* (Burlington, Vt.), n.s., xx (1925): 655–568. Also reprint, pp. 9.

——— "A Protest Against a Protest," *Med. Woman's Jour.* (Cincin.), xxxiii (1926): 70–73.

——— "The Sanitary, Medical, Social and Moral Aspects of Birth Control," *Med. Jour. & Rec.* (New York), cxxiii (1926): 16–20. Also reprinted by Amer. B. C. League under slightly different title.

——— The Medical, Social, Economic, Moral and Religious Aspects of Birth Control. Third edition. New York: S. A. Knopf, 1926, pp. 68, 8°.

——— "Birth Control As It Confronts the Medical Profession in the United States," *Clin. Med. & Surg.* (Chicago), xxxiv (1927): 737–743. Reprint, pp. 7.

——— Various Aspects of Birth Control, Medical, Social, Economic, Legal Moral and Religious. Fourth edition. New York: American Birth Control League, Inc., 1928, pp. [8], 11–92.
[Several editions.]

KNOPF, S. ADOLPHUS, "The Only Effective Famine Relief," *Med. Critic. & Guide*, (Dec. 1928), pp. 4. Also reprint.

―――― "Birth Control Laws, Their Unwisdom, Injustice and Inhumanity," *Med. Jour. & Rec.* (New York), cxxix (1929): 229–234. Also reprint by Amer. B. C. League, pp. 21.

―――― "Puerperal Death Rate, Birth Control and Marriage Advice Stations," *Med. Jour. & Rec.* (New York), cxxxi (1930): 455–458.

―――― "The Myth About Sterility Following Contraceptive Methods and Some New Developments in the Birth Control Movement," *Med. Jour. & Rec.* (New York), cxxxii (1930): 368–371.

―――― "The Dilemma of the Family Physician Regarding Contraception and Sterilization for Race Betterment," *Med. Times* (New York), lviii (1930): 108–115.

―――― "In Memoriam—James Freyer Cooper," *Med. Jour. & Rec.* (New York), (1931): 511–513.

―――― "The Present Status of the Birth Control Movement in England and the United States," *Med. Jour. & Rec.* (New York), cxxiv (1931): 105–109; 171–174; 224–226.

*EDITIONS OF CHARLES KNOWLTON'S FRUITS OF PHILOSOPHY

§1 EARLY AMERICAN EDITIONS

BY A PHYSICIAN, *Fruits of Philosophy, or the private companion of young married people.* New York, Jan. 1832. Probably 32°.

[No copy known to be extant. Known only by a court record.]

KNOWLTON, CHARLES, *The Fruits of Philosophy; or the private companion of young married people. Second edition with additions.* Boston: [A. Kneeland], 1833, pp. iv, 5–158. (H. L. Treas. Room.)

[Harvard copy undoubtedly unique.]

―――― see FRIEND TO FREE ENQUIRY, A.

―――― *Fruits of Philosophy, or the private companion of adult people. Fourth edition, with additions.* Philadelphia: F. P. Rogers, 1839, pp. 128 (112 x 69 mm.) (A. C., N.Y.A.M.)

[Only two copies of the fourth edition are known.]

―――― Fruits of Philosophy.

[Early spurious New York edition not yet located containing the phrase "ought to be" in place of "may be," a phrase used against Abner Kneeland in his blasphemy trial.]

―――― *Fruits of Philosophy, or the private companion of adult people. Tenth edition, with additions.* Boston: Published by Subscription, 1877, pp. 3–128. (H.M.S., A.C.)

[In the absence of any known copy of the ninth American edition, the last authorized edition for which Knowlton was himself responsible, this may be considered the most valuable edition. William James, the philosopher, once owned a copy of this edition, but it seems to have disappeared when his library was dispersed.]

§2 ENGLISH EDITIONS

―――― *Fruits of Philosophy; or, the private companion of young married couples.* London: James Watson, 3 Queen's Head Passage, Paternoster Row, n.d. [1833 ?], pp. 40. (A.C.)

[Probably the first authorized English edition. Note that the title reads *married couples,* not *married people.* Copy probably unique.]

KNOWLTON, CHARLES, *Fruits of Philosophy; or, the private companion of young married people.* Second edition. Reprinted from the American edition. London: J. Watson, 18, Commercial Place, City Road, Finsbury. Adjoining the Mechanics' Hall of Science, n. d., pp. vi, 40. (Yale)

——, —— London: James Watson, 127, Hemingford Road, Islington, n.d. [c. 1838 ?], pp. vi, 7–40.

[Note the use of the sub-title on the first and second American editions. It is possible that this issue rather than the second above is actually the first English issue. This might be determined by tracing Watson's addresses at various dates.]

——, —— Third edition. Reprinted from the American edition. London: J. Watson, 15, City Road, Finsbury, 1841, pp. vi, 7–40. ("P. C.," i.e., Private Cabinet? of the British Museum. Uncatalogued: Field Collection has a copy dated 1844.)

——, —— London: James Watson, 3 Queen's Head Passage, Paternoster Row, 1853, pp. vi, 7–40. (A.C.)

[Bound with newspaper clippings on Bradlaugh trial.]

——, —— London: F. Farrah, 282, Strand, n.d., [c. 1864–1873], pp. vi, 7–40. (A.C.)

[First English preface only. Unique copy. Other copies ought to turn up. In the 'sixties and 'seventies editions were issued by John Brooks, Austin & Co., Holyoake & Co., and either Watts & Co., or Charles Watts. I have never succeeded in locating copies of these editions.]

—— *Fruits of Philosophy. An Essay on the Population Question.* London: Freethought Pub. Co. [i.e., Charles Bradlaugh and Annie Besant], [1876 ?]. (A.C.)

[Annie Besant says in her *Autobiography* (p. 213) that there was an edition on the cover or the title page of which there was printed in red ink: "Recovered from the Police." If any specimen of this edition is extant ten years of search have not revealed its whereabouts.]

——, —— *Second new edition with notes.* London: Freethought Pub. Co., n.d. [1880 ?], pp. vi[2], 9–56. (Advert's of freethought literature.)

—— 70th thousand (A.C.)
—— 90th thousand (A.C., P.H.)
—— 125th thousand (A.C., P.H.)
—— 155th thousand (A.C.)
—— 175th thousand (U.C.)
—— 185th thousand (A.C.)
—— ? thousand (L.C.)

[Watson and first and second Bradlaugh prefaces, original proem, text with "G. R." (George Drysdale) notes, original appendix.]

——, —— *New edition—with notes.* London: Minerva Publishing Co., 1888, pp. 3–49.

[Probably unique copy. Miss Vance, who was more or less of a co-worker with Bradlaugh later in life told me that W. J. Ramsey brought out the Minerva edition, and that he was "not altogether an honorable person." Probably this statement had reference to commercial motives. Reference in the bibliography to the editions of H. A. Allbutt's *The Wife's Handbook* will show that W. J. Ramsey issued an early edition of that title. The footnotes to the present edition of Knowlton's *Fruits* were filched mainly from those by George Drysdale. There are no prefaces as in the other editions, and the original appendix by Knowlton is omitted, but Knowlton's "Philosophical Proem" is here. Some paragraphs in the Bradlaugh edition are absent, and new material has been added. This edition is notable for the inclusion of new material on methods: recommends use of the pessary, quinine soluble pessaries and the combined sheath and pessary. Advert. by Lambert. Minor typographical errors in text.]

KNOWLTON, CHARLES, *Fruits of Philosophy, an essay on the population question.* Sheffield: Printed and Published by J. Taylor, Highfields, n.d. [1881 and later ?], pp. vii, [1] 9–56. (S.G., A.C.)

[My copy has three prefaces, one by Jonathan Taylor. Probably issued shortly after the Bradlaugh-Besant trial during the publicity of that occasion. It has not been possible as yet to collate my copy with that in the Surgeon General's library; but I gather that they are approximately identical.]

——, —— Wakefield: Printed and Published by J. Taylor, n.d. [1881 ?], pp. vii, [1] 9–56. (A.C.)

[Has the same preface as the above edition. Copy unique. This edition virtually identical with edition next above; but different type.]

—— *Fruits of Philosophy* [No sub-title]. n.p. [Newcastle: William Robinson], n.d. [c. 1880], pp. 3–48. (A.C. and elsewhere.)

[This edition has a plain cover and is without all the usual prefaces by the earlier English publishers; but the proem, text and appendix are here. Has G. R. notes. I purchased several copies in mint state from William Robinson, Newcastle bookseller who "did not know" how he came by them. I am reliably informed, however, that they were issued by his father, William Robinson, about the time of the Bradlaugh trial. The extra copies have been distributed among American libraries.]

—— *Fruits of Philosophy. An Essay on the Population Question.* Newcastle-on-Tyne: W. Robinson, bookseller, 18, Book Market, 1886, pp. 3–48. (B.M.L.)

—— *Fruits of Philosophy. An Essay on the Population Question. New Edition, with Notes and Appendix.* London: Forder, 28, Stonecutter Street, 1894, pp. ix, 10–57, advert's. (A.C.)

[Unique. Without the Watson and Bradlaugh prefaces, but containing a new one, the Knowlton proem, text (with G. R. notes). In the place of Knowlton's appendix, there is a new appendix containing "a few observations on modern developments and improvements in 'preventive appliances.' " There is another (second) impression (of 10,000 copies) exactly like the above bearing the date 1898 instead of 1894. Advert's differ. (A.C.)]

——, ——. (Second impression of 10,000 copies.) London: R. Forder, 28 Stonecutter Street, E.C., 1898, pp. ix, 10–57, adverts. (A.C.)

——, —— Newcastle-on-Tyne: J. B. Barnes, 1889, pp. 2–48. (A.C.)

[Another Newcastle edition. Unique. Has G. R. notes, first English preface, Knowlton's proem and appendix.]

—— *Fruits of Philosophy. An Essay on the Population Question. Third* [sic] *new edition with notes.* London: . . . [sic] . . . Publishing Co., n.d. [1880's], pp. iii–vi, [7–9], 10–58. (B.M.L.)

[This copy was probably called the "third new edition with notes" because it was pirated from and published after the "second new edition" issued by the Freethought Publishing Co. It has the two Bradlaugh-Besant prefaces, followed by the original English preface (Watson ?), Knowlton's Philosophical Proem, text with "G. R." notes, and Knowlton's original appendix. The edition, the only copy known to the compiler, bears the names, *as authors,* of Bradlaugh and Besant. We may be quite certain, however, that it was not issued by them. Note that the name of the London Publishing Company is wanting. Though this edition was copyrighted in 1877 in the U. S. A. by the "Excelsior Importing Co." of Covington, Kentucky, it seems quite possible that it was published in the U. S. A., and not imported at all. There is a yellow leaflet pasted near the title page stating that this is "the book the British government is trying to suppress."]

[KNOWLTON, CHARLES], *The Fruits of Philosophy. Translated from the Chinese, an Antidote to the American edition issued by Mr. Bradlaugh and Mrs. Besant*. London: W. Sutton, n.d., pp. 32. (A.C., F.C.)

 [Text not at all related to the Knowlton pamphlet. A personal, irresponsible tirade against Bradlaugh and Besant. Author unknown.]

————— *see* FREETHINKER.

§3 LATER AMERICAN EDITIONS

KNOWLTON, CHARLES, *The Fruits of Philosophy* . . . Chicago: 188? (N.Y.P.L.)

 [One of the few American editions issued after the Bradlaugh-Besant trial.]

————— *Fruits of Philosophy. A Treatise on the Population Question*. By [sic] Charles Bradlaugh and Mrs. Anne [Annie] Besant. Chicago: G. E. Wilson, n.d. [188–], pp. 20. 22½ cm. (L.C., H.M.S.)

————— *Fruits of Philosophy. A Treatise on the Population Question*. By Charles Bradlaugh and Mrs. Annie Besant. Chicago: Wilson Publishing Co., 413 Wabash Avenue, [188– ?], pp. 87. (N.Y.A.M.)

————— *Fruits of Philosophy. An Essay on the Population Question*. New Edition. Chicago: Printed for the Proprietors by W. H. M. Smythe, n.d. (188– ?], pp. 3–32. (A.C.)

 [Unique. Cloth cover. Without English prefaces and Knowlton's Proem and appendix. No English footnotes.]

————— *Fruits of Philosophy. A Treatise on the Population Question by Charles Bradlaugh and Annie Besant*. N.p., International Publishing Co., n.d. [188– ?], pp. iii–vi, 58. (N.Y.P.L.)

 [Has the G. R. footnotes of the Bradlaugh-Besant edition. Pp. 53–56 missing from this copy. 19½ x 12 cm.]

————— *Fruits of Philosophy. A Treatise on the Population Question*. Edited by Charles Bradlaugh and Annie Besant. New York: The Truth Seeker Company, 28 Lafayette Place [188– ?], pp. 58 [and Truthseeker Freethought adverts]. (N.Y.A.M.)

§4 CONTINENTAL EDITIONS

————— *Vruchten der philosophie. Vehandeling over de bevolkings-kwestie en de sexueele moraal, door Charles Knowlton, M.D. . . . Met het Engelsch door Dr. X. Naar het Honderd-zeventigste duizendtal, der tweede met aanteekeningen verrijkte Uitgaaf. Vierde geheel herzien en verbeterde druk med afbeeldingen en vermeerderd met Aphorismen van E. Douwes-Dekker, Jr.* Rotterdam: J. H. H. Rothmeijer, 1880, pp. 62. 5 x 7½ in. (J.C.)

 [This is a scarce Dutch edition based on the Bradlaugh-Besant edition as is clear from the presence of the G. R. footnotes. Has the first English publisher's preface, the Bradlaugh-Besant introduction and a Dutch introduction by the publisher. Has also Knowlton's "Philosophical Proem." On pp. 48–49 are two illustrations of syringes. This is the only edition having illustrations in the *text* that I have seen, though others have appeared with advertisements bearing illustrations. Occasionally there are in this edition original footnotes by the translator.]

[KNOWLTON, CHARLES], Plus d'avortements! Moyens scientifiques, licites et pratiques de limiter la fécondité de la femme. Traduction de l'anglais avec appendice par G. Lennox. Notes du Dr. Z. Édition française [Bruxelles], n.d., pp. 39. (B.M.L.)
    [Loose French trans. of a late edition. Based on the Bradlaugh-Besant edition.]
———, ——— Namur: L. Roman, 1901, pp. 46, 8°. (S.G.)
    [Has the same two appendices as the above edition but the introduction to the ninety-ninth rather than the ninety-second English edition. Appendix signed G. Lennox in this, but not in the above edition. Across the yellow cover one finds printed in red ink the following notice: "Brochure poursuivie et acquittée devant la Cour d'Assises du Brabant 29 octobre 1900." Roman, the publisher ran a general printing shop and was the proprietor-editor of the "Journal [de ?] la Bataille," weekly socialist organ.]

KOLLER, THEO., "Praktische Erfahrungen mit den verschiedenen Methoden der Geburtenregelung," *Schweiz. Med. Wchnschr.*, lxiv (1934): 827–829.

KONIKOW, ANTOINETTE F., Advice to Mothers. Boston: By the author, *c.* 1927, pp. 4.
    [Available also in Hebrew and Italian editions.]
——— [WOMAN PHYSICIAN (Pseud.)], Voluntary Motherhood: A Study of the Physiology and Hygiene of Prevention of Conception. Boston: Published by the author, (Now 11 Keswick St.), [1927], pp. 32.
———, ——— 1928, pp. 37.
*——— *Physicians' Manual of Birth Control.* New York: Buchholz Publishing Co., 1931, pp. xiii, 3–245. [Now Boston: Buchholz Publishing Co., 11 Keswick St.]

*KOPP, MARIE E., "The Development of Marriage Consultation Centers as a New Field of Social Medicine." *Amer. Jour. Obst. & Gyn.*, xxvi: 122–134 (July, 1933).
**——— *Birth Control in Practice.* New York: McBride, 1933.
    [A statistical analysis of 10,000 cases at the Clinical Research Bureau in New York.]

KOSMAK, GEORGE W., "Birth Control: What Shall Be the Attitude of the Medical Profession Toward the Present-day Propaganda?" *Med. Jour. and Rec.* (New York), xci (1917): 268–273. Also *Bull. Lying-In Hosp.*, xi (1917): 88–99. Reprint from *Med. Jour. and Rec.*, pp. 21.
——— "The Attitude and Responsibilities of the Physician in the So-Called Birth Control Movement," *Bull. Lying-In Hosp.* (New York), xi (1917): 181–92.
——— "The Broader Aspects of the Birth Control Propaganda As It Should Interest the Physician," *Amer. Jour. Obst. & Gyn.* (St. Louis), vi (1923): 276–285. Discussion, pp. 351–353.

KOSSMANN, "Die Stellung des Arztes zur Verhinderung der Conception," *Deutsche Med. Press* (Berlin), ii (1898): 153.

KRAFT, HEINRICH, "Die Berechtigung zur Indikation der Konzeptionsverhütung," *Corr. Bl. f. Schweiz. Aerzte*, (Basel), xxxiv (1904): 337–339.
——— "Die Indikationen und Mittel der Schwangerschaftsverhütung," *Münch. Med. Wchnschr.* (München), li (1904): 1748–1749.

KRAUS, EMILE, "Experimenteller Beitrag zur Verhütung der Konzeption durch chemische Mittel," *Zbl. f. Gynäk.* (Leipzig), xxxv (1911): 747–749.

*KRAUSS, FRIEDRICH S., [Ed.] *Anthropophyteia.* Jahrbücher, I–X.
——— [Ed.] *Beiwerke zum Studium der Anthropophyteia.* Band I–XI.

*KRAUSS, FRIEDRICH S., SATOW, TAMIO, and IHM, HERMANN, *Japanisches Geschlechtsleben*, Vol. I, *Das Geschlechtsleben in Sitte, Brauch, Glauben und Gewohnheitsrecht des Japanischen Volkes.* Leipzig: "Anthropophyteia" Verlag für Urtriebkunde, n.d. [1931], pp. 5–432, and plates. Vol. II, *Abhandlungen und Erhebungen über das Geschlechtsleben des Japanischen Volkes. Folklorische Studien von Tamio Satow.* Bearbeitet von Herman Ihm. Leipzig: *Idem,* n.d. [1931], pp. 5–654.

KREBEL, RUDOLPH, *Volksmedizin und Volksmittel . . .* Leipzig, 1858.

KREEMER, J., *Atjeh.* Pt. II, 1922.

KRIEGER, MAXIMILIAN, *Neu-Guinea.* Berlin: Schall, 1899, pp. xii, 1–535.

KROHNE, "Empfängnisverhütung, künstliche Unfruchtbarkeit und Schwangerschaftsunterbrechung vom bevölkerungspolitischen und ärztlichen Standpunkt," *Kriegsärztl. Vortr.* (Jena), 1919: Teil 6, 6–43.

KRÜGER-RETAU, Das Buch über die Ehe der Vernunft oder kinderlose Ehe und Liebe. Stuttgart: Digel, n.d., pp. 80.

KUBE, MINNA, Weniger Menschen aber glücklichere . . . 6 Aufl. Charlottenburg: Published by author, pp. 65.

KUHN, J., ["Attitude of Profession to Birth Control,"] *Ugesk. f. Laeger* (København), lxxxvii (1925): 58–60. (Ab. *Jour. Amer. Med. Asso.,* lxxxiv (1925): 1708.)

KURELLA, HANS, *Geschlecht und Gesellschaft.,* Würzburg, 1911.

KUSTNER, HEINZ, "Das Problem der Verhütung der Empfängnis," *Prakt. Arzt.* (Leipzig), n.f., xiv (1929): 75–82.

KVATER, E. J., *Contraceptive Methods and Their Technique* (In Russian). Moscow: Published by Department of Public Health, 1926.

LABHARDT, ALFRED, "Die Stellungnahme des Arztes zur Frage der Konzeptions-Verhütung," *Schweiz. Med. Wchnschr.* (Basel), liv (1924): 77–81; 101–105.

LACHS, J., "Przerywanie i zapobiegani ciazy w starozytnosci," ["Birth Control in Antiquity,"] *Ginek. Polska,* xiii (1934): 22–55.

LADEWIG, L., Die Verhütung zur reichen Kinderzegens. Kurzgefasste Anweisung unter Angabe der gebräuchlichsten Mittel. Leipzig: Meyer, n.d. [1890 ?], pp. 34.

LAMBERT, EDWARD JOSHUA, The Wife's Adviser. An up-to-date Handbook . . . [containing] also a few notes on contraception. London: Wives Clinic, 1927, pp. 48. [A commercial pamphlet.]

*LAMMERT, G., *Volksmedizin und medizinischer Aberglaube in Bayern . . .* Würzburg: F. A. Julien, 1869, pp. 273.

LAMSON, H. D., "Educated Women and Birth Control in China," *China* [now *Chinese*] *Med. Jour.* (Shanghai), xliv (1930): 1100–1109.

——— "Family Limitation Among Educated Chinese Married Women: A Study of Practice and Attitudes of 120 Women," *Chinese Med. Jour.,* xlvii (May, 1933): 493–503.

LANDTMAN, GUNNAR, *The Kiwai Papuans of British New Guinea.* London: Macmillan, 1927, pp. xxxix, 485.

LANE, WILLIAM ARBUTHNOT, New Health and Birth Control. In *Medical Help,* pp. 63–69.

——— see ch. 9 in Haire [Ed.], *Some More Medical Views.*

*LASCH, RICHARD, "Über Vermehrungstendenz bei den Naturvölkern und ihre Gegenwirkungen," *Ztschr. f. Sozialwisssch.* (Berlin) v (1902): 81–95; 162–169.

*LAUTERBACH, JACOB Z., "Talmudic-Rabbinic View on Birth Control," *Central Conference of American Rabbis, Yearbook,* xxxvii (1927): 369–384.

LEAGUE OF NATIONAL LIFE, *National Life.* 1929 and later.

LEBEHOT, Note sur les injections vaginales au point de vue de la dépopulation présentée à l'Académie de médecine, March, 1892. Caen, 1892.

LEHFELDT, HANS, The Physical and Psychological Aspects of Contraception. In Sanger & Stone, *Practice of Contraception,* pp. 141–149.

LEIPELTS, P., [Ed.?] *Bibl. der Kirchenväter.* liv, 211f.

LE PILEUR, L. *See* PILEUR, L. LE.

LESSER, A., Liebe ohne Kinder. Ein ärztlicher Ratgeber zur Verhütung der Empfängnis. 3 Aufl. Leipzig: Max Spohr, 1896, pp. 31.

*LEUNBACH, J. H., ["Methods of Birth Control. Anti-conceptional Technic,"] *Ugesk. f. Laeger* (København), lxxxvii (1925): 989–990. (Ab. *Jour. Amer. Med. Asso.*, lxxxvi (1926): 160.

———— *Kønslivets Problemer i Nutiden. Kortfattet og populaer fremstilling* [Sexual Life of our Times. A Short and Popular Presentation]. Copenhagen & Oslo: Martins Forlag, 1926, pp. 95.

———— The Technique of Contraception. In *International Medical Group for the Investigation of Contraception.* London, 1930.

———— The Graefenberg Ring. In Sanger & Stone, *Practice of Contraception*, pp. 56–58.

———— My Private Birth Control Clinic. In Sanger & Stone, *Practice of Contraception*, pp. 274–277.

———— "Erfahrungen mit Graefenbergs intrauterinen Silberring," *Arch. f. Gynäk.*, cxliv (1931): 347–352.

———— "The Graefenberg 'Silver Ring' and Inter- and Intra-Uterine Pessaries," *Jour. State Med.* (London), lx (1932): 37–45.

———— and RIESE, HERTHA, *Sexual-Reform-Kongress. Weltliga für Sexualreform. Bericht des 2. Kongresses (in Kopenhagen vom 1. bis 5. Juli 1928).* Kopenhagen: Levin und Munksgaard, 1929; Leipzig: Georg Thieme, 1929.

LEVI, ETTORE, "Natalita ed eugenica (birth control)," *Difesa Sociale*, (Roma), iii (1924): 42–49.

———— "Il controllo delle nascite," *Rassegna di Studi Sessuali* [now *Genesis*] (Roma), iv (1924): 24–30; discussion, 47–50.

———— "Demografia ed eugenics in rapporto al movimento contemporaneo per il razionale controllo delle nascite," *Rassegna di Studi Sessuali* (Roma), vi (1926): xxxviii–xlii.

LEVINSON, MARIE P., "The Problem of Contraception," *Med. Jour. & Rec.* (New York), cxxxi (1930): 300–302.

LEVY, H., "Die Stellung des Arztes zur Verhinderung der Conception," *Aerztl. Praxis* (Würzburg), xi (1898): 353–355.

LEVY-LENZ, LUDWIG, "Eine einfache Methode der Schwangerschaftsverhütung," *Ztschr. f. Sexualwissensch.* (Berlin), xvii (1931): 501–502.

LEWIS, Die Ehe der Gegenwart und Zukunft oder Ehe und Liebe ohne Kinder. Stuttgart u. Hamburg: Wilh. Digel, n.d., pp. 63.

———— *Die Moral-Ehe.* 9 Aufl., Stuttgart: Wilh. Digel, n.d., pp. 95.

LEWITT, M., Liebe und Ehe ohne Kinder. Berlin: Adolph Willdorff, 1899.

LICHKUS, L. G., ["The Rôle of Contraceptive Methods in Prevention of Abortion,"] *J. Akush. i Zhensk. Boliez.* (Leningrad), xxv (1924): 101–116.

LIEPMANN, W., *Gynäkologisches Seminar; praktische Gynäkologie mit besonderer Berücksichtigung der sozialen Frauenkunde.* . . . Berlin: Urban & Swarzenberg, 1931, pp. viii, 368.

———— "Konzeptionsverhütung und klinischer Unterricht," *Zbl. f. Gynäk.* (Berlin), lv (1931): 2551–2555.

LINDER, S., "A sządékos meddöség kérdése," *Gyógyászat* (Budapest), xxxvi (1896): 309–313.

VON LINSERT, Korreferat. In Bendix, *Geburtenregelung*, pp. 38–43.

LISEAUX ISIDORE, *see* KALYĀNAMALLA.

LITTAUER, ARTHUR, "Bemerkungen zu Niedermeyer's Mitteilung 'Präventivverkehr als Ursache schwerer Kolpitis,' in Zbl. f. Gynäk. 1928, Nr. 13." *Zbl. f. Gynäk.* (Leipzig), lii (1928): 1415–16.

*LITTRÉ, ÉMILE [Ed.], *Oeuvres complètes d'Hippocrate.* Paris: J. B. Baillière, 1839–61.

LOCKHART, H., "Practical Aspects of Birth-control," *Jour. Tenn. Med. Asso.* (Nashville), ix (Dec. 1916): 331–334.

LOEB, HEINRICH, "Untersuchungen über Sexualität beim Manne," *Ztschr. f. Sexualwissensch.* (Berlin), xviii (1931): 1–15.

LOEFFLER, LOTHAR, "Sterilisierung, Konzeptionsverhütung und Eugenik," *Arch. f. Gynäk.*, cxliv (1931): 355–360.

LUCRETIUS, *On the Nature of Things.* Trans. by H. A. J. Munro. London: Bell, 1913.

LUDA, G., "Ueber antikonzeptionelle Schutzmittel," *Allg. Med. Centr.-Ztg.* (Berlin), xci (1922): 232.

*LÜNEBURG, H., *Die Gynäkologie des Soranus von Ephesus. Geburtshilfe, Frauen- und Kinder-Krankheiten, Diätetik der Neugeborenen. Übersetzt von Dr. Phil. H. Lüneburg, commentiert und mit Beilagen versehen von Dr. J. Ch. Huber, Medicinalrath.* München: Lehmann, 1894, pp. ix, 1–173.

LURIE, HARRY L., assisted by ROSENTHAL, MINNIE J., and WEBER, EVA MARKMAN, "Adult Sex Hygiene and Family Case Work: A report of the special instruction in the problem of family limitation and in other matters of sexual adjustment available to family clients of the Jewish Social Service Bureau," *Hosp. Soc. Serv.*, November, 1931, pp. 327–369.

———, ——— Reprinted for National Committee on Maternal Health, New York, 1931.

LUSCHAN, F. VON, "Zur anthropologischen Stellung der alten Ägypter," *Globus* (Hildburghauser), lxxix (1901): 197–200.

*LUSE, J. W., The Married Ladies' Private Guide to Health and Happiness giving the Information that Every Married Lady Should Have . . . [Clyde, Ohio, 1883], pp. 12 (L.C. unique copy temporarily lost).

McARDLE, THOMAS E., "The Physical Evils Resulting from the Prevention of Conception," *Trans. Wash. Obst. & Gyn. Soc.* (New York), ii (1890): 159–166. *Idem, Amer. Jour. Obst.*, xxi (1888): 934–939; discussion, 975–977. *Idem*, in transl. *Frauenarzt* (Berlin), iv (1889): 13ff.; 70ff.

——— Die Folgen des ehelichen Präventivverkehrs. 2 Aufl., Leipzig: Spohr, 1916. [Mostly nonsense, but widely reprinted and presumably of some influence. A heavy responsibility for the general prevalence of the notion that modern contraceptive appliances used by the clinics are physically injurious rests upon the shoulders of medical editors who admitted to their pages such irresponsible productions.]

McCANN, FREDERICK J., "The Effect of Contraceptive Practices on the Female Sexual Organs," *Cath. Med. Guard.* (Middlesex, Engl.), v (1927): 48–61.

——— The Dangers of Contraception. London: League of National Life, [1927], pp. 16.

——— "Birth Control (Contraception)," *Med. Press.* (London), n.s., cxxii (1926): 359. [In the same class as McArdle's papers.]

——— Contraception, A Common Cause of Disease. London: Bale, Sons & Danielsson, 1928, pp. 29.

McGEE, ANITA NEWCOMB, "An Experiment in Human Stirpiculture," *American Anthropologist*, 1891.

McILROY, A. LOUISE, "The Harmful Effects of Artificial Contraceptive Methods," *Practitioner* (London), cxi (1923): 25–35.

McNabb, V., "The Ethics and Psychology of Neo-Malthusian Birth-Control," *Cath. Med. Guard.* (Middlesex, Engl.), ii (1924): 12–16.

*McWilliams, William J., Federal and New York State Laws on Contraception. New York: Nat'l Comm. on Maternal Health, 1930, pp. 23.

[A good legal paper. First appeared in the *Birth Control Review*.]

Maack, Martin, Die geschlechtliche Fortpflanzung als Endzweck unsers Daseins.... Leipzig: Max Spohr, 1893, pp. 31.

Mack, Die Gefahren der Mutterschaft und deren Verhütung nach bisheriger und neuester wissenschaftlicher Methode. Berlin: Julius Ohlenschläger, n.d., 12°.

Magnus, Albertus, *De secretis mulierum item de virtutibus herbarum lapidum et animalium.* Amsterdam, 1565, pp. 329.

——— *De mirabile mundi.*

[Magnus, Albertus], *The Secrets of Albertus Magnus. Of the Vertues of Hearbes, Stones and Certaine Beasts.*

*Majima, Kau, Aiji Joseikiokai (Maternity and Child Welfare Centre). In Sanger & Stone, *Practice of Contraception*, 284–287.

——— *"Be Wise Mothers! A Practical Guide to Contraceptive Methods* (in Japanese). Tokyo: Jitsugyono Nippon Sha.

*Malinowski, B., *The Sexual Life of Savages in Northwestern Melanesia* ... London: Routledge, 1929, pp. xxiv, 506. 96 pl., 8°.

——— "Pigs, Papuans, and Police Court Perspective," *Man*, 1932, Art. No. 44.

*Malthusian, The, London: Malthusian League [Organ of], 1879–1921. Continued as *The New Generation.*

*Malthusian League, Committee of, Hygienic Methods of Family Limitation. [First edition. Single sheet 27½ cm. x 37 cm. printed on both sides. London: Malthusian League, 1913.]

———, ——— [Second edition. Single sheet 27½ cm. x 37 cm. London: Malthusian League, 1915.]

———, ——— [Third edition. Single sheet printed on one side only (unlike first and second editions), 46 cm. x 33 cm. London: Malthusian League; n.d. 1920–21.]

———, ——— See later editions catalogued under Dunlop, B. and Haire, N.

Mandelstamm, A. and Tschaikowsky, W. K. ["Hormonal Sterilization of Women; Action of Prolan (Pituitary Preparation) on Ovaries,"] *Arch. f. Gynäk.*, cli (1932): 686–705.

[Marchant, James (Ed.)], *Medical Aspects of Contraception. Being the Report of the Medical Committee Appointed by the National Council of Public Morals* ... London: Hopkinson, 1927, pp. xvi, 1–183.

Marchant, James [Ed.], *The Control of Parenthood.* New York & London: G. P. Putnam's Sons, 1920, pp. xi, 222, 12°.

*——— *Medical Views on Birth Control.* Introd. by Sir Thomas Horder. London: Hopkinson, 1926, pp. xix, 1–175.

[Papers by H. Chrichton-Miller, L. Hill, M. Scharlieb, A. E. Giles, R. C. Buist, L. D. Fairfield, Sir A. Newsholme, J. Robertson.]

*Marcuse, Max, *Die Ehe. Ihre Physiologie, Psychologie, Hygiene und Eugenik. Ein biologisches Ehebuch.* Berlin: Marcus & Weber, 1927.

——— Die sexuologische Bedeutung der Zeugungs- und Empfängnisverhütung und Methodik. Stuttgart: Ferdinand Enke, 1917.

——— *Der Eheliche Präventivverkehr. Seine Verbreitung, Verursachung und Methodik* ... Stuttgart: Ferdinand Enke, 1917.

MARCUSE, MAX, Zur Stellung des Arztes gegenüber der Geburtenbeschränkung," *Deutsche Med. Wchnschr.* (Leipzig), xlii (1916): 259–261.

MARKOV, N., ["Abortion and Its Importance in Prevention of Conception,"] *Russk. Klin* (Mosk.), v (1926): 71–92.

MASCAUX, FERNAND, Thirty Years Practice with Contraceptive Methods.   In Sanger & Stone, *Practice of Contraception*, pp. 17–18.

———— *See* RUTGERS, J.

*MASTERS, WALTER E., "The Prevention of Conception Amongst the Natives of the Kasai Basin, Central Africa," *Jour. Trop. Med.* (London), xix (1916): 90–91.

[MATERNITY AID PUB. ASSOC.], Fallacy of the Customary Means to Prevent Conception. New York: Maternity Aid Pub. Assoc. (33 West 97th St.), [1914?].

MATIGNON, J. J., "Les Eunuques du Palais Impérial à Pékin," *Bull. de la Soc. d'Anthrop. de Paris*, 4ᵉ s., vii (1896): 325–336.

MATRISALUS [Pseud.], Den Frauen Schutz. . . . Leipzig: Spohr, 1897, pp. 38.   2 Aufl., 1898, pp. 45. (A.C.)

*MATSNER, ERIC M., The Technique of Contraception. An Outline.   Foreword by Robert L. Dickinson.   Introduction by Foster Kennedy.   Published for the American Birth Control League by Williams & Wilkins, Baltimore, 1933, pp. 38.

[An able, brief, inexpensive treatise.   Text edited by R. L. Dickinson and Stella Hanau.   Dickinson's drawings from the *Control of Conception*.   Good, short bibliography.]

MATTESON, DAVID E., "Prevention of Conception," *Med. & Surg. Rep.* (Phila.), lix (1888): 759.

MAURICEAU, A. M., *The Married woman's private medical companion, embracing the treatment of menstruation, or monthly turns, during their stoppage, irregularity, or entire suppression.   Pregnancy, and how it may be determined; with the treatment of its various diseases.   Discovery to prevent pregnancy; the great and important necessity where malformation or inability exists to give birth.   To prevent miscarriage or abortion when proper and necessary to effect miscarriage.   When attended with entire safety.   Causes and mode of cure of barrenness, or sterility.*   New York: By the author, 1847, pp. xiii, 238, 16°. (S.G.)

[Earliest known edition.]

————, ———— New York, 1849, 16°. (S. G.)
————, ———— New York, 1851, pp. xiii, 1–238. (P. H.)
————, ———— New York, 1854, 12°. (S. G.)
————, ———— New York, 1855, pp. xiii, 228. (B. M. L., S. G.)
————, ———— New York: Joseph Trow, 1885, pp. xii, 238.

MAXWELL, J. P., "On Contraception," *China Med. Jour.* (Shanghai), xl (1926): 986–994.

MAYER, MAX D., "A Director for the Vaginal Occlusive Pessary," *Amer. Jour. Obst. & Gyn.* (St. Louis), xx (1930): 258–261.

MAZZEO, MARIO, "Igiene e neomalthusianismo," *Folia Medica* (Napoli), xiii (1927): 576–600.

MEDER, FRITZ, "Die Konzeptionsverhütung in der Hand der freipraktizierenden Arztes," *Zbl. f. Gynäk.* (Leipzig), lv (1931): 2561–2564.

———— ["Unreliability of Chemical Contraceptives,"] *Vereinsbl. d. Pfälz. Ärzte*, xliv: 362–364 (Dec. 1, 1932).

MÉLY, F. DE et RUELLE, C. E., *Les lapidaires de l'antiquité et du moyen âge.*   Paris, 1896–1902, 3 vols., 4°.

MEMORANDUM. Memorandum on Birth Control Presented to the Minister of Health by a Deputation on May 9th, 1924. London: Workers' Birth Control Group, [1924], pp. 16.

MENG, HEINRICH, "Der Gegensatz von Arzt und Volk in der Bevölkerungsfrage," *Hippokrates* (Stuttgart), ii (1929): 56–61.

MENGE, C. and OPITZ, E. [Eds.], *Handbuch der Frauenheilkunde fur Ärzte und Studierende.* Wiesbaden: Bergmann, 1913, pp. xvi, 1–802.

**[MENSINGA, WILHELM PETER JOH.], Pseudonym, C. HASSE, Ueber facultative Sterilität beleuchtet vom prophylactischen und hygienischen Standpunkte für practische Aerzte. Neuwied & Leipzig, 1882, 8°. (S. G.)
    [Minor variations in title.]

———, ——— 2 Aufl. Neuwied & Leipzig, 1883. (S.G.)

———, ——— 3 Aufl. Leipzig & Neuwied, 1883. (S.G.)

———, ——— 4 Aufl. Berlin, 1885, pp. 73. (S.G., A.C.)

———, ——— 5 Aufl. Berlin, 1888. (S.G.)

———, ——— 6 Aufl. Berlin & Neuwied, 1892, Part I, pp. 92; Part II, pp. 76. (S.G., A.C.)

———, ——— Das Pessarium Occlusivum und dessen Application. Supplement zu "Über facultative Sterilität, etc." Neuwied & Leipzig, 1882, 8°. (S.G.)

———, ——— 2 Aufl. Berlin, 1883, 8°. (S.G.)

———, ——— 4 Aufl. Berlin, 1885, 8°. (S.G.)

———, ——— 5 Aufl. Berlin, 1888, 8°. (S.G.)

———, ——— 7 Aufl. Berlin, 1900.

MENSINGA, WILHELM PETER JOH., Ein Beitrag zum Mechanismus der Conception (Empfängnis). Leipzig: Ernst Fiedler, 1891, pp. 8.

——— Vom Sichinachtnehmen (congressus interruptus—Zwangsverkehr). Neuwied & Leipzig: Heuser, 1905, pp. 68.

——— 100 Frauenleben in der Beleuchtung des §1354b des bürgerlichen Gesetzbuches. Eine Studie für Kliniker, auch für praktische Ärzte. Neuwied & Leipzig: Heuser. (A.C., F.C. etc.)

——— "Das Schwangerschaftsverbot," *Cbl. f. Gynäk.* (Leipzig), xxii (1898): 140–143.
    [Essentially a discussion of indications with a report of cases.]

——— Meine Lebensaufgabe. Neuwied & Leipzig: L. Heuser, 1907, pp. 25, 8°. (S.G.)

——— Sterilisation durch Hysterokleisis; ein Anhang zu 100 Frauenleben in der Beleuchtung des §1354b des B.G.B. Neuwied & Leipzig: Heuser, [1909], pp. 21, 8°. (S.G.)

MICHIGAN, STATE MEDICAL SOCIETY OF, "Report of Committee on Birth Control. Section on Obstetrics and Gynecology," *Jour. Mich. Med. Soc.*, xxxiii (1934): 140–145.

MIKLUCHO-MACLAY, N. von, "Über die Mika-Operation in Central-Australien," *Ztschr. f. Ethnol.* (Berlin), xii (1880): 85–87 [of Verhandlungen].

——— "Bericht über Operationen australischer Eingeborener," *Ztschr. f. Ethnol*, (Berlin), xiv (1882): 26–29.

*MILLARD, C. K. "The Problem of Birth Control with Special Reference to the Public Health Aspect," *Jour. State Med.* (London), xxvi (1918): 321–337.

——— "Birth Control in Relation to Child Welfare," *Child* (London), ix (1918–19): 392–395.

——— "Birth Control and the Medical Profession," *Rpt. Fifth Int'l Conf.*, pp. 226–234.

——— "Birth Control and Public Health," *Pub. Health* (London), xxxvii (1923–24): 129–133.

——— "Contraception and the Medical Officer of Health," *Jour. State Med.* (London), xxxix (1931): 46–54.

MILLER, A. G., SCHULZ, C. H., and ANDERSON, V. W., "The Conception Period in Normal Adult Women," *Surg. Gyn. & Obst.*, lvi (June, 1933): 1020–1025.

*MOÏSSIDÈS M., "Le Malthusianisme dans l'Antiquité Grecque. Contribution à l'histoire du malthusianisme," *Janus* (Leiden), xxxvi (1932): 169–179.
[An important contribution.]

────── Ο ΜΑΛΘΟΨΣΙΑΝΙΣΜΟΣ. ΑΛΛΟΤΣ ΚΑΙ ΝΨΝ [*Malthusianism: Ancient and Modern*]. Athens: Gerard, 1932, pp. 93
[An able survey with bibliography.]

*MOLL, ALBERT, [Ed.], *Handbuch der Sexualwissenschaften*. Leipzig: F. C. W. Vogel, 1912, pp. xxiv, 1029.

MOONEY, JAMES and OLBRECHTS, FRANS M., *The Swimmer Manuscript. Cherokee Sacred Formulas and Medicinal Prescriptions*. Washington, D. C.: Gov't. Prtg. Off. Smithsonian Institution. Bureau of American Ethnology. Bulletin 99, 1932, pp. 319.

MOORE, MADAME, The Wife's Secret of Power. New York: Madame Moore, [c. 1871], pp. 10[1], 11½ cm. (L.C.)

MOORE, S. G. H., "The Immorality of Family Restriction," *Med. Officer* (London), xx (1918): 145.

MORGHEN, GUGLIELMO, Mezzi preventivi per impedire il concepimento nelle donne deboli malate. Roma: Capaccini, 1900, pp. 61 + advt's.

MOSHER, ELIZA M., "A Protest Against the Teaching of Birth Control," *Med. Woman's Jour.* (Cincin.), xxxii (1925): 320.

MÜLLER, ARTUR, Schwangerschaft? Die Not unserer Zeit und die sichere Verhütung der Empfängnis. Ein Ratgeber für Eheleute. Leipzig, [1931], pp. 70.

MÜLLER, HEINRICH, Ein Beitrag zur Lösung der sozialen Frage. Verhütung der Konception. 2 Aufl. Leipzig: Demme, 1903, pp. 20.

MURPHY, MARGARET C., "Migration of a Gräfenburg Ring," *Lancet*, ii (1933): 1369–1370.
[Found outside uterus.]

MUSITANUS, R. D. CAROLUS, *De morbis mulierum*, 1709.

NACKE, W., Die Unfruchtbarkeit der Frau. Berlin-Grunewald: Dr. Walter Rothschild, 1922, pp. 32.

NAESER, J., ["Measures to Prevent Conception,"] *Ugesk. f. Laeger* (København), lxxxvii (1925): 86–88.

NARDI, D., Dissertatio de onanismo conjugali. Paris & Brussels, 1876.

NATIONAL COMMITTEE ON MATERNAL HEALTH, see COMM. ON MATERNAL HEALTH.

────── Medical Aspects of Human Fertility. A Survey and Report . . . 1932.

NATVIG, H. ["Action of 'steriletten' "], *Norsk. Mag. f. Lægevidensk.* (Kristiania), lxxxvi (1925): 546–549.

NAUJOKS, H., Das Problem der temporären Sterilisierung der Frau. Stuttgart: Ferdinand Enke, 1925.

NAWAZ, M. S., "Indications for Birth Control," *Indian Med. Rec.* (Calcutta), xlvi (1926): 205.

NEFZAOUI, CHEIKH, Le Jardin Parfumé. Trans. in 1850 by Baron R──. Paris: Bibliothèque des Curieux, 1922, pp. 278.

NEISSER-SCHROETER, LOTTE, "Geburtenregelung. Aus den Ergebnissen der Enquete über die Ehe-und Sexual Beratungsstellen Deutschlands," *Neue Generation* (Berlin), xxiv (1928): 432–435.

NEUBAUER, W. and ELKAN, R., "Ein Phantom zur Erlernung der Technik der Kontrazeption," *Ztschr. f. Sexualwissensch.* (Berlin), xviii (1931): 365–368.

NEUFELD, NORBERT, The Breslau Sex Advice Bureau. In Sanger & Stone, *Practice of Contraception*, pp. 244–246.

NEUMANN, HANS OTTO and LANGE, KARL, ["Hormonal Sterilization of Female Rabbits by Repeated Injections of Testicular Substance,"] *Ztschr. f. Geburtsh. u. Gynäk.*, ciii (1932): 257–279.

NEWCOMB, DAN, *How not to and why; or arguments based upon physiological, moral, and social relations, in favor of preventing conception; and giving the "ways and means," in plain language.* Chicago: A. W. Penny & Co., 1872, pp. 92.

NEW GENERATION, 1922 to date. Formerly THE MALTHUSIAN.

NEWSHOLME, ARTHUR, Some Public Health Aspects of "Birth Control." In Marchant [Ed.], *Medical Views*, pp. 132–150.

NEW YORK ACADEMY OF MEDICINE, "Relation of the Medical Profession to 'Birth Control,'" *Bull. N. Y. Acad. Med.*, s. 2 vii (1931): 303–305.

[NEW YORK OBSTETRICAL SOCIETY, SPECIAL COMMITTEE OF], "Summary of the Answers to the Questionnaire Submitted to the Members of the New York Obstetrical Society on the 'Regulation of Conception,'" *Amer. Jour. Obst. & Gyn.* (St. Louis), vii (1924): 266–269. Discussion, 339–342.

NIEBOER, H. J., "Die Bevölkerungsfrage bei den Naturvölkern," *Corresp.-Bl. d. deutsch. Gesellsch. f. Anthrop., Ethnol. u. Urgesch.* (Braunschweig), xxxiv (1903): 143–150.

———— "Der 'Malthusianismus' der Naturvölker," *Ztschr. f. Sozialwiss.* (Berlin), vi (1903): 715–718.

NIEDERMEYER, A., "Präventivverkehr als Ursache schwerer Kolpitis (Colpitis pseudogonorrhoica acuta ex coitu condomato)," *Zbl. f. Gynäk.* (Leipzig), lii (1928): 833–834.

———— see CAPELLMANN.

NORTHCROFT, HILDA M., "Some Suggestions on the Subject of Birth Control," *Med. Woman's Jour.* (Cincin.), xxxi (1924): 252–254.

NOTESTEIN, FRANK W., see STIX, and p. 379, note 65.

NOYES, HILDA H. and NOYES, GEORGE W., "The Oneida Community Experiment in Stirpiculture," *Eugenics, Genetics and the Family* being vol. I of the Proceedings of the Second International Congress of Eugenics, New York, 1921. Baltimore: Williams & Wilkins, 1923.

*NOYES, JOHN HUMPHREY, Male Continence; or Self-Control in Sexual Intercourse. A Letter of Inquiry Answered by J. H. Noyes. Wallingford, Connecticut: Office of the Circular, 1886, pp. 4 (N.Y.A.M.).

**———— Male Continence. Oneida, N. Y.: Office Oneida Circular, 1872, pp. 24.

————, ———— Second edition. Oneida, N. Y.: Office of the American Socialist, 1877, pp. 32.

———— "Essay on Scientific Propagation," *Modern Thinker*, August, 1870. Also reprint in pamphlet form by the Oneida Community.

NOYES, THEODORE R., "Report on the Health of Children in the Oneida Community." Oneida, New York, 1878, pp. 8.

———— "Report on Nervous Diseases in the Oneida Community," *Medical Gazette*, October 22, 1870.

NYSTRÖM, A., "Konzeptionsverhütung," *Sexuale-Probleme* (Frankfort a./M.), iv (1908): 736.

———— "Über Präventivmittel," *Neue Generation* (Berlin), vii (1911): 439–444.

———— The Necessity of Abolishing Laws Against Preventive Measures, *Rpt. Fifth Int'l Conf.*, pp. 240–242.

**OEFELE, FELIX FREIHERR VON, "Anticonceptionelle Arzneistoffe. Ein Beitrag zur Frage der Malthusianismus in alter und neuer Zeit," *Heilkunde* (Wien, etc.), ii (1898): 206–216; 273–284; 409–425; 486–495. Also reprint, Wien, 1898? Pp. 48, 4°.

———— *Over het gebruik van kruiden en dranken ter voorkoming van zwangerschap. Een ethnographische-historische studie.* Derde druk. (On the Custom of Drinking Drugs for the Prevention of Pregnancy.) Trans. from German by Dr. J. Rutgers. Amsterdam: Graauw, [1899 or 1919?] pp. 159.

*OGINO, KYUSAKU, *Conception Period in Women.* Harrisburg, Penn: Medical Arts Pub. Co. [1934?]

[First appeared in Japanese in 1924. Ogino's name has since been much linked with that of Knaus. In 1925 Ogino received the prize of the Japanese Gyn. Soc. for his work.]

OHIO PHYSICIAN, *see* WINDER, DANIEL.

OHNESORGE, V., "Schädigungen durch Silkwormsterilette," *Münch. Med. Wchnschr.* (München), lxxiv (1927): 419–420.

OLBRECHTS, FRANS M., "Cherokee Belief and Practice with Regard to Childbirth," *Anthropos* (Salzburg), xxvi (1931): 17–34.

——— *see* MOONEY, JAMES.

OLOW, JOHN, "Abortprovokation och preventivmedel," [Abortion and the Prevention of Conception,] *Nord. Med. Tidskr.*, viii (1934): 893–898.

OPPENHEIMER, F., "Zum Malthus-Problem," *Arch. f. Sozialwissensch.* (Tübing.), xxxv (1912): 528–543.

*ORIBASIUS, *Oeuvres d'Oribase, texte grec, en grande partie inédit, collationné sur les manuscrits, traduit pour la première fois en français, avec une introduction, des notes, des tables et des planches par les docteurs Bussemaker et Ch. Daremberg.* Paris: À l'Imprimerie nationale, 1851–1876. 6 vols.

OTTO, DR., Künstliche Unfruchtbarkeit des Weibes. 5 Aufl. Leipzig: Spohr, n.d., pp. 79.

OTTO, H., Künstliche Unfruchtbarkeit. Zugleich eine Entgegnung auf Dr. Capellmann's Schrift: Facultative Sterilität ohne Verletzung der Sittengesetze. Leipzig u. Neuwied, 1884.

OTTO, LUISE, Erlösung von der Schwangerschaft. Ein Ratgeber für Eheleute. Magdeburg: W. Pfannkuch, 1923.

OVERBERGH, CYRILLE VAN, *Collection de monographies ethnographiques*, vol. ix.

*EDITIONS OF OWEN'S *MORAL PHYSIOLOGY*

[Arranged by (1) Country, (2) Date]

§1 AMERICAN EDITIONS

OWEN, ROBERT DALE, *Moral physiology; or a brief and plain treatise on the population question.* New York: Wright & Owen, 1831, pp. iv, 5–72, frontis. Orig. tan boards. (B.M.L.)

[Probably unique copy of first American edition.]

———, ——— Second edition. New York: Wright & Owen (359 Broome St.), 1831, pp. [1] iv, 5–72, frontis. Orig. tan boards. (Yale, W.I.)

———, ——— Third edition. New York: Wright & Owen, 1831, pp. vi, 5–72, 12°. (B.M., B.P.L.)

———, ——— Fourth edition. New York: Wright & Owen, 1831, pp. iv, 5–72 (A.C.)

———, ——— Fifth edition. New York: Wright & Owen, 1831, pp. 83. (A.A.S.)

———, ——— Seventh edition. New York: Wright & Owen, 1834, pp. iv, 5–83.

———, ——— New York: Beacon Office (84 Roosevelt St.), n.d. [*c.* 1833–34], pp. vi, 96. 3″ x 5″. (P.H.)

[Only pocket edition known. Probably not an authorized edition. Probably published after Owen left America for England. Contains publisher's notes.

Only edition mentioning chemical contraceptives? Once owned by J. M. Robertson of London. Its present location unknown.]

OWEN, ROBERT DALE, *Moral Physiology; or a brief and plain treatise on the population question*. Eighth edition. New York: G.W. & A.J. Matsell (94 Chatham St.), 1835, pp. i-iv, 5–83, 1 pl. Orig. boards. 18 cm. x 11½ cm. (Ind.).

[Unauthorized?]

—— *The Moral physiology; a treatise on popular questions, or means devised to check pregnancy. By a physician*. New York: Printed for the author [sic?], 1836, pp. vi, 9–76. 15½ cm. (L.C.)

[This copy seems to be unique. Quite possibly another pirated edition.]

[GLOVER, RALPH], *Owen's Moral Physiology; or, a brief and plain treatise on the population question. With alterations and additions*. New York: R. Glover, 1846, pp. v-xii, 2–143. Cloth. (A.C., A.A.S.)

[Probably first issue of the Glover edition. Glover was a New York physician, probably a quack.]

——, —— Third edition, with alterations and additions. New York: R. Glover, 1847, pp. xix, 21–180. Cloth. (A.C., Phil.)

OWEN, ROBERT DALE, —— New York: G. Vale, [1858], pp. iv (5), 88, frontis. pl. 19½ cm. x 11 cm. "Tenth edition with notes by the publisher embodying all modern discoveries; illustrated by anatomical and physiological engravings." (U.C., Ind., N.Y.P.L., W.I., Phil.)

[Ind.St. Lib. copy has no frontispiece. Workingmen's Institute (New Harmony) copy is reported to have 72 pp. Owen was probably not responsible in any way for this edition.]

——, —— Chicago: P. W. Carroll, 1881, pp. 30, illustrated, 12° (The People's Popular Liberal Library, No. 14). (N.Y.P.L.)

[Probably unique copy.]

——, —— Boston, 1881.

——, —— *see* SKIDMORE, THOMAS.

§2 ENGLISH EDITIONS

——, —— "Corrected and reprinted from the sixth American edition." London, 1832. (F.C.)

[One of the first English editions. No other copy traced. Note that it is based on the sixth American edition, of which no copy has been found by the writer. There was also a London: J. Watson, 1832 edition. See Robert Owen's periodical, *The Crisis*, i, 136, (Oct. 27, 1832); i, 140 (Nov. 3, 1832) for a notice of the same. Are we to assume that the Watson edition is the first authorized, and that the Brooks edition below is the unauthorized first English edition? Presumably the Owens would refer to the authorized (Watson) edition. For a portion of its run, Robert Dale Owen assisted his father in editing *The Crisis*.]

——, —— Eighth edition. First English edition. London: John Brooks, 421, Oxford Street, 1832, pp. vi, 63, 8°. (B.M.)

[Unauthorized?]

——, —— Tenth edition. London: John Brooks, 421, Oxford Street, 1833, pp. vi, 64, 8°. (B.M.)

——, —— London: J. Watson, Commercial Place, City Road, Finsbury, 1835, pp. iv, 5–48. (G.L., Yale)

[Contains advertisement of early English edition of Charles Knowlton's *Fruits of Philosophy*. Yale's copy is without date, but otherwise much the same.]

OWEN, ROBERT DALE, *Owen's Moral Physiology; or, a brief and plain treatise on the population question.* London: J. Watson, 15, City Road, Finsbury, 1840, pp. iv, 5–48, 8°. (B.M.)

———, ——— 1841. (Yale)

———, ——— London: J. Watson, 5, Paul's Alley, Paternoster Row, 1842, pp. iv, 5–48. (G.L., A.C.)

———, ——— 1844. (F.C., G.L., S.G., H.L.)

[The copy now in the Goldsmiths' Library, saved by Professor Foxwell, has notes in his hand based on J. A. Field's study. Foxwell's copy was once owned by William Lovett. I think it quite possible that Place gave Lovett this copy, as he is known to have sent a copy to Harriet Martineau and others.]

———, ——— London: J. Watson, 3, Queen's Head Passage, Paternoster Row, 1851, pp. iv, 5–48. (A.C.)

———, ——— London: J. Watson, 3, Queen's Head Passage, Paternoster Row, 1852, pp. iv, 5–48. (A.C., G.L.)

———, ——— A new edition. London: E. Truelove, 256, High Holborn, n.d. 1870?, pp. vi. 7–64. (B.M., A.C., L.C., and elsewhere.)

[Probably the most accessible and common edition. Hence the edition used for quotations and citations herein. Library of Congress card inaccurate: not an "eighth" edition. Though the preface is dated 1832, the approximate date is 1870–76.]

———, ——— London: Austin & Co., 17, Johnson's Court, 1872.

[No copy located by author; known only by an advertisement.]

PACK, ERNEST, Sexual Economics; The Secret of Security. Being a Solution to the Population Problem. [London: Liberator League] n.d., pp. 8.

[Cheap literature.]

PALMER, J. H., *Individual, Family and National Poverty. Reasons why in every family the number should be regulated; the methods that have been proposed, extensively adopted, and found to answer for doing it; together with a few valuable hints for the young.* Second ed. London: Truelove, 1875, pp. 17.

PANNIER, LEOPOLD, *Les Lapidaires français du Moyen Âge des XII*, XIII*, et XIV* Siècles ... Bibliothèques de l'École Hautes Études.* Paris: Vieweg, 1882, pp. xi, 340.

PANNWITZ, K., "Kinderreichtum. Gesundheitsarmut," *Bl. f. Volksgsndhtspfl.* (Berlin), xxi (1921): 129.

PARKER, ROBERT ALLERTON, *A Yankee Saint. John Humphrey Noyes and the Oneida Community.* New York: Putnam, 1935, pp. 322.

PAROLA, E. C., Proposta di un nuovo metodo per evitare la fecondazione; nota preventiva. Avezzano, 1909, 8°.

PARTRIDGE, ERIC, *see* GROSE, FRANCIS.

**PEARL, RAYMOND, "Contraception and Fertility in 2,000 Women," *Human Biology*, iv (1932): 363–407.

[A significant preliminary report.]

——— "Some Data on Fertility and Economic Status," *Human Biology*, iv (1932): 525–553.

——— "Preliminary Notes on a Coöperative Investigation of Family Limitation," *Milbank Memorial Fund Quart. Bull.*, xi (1933): 37–60.

[Abstract of first Pearl paper.]

——— "Contraception and Fertility in 4945 Married Women. A Second Report on a Study in Family Limitation," *Human Biology*, vi (1934): 355–401.

PEARL, RAYMOND, "Second Progress Report on a Study of Family Limitation," *Milbank Memorial Fund Quart.*, xii (1934): 248–269.
[Abstract of above.]

PEFFER, NATHANIEL, *China: The Collapse of a Civilization.* New York: John Day Co., 1930, pp. viii, 3–306.

PEIRCE, ISAAC, "The Prevention of Conception," *Med. & Surg. Rep.* (Phila.), lix (1888): 614–616.

PELLER, SIGISMUND, *Fehlgeburt und Bevölkerungsfrage.* Stuttgart-Leipzig: Hippokrates Verlag, 1931, pp. 9–295.

——— "Abortus und Geburtenrückgang, *Med. Klin.* xxvii (1931): 847.

PERRY, W. J., "Theology and Physiological Paternity," *Man*, 1932, Art. No. 218.

PETERS, "Schädigungen durch Silkwormsterilette," *München. Med. Wchnschr.* (München), lxxiv (1927): 770.

PETERSON, "[Okklusivpessar] Graziella," *Med. Klin.* (Berlin), viii (1912): 541.

PEYER, ALEXANDER, Der unvollständige Beischlaf (Congressus Interruptus, Onanismus Conjugalis) und seine Folgen beim männlichen Geschlecht. Stuttgart, 1890, pp. 64.

PFALZ, G. J., "Antikonzeptionelle Silkwormschlingen als Ursache schwerster Metritis. Kritische Betrachtungen über Wert und Wirkung intrauteriner Schwangerschaftsschutz," *München. Med. Wchnschr.* (München), lxxvi (1929): 1248–1250.

PFEIL, JOACHIM, *Studien und Beobachtungen aus der Südsee* ... Braunschweig: F. Vieweg, 1899, pp. xiii [1], 322.

*PHADKE, N. S., Birth Control. Bombay: Bombay Birth Control League, n.d. [1920?], pp. liv.
[This is probably the first edition. Second edition, n.d., (c. 1929), pp. lx.]

——— *Birth Control. Theory and Practice* (in Marathi dialect). Poona: Vijaya-Sāhitya, 1925, pp. 107.

*LE PILEUR, L., "Les préservatifs de la syphilis à travers les âges," *Annales des Maladies Vénériennes* (Paris), ii (1907): 501–527.

PILLAY, A. P., Birth Control in India with Special Reference to the Work of the Wives' Clinic at Shalapur. In Sanger & Stone, *Practice of Contraception*, pp. 278–282.

——— "The Medical Profession and the Birth Control Movement," *Indian Med. Gaz.*, lxviii: 43–44. (Jan. 1933).

PINÉAS, H., Psychisch-nervöse Auswirkungen der Konzeptionsangst. In Bendix, *Geburtenregelung*, pp. 75–78.

PIRKNER, ERNST H. F., "Remarks on Voluntary Sterility," *Urol. & Cut. Rev.* (St. Louis), xviii (1914): 295–299.

——— "Was Frauen wissen sollen. Etwas über die Unzuverlässigkeit der begräuchlichen antikonzeptionellen Mittel," *Ztschr. f. Sexualwissensch.* (Bonn), i (1914–15): 441–450.

——— "Präventivverkehr und Sterilität der Frau," *Ztschr. f. Sexualwissensch.* (Bonn), x (1923–24): 140–147.

——— "Praktische Erfahrungen über Präventivverkehr," *Ztschr. f. Sexualwissensch.* (Berlin), xiv (1927): 17–20.

PITT-RIVERS, G. H., *The Clash of Culture and the Contact of Races* ... London: Routledge, 1927, pp. xiv, 312.

PLACZEK, S., "Über den Gesetzentwurf betreffend die Unfruchtbarmachung und Schwangerschaftsunterbrechung," *Halbmonatschr. f. Soz. Hyg. etc.* (Berlin), xxvi (1918): 121.

PLACZEK, *Das Geschlechtsleben des Menschen. Ein Grundriss für Studierende, Ärzte und Juristen.* 2 erw. Aufl. Leipzig: Thieme, 1926, pp. 312. [1922 ed., pp. 205.]

PLACZEK, [with the collaboration of others], *Künstliche Fehlgeburt und künstliche Unfrucht-barkeit, ihre Indikationen, Technik und Rechtslage. Ein Handbuch für Ärzte und Bevölkerungspolitiker.* Leipzig: Thieme, 1918, pp. xi, 460.

PLINY, *see* BOSTOCK and RILEY.

PLOETZ, ALFRED, "Neomalthusianismus und Rassenhygiene," *Arch. f. Rassen- u. Gesellsch. Biol.* (Leipzig u. Berlin), x (1913): 166–172.

*PLOSS, HEINRICH and BARTELS, MAX, *Das Weib in der Natur- und Völkerkunde.* 11 Aufl. (neubearbeitet von F. von Reitzenstein) Berlin: Neufeld & Henius, 1927, 3 vols., pp. 790, 866, 630.

PODVIN, E. C., "True Status of Birth Control in England and the United States," *Med. Jour. & Rec.* (New York), cxxxiv (1931): 562–566; 615–617.
[A Catholic replies to Knopf's articles.]

POEHLMANN, A., "Zur Frage der Konzeptionsverhütung," *Zbl. f. Gynäk.* (Leipzig), lv (1931): 3252–3255.

*POLANO, O., "Beitrag zur Frage der Geburtenbeschränkung," *Ztschr. f. Geburtsh. u. Gynäk.* (Stuttgart), lxxix (1916–1917): 567–578.

———— "Die über autochemische Beeinflussung des Cervicalschleims," *Arch. f. Gynäk.* (Leipzig), cxliv (1931): 339–341.

*POPE, THOMAS A., "Prevention of Conception," *Med. & Surg. Rep.* (Phila.), lix (1888), 522–525.

———— "Prevention of Conception," *Critic and Guide* (New York), vii (1906): 83–86.
[Reprint of above]

PORTER, M. F., "The Prevention of Conception," *Cincin. Lancet & Clinic*, n.s., x (1883): 335.

*POWDERMAKER, HORTENSE, *Life in Lesu. The Study of a Melanesian Society in New Ireland.* New York: W. W. Norton, 1933, pp. 352.

PRAGER, Kinderlose Ehen. . . . Leipzig: Rossberg, 1901, pp. vi, 1–38.

**PREUSS, JULIUS, *Biblisch-talmudische Medizin Beiträge zur Geschichte der Heilkunde und der Kultur überhaupt.* Berlin: Karger, 1911, pp. [4] 1–735.

PRITCHARD, ERIC, "Birth Control," *Practitioner* (London), cxi (1923): 56–61.

PROTZ, Die Regulierung der Kinderzahl. 2 Aufl. Berlin: By the Author, 1927, pp. 60.

*PUSEY, WILLIAM ALLEN, Social Problems of Medicine. Address before the American Medical Association at Chicago, June 9th and 10th, 1924. Chicago: A. M. A. Press, 1924, pp. 1–33. See also *Jour. Amer. Med. Asso.*, lxxxiii, 1905–1908, 1960–1964.

———— "Medicine's Responsibilities in the Birth Control Movement," *Birth Control Rev.* (New York), ix (1925): 134–136, 156–158. Also reprint, New York: Amer. Birth Control League, [1925], pp. 8. Also in [Proceedings] Sixth International Neo-Malthusian and Birth Control Conference. New York: Amer. Birth Control League, 1926, iii, 19–30.
[Paper given before Sixth Int'l Neo-Malth. & B. C. Conf.]

PUST, "Ein brauchbarer Frauenschutz," *Deutsche Med. Wchnschr.* (Leipzig), xlix (1923): 952–953.

RABBINOWICZ, ISRAEL-MICHEL, *La médecine du Thalmud ou tous les passages concernant la médecine extraits des 21 traités du Thalmud de Babylone.* Paris: Chez l'auteur, 1880, pp. li, 1–176.

RANSON, R. M., *see* BAKER, JOHN R.

*RANULF, SVEND, "Die moralische Reaktion gegen neomalthusianische Propaganda in Dänemark," *Ztschr. f. Sexualwissensch.* (Berlin u. Köln), xvi (1929): 47–52.

RAPMUND, "Entwurf eines Gesetzes gegen Unfruchtbarmachung und Schwangerschafts-unterbrechung," *Ztschr. f. Med.-Beamte* (Berlin), xxxi (1918): 313–322.

RATZEL, FRIEDRICH, *Völkerkunde*. Leipzig, 1887, 1888, 1895. 3 vols. Eng. trans. by A. J. Butler as *History of Mankind*, London, 1896–98.

REICH, WILHELM, The Socialistic Society for Sexual Advice and Sexual Research. In Sanger & Stone, *Practice of Contraception*, p. 271.

REICHE, ERWIN, Empfängnisverhütung nach geltendem deutschen Recht. In Bendix, *Geburtenregelung*, pp. 17–24.

REISSNER, HANS, "Die Stellung des Judentums zur Frage der Geburtenkontrolle," *Neue Generation* (Berlin), xxvi (1930): 295–299.

REIST, ALFRED, "Die Gefahren der zur Konzeptionsverhütung intrauterin eingeführten sogenannten Sterilette oder Obturatoren, sowie des Fructuletts von Nassauer," *Schweiz. Med. Wchnschr.* (Basel), liv (1924): 650–657.

REITZENSTEIN, F. VON, "Der Kausalzusammenhang zwischen Geschlechtsverkehr und Empfängnis in Glaube und Brauch der Natur-und Kulturvölker," *Ztschr. f. Ethnol.* (Berlin), xli (1909) 644–683.

———— *Das Weib bei den Naturvölkern.* Berlin: Neufeld & Henius, [1923?], pp. 484.

*RENTOUL, ALEX C., "Physiological Paternity and the Trobrianders," *Man* (London) 1931, Art. No. 162.

———— "Papuans, Professors and Platitudes," *Man* (London), 1932, Art. No. 325.

*Report of the Fifth International Neo-Malthusian and Birth Control Conference. London: Heinemann, 1922, pp. 12, 1–308.

Report of the Conference on the Giving of Information on Birth Control by Public Health Authorities held on Friday, April 4th, 1930 at the Central Hall, Westminster. N.p., n.d. [London, 1930], pp. 36.

REYNOLDS, J. P., "The Limiting of Child-bearing Among the Married," *Trans. Amer. Gyn. Soc.* (Phila.), xv (1890): 3–24.

RICHTER, "Zur Bewertung antikonzeptioneller Mittel und Massnahmen. Berichte aus Gynäkologische Gesellschaft zu Dresden," *Zbl. f. Gynäk.* (Leipzig), xlv (1921): 1455.

RICHTER, J., "Zur Geburtenbewegung vor und während des Krieges," *Gynäk. Rundschau* (Berlin u. Wien), x (1916): 37. Discussion, 93.

*RICHTER, PAUL, "Beiträge zur Geschichte des Kondoms," *Ztschr. f. Bekampfg. der Geschlechtskr.* (Leipzig), xii (1911): 35–38.

RICHTER, R., "Ein Mittel zur Verhütung der Konzeption," *Deutsche Med. Wchnschr.* (Leipzig), xxxv (1909): 1525–1527.

*RIESE, HERTHA, "Erfahrungen der Sexualberatungsstelle Frankfurt a. M. nebst Grundsätzlichen Bemerkungen über Geburtenregelungspolitik," *Neue Generation* (Leipzig), xxi (1925): 250–255.

———— "Soziales und Sozialpsychologisches der Geburtenpolitik," *Verhand. I Internat. Cong. f. Sexualforschung* [1926], v, 163–179.

———— Sterilization. In Sanger & Stone, *Practice of Contraception*, pp. 116–122.

———— "Zwei Gerichtsurteile über aktuelle Probleme des Sexuallebens," *Hippokrates*, (Stuttgart), ii (1929–30): 635–654.

———— "Die Technik der Konzeptionsverhütung," *Arch. f. Gynäk* cxliv (1931): 341–342. [Ab. in *Zbl. f. Gynäk.* (Leipzig), lv (1931): 2779–2780.]

———— "Das Verhalten verschiedener antispermatoider Mittel innerhalb des weiblichen Genitalapparates," *Zbl. f. Gynäk.* (Leipzig), lv (1931): 3647–49.

RIESE, WALTER, Continence. In Sanger & Stone, *Practice of Contraception*, pp. 138–141.

RIGLER, LORENZ, *Die Türkei und deren Bewohner in ihren naturhistorischen, physiologischen, und pathologischen Verhältnissen vom Standpunkte Constantinopels.* Wien: C. Gerold, 1852, 2 vols.

RINK, WILL, "Eheberatung und Geburtenregelung," *Aerztl. Rundschau* (München), xl (1930): 71.

RIVERS, W. H. R., *Psychology and Ethnology.* Edited with preface and introduction by G. Eliot Smith. London: Kegan Paul, 1926, pp. xxviii, 3–324.

RIZZACASA, N., "Neomalthusianismo e aborto criminoso," *Med. Prat.* (Napoli), ix (1924): 333–338.

ROBERTS, HARRY, Population and Social Reform. Being a Few Plain Words on a Suppressed Subject. London, 1892.

ROBERTSON, J., "Artificial Birth Restriction," *Cath. Med. Guard.* (Middlesex, Eng.), iv (1926): 6–9.

ROBERTSON, JOHN, The Views of a Medical Officer of Health. In Marchant [Ed.], *Medical Views*, pp. 151–172.

ROBERTSON, WILLIAM, Birth Control and Preventive Medicine. In *Medical Help*, pp. 203–209.

**ROBINSON, CAROLINE HADLEY, *Seventy Birth Control Clinics. A Survey and Analysis Including the General Effects of Control on Size and Quality of Population. Foreword by Robert Latou Dickinson.* Baltimore: Williams & Wilkins, 1930, pp. xx, 351.

*ROBINSON, VICTOR, *Pioneers of Birth Control.* New York: Voluntary Parenthood League, 1919, pp. 107, 11 illus.

―――― *[Ed.], Encyclopedia Sexualis.* New York: Dingwall-Rock, 1936.

*ROBINSON, WILLIAM J., See numerous contributions to the *Critic and Guide* and to *Amer. Jour. Urol.*

―――― "The Limitation of Offspring; the most Important Immediate Step for the Betterment of the Human Race, from an Economic and Eugenic Standpoint," *Amer. Jour. Clin. Med.* (Chicago), xviii (1911): 591; 719.

―――― "Birth Control, or the Regulation of Offspring by the Prevention of Conception," *West. Med. Times* (Denver), xxxv (1915–16): 551–558.

―――― *Practical Prevenception; or, the technique of birth control; giving the latest methods of prevention of conception, discussing their effect, favorable or unfavorable, on the sex act; their indications and contra-indications, pointing out the reasons for failures and how to avoid them. For the medical profession only.* Hoboken, N. J.: Amer. Biol. Soc., 1929, pp. v, 1–170.

―――― [Leaflet without title describing birth control methods.] [1932].

ROBISHAW, RUTH A., Medical Report on Three Years Work of the Maternal Health Association, Inc., of Cleveland, Ohio. Cleveland: Maternal Health Asso., March, 1931.

ROBSON, ALICE L., "Note from a Small Birth Control Centre," *Practitioner* (London), cxxxi (Sept. 1933): 286–287.

RODECURT, M., "Experimentelle Untersuchungen über chemische Antikonzipientien," *Zbl. f. Gynäk.* (Leipzig), lv (1931): 1458–1460.

ROHLEDER, H., Birth Control and Medical Practice. *Rpt. Fifth Int'l Conf.*, pp. 243–5.

―――― Neumalthusianismus (Schwangerschaftsverhütung) und Ärztestand. Reprint from *Die Neue Generation*, xii (1911): 31.

―――― "Hebung der Geburtenziffer nach dem Kriege," *Ztschr. f. Sexualwissensch.* (Bonn), iv (1917–18): 13–22.

ROLLESTON, J. D., "The Medical Interest of Casanova's Mémoires," *Janus*, (Leiden), xxii (1917): 115–130; 205–222.

RONDIBILIS [Pseudonym?], "Quelques considérations historiques sur l'origine et l'usage de la redingote d'Angleterre à travers les siècles," *Progrès Méd.* (Paris), 3 s., xxxiv (1919): 56–58.

*Root, Harry Knox, *The People's Lighthouse of Medicine*, 14th ed., 1856.

*Rosenau, Milton J., *Preventive Medicine and Hygiene*. New York: Appleton-Century. Sixth edition, 1935.
[Has chapter on contraceptive technique by Eric M. Matsner.]

Ross, Edward Alsworth, *Standing Room Only?* New York: Century Co., 1927, pp. xiv, 3–368.

Rossen, Hans, *Die Verhütung der Schwangerschaft betrachtet vom medizinischen und sozialen Standpunkt*. 4 Aufl. (100–150 Taus.) Berlin: Enck, 1921–22, pp. 126.

Rothacker, William A., "The Prevention of Conception," *Cincin. Lancet & Clinic*, n.s., x (1883): 287–290.

Rouyer, Réné, *Les applications jurisprudentielles de la loi du 31 juillet 1920 réprimant la provocation à l'avortement et la propagande anticonceptionnelle*. Paris [thesis], 1923, No. 26, pp. 64, 8°. (B.M.L.)

—— "La loi du 31 juillet 1920 réprimant la provocation à l'avortement et la propagande anticonceptionnelle," *Ann. de Méd. Lég.* (Paris), iii (1923): 186–190.

*Ruben-Wolf, Martha, Birth Control in Soviet Russia. In Sanger & Stone, *Practice of Contraception*, pp. 255–267.

—— The German Birth Control Committee. Report from April, 1928 to August, 1930. In Sanger & Stone, *Practice of Contraception*, pp. 234–239.

—— Mechanische und chemische Verhütungsmittel. In Bendix, *Geburtenregelung*, pp. 29–38.

—— Abtreibung oder Verhütung. Berlin: Internationaler Arbeiter Verlag, n.d. [1930], pp. 16.
[C. H. Robinson says that 100,000 copies were sold six weeks before publication. Circulation stopped by judicial process.]

Rudolphus, Frater, see Franz, Adolph.

Rudolphus, Ioannes Gustav, *Dissertatio medico-ivridica de venenis sterilitatem indvcentibvs qvam praeside christiano godofredo stentzelio*. . . . [Medical and Juristic Dissertation on Drugs to Induce Sterility]. Vitebergae, 1731? (B.M.L.)

Runnalls, H. B., "The Prevention of Conception," *Med. & Surg. Rep.* (Phila.), lix (1888): 710.

Ruppenthal, J. C., "Criminal Statutes on Birth Control," *Jour. Amer. Inst. . . . Criminol.* (Chicago), x (1919–20): 48–50 [pp. 51–61 abstr. of statutes].

—— "Legal Barriers of State and Nation; Criminal Statutes on Birth Control," *Birth Control Rev.* (New York), ii (1928): No. 9, 10–14.

*Rutgers, J., Een Boek voor Jonge Vrouwen en Meisjes Wenken voor het Geslachtsleven (Sexueele Hygiene). 11de en 12de duizendtal. Amsterdam: C. Daniels, 1903. (P.H.)

—— Die Mittel zur Einschränkung der Kinderzahl. Aerztliche Ratschläge für Eheleute. N.p., n.d., pp. 12.

—— *Rassenverbesserung: Malthusianismus und Neumalthusianismus. Einzig berechtige Übersetzung von Martina G. Kramers. Mit Einführing von Marie Stritt*. Dresden u. Leipzig: Verlag von Heinrich Muden, 1908.

—— "The Conscious Limitation of Offspring in Holland," *Med. Pharm. Critic* (New York), xvii (1914): 174–176.

—— *Rasverbetering en bewuste aantalsbeperking. Kritiek van het Malthusianisme en van het Nieuw-Malthusianisme*. Amsterdam: Graauw, 1923, pp. vii, 1–270.

—— *Eugenics and Birth Control*. New and revised ed. Translated by Clifford Coudray. Dresden: R. A. Giesecke [1923].

—— Middelen ter Bewuste Regeling van het Kindertal. Vertrouwelijke Inlichtingen van een Dokter [Means for Regulating Consciously the Number of Children. Confidential Information of a Doctor]. Published by the N.M.B. [1927].

RUTGERS, J., [Ed.], *Het Gelukkig Huizgezin*, (*Organe de la Ligue Neo-Malthusienne Neerlandaise*). Doesstraat, 96, La Haye.

RUTGERS, J. et MASCAUX, F., Moyens d'éviter les grands familles.

SAGE, EARL C., "Birth Control," *Neb. St. Med. Jour.* (Omaha), xv (1930): 79–84.

SANGER, MARGARET H[IGGINS], Magnetation Methods of Birth Control. n.p., n.d. [1915], pp. 3–17 + Adverts.

—— Dutch Methods of Birth Control. n.p., n.d., [1915?], pp. 16.

*—— Family Limitation. Sixth ed. rev. n.p., 1920, pp. 23.
[Continuously reprinted]

—— —— [Yiddish edition] n.p., 1916, pp. 16.

—— Limitazione della Prole [Ital. ed.]. n.d., n.d., pp. 12.

—— Šeimynos Aprybavimas [Lithuanian ed. Family Limitation]. n.p., n.d., pp. 15.

—— Ograniczenie . . . Liczby Dzieci . . . Przez [Polish ed. Family Limitation]. n.p., 1917, pp. 14.

—— Family Limitation, Second Eng. Ed. revised by the author from the ninth Amer. Ed. London, Glasgow: Bakunin Press [i.e., Guy Aldred]. 1920, pp. 16.

—— Family Limitation. Foreword by Leonora Eyles. London: Rose Witcop (Kensington), n.d., pp. 31.
[There are a large number of Witcop editions. In one month in the summer of 1926, the author purchased the 53rd and 60th "editions" (really issues). This suggests the rapidity with which they have been issued.]

—— "Why Not Birth Control Clinics in America?" *Amer. Med.*, n.s. xiv (1919): 164–167.

—— "The Legal Right of Physicians to Prescribe Birth Control Measures," *Amer. Med.*, n.s., xv (1920): 321–323.

—— [Ed.], *Sixth* [1925] *International Neo-Malthusian and Birth Control Conference.* New York: American Birth Control League, 1926. 4 vols. Vol. I, *International Aspects of Birth Control*, pp. xii, 1–244. Vol. II, *Problems of Overpopulation*, pp. 1–208. Vol. III, *Medical and Eugenic Aspects of Birth Control*, pp. 1–247. Vol. IV, *Religious and Ethical Aspects of Birth Control*, pp. 1–240.
[These papers have not been indexed here as in the case of the Fifth (London) International Conference. Material on technique omitted, but these volumes contain general papers by important people.]

**—— [Ed.], *Proceedings of the World Population Conference . . . 1927.* London: Arnold, 1927, pp. 383.

—— "Die erste Beratungsstelle für Geburtenregelung in U. S. A.," *Neue Generation*, (Leipzig), xxiv (1928): 191–197.

—— *My Fight for Birth Control.* New York: Farrar & Rinehart, 1931, pp. vii, 3–360.
[Of autobiographical and historical interest.]

**—— and STONE, HANNAH M. [Eds.], *The Practice of Contraception. An International Symposium and Survey, from the Proceedings of the Seventh International Birth Control Conference, Zurich, Switzerland, September, 1930. With a Foreword by Robert L. Dickinson, M.D.* Baltimore: Williams & Wilkins Co., pp. xviii, 3–316.
[Valuable to the physician.]

SARTON, GEORGE, *Introduction to the History of Science.* Vol. I, *From Homer to Omar Khayyam.* Baltimore: Williams & Wilkins (for the Carnegie Institution of Washington, Pub. No. 376), 1927, pp. xi, 3–839. Vol. II, *From Rabbi Ben Ezra to Roger Bacon*, Part I, 1931, pp. xxv, 1–480; Part II, 1931, pp. xvi, 485–1251.

SATOW, TAMIO, *see* KRAUSS, FRIEDRICH S.

SCHADLITZER, A., Ueber ein neues Anti-Konzeptions.

SCHARLIEB, MARY, The Medical Aspect of Conception Control. In Marchant [Ed.], *Medical Views*, pp. 48–68.

SCHEDEL, J., "Reizmittel im Geschlechtsleben der Japaner," *Anthropophyteia* (Leipzig), vi (1909): 93–95.

SCHEUMANN, F. K., Birth Control and Marriage Advice Bureaus. In Sanger & Stone, *Practice of Contraception*, pp. 249–254.

SCHLEISSNER, FELIX, "Chemische Antikonzipientien als eine Ursache des Minderwuches," ["Use of Chemical Contraceptives as a Cause of Diminished Growth in Children,"] *Kinderärztl. Praxis*, iv (1933): 4–8.

SCHLOSSMANN, A., "Studien über Geburtenrückgang und Kindersterblichkeit unter besonderer Berücksichtigung der Verhältnisse im Regierungsbezirk Düsseldorf," *Ztschr. f. Hyg. u. Infektionskrankh.* (Leipzig), lxxxiii (1917): 177–275.

SCHMEY, F., "Ueber die Folgen des ehelichen Präventivverkehres," *Aerztl. Centr.-Anz.* (Wien), viii (1896): 337.

*SCHMIDT, R[ICHARD], *Liebe und Ehe im alten und modernen Indien.* Berlin: Barsdorf, 1904, pp. 571.

———— *Beiträge zur Indischen Erotik. Das Liebesleben des Sanskritvolkes. Nach den Quellen dargestellt.* 3 Aufl. Berlin: Barsdorf, 1922, pp. xi, 1–691.

SCHMOLL, MME, "La propagande anticonceptionelle," *Soc. Franc. de Prophyl. San. et Mor.* (Paris), ix (1909): 174–179.

SCHOONDERMARK, J., Jr., De voorbehoedmiddelen tegen zwangerschap. (2 ed.) Amsterdam, 1885, 8°.

SCHROEDER, H., *Die Vorbeugung der Empfängnis aus Ehenot.* Leipzig: Spohr, 1892, pp. viii, 1–111.

————, ———— Leipzig, Spohr, n.d., pp. 120.

SCHÜSTER, IRMA, "Prophycols, ein neues Antikonzipiens," *Fortschr. d. Med.* (Berlin) xlv (1927): 308.

SCHWEITZER, A., Über ein neues Anti-Konzipiens. N.d., n.p.

SCOTT, G. RYLEY, *Modern Birth Control Methods.* London: Bale, Sons & Danielsson, 1933, pp. x + 209.

SELIGMANN, C. G., "The Medicine, Surgery, and Midwifery of the Sinangolo," *Jour. Anthrop. Inst. of Gr. Brit. and Ireland* (London), xxxii (1902): 279–304 and plates.

SELITZKY, S. A., —["Intra-uterine Injections as Methods of Prevention of Conception,"] *Mosk. Med. Jour.* (Mosk.), iv, pt. 4 (1924): 17–28.

*———— *Contraceptive Methods in the Light of Modern Science* (in Russian). Moscow: Published by the State Department of Public Health, 1929.

SELLHEIM, HUGO, "Was muss der Arzt von der Regulierung der Fortpflanzung wissen?" *Ztschr. f. Sexualwissensch.* (Berlin), xviii (1931): 341–362.

SEMON, RICHARD, *In the Australian Bush.* London and New York: Macmillan, 1899, pp. xv, 552.

SENFFT, ARNO, "Die Rechtssitzen der Jap-Eingeborenen," *Globus* (Hildburghausen), xci (1907): 153.

SERSON, HANS, *Die Verhütung der Schwangerschaft betrachtet vom medizinischen und sozialen Standpunkt.* 3 Aufl. (60–100th thous.) Berlin: Enck, 1921, pp. 126.

SHROBANSKII, K., ["Abortion and Contraceptive Methods,"] *J. Akush. i Zhensk. Bolêez* (Leningrad), xxxv (1924): 1–13.

SIDDALL, R. S., "The Intrauterine Contraceptive Pessary; Inefficient and Dangerous," *Amer. Jour. Obst. & Gyn.* (St. Louis), viii (1924): 76–79.

SIEBERT, F., "Der Neomalthusianismus und die öffentliche Ankündigung der Verhütungsmittel," *Arch. f. Rassen-u. Gesellsch.-Biol.* (Leipzig u. Berlin), ix (1912): 475–596.

*SKIDMORE, THOMAS, *Moral Physiology exposed and refuted, by Thomas Skidmore, comprising the entire work of Robert Dale Owen on that subject with critical notes showing its tendency to degrade and render still more unhappy than it is now, the condition of the Working Classes, by denying their right to increase the number of their children, and recommending the same odious means to suppress such increase as are contained in Carlile's "What is Love, or Every Woman's Book."* New York: Skidmore and Jacobus, [1831].

[This work is not in the Library of Congress nor the New York Public and Harvard Libraries. No copy has been located. Will anyone locating a copy inform the writer?]

SMEDLEY, AGNES, Birth Control Work in China. In Sanger & Stone, *Practice of Contraception*, pp. 283–284.

DE SMET, [CANON] A., *Betrothment and Marriage.* St. Louis: B. Herder Book Co., 1923.

SMITH, BROUGH, *The Aborigines of Victoria; with notes relating to the habits of natives of other parts of Australia, and Tasmania.* London, 1878.

SMITH, M. HAMBLIN, see ch. 10 in HAIRE [Ed.], *Some More Medical Views.*

SOMMER, KURT, "Konzeptionsverhütung durch Gräfenbergring," *Zbl. f. Gynäk.* (Leipzig), lv (1931): 2547–2549.

SOMMERVILLE, DAVID, Birth Control and Social Work. In *Medical Help*, pp. 173–185.

*SORANOS, see LÜNEBURG.

*SOULE, J., *Science of Reproduction and Reproductive Control.* Stereotype edition. Cincinnati, Ohio, [c. 1856], pp. 72, ill. (Unique copy at L. C. temporarily lost.)

[For full title see ch. xi, n. 12.]

SOUVEUR, ST., Liebe ohne Folgen! Wie verhütet man ungewollte Empfängnis und Schwangerschaft? Zürich: Liga für Menschenrecht und Freiheit.

SOZIAL HARMONIE. [Organ of the Social Harmonische-Verein], Stuttgart.

SPENER, Art. on "Artificial Sterility" in Albert Eulenberg's *Real-Encyclopädie der Gesammten Heilkunde*, i, 456–459. Berlin and Vienna, 1903.

STABEL, H., A New Method of Temporary Sterilization of the Male by Injection of Paraffin into the Vas. In Sanger & Stone, *Practice of Contraception*, p. 127.

STARKMAN, J., "Coitus reservatus," *Medycyna* (Warszawa), xix (1891): 197–199.

STEFKO, W. H. and LOURIÉ, A., "Die pathologisch-anatomischen Veränderungen der Mucosa uteri bei Einführung von Silkwormgut und deren wesentliche antikonceptionelle Wirkung," *Deutsche Ztschr. f. d. ges. gerichtl. Med.* (Berlin), viii (1926): 536–544.

STEFKO, W., "Antikonzeptionelle Mittel als blastophthore Faktoren," *Arch. f. Frauenk.* (Leipzig), xiv (1928): 385–408.

STEIGER-KAZAL, ["Use of Various Contraceptives from Social and Hygienic Viewpoints,"] *Gyógyászat* (Budapest), lxviii (1929): 608–612.

STEINHÄUSER, W., "Über das biologische Verhalten von Spermatozoen gegenüber antikonzeptionellen Mitteln," *Monatschr. f. Geburtsh. u. Gynäk.* (Berlin), lxiii (1923): 146–154.

STERN, BERNARD, *Medizin, Aberglaube und Geschlechtleben in der Türkei* . . . Berlin, 1903.

**STIX, REGINE K. and NOTESTEIN, FRANK W., "Effectiveness of Birth Control. A Study of Contraceptive Practices in a Selected Group of New York Women," *Milbank Memorial Fund Quart.*, xii (Jan. 1934): 57–68. Reprint pp. 12.

——— "Effectiveness of Birth Control. A Second Study of Contraceptive Practice in a

Selected Group of New York Women," *Milbank Memorial Fund Quart.*, xiii (April, 1935): 162–178. Reprint pp. 17.

STIX, REGINE K., "A Study of Pregnancy Wastage," *Milbank Memorial Fund Quarterly*, xiii: 347–365 (October, 1935).

STOCKHAM, ALICE B., *Tokology. A Book for Every Woman.* 29th ed. Chicago: Sanitary Pub. Co., 1885, pp. v, 1–322. (B.M.L.)

——, —— Same rev. ed. Chicago: Sanitary Pub. Co., 1887, pp. xiv, 17–374. (B.M.L.)

——, —— Rev. ed. Chicago: Sanitary Pub. Co., 1897, pp. xiv, 17–373. (B.M.L.)

——, —— Toronto: McClelland, Goodchild and Stewart, 1916, pp. 373. (B.M.)

——, —— London: Fowler, 1918. (B.M.)

—— *Tokologie. Ein Buch für jede Frau.* Aus dem Englischen übersetzt. Verbesserte Aufl. Chicago: Sanitary Pub. Co., 1886, pp. xiv, 17–371. (B.M.L.)

—— *Karezza, Ethics of Marriage.* Chicago: Alice B. Stockham & Co., 1897, pp. viii, 9–136.

—— *Parenthood.* Chicago: Stockham & Co., n.d., pp. 27. (H.L.)

*STOECKEL, W., "Die Konzeptionsverhütung als Gegenstand des klinischen Unterrichts," *Zbl. f. Gynäk.* (Leipzig), lv (1931): 1450–1458.

STÖCKER, HÉLÈNE, "Hundert Jahre Kampf für Geburtenregelung," *Neue Generation* (Berlin), xxiv (1928): 397–405.

—— "Eine Kämpferin für Geburtenregelung in England: Stella Browne," *Neue Generation*, (Leipzig), xxii (1926): 52–54.

—— Zur Geschichte der Geburtenregelung. In Bendix, *Geburtenregelung*, pp. 5–16.

STONE, ABRAHAM, Coitus Interruptus. In Sanger & Stone, *Practice of Contraception*, pp. 131–137.

*STONE, HANNAH M., "Therapeutic Contraception," *Med. Jour. & Rec.* (New York), cxxvii (March 21, 1928): 7–17.— Reprint pp. 18.

—— Contraceptive Methods—A Clinical Survey. New York: Clinical Research Department of the American Birth Control League, [1925], pp. 16.
[Paper read at the contraceptive session of the Sixth Int'l Neo-Mal. and Birth Control Conf.]

—— The Birth Control Clinical Research Bureau, New York. In Sanger & Stone, *Practice of Contraception*, pp. 199–204.

—— The Vaginal Occlusive Pessary. In Sanger & Stone, *Practice of Contraception*, pp. 3–15.

—— *see* ch. 11 in HAIRE [Ed.], *Some More Medical Views.*

—— *see* BLACKER [Ed.], International. . . .

—— "Maternal Health and Contraception: A Study of 2,000 Patients from the Maternal Health Center, Newark, N. J. [Part II], Medical Data," *Med. Jour. & Rec.* (New York), cxxxvii, 7–15 (April 19, 1933) and cxxxvii, 7–13 (May 3, 1933). Reprint pp. 29

—— "Contraception and Mental Hygiene," *Mental Hygiene* (New York), xvii, 417–423, (July 1933).

—— *see* SANGER, MARGARET.

STONE, HANNAH M. and HART, H., Maternal Health and Contraception. A Study of the Social and Medical Data of 2,000 Patients from the Maternal Health Center, Newark, N. J. Part I Social Data. Newark, N. J., 1932, pp. 27.

**STONE, HANNAH M. and STONE, ABRAHAM, *A Marriage Manual. A Practical Guide-Book to Sex and Marriage.* New York: Simon and Schuster, 1935, pp. xi, 334.
[An excellent book for the general public. In the form of a conversation between a physician and patient.]

*STOPES, MARIE C., "The Remedy for Over-population: Some Historical Prejudices Removed," *Cambridge Magazine*, Decennial number, 1912–1921, vol. I, no. 1, pp. 66–73. (B.M., A.C.)

—— Early Days of Birth Control. Third edition. London: Putnam, 1923, pp. 32.

—— [Ed.], *Birth Control News*. 1921, *et seq.*

—— *Wise Parenthood, a Sequel to "Married Love"; a book for married people*. Introd. by Arnold Bennett. 12th edition. (415th thousand) London: G. P. Putnam's Sons, 1919.
[Many editions. Great influence on public opinion.]

—— *Weisheit in der Fortpflanzung. Eine praktische Ergänzung zur "Das Liebesleben in der Ehe." Ein Buch für Ehepaare. Übersetzt von F. Feilbogen.* Zürich: Verlag Arg. Institut Orell Füssli, 1920.

**—— *Contraception (Birth Control): Its Theory, History and Practice. A Manual for the Medical and Legal Professions. With an Introduction by Prof. Sir William Bayliss.* ... London: Bale, Sons & Danielsson, 1923, pp. i–xxiii, 1–417, + plates.
[First important English medical handbook. Later editions and several European translations.]

—— Letter to Working Mothers. On How to Have Healthy Children and Avoid Weakening Pregnancies. London: Mothers' Clinic for Constructive Birth Control, 1924, pp. 15. [First printed in April, 1919. Many later editions.]
[Many editions, some circulated by English retail dealers in contraceptive supplies. Pamphlet very simply written.]

—— The First Five Thousand [being] The First Report of the First Birth Control Clinic in the British Empire .... London: John Bale, Sons & Danielsson, Ltd., 1925, pp. 67.

—— Preliminary Notes on Various Technical Aspects of the Control of Conception. Based on the analysed data from ten thousand cases attending the pioneer Mothers' Clinic, London. London: Mothers' Clinic for Constructive Birth Control, 1930, pp. 44.

—— "Present Day Technique and Clinical Results in Contraception," *Jour. State Med.* (London), xxxix (1931): 352–353.

—— "Positive and Negative Control of Conception in Its Various Technical Aspects," *Jour. State Med.* (London), xxxix (1931): 354–360.

—— "Zur Geschichte der vaginalen Konzeption," *Zbl. f. Gynäk.* (Leipzig), lv (1931): 2549–2551. Reprinted as "Early Vaginal Contraceptives," in *Clin. Med. & Surg.* xxxviii (1931): 889–891.

—— *Roman Catholic Methods of Birth Control.* London: Peter Davies, 1933, pp. 235.

—— see ANONYMOUS.

*STRASSMAN, PAUL, "Wieweit ist der Arzt berechtigt, wieweit verpflichtet, Verordnungen zur Verhütung von Schwangerschaft und welche—zu treffen?" *Arch. f. Frauenk. u. Eugenitik.* (Berlin), viii (1922): 89–98.

*—— "Welche Verordnungen betreffend der verschiedenen Arten der Schwangerschafts-Verhütung müssen wir geben, um unsere Klientel vor Schaden zu bewahren?" *Arch. f. Frauenk. u. Eugenetik.* (Berlin), viii (1922): 98–104.

*—— "Die Gefährlichkeit intrauteriner, empfängnisverhütender Apparate," *Deutsche. Ztschr. f. d. ges. gerichtl. Med.* (Berlin), xii (1928): 278–284.

STRATZ, CARL HEINRICH, *Die Frauen auf Java. Eine gynäkologische Studie.* Stuttgart: Encke, 1897, pp. x, 1–134.

*STREICH, ARTUR, "Zur Geschichte des Condoms," *Arch. für Geschichte d. Med.* (Leipzig), xxii (1929): 208–213.

SUMNER, WILLIAM G., KELLER, ALBERT G., and DAVIE, MAURICE R., *The Science of Society*. New Haven: Yale Univ. Press, 1927, 5 vols.

SUTHERLAND, HALLIDAY GIBSON, *Birth Control Exposed*. [London]: C. Palmer [1925], pp. 255, 12°.

SUTOR, J., *see* JACOBUS X.

SWASEY, GEORGE H., Large or Small Families? Legitimate Methods of Birth Control. [London: Liberator League, 1921], pp. 8.
    [Of little value]

SWIFT, C. E., "Conception: the Fallacy and Evil of Attempted Prophylaxis," *Med. Summary* (Phila.), xix (1897–8): 11–13.

TALKO-HRYNCEWICZ, JULIAN, *La médicine populaire dans la Ruthénie Méridionale* [in Russian]. Krakau, 1893, pp. 461.

TATE, MAGNUS, "Birth Control, Affirmative and Negative Lay Viewpoint and the Attitude of the Medical Profession," *Ohio Med. Jour.* (Columbus), xxi (1925): 245–250.

TAUTAIN, "Étude sur la dépopulation de l'Archipel des Marquises," *L'Anthropologie* (Paris), ix (1898): 298–318; 418–436.

TAYLOR, H., Report on the Hormonic Control of Fertility. In Sanger & Stone, *Practice of Contraception*, pp. 98–104.

TELLING, W. H. MAXWELL, The Family Physician and Birth Control. In *Medical Help*, pp. 3–22.

TERUOKA, G., "Geburtenrückgang in Japan," *Arch. f. Frauenk. u. Eugenetik*. (Berlin), viii (1922): 201–218.

THEILHABER, FELIX A., "Ein deutscher Malthus. Vorschläge aus dem Jahre 1828 gegen die Übervölkerung Europas," *Ztschr. f. Sexualwissensch.* (Berlin), xviii (1931): 45–50.

—— *Das Sterile Berlin. Eine volkswirtschaftliche Studie*. Berlin, 1913, pp. 165, 8°.

THOMPSON, C. J. S., *The Quacks of Old London*. London: Brentano's, 1928, pp. xvi, 19–356.

THOMPSON, D'ARCY, *see* ARISTOTLE.

THOMPSON, J. FORD, in *Amer. Jour. Obst.* (New York), xxi (1888): 976–977.

THOMPSON, JOSEPH, *Through Masai Land*.

THORNDIKE, LYNN A., *History of Magic and Experimental Science*. London & New York: Macmillan, 1923, 2 vols.

TJEENK, WILLINK J. W., "Is vrije Verkoop van Geneeskundige Artikeln gewenscht?" ["Is the Open Sale of Medical Articles Desirable?"] *Nederl. Tijdschr. v. Geneesk.* (Haarlem), lxvii, Pt. II (1923): 1854–1855.

*TOLAND, OWEN J., "Contraception: A Neglected Field for Preventive Medicine," *Amer. Jour. Obst. & Gyn.*, xxvii (1924): 52–59.

TRALL, R[USSELL] T[HACHER], *The Hydropathic Encyclopedia: a system of hydropathy and hygiene* ... New York: Fowlers and Wells, 1853. (L.C.)
    [Stopes mentions an 1852 edition. I have made no attempt to investigate thoroughly the various editions of Trall's works as I have in the instance of those of Knowlton and Owen.]

—— *Hydropathic Encyclopedia*. Glasgow, 1882.

—— *Sexual Physiology: a scientific and popular exposition of the fundamental problems in sociology*. New York: Wood and Holbrook, Hygienic Institute, 15 Laight St., n.d. [1866], pp. xiv, 312. (P.H.)

——, —— Third ed. New York and London, 1866, pp. xiv, 312. (P.H.)
    [Stopes says that the 1884 edition is identical, and that later editions were emasculated.]

TRALL, R[USSELL] T[HATCHER], *Sexual Physiology: a scientific and popular exposition of the fundamental problems in sociology.* Glasgow, 1866.

—— *Sexual Physiology and Hygiene; or, the mysteries of man.* Rev. ed. New York: M. L. Holbrook & Co., [1885], pp. xvi, 17–344. (L.C.)

—— *Sexual Physiology and Hygiene.* Rev. and greatly enl. New York: M. L. Holbrook & Co., 1895, pp. xv, [17]–399. (L.C.)

TREGEAR, EDWARD, *The Maori Race.* Wanganui, N.Z.: Winis, 1904.

TREU, Die Ursache und die Verhütung der Familienlasten und vieler unglücklicher Ehen. Aerztliche Ratgeber zur Beschränkung einer allzureichen Nachkommenschaft. 12 Aufl. Leipzig: Otto Weber, pp. 69.

TRGJIĆ, "Das Geschlechtsleben der Rumänen in Serbien," *Anthropophyteia*, (Leipzig), vi (1909): 150–161.

TSUTSUMI, TATSUO, *Medical Knowledge for the Control of Conception* [in Japanese]. Tokyo: Jitsugyo-no Nippon Sha, 1930, pp. 216.

TURNER, DANIEL, *Syphilis. A Practical Dissertation on Venereal Disease.* London, 1717.

[Tyrer, A. H.], Birth Control and Some of the Simplest Methods. Toronto: Canadian Birth Control League, [1931], unpaged but pp. 9.

UDE, JOHANN, "Hormontabletten und Geburtenrückgang," *Med. Welt.* (Berlin), ii (1928): 959–961.

—— "Zur Frage der Herstellung, der Einfuhr, des Verkaufes, der Anpreisung und des Gebrauches der geburtenverhindernden Mittel," *Med. Welt.* (Berlin), ii (1928): 111–112.

USSHER, R[ICHARD], *Neo-Malthusianism; an Enquiry into That System with Regard to its Economy and Morality.* London; Methuen, 1897, pp. vi, 1–325.
[Very poor material]

VAERTING, M., "Über den Einfluss des Krieges auf Präventivverkehr und Fruchtabtreibung und seine eugenischen Folgen," *Ztschr. f. Sexualwissensch.* (Bonn), iv (1917–18): 137–144; 176–179.
[Of little value]

VALENTA, A., "Über den sogenannten Coitus reservatus als eine Hauptursache der chronischen Metritis und der weiblichen Nervosität," *Memorabilien* (Heilbrunnen), xxv (1880): 481–485. Also reprint.

VAN DE VELDE, TH. H., *Die Fruchtbarkeit in der Ehe und ihre wunschgemässe Beeinflussung.* Horw-Luzern, Leipzig, u. Stuttgart: Montana-Verlag, 1929, pp. 424, 20 tables.

VASILIEVA-TCHEBOTAREVA, A., ["Are Vaginal Douches of Corrosive Sublimate Rational?"] *Vrach. Delo.* (Kharkov), x (1927): 819–824.

[VĀTSYĀYANA], *The Kama Sutra of Vatsyayana. Translated from the Sanskrit. In seven parts, with preface, introduction, and concluding remarks.* Benares: Printed for the Hindoo Karma Shastra Society, 1883. For private circulation only, pp. 198, 8°.

VAUDESCAL, "A propos du pessaire de Grafenburg," *Ann. de Méd. Lég.*, xiii (July, 1933): 444–449.

VERNEY, L., "Per la limitazione delle nascite," *Clin. Ostet.* (Roma), xxvii (1925): 127–129.

VIGDORCHIK, N., "Kvoprosu o neomaltuzianstvie," ["On Neo-Malthusianism,"] *Prakt. Vrach.* (St. Petersb., now Leningrad), vii (1908): 806–810.

*VIGNES, HENRI, "La prophylaxie anticonceptionnelle en U. R. S. S.," *Le Progrès Médical* (Paris), No. 34, Aug. 22, 1931.

**VOGE, C. I. B., "The Relative Value of Contraceptive Methods Presently Employed; with Special Reference to 'Foam Tablets,'" *Proc. Sec. Int'l Cong. [1930] for Sex Research,* London: Oliver & Boyd, 1931, pp. 559–564.

—— Future Research upon Sterilization and Contraception. In Sanger & Stone, *Practice of Contraception,* pp. 76–90.

VOGE, C. I. B., "Natural Infertility. Factors Influencing the Results of Contraceptive Methods," *Eugenics Review* (London), xxv (1933): 85–90.
  [Original, thoughtful, critical.]
——— "Contraception," *Brit. Med. Jour.*, May 27, 1933, p. 918.
——— *The Chemistry and Physics of Contraceptives. Foreword by Robert Latou Dickinson, M.D., F.A.C.S.* London: Jonathan Cape, 1933, pp. 288.
——— *see* WALKER, SIR KENNETH.
——— "Contraceptive Methods. A description of a museum in the London School of Hygiene and Tropical Medicine," *Practitioner* (London), cxxxi (Sept., 1933): 268–277.
——— "The Present Status of the Contraceptive Trade," *Marriage Hygiene* (Bombay, India), i, 52–57 (August, 1934).
——— "The Applicability of Contraceptive Methods," *Marriage Hygiene* (Bombay, India), i, 127–130 (November, 1934).
——— "Further Progress in Contraception," *Marriage Hygiene* (Bombay, India), i, 346–349 (May, 1935).
VOGTHERR, K., "Über die moralische Beurteilung der willkürlichen Verhütung und Unterbrechung der Schwangerschaft," *Med. Klin.* (Berlin), xxii (1926): 195–198.
DE VRIES, STELLA, Het niewste en volmaakste voorbehoedmiddel tegen zwangerschap door de uitvinsler [The Newest and Most Perfect Means for Preventing Pregnancy by Means of Apparatus]. Amsterdam, 1905.
*W., W. S., Conditions of the Female Organs of Generation in Which Pregnancy Endangers Life. N.d., n.p., pp. 3–41. (S.G., B.M.L.)
WALD, E., Die Vorbeugung der Empfängnis. (Sonderdruck d. Gemeinschaft d. Bücherfreunde.) Berlin: Lilien [Komm: Karl Emil Krug, Lpz.], 1929, pp. 56.
——— *Lehrbuch der Liebe. Ein intimer Ratgeber f. Braut-u. Eheleute. Sonderdr. d. Gemeinschaft d. Bücherfreunde.* Berlin: Lilien-Verlag [Komm: Karl Emil Krug, Lpz.], 1929, pp. 219, 56.
WALES, GEORGE H., Methods of Birth Control Explained. Prefaced by Dr. G. Courtenay Beale. London: The George H. Wales Pub. Co., [1930], pp. 62.
  [Intended for the layman.]
WALKER, SIR KENNETH, *Preparation for Marriage, A Handbook for Leaders*. London: Cape, 1932.
  [First attempt at a leader's handbook. Issued by the British Social Hygiene Council. Originally planned as a symposium, but entirely rewritten by Sir Kenneth. Voge has done the section on contraception, sterility, eugenics, and heredity.]
———, ——— New York: W. W. Norton Co., 1933, pp. 159.
  [With an introduction by Logan Clendenning. No sub-title, no reference to British Social Hygiene Council.]
WALSHE, F. M. R., "Medical Views on Birth Control; Facts and Speculations," *Cath. Med. Guard.* (Middlesex, Eng.), v (1927): 82–88.
WALTHARD, M., "Zur Pathogenese der Sterilettinfektion," *Schweiz. Med. Wchnschr.* (Basel), liv (1924): 649–650.
*WARNER, W. LLOYD, "Birth Control in Primitive Society," *Birth Control Rev.* (New York), xv (1931): 105–107.
*WARREN, G. W., A confidential letter to the married. Cleveland, Ohio, 1854, pp. 28, 12½ cm. (L.C.)
  ["Lost" at Library of Congress. Unique.]
WASSERMANN, RUDOLF, "Die Verhütung der Empfängnis im Wandel der Zeiten," *Ztschr. f. Sexualwissensch.* (Berlin u. Köln), xvi (1929–1930): 555–564.

[WATERS, DR.], see CARLILE, R.

WATTAL, P. K., The Population Problem in India. A Census Study. Bombay: Bennett, Coleman, & Co., 1916, pp. iii, 1–83.

WEINHOLD, C. A., see Theilhaber.

WEISL, "Über Präservativa und Demonstration eines weiblichen Condoms," *Allg. Wien. Med. Ztg.*, xl (1895): 528–529.

WERNER, B., Ratgeber für Frauen. Berlin: A. Stephan, n.d., pp. 70.

―――― Physiologie der Flitterwochen. Berlin: A. Stephan, n.d., pp. 39.

―――― Die Verhütung der Empfängnis. Berlin: A. Stephan.

*WERSHOW, MAX, A Social Experiment in Birth Control. An analysis of over 1000 cases from the records of the Mothers' Clinic of Detroit. Detroit: Mothers' Clinic for Family Regulation, [1931], pp. 16.

WESTERMARCK, EDWARD, *Marriage Ceremonies in Morocco.* London: Macmillan, 1914, pp. xii, 1–422.

―――― *Ritual and Belief in Morocco.* London: Macmillan, 1926, 2 vols. i, v–xxxii, 1–608; ii, v–xvii, 1–629.

WEULE, KARL, "Wissenschaftliche Ergebnisse meiner ethnogr. Forschungsreise in den Südosten Deutsch-Ostafrikas," *Mitt. a. d. D. Schutzgeb. Erg.*, Heft I.

WHITEHOUSE, BECKWITH, "The Problem of Birth Control," *Practitioner* (London), cxi (1923): 43–48.

WHITING, P. W., "The Relation of Recent Advances in Genetics to Birth Control," *Rpt. Fifth Int'l Conf.*, 154–158.

WICKSELL, K., "The Crux of Malthusianism," *Rpt. Fifth Int'l Conf.*, 64–69.

**WILDE, FRIEDRICH ADOLPH, *Das weibliche Gebär-unvermögen. Eine medicinisch-juridische Abhandlung zum Gebrauch für practische Geburtshelfer, Aerzte, und Juristen.* Berlin: In der Nicolai'schen Buchhandlung, 1838, pp. xvi, 413.

*WILLIAMS, J. WHITRIDGE, "Indications for Therapeutic Sterilization in Obstetrics. When is Advice Concerning the Prevention of Conception Justifiable? *Jour. Amer. Med. Asso.* (Chicago), xci (Oct. 27, 1928): 1237–1242. Also reprint, pp. 16.

WILLCOX, WALTER S., "Changes Since 1900 in the Fertility of Native White Wives," *Milbank Memorial Fund Quar. Bull.* (New York), x (1932): 191–202.

*[WINDER, DANIEL], By an Ohio Physician, A Rational or Private Marriage Chart. For the Use of all who wish to Prevent an Increase of Family. Mansfield, Ohio, 1858.

WINKLER, MAX, Das Geburtenproblem und die Verhütung der Schwangerschaft. Amsterdam: Verlag "Roode Bibliotheek," 1925, pp. 48.

WINTERBERG, J., see BRAUN and WINTERBERG.

WISHARD, W. N., "Contraception; Are Our County Societies Being Used for the American Birth Control League Propaganda?" *Jour. Indiana Med. Asso.* (Fort Wayne), xxii (1929): 187–189.

WITKOWSKI, GUSTAVE JULES A., *Histoire des Accouchements chez tous les Peuples.* Paris, n.d., pp. xii, 714, + App. 182, (1584 figs.).

WOLF, H. DE, Birth Control Work in Holland. In Sanger & Stone, *Practice of Contraception*, pp. 272–274.

WOLFF, LOTTE, The Sex Advice Bureaus of the Berlin Krankenkassen. In Sanger & Stone, *Practice of Contraception*, pp. 242–244.

WOLFHEIM, M., "Über ein neues Mittel zur Verhütung der Gravidität," *Frauenarzt* (Leipzig), xxvii (1912): 56–59.

A WOMAN PHYSICIAN OF TWENTY YEARS' EXPERIENCE, see KONIKOW, ANTOINETTE F.

[WORKERS' BIRTH CONTROL GROUP], Memorandum on Birth Control presented to the

Minister of Health by a Deputation on May 9th, 1924. London: Workers' Birth Control Group, n.d. [1924], pp. 16.

WOROSCHBIT, A. J., see GUREWITSCH, Z. A.

WORTHINGTON, G. E., "Statutory Restrictions on Birth Control," *Jour. Soc. Hyg.* (New York), ix (1923): 458–465.

WRIGHT, HELENA, Indications for the Use of the Dumas and Pro-Race Cervical Caps. In Sanger & Stone, *Practice of Contraception*, pp. 15–16.

WURZBERGER, ANNA, Verhütung der Schwangerschaft. Leipzig: Wilhelm Besser, 1901, pp. 31.

——— Die Verhütung der Empfängniss. Berlin: A. Stephan.

WYNNE, FRED E., Birth Control and Population. In *Medical Help*, pp. 213–225.

YANG, MARION, "Birth Control in Peiping. First Report of the Peiping Committee on Maternal Health," *Chinese Med. Jour.*, xlviii (1934): 786–791.

*YARROS, RACHELLE S., "Practical Aspects of Birth Control," *Surg., Gyn., & Obst.* (Chicago), xxiii (1916): 188–190.

——— "Birth Control and Its Relation to Health and Welfare," *Med. Woman's Jour.* (Cincin.), xxxii (1925): 268–272. Reprinted [changes?] Chicago: Illinois Birth Control League, 1925, pp. 16.

——— "Significance of Birth Control for Race Betterment," *Med. Woman's Jour.* (Cincin.), xxxv (1928): 194–197.

——— Experience with the Cervical Pessary. In Sanger & Stone, *Practice of Contraception*, p. 17.

YONGE, C. D. see ATHENAEUS.

*YOUNG, JAMES, "The Medical Profession and Birth Control," *Brit. Med. Jour.* (London), i: 213–217, (Feb. 11, 1933).

YOUNG, M., "The Volitional Regulation of Families," *Pub. Health* (London), xxxvi (1922–23): 185–188.

ZACHARIAS, E., "Chininexanthem durch Contrapan," *Med. Klin.* (Berlin), xxii (1926): 373–374.

ZADEK, F., Frauenleiden, nebst einem Anhang: Die Verhütung der Schwangerschaft. Mit 9 Textillustrationen. Berlin: Buchhandlung Vorwärts, 1912, pp. 20.

ZEIDLER, P., "Dopustimïli pri nïekotorïkh patologicheskikh protsessakh mïerï, klonyashtshiya sya k vremennomu predotvrashtsheniyu beremennosti?" *J. Akush. i. Zhensk. Boližez* (St. Petersb. now Leningrad) iii (1889): 321–331.

ZEILER, A., "Die Zweikinderehe; ihre Gefahren und ihre Abwehr," *Ztschr. f. Bevölkrngspolit., etc.* (Leipzig), ix (1916–17): 359–367.

——— "Ein Ende der Angst vor dem Kinde," *Bl. f. Volksgsndhtspfl.* (Berlin), xvii (1917): 78–80.

——— "Die Wirtschaftslage der Familie und die Bevölkerungsfrage," *Ztschr. f. Bekampf. d. Geschlechtskrankh.* (Leipzig), xviii (1917–18): 188–191.

*ZERVOS, SKEVOS, [Ed.], AËTIOS, *Maladies des Femmes*, Leipzig, 1901.

ZIKEL, HEINZ, Die Verhinderung der Empfängnis vom medizinischen u. sozialen Standpunkt. Berlin u. Leipzig, 1912, pp. 56.

ZSCHOMMLER, OLGA, Malthusianismus. Verhütung der Empfängnis und ihre gesundheitlichen Folgen. Berlin: Möller, 1891.

INDEX OF NAMES AND AUTHORS

(Note: The bibliography is not indexed here.   This Index contains names of organizations as well as of individuals, but not names of geographic places.)

INDEX OF SUBJECTS

N